THIRD
EDITION

THE EYE

BASIC SCIENCES IN PRACTICE

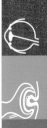

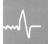

To Anne, Lindsay, Christine and Craig

Commissioning Editor: Michael Parkinson
Project Development Manager: Lulu Stader
Project Manager: Jess Thompson
Designer: Erik Bigland
Illustrator: Oxford Illustrators

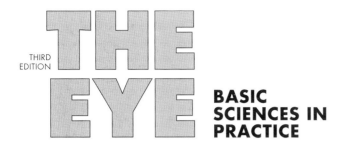

THIRD EDITION

THE EYE

BASIC SCIENCES IN PRACTICE

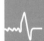

John V. Forrester MB ChB MD FRCS(Ed) FRCS(Glasg) FRCOphth FRCP FMedSci FRSE

Professor of Ophthalmology and Head of Department of Ophthalmology
University of Aberdeen
Aberdeen, UK

Andrew D. Dick BSc MB BS MD FRCP FRCS FRCOphth FMedSci

Professor of Ophthalmology and Head of Academic Unit of Ophthalmology
University of Bristol
Bristol, UK

Paul G. McMenamin BSc MSc(MedSci) PhD

Professor, School of Anatomy and Human Biology
Associate Dean (Teaching and Learning)
Faculty of Medicine, Dentistry and Health Sciences
The University of Western Australia
Perth, Australia

Fiona Roberts BSc MB ChB MD FRCPath

Consultant Ophthalmic Pathologist and Honorary Senior Lecturer in Pathology
University Department of Pathology
Western Infirmary
Glasgow, UK

SAUNDERS

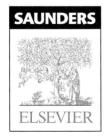

ELSEVIER

EDINBURGH   LONDON   NEW YORK   OXFORD   PHILADELPHIA   ST LOUIS   SYDNEY   TORONTO
2008

SAUNDERS
ELSEVIER

© Elsevier Limited 2002, 2008. All rights reserved.

No part of this publication may be reproduced, stored in a retrieval system, or transmitted in any form or by any means, electronic, mechanical, photocopying, recording or otherwise, without the prior permission of the Publishers. Permissions may be sought directly from Elsevier's Health Sciences Rights Department, 1600 John F. Kennedy Boulevard, Suite 1800, Philadelphia, PA 19103-2899, USA; phone: (+1) 215 239 3804; fax: (+1) 215 239 3805; or e-mail: *healthpermissions@elsevier.com*. You may also complete your request on-line via the Elsevier homepage (www.elsevier.com), by selecting 'Support and contact' and then 'Copyright and Permission'.

First edition 1996
Second edition 2002
Reprinted 2003, 2004
Third edition 2008
  Reprinted 2008

ISBN 9780702028410

British Library Cataloguing in Publication Data
A catalogue record for this book is available from the British Library

Library of Congress Cataloging in Publication Data
A catalog record for this book is available from the Library of Congress

The
publisher's
policy is to use
**paper manufactured
from sustainable forests**

Printed in China

CONTENTS

PREFACE

It is our great pleasure to write a few words of introduction to this the third edition of *The Eye*. The book was originally conceived as an aid to many different types of individual, all with a common need to rapidly acquire information about our present understanding of the basic scientific principles of the vegetative functions of the eye and how these can be altered through the general mechanisms that affect all other systems in the organism. After all, despite the unique anatomical and physiological organization of the eye, the processes that modify its workings are not different in principle from those affecting other organs and tissues. Of course, much of this information is available in general texts, but rarely is it described in the context of the eye. Indeed, the mainstream geneticist, microbiologist or immunologist, for example, is unlikely to consider ocular effects unless as an interesting curiosity.

Accordingly, the nascent vision scientist, ocular immunologist or geneticist has a difficult experience trying to gather information about the eye generally while developing their specific interest in their chosen field. This book is aimed at such individuals as a basic science handbook, mainly to get them 'up to speed' with aspects of ocular and non-ocular basic science. The book is also aimed at several other groups of individuals: for instance the trainee ophthalmologist at the start of his or her career needs a primer on the basic science of the eye as does the trainee optometrist. It is hoped that this book provides such a utility.

For this reason the book is organized in such a way that it provides simple descriptions of our current knowledge in various fields including anatomy, embryology, genetics, biochemistry and cell biology, ocular neurophysiology, pharmacology, microbiology and pathology. Intentionally, optics is omitted as this subject is dealt with admirably in many other texts and is outside the remit of the above more 'vegetative' ocular functions that are the core of *The Eye*.

This current edition has been extensively revised and updated in accordance with many of the fast-developing fields such as genetics and immunology. An attempt has been made to minimize complexity and present concepts as simply as possible to the reader, particularly those who may be newcomers to any of the specific fields. Material from several other texts has been drawn upon extensively in order to synthesize the information and these contributions are gratefully acknowledged throughout the text.

John V. Forrester
Andrew D. Dick
Paul G. McMenamin
Fiona Roberts

ACKNOWLEDGEMENTS

We would like to thank Professor William R. Lee, who co-authored the first two editions of *The Eye*, for his guidance and support and generous provision of material for the current edition. We are also grateful to the anonymous reviewers who commented on the draft text.

Paul McMenamin would like to thank the following for discussions relating to the revisions for this third edition: Professor Alan Harvey (the anatomy of the visual pathways), Dr Joseph Demer (anatomy of extraocular muscles) and Professor Brian Hall (embryology of the head and neck). He also wishes to thank Martin Thompson for preparation of the artwork in Chapters 1 and 2, Dorothy Aitken for providing several micrographs of cornea and conjunctiva, Professor Turab Chakera for some of the radiographs in Chapter 1, and Dr Dipika Patel for the in vivo confocal microscopy images of the human cornea.

John V. Forrester
Andrew D. Dick
Paul G. McMenamin
Fiona Roberts

1 ANATOMY OF THE EYE AND ORBIT

- ■ Anatomical terms of reference
- ■ Osteology of the skull and orbits
- ■ Structure of the eye
- ■ Orbital contents
- ■ Cranial nerves associated with the eye and orbit
- ■ Ocular appendages (adnexa)
- ■ Anatomy of the visual pathway

ANATOMICAL TERMS OF REFERENCE

Anatomy and histology obviously require internationally accepted terminology for description of the relations and position of structures. The body is divided by a series of imaginary *planes* (Fig. 1.1). That which divides the body into right and left halves is known as the *median* or *mid-sagittal plane*. Anything parallel to this plane is said to be *sagittal*. The plane that is at right angles, and therefore divides the body into front and back, is *coronal* and that which is at right angles to both of the above planes is the *horizontal*.

Relative positions of anatomical structures are referred to in terms of: *medial* (nearer the median or mid-sagittal plane) and *lateral* (away from this plane); *anterior* and *posterior* refer to the front and back surfaces of the body; *superior* (cranial or rostral) or *inferior* (caudal) refer to position in the vertical; *superficial* and *deep* specify distance from the surface of the body. A combination of terms can be used to describe the relative position of structures that do not fit exactly any of the other terms, e.g. ventrolateral, posteromedial, etc.

OSTEOLOGY OF THE SKULL AND ORBITS

GENERAL ARRANGEMENT OF THE SKULL

The skull, including the mandible (or more correctly the dentary), is comprised of a mixture of highly modified axial skeletal elements (occipital bone) and craniofacial skeleton. The latter is divided into two parts, an upper part shaped like a bowl, which contains the brain, known as the *cranium* or

1

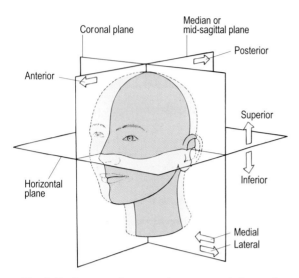

Fig. 1.1 Diagram illustrating the anatomical planes of reference.

neurocranium, and a lower part, the *facial skeleton* or *viscerocranium*. The cranium can be further subdivided into the cranial vault and cranial base.

FEATURES OF THE SKULL

The skull is composed of a large number of separate bones that are united by *sutures* (fibrous immovable joints). The cranium consists of eight bones (only two are paired), the facial skeleton consists of 14 bones, of which only two are single (Fig. 1.2A,B). The skull contains a number of cavities that reflect its multiple functions:

- *Cranial cavity* – houses, supports and protects the brain
- *Nasal cavity* – concerned with respiration and olfaction
- *Orbits* – contain the eyes and adnexa
- *Oral cavity* – start of gastrointestinal tract, responsible for mastication and initial food processing; houses taste receptors.

Many of the cranial bones are hollow and contain air-filled spaces, the paranasal sinuses (Fig. 1.3). The main anatomical features of the whole skull are indicated in Figure 1.2A and B, which shows views of the skull (*norma frontalis* and *norma lateralis*). These illustrate most of the features relevant to the study of the eye and orbits.

OSTEOLOGY OF THE ORBIT

The two orbital cavities are situated between the cranium and facial skeleton and are separated from each other by the nasal cavity and the ethmoidal and sphenoidal air sinuses (Fig. 1.3A–C). Each orbit is a socket that accommodates and protects the eye and adnexa, and serves to transmit the nerves and vessels that supply the face around the orbit. Parts of the following bones contribute to the walls of the orbit: maxilla, frontal, sphenoid, zygomatic, palatine, ethmoid and lacrimal (Figs 1.4 and 1.5A,B). The orbit is roughly the shape of a quadrilateral pyramid whose base is the *orbital margin* and whose apex is the *optic canal*. It has a floor, roof, medial wall and lateral wall (Fig. 1.4). The floor tapers off before the apex; therefore the apex of the pyramid is triangular. The orbit is widest approximately 1.5 cm behind the orbital margin. The walls are mostly triangular, except the medial wall, which is oblong. The medial walls are approximately parallel to the mid-sagittal plane, while the lateral walls are oriented at an angle of approximately 45° to this plane. The *orbital aperture* is directed forwards, laterally and slightly downwards. Thus nerves and muscles passing from the apex into the orbit pass forward and laterally (Fig. 1.3A,B). The orbit is approximately 40 mm in height, 40 mm in width and 40 mm in depth. The volume is approximately 30 ml, of which one-fifth is occupied by the eye.

The walls of the orbit

The bones that make up the roof, floor, medial and lateral walls are summarized in Figure 1.4.

Features of the orbital roof
- *Fossa for the lacrimal gland* The fossa lies in the anterolateral aspect of the roof behind the zygomatic process of the frontal bone.
- *Trochlear fossa (fovea)* This lies in the anteromedial aspect of the roof, 4 mm from the margin, and is the site at which the trochlea (small pulley) is attached. The tendon of the superior oblique passes through the trochlea.
- *Anterior and posterior ethmoidal canals* Positioned at the junction of roof and medial wall above the frontoethmoidal suture (Fig.1.5A). They transmit the anterior and posterior ethmoidal nerves and vessels.

Relations The roof, which is thin and translucent except at the lesser wing of the sphenoid, separates the orbit from the anterior cranial fossa and frontal lobes of the brain. Anteriorly the frontal sinus lies above the orbit.

A

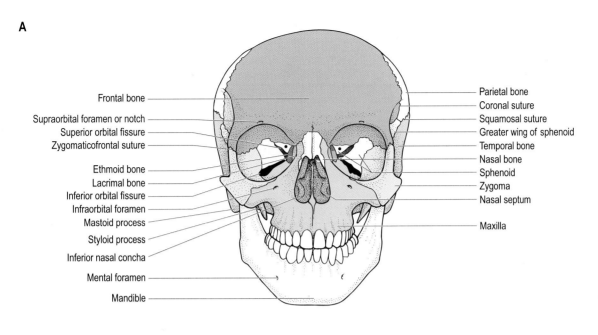

Frontal bone

Supraorbital foramen or notch
Superior orbital fissure
Zygomaticofrontal suture

Ethmoid bone
Lacrimal bone
Inferior orbital fissure
Infraorbital foramen
Mastoid process
Styloid process
Inferior nasal concha

Mental foramen

Mandible

Parietal bone
Coronal suture
Squamosal suture
Greater wing of sphenoid
Temporal bone
Nasal bone
Sphenoid
Zygoma
Nasal septum

Maxilla

B

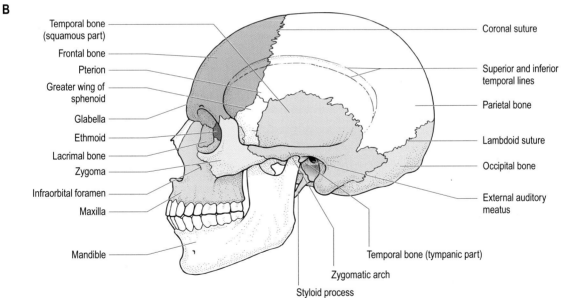

Temporal bone
(squamous part)
Frontal bone
Pterion
Greater wing of
sphenoid
Glabella
Ethmoid
Lacrimal bone
Zygoma
Infraorbital foramen
Maxilla

Mandible

Coronal suture

Superior and inferior
temporal lines

Parietal bone

Lambdoid suture

Occipital bone

External auditory
meatus

Temporal bone (tympanic part)
Zygomatic arch
Styloid process

Fig. 1.2 Osteology of the skull. Two views of the skull: (**A**) norma frontalis; and (**B**) norma lateralis to illustrate the individual bones and important anatomical landmarks.

Features of the medial orbital wall
- This wall is oblong in shape and thin (0.2–0.4 mm). The four bones that comprise this wall are separated by vertical sutures (Figs 1.4 and 1.5A).
- *Lacrimal fossa* for the lacrimal sac: it is bound by anterior and posterior lacrimal crests and is con-

tinuous below with the *nasolacrimal canal* (Fig. 1.5B).

Relations This is the thinnest of the walls and is largely transparent or semitransparent – the ethmoidal air sinuses can easily be seen through this

3

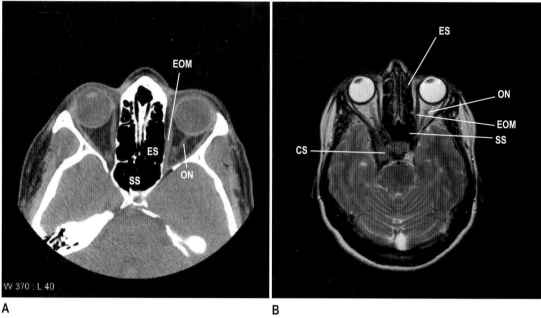

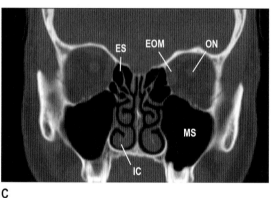

Fig. 1.3 Transverse (**A,B**) and coronal (**C**) computed tomography (CT) and magnetic resonance imaging (MRI) scans of the head displaying the major relations of the orbits. Features identifiable in the scans include ethmoid air cells/sinuses (ES), frontal sinus (FS), maxillary sinus (MS), sphenoid sinus (SS), nasal cavity (NC), inferior nasal concha (IC), extraocular muscle (EOM), optic nerve (ON) and cavernous sinus (CS).

wall in a dried skull (Fig. 1.5A,B). Medial to this wall in an anterior to posterior sequence lie the anterior, middle, posterior ethmoidal air cells and the sphenoidal sinus.

Orbital cellulitis

This condition may be a consequence of infection spreading from the air sinuses to the orbit via the paper-thin medial wall (lamina papyracea) that separates the two.

Features of the orbital floor
- The floor slopes slightly downwards from the medial to the lateral wall.
- It is crossed by the *infraorbital groove*, which runs forward from the *inferior orbital fissure*. Before it reaches the orbital margin it becomes the *infraorbital canal*, which opens as the *infraorbital foramen* 4 mm below the orbital margin on the anterior surface of the maxilla (Figs 1.3C, 1.4 and 1.5A).

Relations Below the floor lies the maxillary sinus, the bone being only 0.5–1 mm in thickness (Fig. 1.3C).

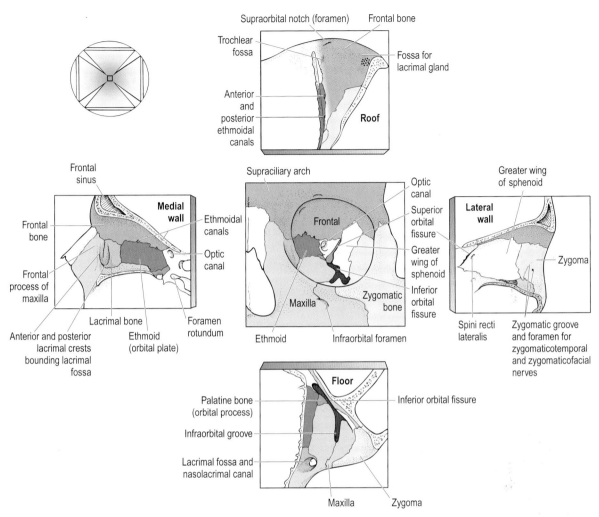

Fig. 1.4 Osteology of the orbit. The central diagram illustrates the anterior view of the intact orbit: the four surrounding diagrams ('exploded orbit' – see inset, top left) show the individual bones which form the roof, floor, medial and lateral walls and other noteworthy features. *Roof:* orbital plate of the frontal bone and small area of lesser wing of the sphenoid. *Medial wall:* frontal process of the maxilla, lacrimal bone, orbital plate of the ethmoid and the body of the sphenoid. *Floor:* orbital plate of the maxilla, orbital surface of the zygoma and the orbital process of the palatine bone. *Lateral wall:* orbital surfaces of greater wing of sphenoid posteriorly and zygomatic bone anteriorly.

The floor, although thicker than the medial wall, is more often involved in orbital blow-out fractures, probably because it lacks the buttress-like supports of the ethmoidal air cells and the protection of the nose. Tumour spread to or from the maxillary sinus may occur via the floor of the orbit.

Features of the lateral orbital wall (Fig. 1.4)

- *Spina recti lateralis* A small bony spine near the apex of the orbit on the greater wing of the sphenoid gives origin to part of the lateral rectus.
- *Zygomatic foramen* Transmits zygomatic nerve and vessels to temporal fossa and cheek (zygomaticotemporal nerve and zygomaticofacial nerve) (Fig. 1.5B).
- *Lateral orbital tubercle* The origin of the check ligament of the lateral rectus, suspensory ligament of

5

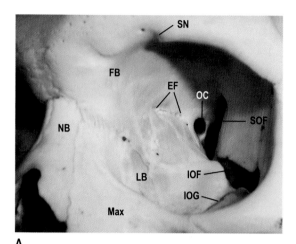

A

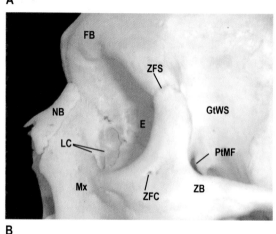

B

Fig. 1.5 (**A**) Anterior view of the bony orbit showing important osteological features of the apex including the relation of the superior orbital fissure (SOF), optic canal (OC) and inferior orbital fissure (IOF). IOG, inferior orbital groove; LB, lacrimal bone; EF, anterior and posterior ethmoidal foramina; SN, supraorbital notch; FB, frontal bone; NB, nasal bone; Max, maxilla. (**B**) Lateral view of the orbit. ZB, zygomatic bone; PtMF, pterygomaxillary fissure; GtWS, greater wing of the sphenoid; ZFS, zygomaticofrontal suture; ZFC, zygomaticofacial canal; LC, lacrimal crest; E, ethmoid bone; Mx, maxilla.

the eye, and aponeurosis of levator palpebrae superioris.
• Foramina for small veins that communicate with middle cranial fossa.

Relations Laterally–skin, temporal fossa and middle cranial fossa in an anterior–posterior sequence (Fig. 1.3A).

Orbital margin, fissures and optic canal

Orbital margin
This is a thickened rim of bone that helps protect the orbital contents. It is made up of three bones: the frontal, zygomatic and maxilla (Figs 1.4 and 1.5A,B). The lateral margin is thickest because it is the most exposed and therefore prone to trauma. It is also concave forward; thus it does not reach as far anteriorly as the medial margin (see Figs 1.2B and 1.5B). The medial margin is sharp and distinct in its lower half because of the anterior lacrimal crest, but is indistinct superiorly (Figs 1.4 and 1.5B).

Superior orbital fissure
This gap lies between the roof and lateral wall of the orbit and is bounded by the lesser and greater wings of sphenoid (Figs 1.4 and 1.5A,C). It is the largest communication between the orbital and cranial cavities. It is comma-shaped, being wider at its medial end and narrowest at its lateral end. It is around 22 mm long and is separated from the optic foramen above by the posterior root of the lesser wing of the sphenoid. The part of the *common tendinous ring* that gives origin to the lateral rectus spans between the narrow and wide parts of the fissure. Structures passing above or outside the tendinous ring or annulus include the lacrimal nerve, frontal nerve, trochlear nerve, superior ophthalmic vein and recurrent branch of the lacrimal artery. The latter anastomoses with the orbital branch of the middle meningeal artery and may more commonly travel in a small cranio-orbital foramen lateral to the superior orbital fissure. Structures passing within the ring, and thus within the apex of the muscle cone, include the oculomotor nerve (superior and inferior divisions), abducent nerve, nasociliary nerve, sympathetic root of the ciliary ganglion, and variably the inferior ophthalmic vein (Fig. 1.5C).

Inferior orbital fissure
This fissure lies between the lateral wall and floor of the orbit. It forms a communication between the orbit and the infratemporal fossa and pterygopalatine fossa. Its posterior end lies below and lateral to the optic foramen near the superior orbital fissure. It runs forward and laterally for approximately 20 mm and ends 20 mm from the orbital margin (Figs 1.4 and 1.5A). The fissure is narrowest in the middle section and in life is covered by periorbita and a sheet of smooth muscle of unknown function, the orbitalis or 'muscle of Müller'. It transmits the infraorbital nerve, zygomatic nerve and branches from the pterygopalatine ganglion.

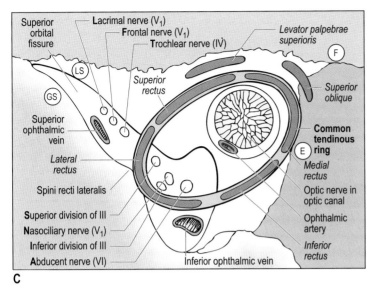

Fig. 1.5 *Continued* **(C)** Diagram of the superior orbital fissure and optic canal in the right orbit. Note the origins of the extraocular muscles from the common tendinous ring and the relative position of the cranial nerves and vessels as they enter or exit the orbit. GS, greater wing of sphenoid; LS, lesser wing of sphenoid; F, frontal bone; E, ethmoid. The positions of the veins are variable. The first letters of each of the structures passing through the superior orbital fissure (LFTSNIA) form a well-known mnemonic.

Optic canal

This is a bony channel in the sphenoid that passes anteriorly, inferiorly and laterally (36°) from the middle cranial fossa to the apex of the orbit. It is formed by the two roots of the lesser wing of the sphenoid. The two optic canals are 25 mm apart posteriorly and 30 mm anteriorly. Each is funnel-shaped, narrowest anteriorly where its opening into the orbit is oval with sharp upper and lower borders and a prolonged roof (10–12 mm in length). The opening at the cranial aspect is oval with a prolonged floor. The sphenoidal and posterior ethmoidal air sinuses are important medial relations, and the olfactory tracts are superior relations of the canal. The canal transmits the *optic nerve* with its meningeal coverings and the *ophthalmic artery*, which lies below and then lateral to the nerve within the dural sheath for part of its course (Fig. 1.5C). Sympathetic nerve fibres accompany the artery.

PARANASAL SINUSES

The paranasal sinuses comprise the frontal, ethmoidal, sphenoidal and maxillary sinuses. They are air-filled cavities in the skull that are in communication with the nasal cavity via a series of apertures. Mucus secreted by the mucous membrane lining the sinuses is swept towards these apertures by the motion of cilia on the epithelium, which closely resembles that lining the main airways. Infection commonly spreads from the nasal cavity into the sinuses and mucus may accumulate and become secondarily infected. The sinuses function to warm and moisten the air, add resonance to the voice and lighten the skull. They vary in size and shape between individuals.

Frontal sinuses (Figs 1.4 and 1.6)

The frontal sinuses are paired and lie behind the superciliary arches within the frontal bone. They are separated from each other or further subdivided by thin bony septa that are not necessarily in the midline. The sinuses may extend as far laterally as the zygomatic process of the frontal bone. Each is approximately triangular and extends highest above the medial end of the eyebrow (Fig. 1.6). Each sinus opens into the middle meatus of the nasal cavity, either through the ethmoidal infundibulum or directly via the frontonasal duct. The mucosal lining is supplied by the supraorbital nerves and vessels; hence referred pain from frontal sinusitis is experienced along the course of the supraorbital nerve.

Recent geometric morphometric studies (elliptic Fourier analysis) of the outlines of frontal sinuses from large numbers of radiographic images have confirmed a long-held belief that each individual's frontal sinus is distinct and unique. This may have important applications for personal identification in the context of forensics (Christensen, 2004).

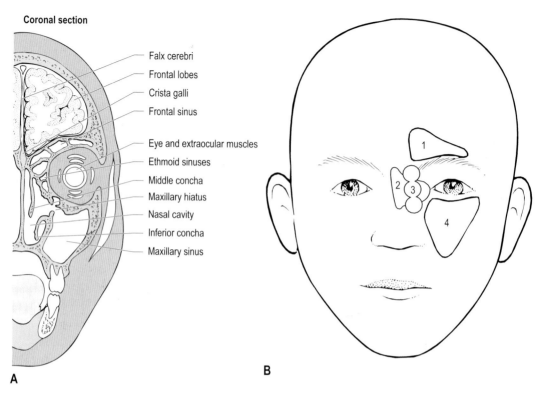

Coronal section

- Falx cerebri
- Frontal lobes
- Crista galli
- Frontal sinus

- Eye and extraocular muscles
- Ethmoid sinuses
- Middle concha
- Maxillary hiatus
- Nasal cavity
- Inferior concha
- Maxillary sinus

A

B

Fig. 1.6 (**A**) Diagram of a coronal section of the head revealing most of the paranasal sinuses except the sphenoid sinus. (**B**) Diagram to show the surface anatomy of the head and the relative positions of the paranasal air sinuses: 1, frontal sinus; 2, sphenoidal sinus; 3, ethmoidal sinus; 4, maxillary sinus.

Ethmoidal sinuses (air cells)
(Figs 1.3A–C and 1.6)
These thin-walled sinuses are for the most part situated in the lateral mass of the ethmoid, although frontal, maxillary, lacrimal, sphenoidal and palatine bones contribute to the walls. They are variable in number and are grouped into anterior, middle and posterior. The general pattern of drainage of the sinuses is as follows: the anterior opens into the hiatus semilunaris, the middle onto the bulla ethmoidalis (both middle meatus), and the posterior into the superior meatus. They are related to the frontal sinus anteriorly, the sphenoidal sinus posteriorly, the nasal cavity medially and below, and laterally the orbit (Fig. 1.6A).

Sphenoidal sinus (Figs 1.3A,B and 1.6)
This sinus lies within the body of the sphenoid bone and possesses an indented roof because of the pitu-

itary fossa that lies above and houses the pituitary gland (Fig. 1.7). It may be divided by a variable midline septum. A transverse ridge in the lateral wall marks the position of the internal carotid artery (within the cavernous sinus). Other important relations of the sinus include the optic chiasma and nerves above, the nasal cavity below, the ethmoidal sinuses anteriorly, and the paired cavernous sinuses laterally (Fig. 1.8E). The sphenoidal sinus drains into the superior meatus or sphenoethmoidal recess. Surgical access to the pituitary gland may be gained via the nasal cavity and sphenoidal sinus; hence surgeons must be aware of the above-mentioned relations.

Maxillary sinus (Figs 1.3C and 1.6)
These are the largest of the paranasal air sinuses. They are pyramidal in shape and lie within the body of the maxilla. The *base* forms part of the lateral wall of the nasal cavity and the *apex* is within the zygo-

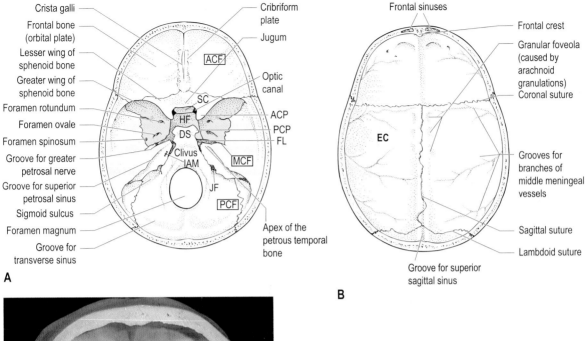

Crista galli

Frontal bone
(orbital plate)

Lesser wing of
sphenoid bone

Greater wing of
sphenoid bone

Foramen rotundum

Foramen ovale

Foramen spinosum

Groove for greater
petrosal nerve

Groove for superior
petrosal sinus

Sigmoid sulcus

Foramen magnum

Groove for
transverse sinus

Cribriform
plate

Jugum

ACF

Optic
canal

ACP

PCP

FL

MCF

JF

PCF

SC

HF

DS

Clivus
IAM

Apex of the
petrous temporal
bone

A

Frontal sinuses

Frontal crest

Granular foveola
(caused by
arachnoid
granulations)

Coronal suture

EC

Grooves for
branches of
middle meningeal
vessels

Sagittal suture

Lambdoid suture

Groove for superior
sagittal sinus

B

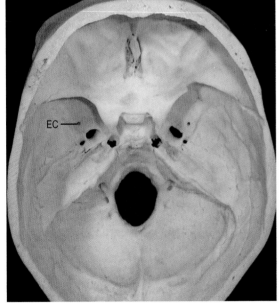

EC

C

Fig. 1.7 Osteology of the cranial cavity. (**A**) The
boundaries of the anterior (ACF), middle (MCF) and posterior
(PCF) cranial fossae together with major foraminae and
important landmarks on the base of the skull. HF,
hypophyseal fossa; DS, dorsum sella; SC, sulcus chiasmatis;
IAM, internal auditory meatus; JF, jugular foramen and fossa;
ACP, anterior clinoid process; PCP, posterior clinoid process;
FL, foramen lacerum. (**B**) Features of the vault interior.
(**C**) Photograph of cranial cavity to illustrate features shown
in (**A**): EC, emissary canal.

matic process. Each sinus is in communication with
the middle meatus of the nasal cavity via an aperture, the maxillary hiatus, on its base, which empties
into the lower part of the hiatus semilunaris. The
opening is positioned high on this wall and therefore does not facilitate gravitational drainage in the
upright position. The *nasolacrimal duct* lies in a thin
bony canal in the anterior part of the base. The
orbital plate forms the *roof* of the sinus and floor of
the orbit.

Orbital floor fractures

Rapid traumatic compression of the orbital contents, such as occurs during squashball injuries, can lead to blow-out fractures; orbital contents may herniate into the maxillary sinus. It was once thought that orbital contents, including extraocular muscles, became trapped in the fractured floor, thus restricting range of movement and explaining the diplopia suffered by these patients. However, recent studies have indicated that in many cases only orbital fibroadipose tissue is trapped in the damaged floor of the orbit (see p. 64).

The *floor* of the maxillary sinus is formed by the alveolar process housing a variable number of the roots of the first and second molars that protrude into the sinus, and may be separated from the sinus by only a thin covering of bone or mucous membrane. Thus sinusitis may present as referred pain such as toothache and vice versa. In addition, abscesses in the maxillary sinus may result from infection of these roots. The *anterior/lateral wall* is directed onto the face, and access for drainage of maxillary obstructions or other surgical procedures in the sinus may be gained by this route. The *posterior wall* faces the infratemporal fossa.

CRANIAL CAVITY (Fig. 1.7A–C)

The cranial cavity houses the brain and its meninges and their associated vessels, in addition to the intracranial portions of the cranial nerves. The base of the cranial cavity can be subdivided into three fossae: anterior, middle and posterior. Accounts of the detailed anatomy of these fossae can be found in any standard anatomy text; therefore only features of relevance to the eye and orbit will be described.

Cranial fossae

Anterior cranial fossa

The anterior cranial fossa is limited in front and laterally by the frontal bone and posteriorly by the lesser wing of the sphenoid. Its floor is formed by the orbital plate of the frontal bone, the cribriform plate of the ethmoid (with a median crest-like ridge, the crista galli, which forms the anterior attachment of the falx cerebri), and the lesser wings and anterior part of the body (jugum) of the sphenoid. The perforations of the cribriform plate transmit the olfactory nerves. The orbital plate of the frontal bone separates the orbit below from the frontal lobes of the cerebral hemispheres, whose sulci and gyri

cause surface impressions on the bone. Projecting posteriorly from the lesser wings of the sphenoid are the anterior clinoid processes that overhang the middle cranial fossa and give attachment to the free edge of the tentorium cerebelli.

Middle cranial fossa

The middle cranial fossa lies at a lower plane than the anterior cranial fossa but is higher than the posterior cranial fossa. Its floor is shaped like a butterfly, namely it consists of a narrow central or median part and expanded lateral parts ('wings'). It is bound anteriorly by the posterior free edge of the lesser wing of the sphenoid, the anterior clinoid processes, and the anterior margin of the sulcus chiasmatis (Fig. 1.7A,C). Posteriorly it extends to the superior borders of the petrous temporal bones and dorsum sellae of the sphenoid, and laterally it is bound by the squamous part of the temporal bone, part of the parietal bones, and the greater wings of the sphenoid. Features and foramina of the floor of the middle cranial fossa and the structures that they transmit are summarized in Table 1.1.

Pituitary fossa

The *pituitary fossa* (hypophyseal fossa) is an indentation in the roof of the body of the sphenoid bone in the middle cranial fossa. It is bound anteriorly by the *tuberculum sellae*, in front of which lies the *sulcus chiasmatica*, and posteriorly by the *dorsum sellae*, a ridge of bone at either end of which lies the *posterior clinoid processes*. The pituitary fossa houses the pituitary gland or *hypophysis cerebri*. This is connected by a thin stalk – the pituitary stalk (or tuber cinereum) – to the brain. The fossa is roofed by a sheet of dura mater, the diaphragma sella (Fig. 1.8E,F) which is attached in front to the tuberculum and behind to the dorsum sellae. The pituitary stalk passes through a small opening in the roof. Laterally lie the two cavernous sinuses (Fig. 1.8E).

Posterior cranial fossa

This is the deepest of the three cranial fossae, its floor lying below the level of the middle fossa. Its roof is formed by the tentorium cerebelli. It lodges the hindbrain: the cerebellum, pons and medulla oblongata. The fossa is bound anteriorly by the superior border of the petrous temporal bone and the dorsum sella, and surrounds the foramen magnum, the cerebellum being housed in the cerebellar fossae on the squamous part of the occipital bone. Features and openings on the floor of the posterior cranial fossa are not as relevant to the eye and orbit as those in the anterior or middle fossae; however, readers

Table 1.1 Summary of features on the floor of the middle cranial fossa

Feature/foramen	Position	Relevance
Sulcus chiasmatis	Between the two optic canals anterior to tuberculum sella	Only rarely does optic chiasma lie in contact with this region
Sella turcica ('Turkish saddle')	Central part of sphenoid body between the two cavernous sinuses	The central hollow, the hypophyseal fossa, houses the pituitary gland. Anterior and posterior clinoid processes give attachment to the free and attached margins of the tentorium cerebelli
Optic canal	Between the two roots of the lesser wing of the sphenoid	Transmits optic nerve, ophthalmic artery, sympathetic nerves and meningeal coverings
Superior orbital fissure	Between the lesser and greater wings of the sphenoid. Lies at apex of cavernous sinus	Transmits trochlear, abducent and oculomotor nerves and terminal branches of ophthalmic nerve
Foramen rotundum	Pierces greater wing of sphenoid	Transmits maxillary nerve and small veins from cavernous sinus
Foramen ovale	Pierces greater wing of sphenoid	Transmits mandibular nerve, accessory meningeal artery and occasionally the lesser petrosal nerve
Foramen spinosum	Posterolateral to foramen ovale	Transmits middle meningeal artery and vein and meningeal branch of the mandibular nerve
Foramen lacerum	At apex of petrous temporal bone	The upper end transmits the internal carotid artery before it enters the cavernous sinus. Also trasmits sympathetic nerves and a small plexus of veins. The lower end is covered by connective tissue and pierced only by small branches of the ascending pharyngeal artery
Trigeminal impression	Anterior surface of petrous temporal bone behind foramen lacerum	Occupied by trigeminal ganglion in trigeminal cave. Joined on lateral aspect by grooves for the greater and lesser petrosal nerves
Tegmen tympani and arcuate eminence	Tegmen is a thin plate of temporal bone over middle ear cavity. Arcuate eminence is produced by superior semicircular canal in petrous temporal bone	Infections in middle ear may spread through thin plate of bone to middle cranial fossa and temporal lobe of the brain

should be able to identify the following: foramen magnum, jugular foramen, hypoglossal canal, internal acoustic meatus, grooves for the sigmoid and transverse sinuses, internal occipital protuberance and the clivus (Fig. 1.7A,C).

The meninges (Fig. 1.8A–C)
The brain and spinal cord are surrounded by three layers of meninges: a tough *pachymeninx*, the dura mater, and the *leptomeninges* consisting of the arachnoid mater and pia mater. Between the arachnoid and pia is the *subarachnoid* space filled with cerebrospinal fluid.

Dura mater
The *dura mater* is theoretically 'divided' into an endosteal layer (really the periosteum on the inner surface of the skull) and a meningeal layer; however, on the whole they are fused except where they separate to form *dural venous sinuses* and *dural folds* (Fig. 1.8A,B). The latter are connective tissue septae that extend into the cranial cavity and serve to subdivide it into compartments. In association with the cerebrospinal fluid they aid in providing physical support and protection for the brain. The position and form of the dural folds are summarized diagrammatically in Figure 1.8A.

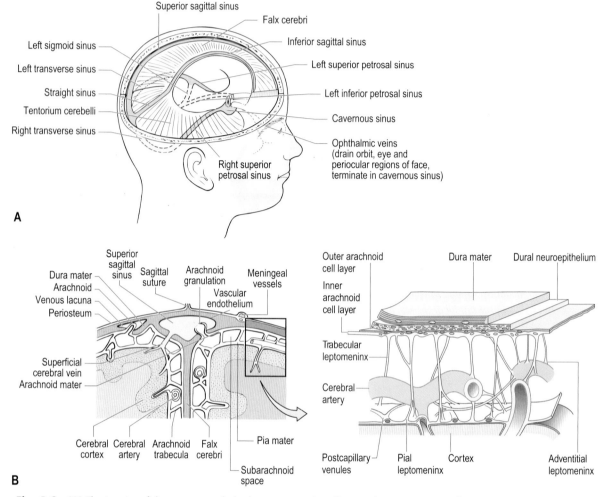

Fig. 1.8 (**A**) The interior of the cranium with the brain removed to illustrate the arrangement of the dural folds and some of the related dural venous sinuses. (**B**) The meninges as seen in coronal section in the region of the superior sagittal sinus (modified from Fitzgerald). Inset higher-power diagrammatic representation of the meningeal layers. (Modified from Fitzgerald 1992.)

The *dural venous sinuses* are valveless, highly specialized, firm-walled veins within the cranial cavity, which drain venous blood from the brain and cranial bones (Fig. 1.8B). In common with other veins the sinuses are lined by endothelial cells; however, their walls contain no smooth muscle cells. The arrangement of the sinuses is summarized in Figure 1.8A and D. Of particular note to those studying the eye and orbit is the pair of cavernous sinuses lying either side of the body of the sphenoid (Fig. 1.8E,F).

The importance of the *cavernous sinuses* (Fig. 1.8E,F) lies in their *position*, *relations* and extensive *communications*. Each cavernous sinus is around 2–3 cm

long in the sagittal plane and consists of a series of incompletely fused venous channels or a single venous channel partially subdivided by *trabeculae*. It has walls of dura mater, like other venous sinuses.

Position There is one cavernous sinus on either side of the body of the sphenoid. The sinus extends from the superior orbital fissure in front to the apex of the petrous temporal bone behind.

Relations These are summarized in Figure 1.8E and F (coronal section).

Communications The sinuses communicate with each other via the anterior and posterior intercavern-

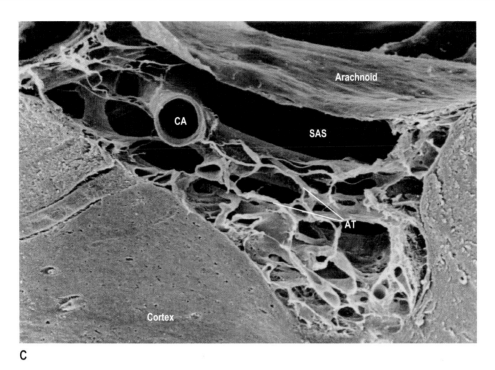

C

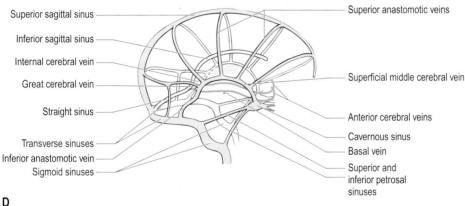

Superior sagittal sinus

Inferior sagittal sinus

Internal cerebral vein

Great cerebral vein

Straight sinus

Transverse sinuses

Inferior anastomotic vein

Sigmoid sinuses

Superior anastomotic veins

Superficial middle cerebral vein

Anterior cerebral veins

Cavernous sinus

Basal vein

Superior and
inferior petrosal
sinuses

D

Fig. 1.8 *Continued* (**C**) Scanning electron micrograph of the meninges and cortex of the brain showing the arrangement of the arachnoid trabeculae (AT) supporting the cerebral arteries (CA) as they course through the subarachnoid space (SAS) (× 100). (**D**) Schematic diagram of the dural venous sinuses and their connections with cerebral veins.

ous sinuses. Tributaries draining into the sinuses anteriorly include the superior and inferior ophthalmic veins (which drain the eye and orbit as well as areas of skin around the periorbital region of the face and nose), and the sphenoparietal sinuses. The superficial cerebral vein from the brain drains into the sinus from above (Fig. 1.8D). Blood from each sinus may, depending on relative pressures, drain via the superior and inferior petrosal sinuses either directly to the internal jugular veins (inferior petrosal) or to the transverse sinuses and thus to the internal jugular veins. Other exits include venous plexi around the internal carotid artery or veins traversing the foramen ovale or sphenoidal emissary foramen to communicate with the pterygoid plexus and other veins in the region of the skull base. Communications with the vertebral venous plexus in the epidural space also exist via the basilar venous plexus on the clivus.

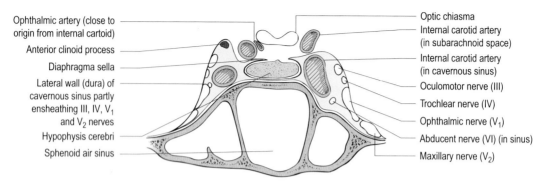

Ophthalmic artery (close to origin from internal cartoid)
Anterior clinoid process
Diaphragma sella
Lateral wall (dura) of cavernous sinus partly ensheathing III, IV, V₁ and V₂ nerves
Hypophysis cerebri
Sphenoid air sinus

Optic chiasma
Internal carotid artery (in subarachnoid space)
Internal carotid artery (in cavernous sinus)
Oculomotor nerve (III)
Trochlear nerve (IV)
Ophthalmic nerve (V₁)
Abducent nerve (VI) (in sinus)
Maxillary nerve (V₂)

E

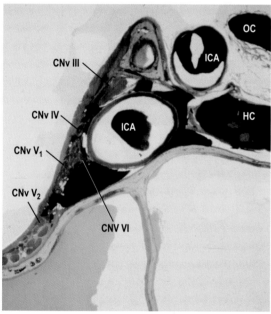

F

Fig. 1.8 *Continued* (**E**) Coronal section approximately midway along the body of the sphenoid bone to reveal the paired cavernous sinuses, one on either side. Note the position of the cranial nerves (II, III, IV, V₁, V₂ and VI), internal carotid artery (cut in two places, within and above the sinus) and hypophysis cerebri (pituitary gland). (**F**) High-power view of the left cavernous sinus (coronal plane, 100-μm thick section of low-viscosity nitrocellulose resin-embedded specimen) upon which (**D**) was based. OC, optic chiasma; HC, hypophysis cerebri; ICA, internal carotid artery.

Fistulas and thrombosis in the cavernous sinus

Arteriovenous fistulas These cause a variety of symptoms including pulsating protrusion of the globe and congestion of the vessels of the lids and conjunctiva owing to raised venous pressure. Patients complain of hearing noises like rushing water, probably because of increased flow rates in the labyrinthine plexus, which is in communication with the cavernous sinus via the superior petrosal sinus.

Cavernous sinus thrombosis as a sequel to infection spreading to the sinus, from such diverse initial sites as the nose, lids, behind the ear, bony labyrinth, pharynx and temporomandibular joint, can give rise to a variety of symptoms explainable on the basis of structures affected in and around the sinus. Facial pain may be the result of the involvement of the ophthalmic nerve (V₁).

Lateral rectus paralysis may follow involvement of the abducent nerve. Involvement of the other oculomotor nerves is less common because they are more protected in the lateral wall of the sinus. Thrombosis is usually bilateral because of the communications via the intercavernous sinuses. Papilloedema may result from obstruction of central retinal venous return.

The major *dural folds* (Fig. 1.8A) are as follows:

• *Falx cerebri* A sickle-shaped fold with its attached border in the mid-sagittal plane from the crista galli to the tentorium cerebelli behind. It lies in the vertical fissure between the two cerebral hemispheres, its lower border lying above the corpus callosum. The superior sagittal sinus is situated in the attached border and the inferior sagittal sinus is in the lower free border of the falx cerebri.

- *Tentorium cerebelli* This fold lies approximately in a horizontal plane at 90° to the falx, although it is elevated centrally (hence 'tent-like'). It separates the occipital lobe of each cerebral hemisphere above from the cerebellum in the posterior cranial fossa below. The free edge forms the boundary of the *tentorial notch*, which separates the forebrain from the hindbrain and 'houses' the midbrain. Sinuses related to the tentorium include the straight sinus, right and left transverse sinuses, superior petrosal sinuses, and cavernous sinuses.
- *Cavum trigeminale* A blind-ended dural recess whose entrance is in the posterior cranial fossa. It is formed by an invagination of the dura beneath the free edge of the tentorium and is roofed by dura on the floor of the middle cranial fossa. It houses the trigeminal ganglion, which sits in a shallow hollow on the apex of the petrous temporal bone, and some accompanying vessels. The ganglion is surrounded by cerebrospinal fluid continuous with the subarachnoid space of the posterior cranial fossa.
- *Diaphragma sella* A small circular fold of dura over the sella turcica that is pierced centrally by the infundibulum (Fig. 1.8E). It blends laterally with the roof of the cavernous sinus (Fig. 1.8F).

The area above the tentorium is known as the *supratentorial compartment*; that below is the *infratentorial compartment*. The cranial dura of the supratentorial compartment is innervated by sensory branches of the trigeminal nerve, and stimulation of these nerves (stretching, inflammation, compression) gives rise to frontal or parietal headache. The infratentorial compartment is supplied by branches of the upper cervical nerves, and stimulation of these sensory nerves may therefore manifest as occipital and neck pain.

> The *neck rigidity* accompanying *acute meningitis* of the infratentorial region is most likely the result of reflex contractions, or spasm, of posterior neck musculature in response to stretching of the inflamed cranial and spinal cord meninges.

The *meningeal arteries* lie within the inner (or periosteal) layer of dura with their accompanying veins (Fig. 1.8B) and are responsible for the many fine grooves that ramify over the inner surface of the cranium (see Fig. 1.7B,C). The largest and most important of these is the middle meningeal artery, which enters the skull through the foramen spinosum. These arteries supply the meninges and diploë (bone marrow of cranial bones), but they *do not* supply the brain.

> Damage to middle meningeal vessels, especially the frontal branch of the middle meningeal artery and vein (the latter lying closest to the bone), may result from blows to the head, especially in the temporal region (the pterion; see Figs 1.2B, 1.5B, 1.7C) where the bones are thinnest and most likely to fracture. Slow venous, and possibly then later arterial, bleeding will lead to an extradural haematoma with a resultant rise in intracranial pressure. Coma and death will occur if such a haematoma is not drained as soon as possible after symptoms of raised intracranial pressure manifest. A subdural haematoma may occur if the trauma results in brain laceration or tearing of intradural veins.

Arachnoid mater (Fig. 1.8C)

The arachnoid (*Gk.* spider) is a delicate fibrocellular layer beneath the dura (separated by potential subdural space) that is connected to the pia mater covering the brain by numerous fibrocellular bands that cross the cerebrospinal fluid-filled subarachnoid space. This arrangement has led some to state that the leptomeninges should be considered as a conjoined pia–arachnoid membrane. The arachnoid bridges over the sulci, gyri and other irregularities on the brain surface thus creating the *subarachnoid cisterns* or enlargements in the subarachnoid space (Fig. 1.8B, inset and C). Specialized regions of arachnoid, the *arachnoid villi* and *granulations* (fibrous aggregations of villi), project into several of the dural venous sinuses (Fig. 1.8B) and act as one-way pressure-sensitive valves allowing cerebrospinal fluid to drain from the subarachnoid space into the dural venous sinuses. Structures passing to and from the brain to the skull or its foramina, such as cranial nerves, must traverse the subarachnoid space. In addition, all cerebral arteries and veins lie in this space (Fig. 1.8C). Since the arachnoid fuses with the perineurium of cranial nerves, the cerebrospinal-fluid-containing subarachnoid space extends for a short distance around all cranial nerves and surrounds the optic nerve in a cuff-like manner as far as the posterior surface of the eye.

Pia mater (Fig. 1.8B,C)

The pia mater, a vascular fibrocellular membrane that is thicker than the arachnoid, follows closely the

15

contours of the brain. Vessels entering or leaving the brain substance carry a pial sheath with them. Pial tissue is rich in astrocytes, which extend along the vessel walls.

STRUCTURE OF THE EYE

The eye (Fig. 1.9) is a highly specialized organ of photoreception, the process by which light energy from the environment produces changes in specialized nerve cells in the retina, the rods and cones. These changes result in nerve action potentials, which are subsequently relayed to the optic nerve and then to the brain, where the information is processed and consciously appreciated as vision. All the other structures in the eye are secondary to this basic physiological process, although they may be part of the system necessary for focusing and transmitting the light on to the retina, for example cornea, lens, iris and ciliary body, or they may be necessary for nourishing and supporting the tissues of the eye, for

example the choroid, aqueous outflow system and lacrimal apparatus.

GENERAL SHAPE, SIZE AND POSITION OF THE EYE

The eye is approximately a sphere 2.5 cm in diameter with a volume of 6.5 ml. However, in reality it is the parts of two spheres, a smaller one anteriorly, the cornea, that has a greater curvature than the sclera, which constitute the large sphere. The cornea forms one-sixth of the circumference of the globe and has a radius of 7.8 mm; the remaining five-sixths is formed by the sclera, which has a radius of 11.5 mm. There is variation in size between individuals but the average axial length of the globe is 24 mm (range 21–26 mm). The diameter is 23 mm and the horizontal length approximately 23.5 mm. Small eyes (< 20 mm) are hyperopic or hypermetropic, while large eyes (26–29 mm) are myopic. The eye is situated in the anterior portion of the orbit, closer to the lateral than the medial wall and nearer the roof than the floor. The eye is made up of three

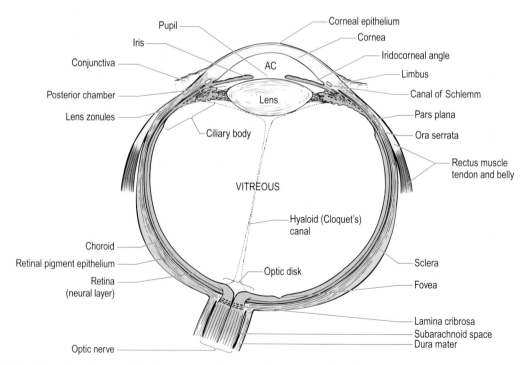

Fig. 1.9 Schematic diagram of the human eye in horizontal section revealing the major components and the arrangement of the three layers. AC, anterior chamber. The corneoscleral envelope (blue), the uveal tract (orange/red) and the inner neural layer (purple).

basic layers or coats, often known as tunics (Fig. 1.9). These are the fibrous (corneoscleral) coat, the uvea or uveal tract (composed of choroid, ciliary body and iris), and the neural layer (retina). The coats surround the contents, namely the lens and the transparent media (aqueous humour and vitreous body).

The cornea and sclera (see below) together form a tough fibrous envelope that protects the ocular tissues. The fibrous coat also provides important structural support for intraocular contents and for attachment of extraocular muscles. The cornea meets the sclera at a region known as the limbus or corneoscleral junction (see below).

THE CORNEA

The surface of the cornea (air–tissue interface) and associated tear film is responsible for most of the refraction of the eye; the refractive index changes little with age. The transparency of the cornea is its most important property, although because of its highly exposed position it must also present a tough physical barrier to trauma and infection. Corneal transparency is the result of a number of related factors: the regularity and smoothness of the covering epithelium; its avascularity; and the regular arrangement of the extracellular and cellular components in the stroma, which is dependent on the state of hydration, metabolism and nutrition of the stromal elements (see p. 209).

Shape
The cornea is smaller in the vertical diameter (10.6 mm) than in horizontal diameter (11.7 mm); however, viewed from behind, the circumference appears circular. The central radius is 7.8 mm with the peripheral corneal curvature being less marked. The cornea is also thicker at the periphery (0.67 mm) than in the centre (0.52 mm).

> Astigmatism is usually the result of differences in the radius of curvature in the vertical and horizontal meridians. Abnormalities in corneal curvature can be readily demonstrated by computerized video keratography, which applies the principle of projecting placido rings onto the corneal surface from which topographic maps can be constructed (Fig. 1.10).

Structure
The cornea is composed of five layers (Fig. 1.11A).

Corneal epithelium (Fig. 1.11B)
The corneal epithelium is a *stratified* (possessing five or six layers) *squamous non-keratinized* epithelium (the superficial cells are flattened, nucleated and non-keratinized). It is 50–60 μm in thickness and adjacent cells are held together by numerous *desmosomes* and to the underlying basal lamina by *hemidesmosomes* and anchoring filaments (Fig. 1.11B). The anterior surface of the corneal epithelium is characterized by numerous microvilli and microplicae (ridges) whose glycocalyx coat interacts with, and helps stabilize, the precorneal tear film. New cells are derived from mitotic activity in the limbal basal cell layer and these displace existing cells both superficially and centripetally. The corneal epithelium responds rapidly to repair disruptions in its integrity by amoeboid sliding movements of cells on the wound margin followed by cell replication.

The basal epithelial cells rest on a thin, but prominent, *basal lamina* (lamina lucida, 25 nm; lamina densa, 50 nm). Corneal epithelial adhesion is maintained by a basement membrane complex, which anchors the epithelium to *Bowman's layer* via a complex mesh of anchoring fibrils (type VII collagen) and anchoring plaques (type VI collagen), which interact with the lamina densa and the collagen fibrils of Bowman's layer. The corneal epithelium is devoid of melanocytes. Immunocompetent cells, including major histocompatibility complex (MHC) class II antigen-positive dendritic cells (Langerhans cells) are rare in the central cornea. While present in the limbus and peripheral cornea, dendritic cells decline sharply in density in a centripetal gradient. The recent discovery of MHC class II-negative dendritic cells in the mouse central cornea (Hamrah et al., 2002) has yet to be confirmed in the human eye. The paucity of potential antigen-presenting cells, such as dendritic cells, and the avascular nature of the cornea are of crucial importance to the success of corneal grafting (see Ch. 7).

Anterior limiting lamina (Bowman's layer)
Bowman's layer (a modified acellular region of the stroma) (8–12 μm thick) consists of fine, randomly arranged, collagen fibrils (20–30 nm diameter, types I, III, V and VI). The anterior surface is well delineated and is separated from the epithelium by the thin basal lamina, while the posterior boundary merges with the stroma (Fig. 1.11A). Bowman's layer terminates abruptly at the limbus.

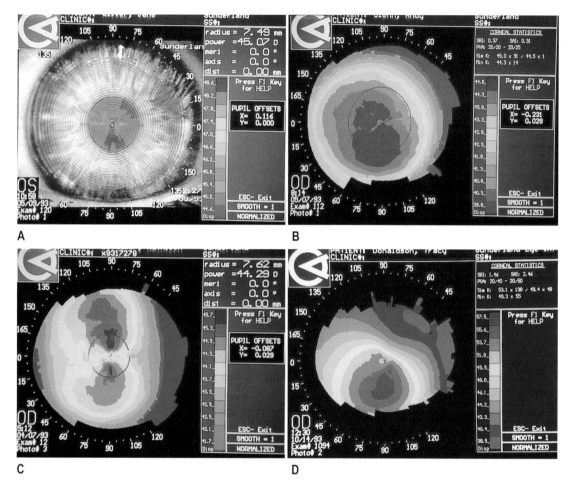

Fig. 1.10 Computerized video keratography (CVK). (**A**) This method involves the projection of over 6000 points of light onto the corneal surface in the form of placido rings. The images are analysed by the computer and complex colour-coded topographical/dioptric maps can be constructed. The scale or key is shown alongside: 'hotter' colours represent higher dioptric values. (**B**) A normal or round topographic map. (**C**) Regular 'with the rule' astigmatism in a normal healthy cornea with + 1.5 diopters of astigmatism at 90°. (**D**) Corneal topographic map of a patient with early keratoconus. CVK analysis is particularly useful in identifying early keratoconus. In this case the higher dioptric values are concentrated in the infratemporal region. (Photographs kindly provided by Prof. C. McGhee.)

In vivo confocal microscopy (IVCM)

This is a powerful non-invasive instrument used in the clinical evaluation of corneal abnormalities and normal structure of the tear film, cornea and conjunctiva. IVCM images are obtained by performing 'optical sections' of the cornea using non-coherent white light. Cells and matrix components with differing reflective properties within the transparent cornea can be imaged. The advantage of a 'confocal' approach is that only information in a narrow focal plane, approximately 4–25 μm in thickness, is analysed or collected by the microscope and scattering of light from structures outside the focal plane is thus minimized. The optics allow the light beam to be scanned (in the x and y axes) in a narrow area at one focal plane before shifting in depth to another plane of 'focus'(z axis) where the scan is repeated. Thus a series of optical 'slices' of high lateral resolution (1–2 μm) can be obtained from the entire cornea and, because of small differences in brightness/contrast, cellular detail can be visualized. This provides information that is normally the realm of conventional light microscopic and *ex vivo* laser scanning fluorescence confocal microscopic studies of processed tissues and wholemounts.

The images below are 'slices' at differing depths in the cornea from superficial to deep. (A) epithelium, (B) subbasal nerve plexus and dendriform cells, which may represent Langerhans cells, (C) keratocytes in the posterior stroma (D) corneal endothelial cells.

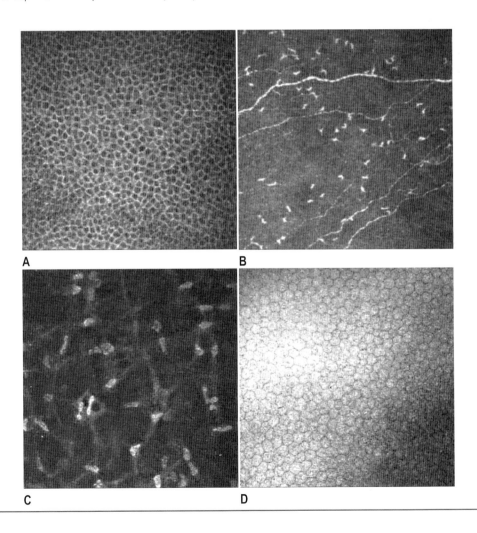

A B

C D

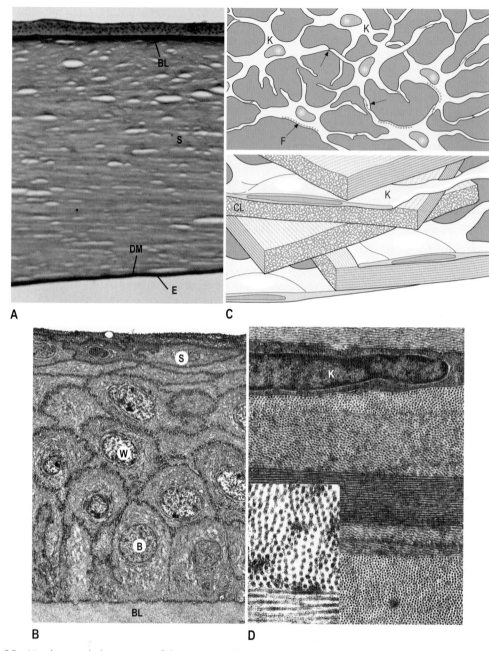

Fig. 1.11 Histology and ultrastructure of the cornea and its constituent layers. (**A**) Low-power light micrograph showing the five layers of the human cornea. Ep, epithelium; BL, Bowman's layer; S, substantia propria or stroma; DM, Descemet's membrane; E, endothelium. (**B**) Electron micrograph of the corneal epithelium. B, basal cell layer; W, wing cells; S, superficial cells; BL, Bowman's layer. (**C**) Schematic diagram showing the arrangement of the collagenous lamellae (CL) and the interposed keratocytes (K); arrows, gap junctions; F, fenestrations. (**D**) Electron micrograph illustrating a keratocyte among regularly spaced collagenous lamellae. [Inset – higher power to show collagen fibres.]

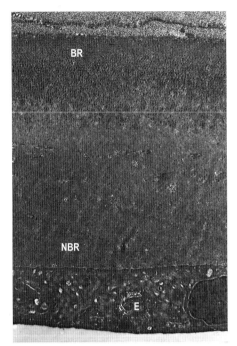

E

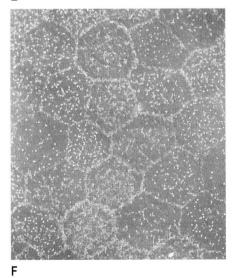

F

Fig. 1.11 *Continued* (**E**) Electron micrograph of Desçemet's membrane and corneal endothelium (E) to illustrate the banded region (BR) and non-banded region (NBR). (**F**) An 'en face' view of the inner surface of the corneal endothelium as seen by scanning electron microscopy. Note the homogeneous hexagonal array of endothelial cells. A similar but less detailed view of the endothelium can be achieved in the living patient with the aid of specular microscopy. Original magnifications: **A**, × 80, **B**, × 3000, **D**, × 20 000, **E**, × 7000, **F**, × 1200. (Parts B, D, E, and F courtesy of W.R. Lee and D. Aitken; Part E courtesy of Springer-Verlag.)

Substantia propria or corneal stroma (Fig. 1.11C,D)

The corneal stroma is a dense connective tissue of remarkable regularity. It makes up the vast majority of the cornea and consists predominantly of 2-µm thick, flattened, *collagenous lamellae* (200–250 layers) oriented parallel to the corneal surface and continuous with the sclera at the limbus. Between the lamellae lie extremely flattened, modified fibroblasts known as *keratocytes*. These cells are stellate in shape with thin cytoplasmic extensions containing conspicuously few distinctive organelles (Fig. 1.11C,D) when viewed in conventional cross-sections. However, recent studies (Muller et al., 1995) using frontal sections have revealed an abundance of organelles and a novel network of fenestrations on their surface which may facilitate the diffusion of metabolites or the mechanical 'anchoring' or attachment of collagen bundles (Fig. 1.11C). Recent *in vivo* confocal microscopy (see box, p. 19) data suggest that the density of keratoctyes in the anterior stroma is 20 000–24 000 cells/mm^2 and that the density decreases posteriorly before increasing again near Desçemet's membrane. Keratocytes are connected by gap junctions to their neighbouring cells and arranged in a corkscrew pattern (Muller et al., 1995). The collagenous lamellae form a highly organized orthogonal ply, adjacent lamellae being oriented at right angles, with the exception of the anterior third in which the lamellae display a more oblique orientation. The collagen fibres (Fig. 1.11D, inset) are predominantly of type I (30 nm diameter, 64–70 nm banding) with some type III, V and VI also present. The transparency of the cornea is highly dependent on the regular diameter (influenced by the presence of type V collagen in particular) and spacing of the collagen fibres (interfibrillary distance), which in turn is regulated by glycosaminoglycans (GAG) and proteoglycans forming bridges between the collagen fibrils. The GAGs in the human cornea are predominantly keratan sulphate and chondroitin (dermatan) sulphates (see Stiemke et al., 1995, and Ch. 4). The corneal stroma normally contains no blood or lymphatic vessels, but sensory nerve fibres are present in the anterior layers 'en route' to the epithelium (see below and box on p. 19). Recent data, obtained using transgenic mice in which eGFP (enhanced green fluorescent protein) is expressed on all CX3CR1 positive monocyte derived cells, has revealed extensive populations of resident tissue macrophages throughout the corneal stroma (Chinnery et al., 2007).

Posterior limiting lamina (Desçemet's membrane) (Fig. 1.11A,E)

This is a thin, homogeneous, discrete, periodic acid–Schiff-positive layer between the posterior stroma and the endothelium, from which it can become detached. It is 8–12 μm in thickness and represents the modified basement membrane of the corneal endothelium. It consists of two parts, an anterior third that is banded and a homogeneous or non-banded posterior two-thirds. It is rich in basement membrane glycoproteins, laminin and type IV collagen. The anterior banded region is reported to contain type VIII collagen. Types V and VI collagen may be involved in maintaining adherence at the interface of Desçemet's membrane with the most posterior lamellae of the stroma. Desçemet's membrane is continuous peripherally with the cortical zone of the trabeculae in the trabecular meshwork. Microscopic wart-like protuberances (Hassall–Henle bodies) containing 'long banded' (100 nm) deposits of unknown nature appear in the periphery of Desçemet's membrane with age. It is frequently thickened at its peripheral termination (Schwalbe's line, the anterior limit of the trabecular meshwork). If disrupted, Desçemet's membrane tends to curl inwards towards the anterior chamber.

Corneal endothelium

Fluid is constantly being lost via evaporation at the ocular surface, a fact illustrated by increased corneal thickness after a night of lid closure and when an impermeable lens is placed over the epithelium. The corneal endothelium, a *simple squamous epithelium* on the posterior surface of the cornea, has a critical role in maintaining corneal hydration and thus transparency. The endothelial cells rest on Desçemet's membrane (Fig. 1.11E) and form an uninterrupted polygonal or hexagonal array, or mosaic (Fig. 1.11F), which can be clearly seen *in vivo* with the aid of *specular microscopy* and *in vivo confocal microscopy* (see below and box on p. 19). The cells are 5–6 μm in height and 18–20 μm in diameter. Their lateral surfaces are highly interdigitated and possess apical junctional complexes that, together with cytoplasmic organelles such as very large numbers of mitochondria (Fig. 1.11E), are indicative of their crucial role in active fluid transport. These cells in the normal human cornea have low regenerative capacity and lost cells are quickly replaced by spreading of adjacent cells. There are approximately 350 000 endothelial cells per cornea (3–4000 cells/mm^2 at birth, falling to 2500 cells/mm^2 in middle age and 2000 cells/mm^2 in old age; see review, Waring et al., 1982). Consequently, with age, the dense, regular hexagonal arrangement typical of the young cornea is replaced by fewer cells of more heterogeneous size and shape. Damage to corneal endothelial cells and density below 800 cells/mm^2 leads rapidly to oedema and swelling of the stroma with resultant loss of transparency (see Ch 9, p. 487). A density lower than 1500 cells/mm^2 in a potential donor cornea is considered unsuitable for transplantation.

Nerve supply of the cornea

The cornea is richly supplied by sensory fibres derived from the ophthalmic division of the *trigeminal nerve*, mainly via the *long ciliary* nerves. Occasionally the inferior cornea receives some branches from the maxillary division of the trigeminal. Nerve bundles enter the peripheral cornea in a radial manner and as they travel centrally below the anterior one-third of the stroma and approximately 1 mm from the limbus they lose their perineurium and myelin sheaths. This alteration in myelination is thought to be related to the importance for transparency. They divide into smaller branches and begin to change direction towards the epithelium where they must pierce Bowman's layer, whereupon they further divide into smaller bundles to form the *subepithelial* or *sub-basal plexus* in the interface between Bowman's layer and the basal aspect of the corneal epithelium (Fig 1.11G). There are apparently no specialized end-organs associated with these terminal axons, which are predominantly within the size range 0.1–0.5 μm consistent with A-delta and C-fibres that function to transmit the sensory modalities of pain and temperature. Individual beaded fibres penetrate the epithelial layers and terminate in the superficial layers in the form of an intra-epithelial plexus. It is estimated that there are approximately 7000 nociceptors per mm^2 in the human corneal epithelium (Muller et al., 2003).

> Larger myelinated nerve fibres can often be seen during slit-lamp examination as fine whitish fibres radiating into the cornea from the limbus. Reflected light *in vivo confocal microscopy* has greatly added to our understanding of the distribution of corneal nerves in healthy and diseased corneas (see box, p. 19) (Muller et al., 2003). Due to their position in the anterior stroma and their radial arrangement, many are damaged during refractive procedures such as *LASIK* (Excimer laser *in situ* keratomileusis). Damage to the corneal epithelium and intraepithelial nerve terminals can cause a great deal of pain.

Reactivation of latent herpes simplex virus in the trigeminal ganglion occurs following damage to nerve terminals (cold, exposure to ultraviolet light, trauma, corticosteroids), and activated virus is transmitted to the cornea along sensory nerve branches, leading to recurrent herpes simplex keratitis and superficial corneal ulceration.

THE SCLERA

The sclera (Fig. 1.12A–E) forms the principal part of the outer fibrous coat of the eye and functions both to protect the intraocular contents and to maintain the shape of the globe when distended by intrinsic intraocular pressure. The globe shape is maintained even during contraction of the extraocular muscles, whose tendons insert on its surface. The sclera is relatively avascular and in adults appears white externally. The viscoelastic nature of the sclera (great tensile strength, extensibility and flexibility) allows only limited distension and contraction to accommodate minor variations in intraocular pressure.

Buphthalmos

The corneoscleral envelope of children with congenital glaucoma responds to raised intraocular pressure by irreversibly stretching, owing to the immaturity of the collagen fibres, thus producing the characteristically enlarged buphthalmos ('ox-eye') of this condition.

The sclera is thickest posteriorly (1 mm) and thinnest (0.3–0.4 mm) behind the insertions of the aponeurotic tendons of the extraocular muscles. It is covered by the *fascia bulbi* posteriorly and the conjunctiva anteriorly. The sclera consists of dense irregular connective tissue comprising extracellular matrix and matrix-secreting fibroblasts. The matrix consists principally of collagen type I although types III, IV, V, VI, VIII, XII and XIII have been identified (Rada et al., 2006). Unlike the cornea, the scleral collagenous lamellae are irregularly arranged (Fig. 1.12D) and are interspersed with elastic fibres, each consisting of an elastin core surrounded by longitudinally arranged microfibrils composed of a number of glycoproteins including fibrillin. The opaque nature of the sclera, in contrast to the transparency of the cornea, can be partly ascribed to this irregular arrangement of the collagen fibres (Fig. 1.12D), but also to the variable fibre diameter (25–250 nm), variable and irregular fibrillar spacing, higher water content, and the reduced coating of GAGs on collagen fibres. Indeed, the sclera contains one-quarter of the proteoglycan and GAG content of the cornea.

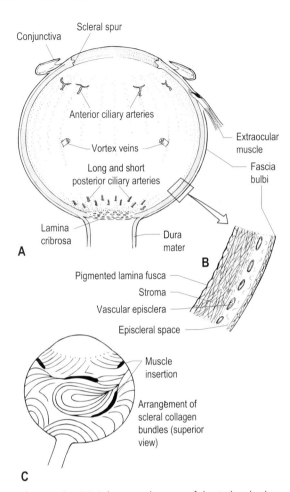

Fig. 1.12 (**A**) Schematic diagram of the isolated sclera and structures that blend with it (muscle tendons and optic nerve dura) or traverse its substance. (**B**) The scleral layers. (**C**) The pattern of orientation of the collagen bundles in the scleral stroma in relation to the extraocular muscle tendinous insertions.

Dermatan sulphate and chondroitin sulphate proteoglycans are the most abundant in the sclera (Watson and Young, 2004).

Collagen fibrils take up tensile force and are aligned with the direction of greatest tensile strength. The arrangements of scleral collagen can be studied using the 'split-line' technique, which has revealed that the collagen fibrils in the outer sclera are arranged in bundles that course in whorls, loops and arches, particularly around the muscle insertions and optic nerve (Fig. 1.12C). The collagen fibrils on the internal aspect of the sclera are arranged in a rhombic pattern (Thale and Tillman, 1993) (Fig. 1.12D).

23

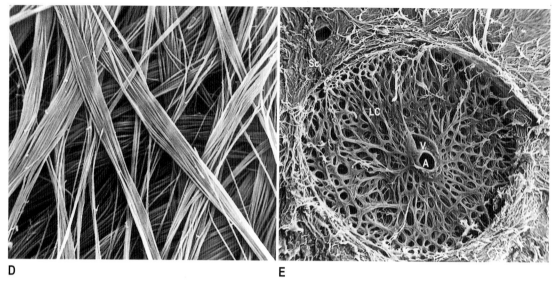

D
E

Fig. 1.12 *Continued* (**D**) Collagen bundles in sclera. (**E**) Arrangement of the collagen bundles in the lamina cribrosa (LC). A and V, apertures for the central retinal artery and vein. Original magnifications: **D**, ×7000; **E**, ×75. (Parts D and E courtesy of Dr A. Thale, from Thale and Tillmann, 1993.)

The sclera commences anteriorly at the *limbus* and ends posteriorly where the optic nerve perforates the sclera in the region known as the *lamina cribrosa* (Fig. 1.12A,E). The scleral collagen fibrils are arranged in circles or figure-of-eight patterns at the lamina cribrosa. Structures that transverse the sclera are shown in Figure 1.12A. The three histological layers of the sclera – the lamina fusca, stroma and episclera – are summarized in Figure 1.12B.

The 'blue' sclera of infants is the result of the underlying choroidal pigment showing through the thin collagenous stroma. In elderly individuals, fat deposition in the sclera may produce a yellowish hue. The yellowing of the eyeball in jaundice is the result of bilirubin deposition in the conjunctiva and not the sclera. Abnormal thinning of the sclera, such as occurs in some connective tissue disorders, e.g. Ehlers–Danlos syndrome, may also lead to a blue tinge. Localized thinning of the stromal collagenous layers may lead to *staphyloma* (bulging).

LIMBUS AND AQUEOUS OUTFLOW PATHWAYS (Fig. 1.13)

It is becoming increasingly appreciated that the *limbus* (Fig. 1.13A–C) is more than the border zone between the cornea and sclera; it has multiple func-

tions including nourishment of the peripheral cornea, corneal wound healing, immunosurveillance of the ocular surface and hypersensitivity responses; it contains the pathways of aqueous humour outflow and is thus involved in the control of intraocular pressure. It is also the site of surgical incisions into the anterior chamber for cataract and glaucoma surgery (see review by Van Buskirk, 1989). The limbus is 1.5–2.0 mm in width and the change in the radius of curvature between the sclera and cornea produces a shallow *external scleral sulcus* and an *internal scleral sulcus*; the latter is deepened by the *scleral spur* and houses the canal of Schlemm and trabecular meshwork. The longitudinal ciliary muscle fibres attach to the posterior aspect of the *scleral spur*, and its anterior surface gives rise to the corneoscleral trabeculae.

Several important transitions take place at the limbus (Fig. 1.13A–C).

- The regularly arranged corneal lamellae give way to the more random array of lamellae in the sclera. The corneal termination is V-shaped (Fig. 1.13B,C).
- The stratified squamous non-keratinized corneal epithelium with its parallel internal and external surfaces gives way to conjunctival epithelium, characterized by a folded basal surface and interdigitating subepithelial connective tissue (sometimes forming distinct *papillae*) (Fig. 1.13C).

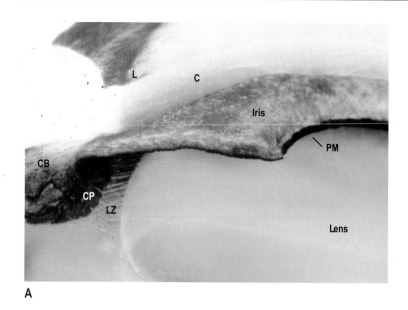

A

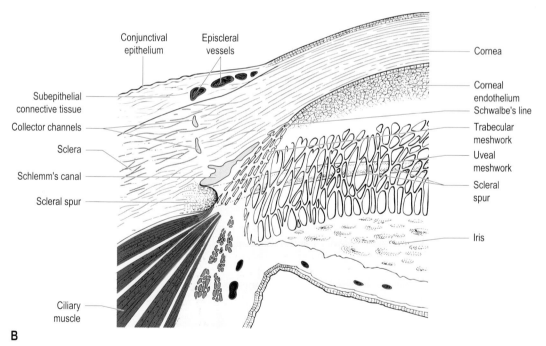

B

Fig. 1.13 (**A**) Macroscopic photograph of the anterior segment of a primate eye, which is almost identical to the human eye. Note the heavily pigmented limbus (L) characteristic of primates: C, cornea; CB, ciliary body; CP, ciliary processes; LZ, lens zonules; PM, pupillary margin. (**B**) Three-dimensional schematic diagram of important features in and around the iridocorneal angle and corneoscleral limbus.

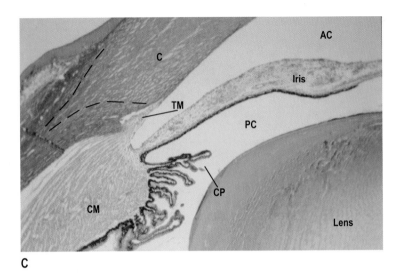

C

Fig. 1.13 *Continued* **(C)** Histology section of the primate anterior segment (Van Gieson stain). Dotted line indicates the corneoscleral junction: AC, anterior chamber; CM, ciliary muscle; PC, posterior chamber; TM, trabecular meshwork; C, cornea; CP, ciliary processes. Original magnifications: **A** and **C**, × 50.

- The conjunctival epithelium contains goblet cells and a network of MHC class II+ dendritic (Langerhans) cells (see section on conjunctiva, p. 87); the density of these cells declines sharply at the limbus, extending only a short distance into the corneal epithelium (see p. 17).
- Loops or arcades of conjunctival capillaries (derived from the anterior ciliary arteries) and lymphatic capillaries terminate at the limbus. The smaller vessels are not under neuronal control and are particularly susceptible to the effects of vasoactive amines (e.g. histamine, leukotrienes, prostaglandins) released by local immune cells (see below).
- Descemet's membrane and Bowman's layer terminate in this region.
- The loose conjunctival subepithelial vascularized connective tissue (substantia propria), containing immunocompetent cell types such as mast cells, plasma cells and lymphocytes, tapers off at the limbus and is absent in the cornea (Fig. 1.13C).

Anatomical and surgical limbus

Definitions of the limits and markings of the limbus vary among anatomists, pathologists and surgeons. The anatomical (histological) limbus is defined by a line that follows the V-shaped transition of corneal lamellae to scleral lamellae (Fig. 1.13C). Pathologists define the limbus as a block of tissue bordered anteriorly by a line passing through the termination of Schwalbe's line and the junction of the conjunctival and corneal epithelium (corneolimbal junction), and posteriorly by a line from the scleral spur perpendicular to the tangent of the external surface. Surgeons usually cut close to the blue–grey transition zone seen on external examination, and incisions made here will pass anterior to the trabecular meshwork and Schlemm's canal (Fig. 1.13B,C).

Aqueous outflow pathways

In the chamber or iridocorneal angle, partially nestled in the internal scleral sulcus, lies a complex wedge-shaped circumferential band of specialized, sponge-like, connective tissue, the *trabecular meshwork*, with the *canal of Schlemm* (sinus venosus sclerae) on its outer aspect (Figs 1.13B,C and 1.14A). The base of the trabecular meshwork is formed posteriorly by the scleral spur, the anterior face of the ciliary muscle and the iris root. The apex of the meshwork terminates anteriorly at Schwalbe's line and the adjacent innermost corneal lamellae (Figs 1.13 and 1.14A). The trabecular meshwork can be further subdivided into three anatomical zones: the innermost *uveal meshwork* with cord-like trabeculae; the *corneoscleral meshwork* with flattened sheet-like trabeculae (Fig. 1.14D); and the outermost *cribriform meshwork* beneath the inner wall of Schlemm's canal (Fig. 1.14E). The cribriform meshwork, unlike the rest of the trabecular meshwork, is not arranged in lamellae but consists of trabecular cells enmeshed in a loose extracellular matrix of collagen (types I, III and IV), elastic-like fibres and proteoglycans. This layer is thought to be the main site of resistance to aqueous outflow. The elastic cores of the trabeculae are continuous with the elastic fibres in the cribriform meshwork, which are in turn connected to the inner wall of Schlemm's canal via 'connecting fibres'. The anterior ciliary muscle fibres terminate in the elastic cores of the trabeculae. As the cilary muscle contracts and moves inwards, the three-dimensional trabecular meshwork can be expanded, which results in an increase in the amount of 'free' spaces in the cribriform meshwork. This in turn allows greater aqueous outflow thus increasing aqueous outflow facility (see review, Lütjen-Drecoll, 1998).

Aqueous humour passes from the anterior chamber through the *intertrabecular* and *intratrabecular spaces*, which are lined by trabecular cells. These cells envelop the trabeculae (Fig. 1.14D) and maintain the state of hydration of the connective tissue core in a similar manner to corneal endothelium. In addition, trabecular cells are also phagocytic, trapping and removing debris from the aqueous humour as it percolates through the tortuous intertrabecular and intratrabecular spaces which narrow as Schlemm's canal is approached (Fig 1.13B and 1.14A).

Schlemm's canal (sinus venosus sclerae) is an endothelium-lined 36 mm long circumferential channel filled with aqueous humour. It measures 200–400 μm in the anteroposterior axis, is seldom more than 50–60 μm deep and is often septate. The canal is drained by 25–35 *collector channels* (20–90 μm in diameter) and between two and eight *aqueous veins* (of Ascher) (up to 100 μm in diameter). These either join deep, intrascleral and episcleral venous plexuses which drain into conjunctival veins or, in the case of aqueous veins, may drain directly into superficial conjunctival veins. The majority of aqueous humour (70–90%) leaves the anterior chamber through the trabecular meshwork and Schlemm's canal ('*conventional*' outflow pathways). The inner wall of the canal is characterized, in well-preserved

and properly fixed eyes, by transcellular channels or giant vacuoles (Fig. 1.14B,C). There is good evidence to suggest that these intracellular vacuoles, with openings on both the trabecular and luminal aspects, function to drain the great bulk of aqueous humour. The number and size of vacuoles and their openings or pores vary in a pressure-sensitive manner. Small quantities of aqueous may also pass between endothelial cells in the canal wall.

A proportion (10–30%) of aqueous humour drains via the '*nonconventional*' *aqueous outflow pathways*. This route is not pressure sensitive and consists of the intercellular spaces between ciliary muscle fibres and the loose connective tissue of the suprachoroidal space. From here, aqueous traverses the sclera via the connective tissue sheaths of nerves and vessels that pierce its substance (see Fig. 1.12A).

Glaucoma

Glaucoma is defined as a progressive optic nerve neuropathy. For most forms of glaucoma, elevated intraocular pressure and ageing remain important risk factors, although low tension or normal tension forms of glaucoma do exist. However, in many forms of this condition pathological changes in the trabecular meshwork and Schlemm's canal may be responsible for increased resistance to aqueous outflow and raised intraocular pressure. In *congenital glaucoma* there is malformation of the complex three-dimensional arrangement of the trabeculae and excess extracellular matrix in the outer meshwork. Physical blockage of the inner surface of the chamber angle by the iris occurs in *closed-angle glaucoma*; this may be a primary or a secondary process (see p. 492). Various forms of obstruction in the trabecular meshwork may give rise to *open-angle glaucoma* (see p. 491); the cause of the primary form of this condition is unknown, although there is evidence to indicate that excessive deposition of extracellular elements may occur in the cribriform meshwork. Secondary forms of open-angle glaucoma may be the result of debris such as lens proteins, melanin, macrophages and haemorrhagic products physically obstructing the intertrabecular and intratrabecular spaces (see p. 492).

Uveal tract or uvea

The uveal tract (L. *uva* = grape), the middle vascular pigmented layer of the eye, consists of, from anterior to posterior: the *iris, ciliary body* and *choroid* (see Fig. 1.9). These three components are continuous with one another and have an opening anteriorly, the *pupil*, and posteriorly, the *optic nerve canal*. The uveal tract is analogous to the vascular pia–arachnoid of

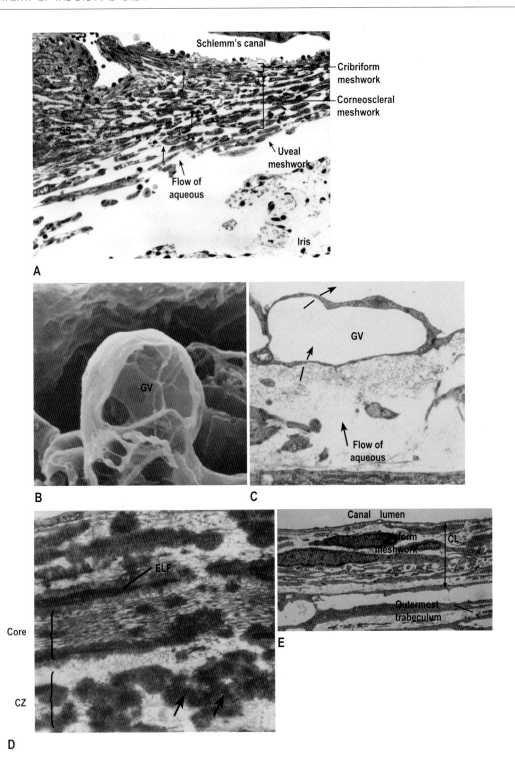

the brain and optic nerve, with which it anastomoses at the optic nerve head. The choroid is described on p. 57; the iris and ciliary body are described below.

THE IRIS

The iris (Fig. 1.15A,B) is a thin, heavily pigmented, contractile, circular disk analogous to the diaphragm of a camera. It is suspended in the frontal or coronal plane anterior to the lens and ciliary body, and is surrounded by aqueous humour. The iris separates the anterior and posterior chambers, which are in continuity through an opening, the *pupil*, which lies slightly inferonasal to the centre of the iris. The iris is attached by its *root* at the angle (iridocorneal) of the anterior chamber where it merges with the ciliary body and trabecular meshwork. The free edge is known as the *pupillary margin*.

The iris is 12 mm in diameter with a circumference of 37 mm. It is cone-shaped with the pupil margin positioned more anteriorly than the root. The pupil margin rests on the lens without whose support, for example in aphakic patients, it becomes tremulous (iridonesis). The size of the pupil regulates the amount of light entering the eye and is dependent on the state of contraction of the intrinsic pupillary muscles, the *dilator* and *sphincter* pupillae. The pupil may vary from 1 to 8 mm in diameter and there may be a slight degree of asymmetry between right and left eyes in normal individuals.

Structure (Fig. 1.15A,B)
The pupil margin and iris root are thin, and hence more susceptible to tearing in contusion injuries (iridodialysis). The anterior surface is divided into two zones, the *ciliary zone* and *pupil zone*, by the thickened region known as the *collarette*. The collarette marks the embryonic site of the minor vascular circle from which the pupillary membrane originated (see Ch. 2). The anterior surface is characterized by *radial streaks* (straight when the pupil is

contracted and wavy when dilated) and *contraction furrows* (more noticeable in dilated irides). The surface of the iris appears smooth in dark irides, in which the intrastromal melanocytes are heavily pigmented, and more irregular in blue irides, which have a less heavily pigmented stroma. The blue appearance of some irides is because of absorption of long wavelengths and reflectance of shorter wavelengths, especially by the collagenous stroma.

Microscopic anatomy
The iris consists of four layers: anterior border layer, stroma, dilator pupillae muscle and posterior pigment epithelium.

Anterior border layer (Fig. 1.15B,C)
This layer is not covered by a layer of epithelial cells, as early anatomists believed, but is in fact made up of modified stroma consisting of a dense collection of fibroblasts, melanocytes, and a few interspersed collagen fibres. This layer is deficient in areas; therefore the iris stroma is in free communication with the aqueous humour in the anterior chamber. Larger deficiencies in the anterior border layer are evident macroscopically as *crypts*. Aggregates of heavily pigmented melanocytes in this layer appear as *naevi*.

Stroma (Fig. 1.15C,D,E)
This consists of loose connective tissue containing fibroblasts, melanocytes and collagen fibres (types I and III). The loose nature of this tissue, and its free communication via openings in the anterior border layer, allows fluid to move in and out of the stroma quickly during dilation and contraction. The iris stroma in humans contains numerous mast cells and macrophages, many of which are perivascular (see Ch. 7). Many of the macrophages are heavily pigmented, and a subgroup may form large ovoid 'clump cells' (of Koganei) which tend to accumulate near the iris root and sphincter pupillae muscle (Fig. 1.15B,E). Lying free within the stroma close to the

Fig. 1.14 Histology and ultrastructure of the trabecular meshwork and Schlemm's canal. (**A**) Light micrograph showing the scleral spur (SS), Schlemm's canal and the three zones of the meshwork: the uveal, corneoscleral and cribriform meshworks. The path of aqueous through the inter- and intratrabecular spaces is indicated by arrows. (**B**) 'Giant vacuole' (GV) in the inner wall of Schlemm's canal as seen by scanning electron microscopy. (**C**) Transmission electron micrograph of a 'giant vacuole'. The flow of aqueous is indicated by the arrows. This particular section does not include the basal or luminal pores seen in some 'giant vacuoles'. (**D**) Electron micrograph of a trabecula cut in cross-section showing the layered arrangement of the extracellular components: CZ, cortical zone; ELF, elastic-like fibres; arrows, 'long spacing collagen'. (**E**) High-power micrograph of the cribriform meshwork or layer showing the lack of trabecular organization. Fibrocyte-like cells are loosely arranged in various types of extracellular matrix. Original magnifications: **A**, × 340, **B** and **C**, × 7000, **D**, × 13 000, **E**, × 5000. (From McMenamin, Lee and Aitken, 1986, *Ophthalmology*, with permission.)

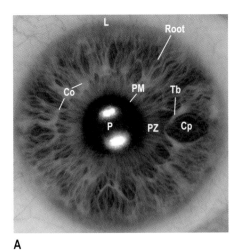

A

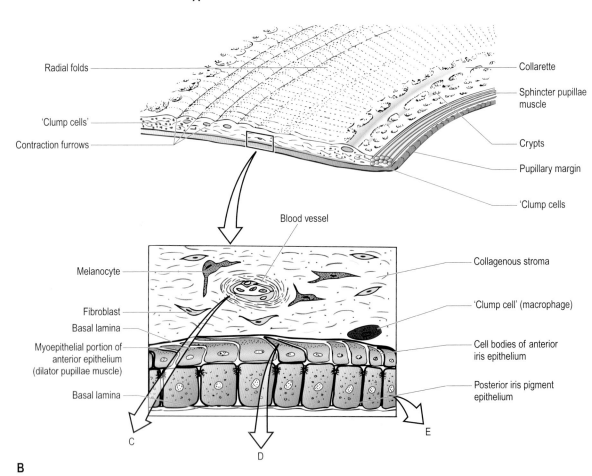

B

Fig. 1.15 The structure of the iris. (**A**) Clinical macroscopic image of a blue iris. Note the pupil (P), pigmented pupil margin (PM) and pupillary zone (PZ) separated from the ciliary portion by the collarette (Co). The root from the iridocorneal angle at the limbus (L). Note the fine collagenous trabecula (Tb), some of which form the boundaries of ovoid crypts (Cp). (**B**) Top diagram: surface features of a portion of the iris. Bottom diagram: high-power exploded view summarizing the arrangement of the pigmented (posterior) and non-pigmented (anterior) layers.

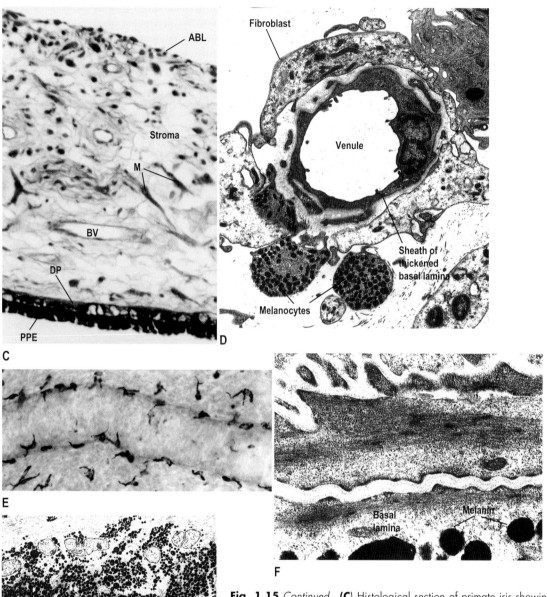

Fig. 1.15 *Continued* **(C)** Histological section of primate iris showing the anterior border layer (ABL), stroma containing melanocytes (M), blood vessels and collagenous matrix (red) and posterior portion characterized by dilator pupillae muscle (DP) and posterior pigmented epithelium (PPE). **(D)** Electron micrograph of an iris stromal vessel surrounded by fibroblasts and melanocytes. **(E)** Immunohistochemical staining of iris wholemount (rat) demonstrating networks of resident tissue macrophages (red) and MHC class II dendritic cells (blue). Note the macrophages are more perivascular in their distribution. **(F)** Ultrastructure of the contractile myoepithelial portion of the anterior iris epithelium, namely the dilator pupillae muscle: note the cytoplasmic microfilaments and membranous densifications, both characteristic features of smooth muscle cells. **(G)** Electron micrograph of the posterior iris epithelium illustrating the size, columnar shape and heavily pigmented nature of these cells. Original magnifications: C, × 300; D, × 7100; F, × 16 000; G, × 1400. (Part E from McMenamic *et al.* 1986, *Ophthalmology*, with permission.)

pupil margin is the *sphincter pupillae* muscle, a circumferential ring of smooth muscle fibres about 1 mm in width. The sphincter muscle consists of muscle bundles, each comprising six to eight smooth muscle cells, which are continuous via gap junctions and surrounded by a basal lamina. The muscle is innervated by parasympathetic nerve fibres derived from the oculomotor nerve (postganglionic fibres travel to the eye from the ciliary ganglion via the short ciliary nerves) although sympathetics also terminate in this muscle. The unusual embryological origin of this muscle from the neuroectoderm is described in Chapter 2.

Dilator pupillae muscle

This is a layer of myoepithelial cells derived from the *anterior iris epithelium*. The basal processes of this epithelium are 4 μm in thickness and extend up to 50–60 μm in a radial direction, while the apices of the myoepithelial cells are lightly pigmented and closely apposed to the apical aspect of the *posterior pigment epithelium* (Fig. 1.15B,C,F). The *dilator pupillae muscle* is innervated by non-myelinated sympathetic fibres whose cell bodies are situated in the superior cervical sympathetic ganglion. Its parasympathetic innervation seems less significant. The dilator pupillae extends only as far centrally as the outer margin of the sphincter pupillae.

Posterior pigment epithelium (Fig. 1.15G)

This heavily pigmented layer consists of large cuboidal epithelial cells that appear black macroscopically on examination of the posterior surface of the iris. The posterior layer is derived from the inner neuroectodermal layer of the optic cup (see Ch. 2). The cells extend for a short distance onto the anterior iris surface at the pupillary margin; this forms the black ruff seen on the pupil margin during slit-lamp examination of the eye (Fig. 1.15A). The posterior pigmented epithelial layer forms a series of radially arranged furrows (most evident near the pupil margin) and circumferential contraction folds (most evident in the periphery).

Pupil movements

Mydriasis (dilation) occurs in conditions of low light intensity and in the states of excitement or fear. It is a result of the action of the dilator pupillae muscle.

Miosis (contraction) occurs in more illuminated conditions, during convergence, and while sleeping. It is the result of the action of the sphincter pupillae.

Blood supply of the iris

The iris has a rich blood supply and extensive anastomoses. At the root there is an incomplete major 'circle' of the iris that is derived from anterior rami of the anterior ciliary arteries. Branches from here pass centripetally and form an incomplete minor arterial 'circle' at the level of the collarette.

The arteries have an unusual coiled form to accommodate the variable states of contraction of the iris. Veins lie close to the arteries, with larger veins primarily in the anterior stroma and smaller veins in the deeper layers. Veins drain posteriorly/centrifugally into the ciliary body and eventually the vortex veins (Fig. 1.33A).

Iris capillaries are characterized by non-fenestrated endothelial cells that have a high density of endocytotic vesicles and tight junctions. This makes them less permeable to a variety of solutes than normal somatic vessels (hence they do not normally leak in fluorescein angiography). These vessels thus constitute an important component of the *blood–ocular barrier*. The basal lamina of the endothelial cells is thickened (0.5–3 μm) and further strengthened by perivascular collagenous/hyalinized layers (Fig. 1.15C,D). Periarteriolar smooth muscle cells are rare and elastic fibres are absent.

Nerve supply

The iris possesses a rich three-dimensional nerve plexus of myelinated and non-myelinated nerves. The sensory nerves are branches of the long and short ciliary nerves, themselves branches of the nasociliary nerve (ophthalmic division of the trigeminal). The autonomic innervation of the muscles is discussed above.

THE CILIARY BODY

The ciliary body (Fig. 1.16A–D) is an approximately 5- to 6-mm wide ring of tissue that extends from the scleral spur anteriorly to the ora serrata posteriorly. Temporally it measures 5.6–6.3 mm, and nasally 4.6–5.2 mm. It is divided into two zones, an anterior *pars plicata* (corona ciliaris) and a posterior *pars plana* (Fig. 1.16A). The ciliary body is approximately triangular in cross-section; its base faces the anterior chamber and the apex blends posteriorly with the vascular choroid. The pars plicata is 2 mm wide and consists of 70 radially arranged folds known as *ciliary processes* (Fig. 1.16B), each of which is 0.5–0.8 mm high and 0.5 mm wide. The tips are paler as a result of decreased pigmentation. Minor ciliary

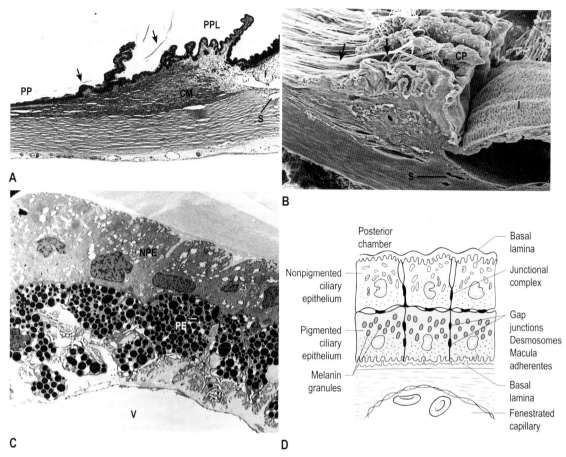

Fig. 1.16 (**A**) Histological section of the ciliary body showing the two major regions; the pars plana (PP) and the pars plicata (PPL) which includes the ciliary processes: CM, ciliary muscle; I, iris; S, Schlemm's canal. (**B**) Scanning electron micrograph of the inner surface of the ciliary processes (CP) and iris (I). Arrows in (**A**) and (**B**), zonular fibres. (**C**) Low-power electron micrograph of the pigmented (PE) and non-pigmented ciliary epithelia (NPE) of a ciliary process. Note the large fenestrated blood vessel (V) and the lens zonules blending with the basal lamina of the non-pigmented epithelium. (**D**) Diagrammatic representation of this double layer of epithelium, which constitutes the major site of the blood–aqueous barrier. Original magnifications: **A**, × 40; **B**, × 45; **C**, × 1600. (Part A courtesy of W.R. Lee and Springer-Verlag.)

processes may be present in the valleys between the major processes. The pars plana is an approximately 4-mm wide zone stretching from the posterior limits of the ciliary processes to the *ora serrata*, the sharp serrated or dentate junction where non-pigmented ciliary epithelium undergoes a sharp transition to become the neural retina.

The ciliary body can be divided histologically into the ciliary epithelium, ciliary body stroma and ciliary muscle (Fig. 1.16A). Each is described below in the context of the three principal functions of the ciliary body: (1) accommodation; (2) aqueous humour production; and (3) production of lens zonules, vitreal glycosaminoglycans and vitreal collagen.

Accommodation

The anterior two-thirds of the ciliary body is occupied by the *ciliary muscle* which, in conjunction with the *lens zonules* (suspensory ligament) and the natural elastic nature of the lens capsule, functions to alter the refractive power of the lens. Histologically, the ciliary muscle in meridional sections consists of three groups of smooth muscle fibre bundles embedded in a vascular connective tissue stroma (Figs 1.13 and 1.16A). The stroma contains melanocytes, fibroblasts, and occasional immune cells such as mast cells, macrophages and lymphocytes.

The *outer longitudinal muscle fibres* are attached to the scleral spur and therefore indirectly to the

33

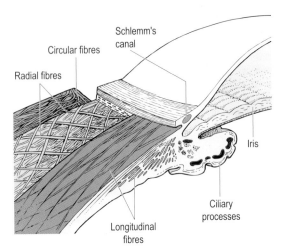

Fig. 1.17 Arrangement of the ciliary muscle fibres as seen on external view with the sclera removed. (After Rohen and Ciliankorpër, 1964.)

corneoscleral trabeculae anteriorly; posteriorly they are anchored to the inner aspect of the sclera. The *middle oblique* or *radial muscle fibres* are continuous with inner corneoscleral trabeculae. The *inner circular muscle fibres* (one of the three so-called 'Müller's muscles' associated with the eye and adnexa) appear as cross-sectional profiles in conventional meridional sections of the ciliary body (Figs 1.13B and 1.16A). A three-dimensional scheme has been proposed to explain the interrelationship between all three groups of muscle bundles; it appears that the fibres are all components of one interwoven fibre network (see Fig. 1.17 for summary).

The mode of action of the ciliary muscle is still controversial; however, it is generally agreed that during accommodation there is some degree of forward and inward shift of the ciliary body, which serves to slacken the tension on the zonules, thus increasing the refractive power of the lens (see p. 38).

Action of the ciliary muscle on aqueous outflow

There is some evidence that contraction of the longitudinal ciliary muscle fibres causes an inwards and posterior movement of the scleral spur, hence distending the inter- and intratrabecular spaces of the trabecular meshwork. This has been proposed as one of the modes of action of miotic drugs such as pilocarpine, which are used to increase aqueous outflow facility in patients with *glaucoma*.

Production of aqueous humour

Aqueous humour is a clear colourless fluid actively secreted by the ciliary processes (for details of aqueous constituents see Ch. 5). The ciliary processes consist essentially of delicate finger-like protrusions of loose vascular connective tissue covered by a bilaminar cuboidal/columnar neuroepithelium, the outer pigmented and inner non-pigmented ciliary epithelium, both derived embryologically from the double neuroectoderm of the optic cup (see Ch. 2). The morphological basis of the blood–aqueous barrier is depicted in Figure 1.16B. Aqueous humour is actively secreted by the inner non-pigmented ciliary epithelium whose apices are connected by junctional complexes including tight junctions. Macromolecules, having filtered through the highly permeable fenestrated stromal capillaries, pass between pigment epithelium cells held together only by punctate adherentes (macula adherentes)-like junctions or permeable band-like junctions (zonula adherentes), and are prevented from passing into the posterior chamber. The non-pigmented ciliary epithelium has morphological features characteristic of secretory epithelium, namely numerous mitochondria, and histochemically can be shown to contain enzymes, such as carbonic anhydrase, necessary for active fluid transport (see Ch. 4, p. 220).

Production of zonules, vitreal collagen and vitreal hyaluronic acid

The non-pigmented ciliary epithelial cells of the pars plana are cuboidal, columnar or irregular, depending on age and location. It is likely that these cells play a role in secretion of zonular fibres, the extracellular vitreal components, i.e. collagen and hyaluronic acid, and the inner limiting membrane, especially during embryonic development (Halfter et al., 2005).

Some inner non-pigmented cells 'tilt' anteriorly, suggesting traction by the zonular fibres. The lens zonules (of Zinn) or suspensory ligament of the lens merge with the fibrous basal lamina material of the non-pigmented ciliary epithelium (Fig. 1.16C). The precise mode of zonule synthesis is still unclear. Tall non-pigmented ciliary epithelial cells in the pars plana have ultrastructural and histochemical features that indicate active hyaluronic acid secretion.

Blood supply of the ciliary body

The blood supply of this region is derived from long posterior ciliary arteries and anterior ciliary arteries. The two long posterior ciliary arteries arise from the ophthalmic artery and after piercing the sclera near the optic nerve head they travel forward in the choroid in the medial and lateral horizontal plane and divide in the ciliary body before anastomosing with anterior ciliary branches, thus forming the major 'circle' of the iris (see p. 219, and Fig. 1.33). From this circle arises muscular and recurrent choroidal branches and the numerous branches that form the vascular plexus in the ciliary processes. Venous return occurs predominantly posteriorly through the system of vortex veins and less so through the anterior ciliary veins.

Nerve supply of the ciliary body

The ciliary body has rich parasympathetic, sympathetic and sensory innervations.

Parasympathetic innervation

Preganglionic neurone cell bodies are located in the Edinger–Westphal nucleus. Their axons travel in the oculomotor (III) nerve and synapse with postganglionic cell bodies located in the ciliary ganglion. The postganglionic fibres travel to the eye in the short ciliary nerves and terminate as an extensive plexus in the ciliary muscle. The action is mediated by acetylcholine on muscarinic receptors (see Ch. 6, p. 337).

Sympathetic innervation

Preganglionic neurone cell bodies are situated in the lateral grey horn of the first thoracic segment of the spinal cord. Preganglionic fibres relay in the superior cervical ganglion (adjacent to vertebrae C2 and C3, behind the internal carotid artery). Postganglionic fibres leave the ganglions as the internal carotid nerve and plexus. These fibres may reach the orbit as either direct branches of the internal carotid plexus or by joining the ophthalmic division of the trigeminal and its main branch in the orbit, the nasociliary nerve. Sympathetic fibres may either pass directly to the retrobulbar plexus behind the eye or through the ciliary ganglion uninterrupted. From the ciliary ganglions, fibres are distributed via the short ciliary nerves to the blood vessels of the eye, including the ciliary body. Some terminal filaments of the internal carotid plexus may also be distributed via the ophthalmic artery and its branches. The sympathetic action is mediated by the action of norepinephrine on two subclasses of receptors, α1- and β2-adrenoceptors, both of which are inhibitory (see Ch. 6, p. 337).

Sensory innervation

Sensory innervation is derived from the nasociliary nerve; however, the function of these fibres is unknown.

THE LENS AND ZONULAR APPARATUS

The lens (Fig. 1.18) is a highly organized system of specialized cells (so-called lens 'fibres'), which constitutes an important component of the optical system of the eye and fulfils the important function of altering the refractive index of light entering the eye to focus on the retina. While it has less refractive power (15 dioptres) than the cornea, the lens has the ability to change shape, under the influence of the ciliary muscle, and thus alter its refractive power. The range of dioptric power diminishes with age (8 at 40 years, 1–2 by 60 years). The transparency of the lens is due to the shape, arrangement, internal structure and biochemistry of the lens cells or lens fibres.

Position, size and shape

The lens, enclosed in its capsule, lies behind the iris and in front of the vitreous body. It is encircled by the ciliary processes and held in position by the zonular fibres laterally, the anterior vitreous face posteriorly (patellar fossa), and the iris anteriorly (see Fig. 1.9). It is normally transparent and avascular following regression of the tunica vasculosa lentis late in fetal development (see Ch. 2). It receives its nourishment from the aqueous and vitreous humours. It is a biconvex, ellipsoid structure with differing radius of curvature on the anterior and posterior surfaces. The anterior curvature is approximately 10 mm (range 8–14 mm) and the posterior curvature is approximately 6 mm (range 4.5–7.5 mm). The centre points of these surfaces, described as the *anterior* and *posterior poles*, are connected by an imaginary *axis*. The anterior pole lies 3 mm from the posterior corneal surface. The anterior and posterior surfaces are separated by the *equator*, which has a ridged (indented) appearance caused by the zonular fibres. In the adult the lens measures approximately 10 mm in diameter and has an axial length of 4 mm. The lens continues to grow (0.023 mm per year) and alters shape throughout life. It becomes rounder with age, especially after the age of 20 years.

Structure

The lens comprises three parts: (1) the capsule; (2) anterior or lens epithelium; and (3) the lens fibres (Fig. 1.18A,D).

Lens capsule

The *lens capsule* is a thickened, smooth, basement membrane produced by the lens epithelium and

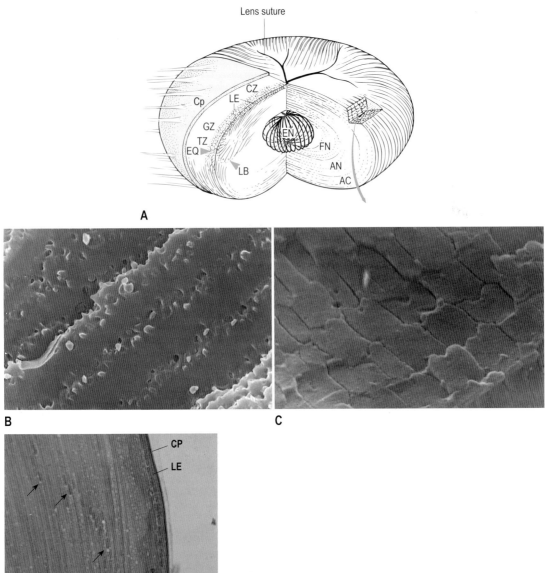

Fig. 1.18 (**A**) The structure of the lens: CZ, central zone; GZ, germinative zone; TZ, transitional zone; LE, lens epithelium; EQ, equator; LB, lens bow; Cp, capsule; AC, adult cortex; AN, adult nucleus; FN, fetal nucleus; EN, embryonic nucleus. (**B** and **C**) Scanning electron micrographs of lens fibres in longitudinal section (**B**) and in cross-section (**C**). Note the 'tooth and peg' arrangement interlocking the adjacent lens fibre surfaces. (**D**) Histological section of the equatorial region of the lens showing the orientation of the lens fibres, the lens capsule, lens epithelium and lens bow (arrows). Original magnifications: **B**, × 2500, **C**, × 5000, **D**, × 150.

lens fibres. It completely envelops the lens and has regions of variable thickness, being thickest pre- and post-equatorially (17–28 μm) and thinner at the posterior (2–3 μm) than at the anterior pole (9–14 μm). Ultrastructural examination reveals a fibrillar or lamellar appearance. The interfibrillar matrix consists of basement membrane glycoproteins (type IV collagen) and sulphated GAGs which are responsible for its prominent periodic acid–Schiff-positive staining properties in histological sections. It possesses elastic properties and, when not under tension of the zonules, the capsule together with the cortex causes the lens to assume a more rounded shape.

Lens epithelium
This is a simple cuboidal epithelium (Fig. 1.18A,D) restricted to the anterior surface of the lens. The cells become more columnar at the equator. As they elongate, the apical portion comes to lie deeper to other, more anteriorly positioned, lens cells. These elongated lens cells are known as lens 'fibres' (Fig. 1.18D). The manner in which equatorial lens epithelial cells are transformed into lens fibres is depicted in Figure 1.18A. The cell nucleus and cell body sink deeper into the lens as further cells are laid down externally. Mitotic activity is maximal in the pre-equatorial and equatorial lens epithelium, known as the germinative zone (Fig. 1.18A).

Lens fibres
While each lens fibre is only a 4×7 μm hexagonal prismatic band in cross-section (Fig. 1.18C), it may be up to 12 mm in length. The apical portion of the elongated lens cell (or lens 'fibre') passes anteriorly, the basal portion posteriorly. The cell nucleus migrates anteriorly as the cell is pushed deeper in the lens, hence creating the anteriorly oriented *lens bow* (Fig. 1.18D). The meridionally oriented lens fibres extend the full length of the lens, meeting at the anterior and posterior sutures (Fig. 1.18A). Deeper (hence older) lens fibres are anucleate. Continual growth of the lens, by addition of superficial strips of new cells, produces a series of concentrically arranged laminae, similar to the layers of an onion (best seen by dissecting a fixed or frozen lens). In life, the outer *cortex* of the lens has a softer consistency than the hard central *nucleus*.

Lens fibres are tightly packed with little intercellular space. Neighbouring cells are linked by ball-and-socket cytoplasmic interdigitations (Fig. 1.18B,C) and numerous gap junctions. The junctions may aid maintenance of centrally positioned cells (via intercellular and molecular coupling or metabolic coop-

eration) some distance from the source of nutrition (aqueous humour). Superficially located lens fibres are rich in ribosomes, polysomes and rough endoplasmic reticulum, and actively synthesize unique lens proteins, lens crystallins (see Ch. 4); however, the cytoplasm of mature lens fibres appears homogeneous. Lens fibres are rich in cytoskeletal elements (5 nm microfilaments, 25 nm microtubules, 10 nm intermediate filaments) oriented parallel to the long axis of the cell.

Cataract
This is the loss of normal lens transparency, besides the normal age-related yellowing, and may be caused by radiation such as X-rays, or, more commonly, ultraviolet light. As well as the biochemical changes in cataractous lenses, opacification may be the result of damage or disruption of the capsule, the lens fibre configuration, or the lens epithelium (see Ch. 9).

Lens zonules (zonular apparatus)
The lens is held in position by a complex three-dimensional system of radially arranged zonules (zonules of Zinn or the suspensory ligament of the lens) (Fig. 1.19). These delicate fibres are attached to the lens capsule 2 mm anterior and 1 mm posterior to the equator, and arise from the region of the pars plana ciliary epithelium and pass forward closely related to the lateral surfaces of the ciliary processes (Fig. 1.19A,B).

The zonules consist of dense, glassy bundles 5–30 μm in diameter. Each bundle consists of a series of fine fibres (0.35–1 μm in diameter), themselves composed of 8–12 nm fibrils. Biochemical analysis has revealed that the zonules are a unique fibrous non-collagenous protein with properties (α-chymotrypsin-sensitive) and ultrastructure similar to elastin. The microfibrils are surrounded by a layer of glycoproteins and GAGs and also contain fibrillin (see p. 223). The definitive site of synthesis of the lens zonules is not known; however, they are probably synthesized and maintained by the non-pigmented ciliary epithelial cells in the pars plana where their attachment can be traced to basal lamina material of the neuroepithelial cells close to the ora serrata (Fig. 1.19C).

The fibrous lens zonules blend with the basal lamina material of the lens capsule. The anterior and posterior zonules insert obliquely into the superficial 1–2 μm of the pre- and post-equatorial lens capsule, while the equatorial zonules insert at right angles.

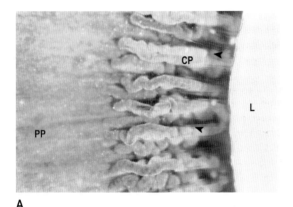

A

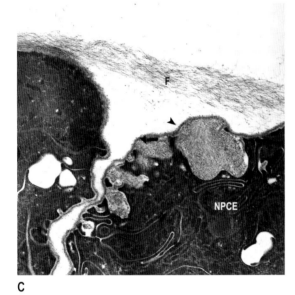

C

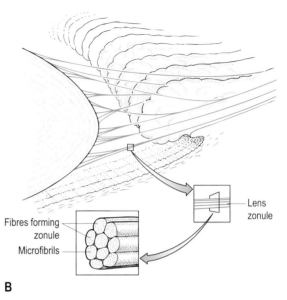

B

Fig. 1.19 Arrangement of the zonular fibres.
(**A**) Macroscopic view of ciliary processes (CP) and intervening lens zonules (arrowheads) inserting into the lens capsule in a monkey eye: PP, pars plana; L, lens.
(**B**) Arrangement of the different groups of lens zonules.
(**C**) Electron micrograph showing the close association of zonular fibres (F) to the non-pigmented epithelial cells (NPCE) of the ciliary processes. Note the material similar to zonular fibres beneath the basal lamina of the epithelium (arrowheads). Original magnifications: **A**, × 24, **C**, × 10500.

Accommodation

The zonules, besides holding the lens in place, also transmit accommodative movements of the ciliary muscle to the lens. In the non-accommodated state, the ciliary body maintains tension on the zonules. During accommodation, movement of the ciliary body causes slackening of the zonules, which take on a wavy appearance. Without the zonules pulling on the lens equator, the lens assumes an increased anterior curvature, with resultant increase in refractive power, owing to elasticity of the lens capsule and the outer cortical layers. Some authorities believe that there are two sorts of zonules: main zonules and 'tension' zonules, the latter being placed under tension during accommodation.

Posterior zonules are closely associated with the collagenous material of the anterior hyaloid membrane. Zonules running perpendicular to the main zonule stream form circumferential bands near the base of the ciliary processes or in the pars plana (posterior zonular girdle) and over the apices of the ciliary processes (anterior ciliary girdle).

Presbyopia

This condition may develop around the age of 40–50 years when the elasticity of the lens markedly decreases and there is associated atrophy of the ciliary muscle fibres; consequently the lens fails to change shape sufficiently during accommodation. This becomes evident as decreasing ability to read, i.e. use near vision.

ANTERIOR AND POSTERIOR CHAMBERS

The cavity anterior to the lens and lens zonules is divided into two chambers by the iris. These two chambers, the larger anterior and smaller posterior, communicate through the pupil. The boundaries of these two chambers are shown in Figure 1.20.

Posterior chamber

This is a very small irregularly shaped space whose size varies during accommodation. It is approximately triangular with its apex at the pupil margin; the base is formed by the ciliary processes; the posterior border is the lens and zonular apparatus; and the anterior border is the posterior surface of the iris. Aqueous humour secreted by the ciliary processes continually enters this chamber before passing through the pupil into the anterior chamber.

Anterior chamber

The anterior chamber is bound in front by the cornea and posteriorly by the anterior iris surface and the pupillary portion of the lens. The lateral recess of the anterior chamber is formed by the iridocorneal angle occupied by the trabecular meshwork. The anterior chamber is deepest centrally (3 mm) and contains approximately 250 µl of aqueous humour. Aqueous humour is produced at around 2–4 µl/minute. A little passes back into the vitreous; however, the bulk flow of aqueous is from the posterior chamber through the pupil into the anterior chamber. The aqueous humour is drained from the anterior chamber via the conventional and non-conventional routes (see p. 26).

Aqueous humour has two principal functions. It is the medium by which the necessary metabolites are transported to the avascular lens and cornea. It also removes toxic metabolic waste products of the cornea and iris. Second, it has a hydromechanical function in maintenance of intraocular pressure. This pressure depends on the balance between the *rate* of production of aqueous humour and its *resistance* to drainage. These two properties of aqueous humour, together with the fact that it is transparent, are necessary for the normal functioning of the eye (see p. 223).

THE VITREOUS

The vitreous cavity (Fig. 1.21) is the largest cavity of the eye (two-thirds the volume of the eye, weight 3.9 g) and contains the vitreous humour or vitreous. It is bound anteriorly by the lens, posterior lens zonules and ciliary body, and posteriorly by the retinal cup. The vitreous is a transparent viscoelastic gel that is more than 98% water with a refractive index of 1.33. Its viscosity is two to four times that of water. The main constituents of the vitreous, besides water, include hyaluronan (hyaluronic acid), collagens type II and IX, fibronectin, fibrillin and opticin (Bishop, 2000). The gel structure of the vitreous body is dependent on the collagenous constituents and not the hyaluronan. The fine-diameter type II collagen fibres (8–12 nm in diameter) entrap large coiled hyaluronan molecules (see p. 238).

The vitreous is shaped like a sphere with an anterior depression, the *hyaloid fossa* (also known as the patellar or lenticular fossa) (Fig. 1.21A). The vitreous is traditionally regarded as consisting of two

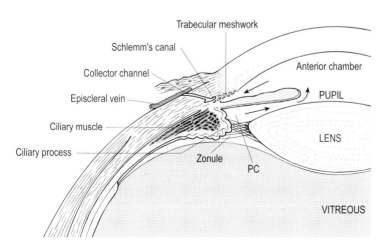

Trabecular meshwork
Schlemm's canal
Collector channel
Episcleral vein
Ciliary muscle
Ciliary process
Zonule
PC
Anterior chamber
PUPIL
LENS
VITREOUS

Fig. 1.20 Diagram of the anterior segment of the eye. The major pathway followed by aqueous humour from the posterior chamber (PC) to the anterior chamber and outflow pathways is shown by arrows.

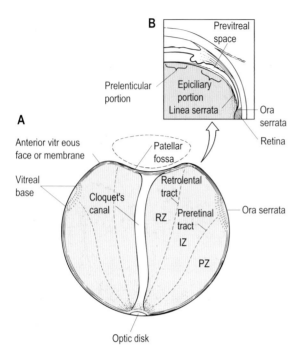

Fig. 1.21 (**A**) Diagram summarizing the anatomical zones of the vitreous (PZ, preretinal zone; IZ, intermediate zone; RZ, retrolental zone) and the major vitreal condensations (the retrolental tract, preretinal tract, vitreous base, anterior hyaloid face, vitreous cortex). (**B**) Higher power of the anterior vitreous face and its relation to the ciliary body and iris.

portions: a *cortical zone*, characterized by more densely arranged collagen fibrils, and a more liquid *central vitreous*. The vitreous can be further subdivided for descriptive purposes into three major topographical zones, namely preretinal, intermediate and retrolental zones, by two tracts, the preretinal and the retrolental tracts (Fig. 1.21A).

The cortical vitreous is attached by condensation of fine collagen fibrils at several points around its margin to (Fig. 1.21A,B):

- the peripheral retina and pars plana via the *vitreous base*, a 3- to 4-mm wide band
- the posterior lens capsule (ligamentum hyaloide capsulare)
- the retina along the margins of the optic disk (base of the hyaloid canal); although this is disputed (Sebag, 2004)
- the inner limiting membrane of the retina especially near retinal vessels (most variable and weakest of attachments).

Surgical removal of the posterior lens capsule can lead to disruption of the anterior hyaloid membrane and leakage of hyaluronate into the anterior chamber.

The *central vitreous* possesses less collagen than cortical vitreous. It is traversed by a central fluid-filled canal (hyaloid or Cloquet's canal), which represents the remnants of the course taken by the hyaloid artery that supplied the vitreous and lens in the fetal eye (see Ch. 2). The retrolental and intermediate zones in the human eye are semiliquid. The existence of an ordered, organized, vitreal structure is still controversial owing to the problems of studying a gel that is 98.5–99.7% water (see review; Sebag, 2004).

The human vitreous begins to degenerate at adolescence, leading to the appearance of liquid-filled cavities and fibrillar strands, such as the retrolental, preretinal and other named tracts of significance only to vitreal specialists. Most of the central tracts (except preretinal) are mobile and change during eye movements. The posterior vitreous cortex may possess zones of reduced density or 'cortical holes' or pockets that, if present, occur close to the fovea, retinal vessels and any developmental anomalies. While these are normal features, secondary pathological holes may develop following various disease processes.

Posterior vitreous detachment

The thin potential (subhyaloid or sublaminar) space between the surface of the cortical vitreous and the retina may fill with fluid in cases of vitreous detachment. The vitreous may detach relatively easily in the posterior segment where it is less weakly bound to the retina. The fluid may accumulate rapidly in the case of rhegmatogenous vitreous detachment and more slowly where the cortex is not ruptured (arrhegmatogenous vitreous detachment). The former is an age-related change in the vitreous. Vitreous detachment may predispose to retinal detachment (see Ch. 9).

Vitreous cells (Fig. 1.22)
The vitreous is essentially acellular; however, occasional isolated cells may occur in the cortex, particularly near the vitreous base, optic disk and retinal vessels. Cells known as hyalocytes, which bear the morphological, immunophenotypic and functional characteristics of bone-marrow-derived macrophages (Qiao et al., 2005) are the main cell types in

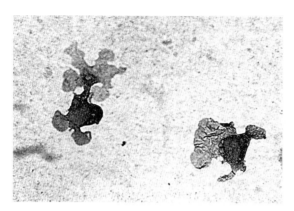

Fig. 1.22 Light micrograph of hyalocytes in the rat subhyaloid space stained with an anti-macrophage monoclonal antibody ED2 (plan view, retinal whole mount). Magnification: ×900.

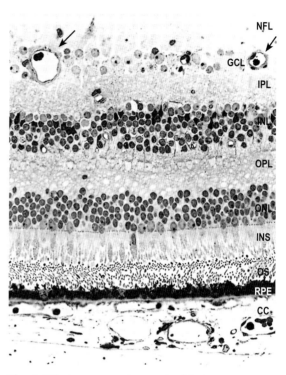

Fig. 1.23 Low-power micrograph of the human retina (wax histology): arrows, retinal vessels. Original magnification: ×150. Abbreviations: see Fig. 1.26A.

the vitreous. Their ability to produce hyaluronan is controversial. A marked vitreal cellular infiltrate is indicative of pathological or inflammatory processes in adjacent tissues, e.g. uveoretinitis.

Origin of the vitreous

The precise origin of the vitreous is still unclear. Suggestions include hyalocytes, ciliary epithelium, mesenchymal cells at the rim of the optic cup, hyaloid vessels during fetal development and retinal glial cells (Müller cells).

RETINA AND RETINAL PIGMENT EPITHELIUM (Fig. 1.23)

The retina is the innermost of the three coats of the eye. This layer is in the image plane of the eye's optical system and is responsible for converting relevant information from the image of the external environment into neural impulses that are transmitted to the brain for decoding and analysis. It consists of two primary layers: an *inner neurosensory retina* and an outer simple epithelium, the *retinal pigment epithelium* (RPE). These two layers can be traced embryologically to the inner and outer layers of the invaginated optic cup (see Ch. 2). In the adult they are continuous anteriorly with the epithelial layers over the ciliary processes and posterior iris surface (see pp. 32 and 33). Between the neural retina and RPE is a potential space, the *subretinal space*, across which the two layers must adhere. The neural retina is firmly attached only at its anterior termination,

the ora serrata, and at the margins of the optic nerve head.

Retinal detachment

In this condition the neural retina separates from the RPE, thus reopening the embryonic intraretinal space or optic ventricle (analogous to the ventricles of the brain), known in the adult as the *subretinal space*. Proteinaceous exudate tends to accumulate in the newly formed space (see Ch. 9). Adhesion of the neural layer and RPE is normally maintained by negative pressure, viscous proteoglycans in the subretinal space, and electrostatic forces.

The retina is bound externally by Bruch's membrane and on its internal aspect by the vitreous (Fig. 1.23). It is continuous with the optic nerve posteriorly, the site of exit of ganglion cell axons from the eye.

Regions of the retina

Before considering the histological structure of the individual retinal layers (Fig. 1.23) and their constituent cell types, it is important that the reader appreciates the regional or topographical variations of the human retina (Fig. 1.24A,B).

41

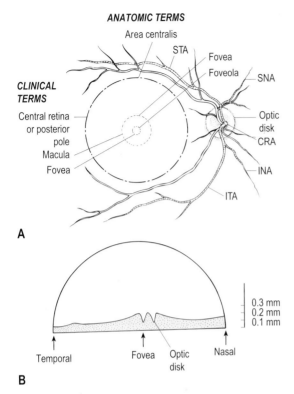

ANATOMIC TERMS

Area centralis

STA

Fovea

Foveola

SNA

CLINICAL TERMS

Central retina or posterior pole

Macula

Fovea

Optic disk

CRA

INA

ITA

A

0.3 mm
0.2 mm
0.1 mm

Temporal

Fovea

Optic disk

Nasal

B

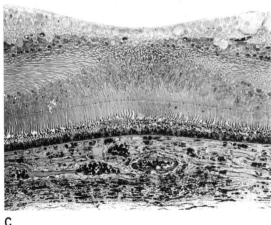

C

Fig. 1.24 (**A**) Anatomical and clinical terminology used to describe the regions of the retina: STA, superior temporal artery; ITA, inferior temporal artery; SNA, superior nasal artery; INA, inferior nasal artery; CRA, central retinal artery. (**B**) Regional variations in retinal thickness. (**C**) Section of the retina at the fovea. (Courtesy of D. Aitken and W.R. Lee.) Original magnification: × 150.

Clinical and anatomical terms

There is often confusion regarding the terminology of the regions of the retina owing to the use of differing terms by clinicians and anatomists. Figure 1.24A gives a summary of both terminologies.

1. The *posterior pole* or *central retina* (anatomically, area centralis) is a 5- to 6-mm diameter circular zone of retina situated between the superior and inferior temporal arteries. This region is cone-dominated and is characterized histologically by the presence of more than a single layer of ganglion cell bodies.
2. The *macula lutea* (anatomically, fovea) is a 1.5-mm diameter area in the posterior pole, 3 mm lateral to the optic disk. It is partly yellow as a result of yellow screening xanthophyll carotenoid pigments (zeaxanthin and lutein) in the cone axons. This may serve to act as a short wavelength filter protecting against UV irradiation.
3. The *fovea centralis* (anatomically, foveola) is a central 0.35-mm wide zone in the macula, consisting of a depression surrounded by slightly thickened margins. It is where cone photoreceptors are concentrated at maximum density to the exclusion of rods. The inner retinal layers in the margins of the pit (clivus) are displaced laterally and the outer retina consists purely of cones (Fig. 1.24C). The foveal retina is avascular and relies on the choriocapillaris for nutritional support.
4. The *optic disk* lies 3 mm medial to the centre of the macula (fovea). There are no normal retinal layers in this zone (blind spot) where ganglion cell axons from the retina pierce the sclera to enter the optic nerve. This pale pink/whitish area is 1.8 mm in diameter with a slightly raised rim. The central retinal vessels emerge at the centre of the optic disk, pass over the rim, and radiate out to supply the retina (Figs 1.24A and 1.31). The vein usually lies lateral to the artery.
5. The *peripheral retina* is the remainder of the retina outside the posterior pole. The distance from the optic disk to the ora serrata is 23–24 mm on the temporal aspect and approximately 18.5 mm on the nasal aspect. The peripheral retina is 110–140 µm in thickness, rich in rods, and possesses only one layer of ganglion cell bodies.
6. The *ora serrata* is the scalloped or dentate anterior margin of the sensory retina. At this transition zone, the neuroretina is continuous with the columnar non-pigmented epithelial cells of the

pars plana. The ora serrata is around 1 mm closer to the limbus on the nasal than on the temporal side.

For descriptive purposes, the retina is divided into nasal and temporal halves by a vertical line through the fovea. The optic nerve head is often used as a central point to describe the retina as having supero- and inferonasal and supero- and inferotemporal quadrants. The area of the retina is approximately 1250 mm^2 and varies in thickness from 100 μm (periphery) to 230 μm (near the optic nerve head) (Fig. 1.24B).

Retinal pigment epithelium (RPE)

The RPE (Fig. 1.25) is a continuous monolayer of cuboidal/columnar epithelial cells, which extends from the margins of the optic nerve head to the ora serrata, where it is continuous with the pigment epithelium of the pars plana. This cell layer has many physical, optical, metabolic/biochemical and transport functions, which play a critical role in the normal visual process (Fig. 1.25A). These include: maintaining adhesion of the neurosensory retina; providing a selectively permeable barrier between the choroid and neurosensory retina; phagocytosis of rod, and to a lesser extent cone, outer segments; synthesis of interphotoreceptor matrix; absorption of light and reduction of light scatter within the eye, hence improving image resolution; and transport plus storage of metabolites and vitamins (especially vitamin A). The complex morphology of this neuro-ectoderm-derived epithelium reflects these multiple functions.

Cell size, shape and structure (Fig. 1.25)

The RPE cells vary in size and shape depending on age and location, being more columnar in the central retina (14 μm tall, 10 μm wide) and more flattened (10–14 μm tall, 60 μm wide) in the peripheral retina. The basal aspect of the cells lies on *Bruch's membrane* and their apical surface is intimately associated with the photoreceptor outer segments (Fig. 1.25A,B). When examined *en face* they form a highly organized hexagonal pattern of homogeneously sized cells (Fig. 1.25C). The RPE has low regenerative capacity in the normal eye; therefore, cell loss is accommodated by hyperplasia of adjacent cells. Thus, in older eyes, the regular hexagonal array is lost and a heterogeneous mixture of sizes and shapes is more evident. The number of RPE cells per eye varies from 4.2 million to 6.1 million. The correlation between structure and function of this monolayer is summarized diagrammatically in Figure 1.25A.

Neurosensory retina (Figs 1.23 and 1.26)

The neurosensory retina is a thin transparent layer of neural tissue that in life has a red/purple tinge because of the presence of visual pigments; however, after death and in fixed specimens, it is white or opaque and often detached from the underlying RPE. Light stimuli are converted into neural impulses in the retina. These impulses are then partially integrated locally before transmission to the brain via the ganglion cell axons in the optic nerve. An appreciation of the anatomy of the neurosensory retina is crucial to an understanding of the physiology of vision (see Ch. 5).

The retina consists of several cell types of which neural cells predominate; other cell types include glial cells, vascular endothelium, pericytes and microglia. The three principal neurone cell types that relay impulses generated by light are photoreceptors, bipolar cells and ganglion cells, and their activity is modulated by other cell types such as horizontal cells, amacrine cells, and possibly by non-neuronal elements. It is the culmination of this neural processing concerning the visual image that is eventually transmitted to the brain along the optic nerve. Retinal cells are arranged in a highly organized manner, and in histological sections appear as eight distinct layers that include three layers of nerve cell bodies and two layers of synapses. The arrangement as seen in conventional histological section is shown in Figure 1.23 and the ultrastructural appearance is shown in Figure 1.26A. A simplified schematic diagram of retinal circuitry is shown in Figure 1.26B. Each of the principal cell types is described briefly below.

> *Weblink* Readers are recommended to visit the following website for more detailed description of retinal anatomy and function: http://webvision.med.utah.edu (Kolb, Fernandez and Nelson).

Photoreceptors (Fig. 1.27)

There are two types of photoreceptor in the human eye: rods and cones. They are situated on the outer or 'sclerad' aspect of the retina. There are approximately 115 million rods and 6.5 million cones in the human eye. Rods are responsible for sensing contrast, brightness and motion, while cones subserve fine resolution, spatial resolution and colour vision (see Ch. 5). The density of rods and cones varies in different regions of the retina, the periphery being rod-dominated (30 000/mm^2) while cone density

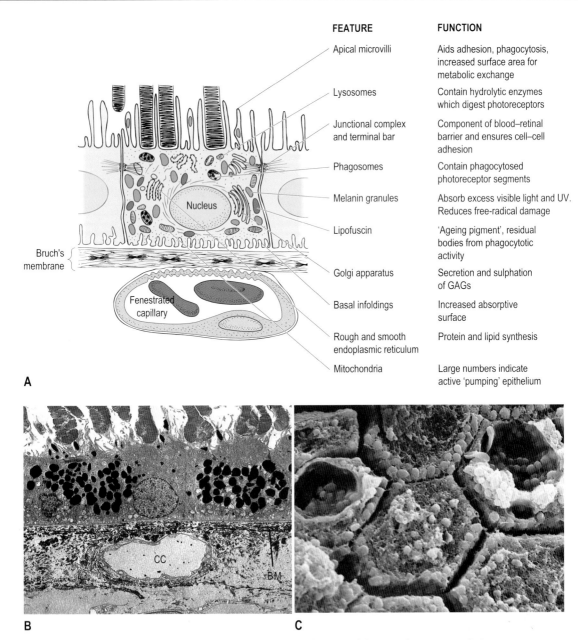

FEATURE	FUNCTION
Apical microvilli	Aids adhesion, phagocytosis, increased surface area for metabolic exchange
Lysosomes	Contain hydrolytic enzymes which digest photoreceptors
Junctional complex and terminal bar	Component of blood–retinal barrier and ensures cell–cell adhesion
Phagosomes	Contain phagocytosed photoreceptor segments
Melanin granules	Absorb excess visible light and UV. Reduces free-radical damage
Lipofuscin	'Ageing pigment', residual bodies from phagocytotic activity
Golgi apparatus	Secretion and sulphation of GAGs
Basal infoldings	Increased absorptive surface
Rough and smooth endoplasmic reticulum	Protein and lipid synthesis
Mitochondria	Large numbers indicate active 'pumping' epithelium

Fig. 1.25 (**A**) Diagram summarizing the main ultrastructural features of the retinal pigment epithelium (RPE). (**B**) Transmission electron micrograph of human RPE layer: CC, choriocapillaris; BM, Bruch's membrane. (**C**) Scanning electron micrograph of the apical surface of the retinal pigment epithelium. Note the hexagonal shape and the ovoid melanin granules, only visible because of post-mortem-induced disruption of the apical cell membrane. Original magnifications: **B**, × 2600; **C**, × 3600. (Parts B and C courtesy of D. Aitken and W.R. Lee.)

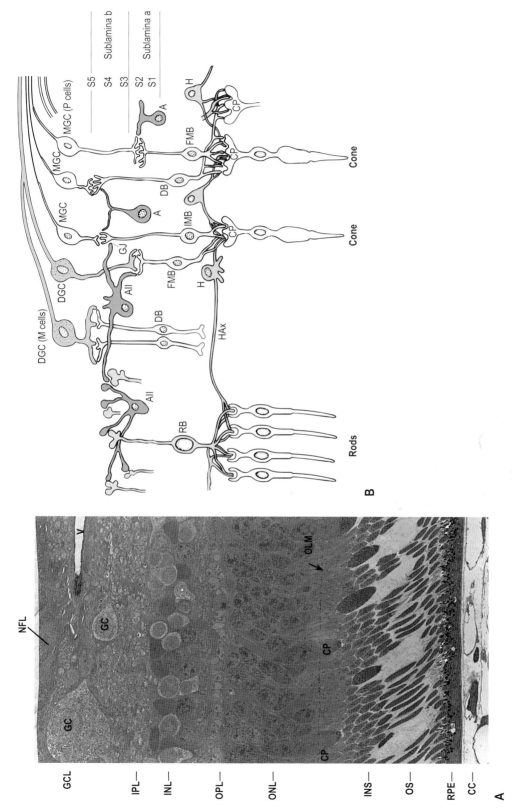

Fig. 1.26 **(A)** Low-power transmission electron micrograph of the primate retina demonstrating the layered arrangement: CC, choriocapillaris; RPE, retinal pigment epithelium; OS, outer segments; INS, inner segments; ONL, outer nuclear layer; OPL, outer plexiform layer; INL, inner nuclear layer; IPL inner plexiform layer; GCL, ganglion cell layer; GC, ganglion cell; NFL, nerve fibre layer; V, retinal vessel; OLM, outer limiting membrane; CP, cone pedicle. Original magnification: × 930. **(B)** Schematic diagram showing the arrangement and relations of the major cell types in the retina: RB, rod bipolar cell; CP, cone pedicle; H, horizontal cell; HAx, horizontal cell axon; A, cone amacrine cell; AII, AII (rod) amacrine cell; IMB, invaginating midget bipolar cell; FMB, flat midget bipolar cell; DB, diffuse bipolar cell; MGC midget ganglion cell. DGC, diffuse ganglion cell; GJ, gap junction.

45

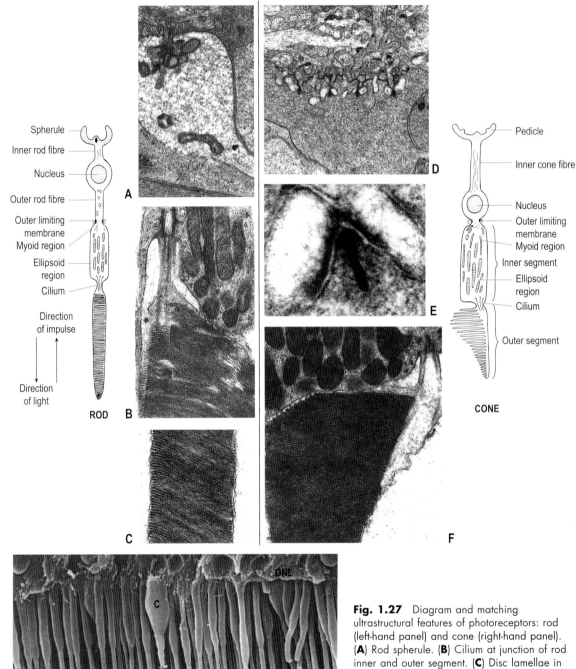

Fig. 1.27 Diagram and matching ultrastructural features of photoreceptors: rod (left-hand panel) and cone (right-hand panel). (**A**) Rod spherule. (**B**) Cilium at junction of rod inner and outer segment. (**C**) Disc lamellae in rod outer segment. (**D**) Cone pedicle with rows of synaptic ribbons or triads. (**E**) High power of triad-type synapse in a cone pedicle. (**F**) Cone outer segment and connecting cilium. (**G**) Scanning electron micrograph of human photoreceptors: C, cone; ONL, outer nuclear layer. Original magnifications: **A**, ×14000; **B**, ×28000; **C**, ×34000; **D**, ×10000; **E**, ×92000; **F**, ×28000; **G**, ×1700.

increases nearer the macula (150 000/mm² at the fovea), the fovea being exclusively cones.

Each photoreceptor consists of a long narrow cell with an inner and outer segment joined by a connecting stalk consisting of a modified cilium (Fig. 1.27). These inner and outer segments are 'separated' from the cell body by the outer limiting membrane. The nucleus is situated in the outer nuclear layer of the retina and axons pass into the outer plexiform layer where they form synaptic terminals (cone pedicle or rod spherule) with bipolar cells and interneurones (horizontal cells) (Fig. 1.26B). The outer segments of rods and cones are shaped precisely as their name implies. They contain the visual pigments that are responsible for absorption of light and initiation of the neuroelectrical impulse.

Rod cells

Rods are long (100–120 μm) slender cells whose outer segment contains the visual pigment rhodopsin sensitive to blue-green light (maximal spectral sensitivity 496 nm). Rods are highly sensitive photoreceptors and are used for vision in dark-dim conditions. The rhodopsin is contained within the membrane-bound lamellae or disks (up to 1000 per cell, 10–15 nm thick) that are enclosed by a single cell membrane (a conceptually useful analogy is to liken them to coins stacked inside a stocking). Each outer segment is only 1–1.5 μm in width (Fig. 1.27A–C,G) and 25 μm in length. The disks are produced at the base of the outer segment (the ciliary connection) and over the course of 10 days travel to the tips, which are enclosed by the apical microvilli of the RPE. Here they are phagocytosed by the RPE cells in a circadian manner (predominantly shed in the early morning) (Young, 1967). The rods are separated by a modified extracellular ground substance known as interphotoreceptor matrix, which contains a 135 kDa glycolipoprotein, interphotoreceptor binding protein (IRBP). The inner half of the inner segment is known as the *myoid*, the outer half the *ellipsoid* (3 μm in length). The ellipsoid is connected to the outer segment by a modified cilium (nine doublet microtubules without a central pair) (Fig. 1.27B) whose basal body is situated in the ellipsoid. The cilium represents the embryological vestige of the ciliated neuroepithelial cells that line the primitive retinal or optic ventricle (see Ch. 2). The cilium acts as a conduit for metabolites and lipids between the inner and outer segments. The remainder of the ellipsoid contains numerous mitochondria, indicative of the high metabolic activity of these cells. The myoid region contains numerous organelles includ-

ing Golgi apparatus, smooth endoplasmic reticulum, microtubules and glycogen, evidence of a metabolically and synthetically active cell.

Metabolic disturbances in the photoreceptors may lead to disturbances in visual pigment or photoreceptor membrane (lipid) synthesis and therefore specific abnormalities in vision. In addition, dysfunction in the hydration state of interphotoreceptor matrix can lead to retinal detachment as a result of loss of adhesive forces between the outer segments and the RPE (see Ch. 9).

Cones (Fig. 1.27D–F)

In most diurnal animals two spectrally distinct cone types exist (one maximally sensitive to short wavelengths and one to long wavelengths); however, in diurnal Old World primates, apes and humans, a third type exists. The three types are generally referred to as blue, green and red (or the short, medium and long wavelength) sensitive cones (see Ch. 6). Cone outer segments are generally shorter than rods and are so called because they are generally conical (6 μm at the base, 1.5 μm at the tip); however, in the fovea they are long, slender and tightly packed (see Fig. 1.24C). The lamellae or disks in cones are not surrounded by a plasma membrane in the same manner as rods but are in free communication with the interphotoreceptor space. Cone disks have a greater lifespan than rods and are not produced in the same manner; in addition, they do not undergo circadian phagocytosis by the RPE cells. They are surrounded by the long villous melanin-containing apical processes of the RPE.

Cones are about 60–75 μm in length. The outer segment is connected to the mitochondria-rich ellipsoid region (containing around 600 mitochondria per cell) of the inner segment by a cilium similar to that described in rods (Fig. 1.27F). The cell body of the cone can be easily identified histologically in the sclerad aspect of the outer nuclear layer because of its large pale-staining nucleus and perinuclear cytoplasm (Figs 1.23 and 1.26A).

The cell bodies of rods and cones are connected by an *inner fibre* to specialized expanded synaptic terminals, known as *spherules* and *pedicles* respectively. These synapse with bipolar and horizontal cells and contain many highly specialized presynaptic vesicles.

Rod spherules lie more sclerad than the cone pedicles and are deeply indented by bipolar and horizontal cell processes (telodendria). A specialized region known as a *synaptic ribbon* is present between two adjacent nerve fibres. The horizontal cell telodendria penetrate deeply into the spherule, the bipolar cell dendrites (from one to four cells) have a shallower penetration. Up to five processes may be embedded in one spherule (Fig. 1.27A). There is no apparent contact between rod spherules; however, cone pedicles may be connected by gap junctions.

Cone pedicles are broader than rod spherules (7–8 µm) and have a pyramidal shape. In the cone pedicle there are up to 12 indentations, each of which contains three neuronal terminals (*triad*) (Fig. 1.27D,E). The central process in each triad is a midget bipolar cell dendrite (each may have multiple contacts with the same pedicle; Fig. 1.26B). The laterally disposed processes in the triad are horizontal cell processes that may also be involved in several triads on the one pedicle. Thus there may be up to 25 synaptic ribbons in each pedicle (Figs 1.26B and 1.27D,E). Each cone is usually contacted by all the horizontal cells (four to six) in the immediate area or field. Each pedicle also has numerous shallow indentations or synapses with flat diffuse bipolar cells (Fig. 1.26B).

Bipolar cells (Figs 1.26B and 1.28A)

The retina contains approximately 35.7 million bipolar cells, which comprise several functional and morphological subtypes. They are primarily responsible for transmitting signals from photoreceptors to ganglion cells, between which they are interposed. Their cell bodies lie in the *inner nuclear layer* and are oriented in a radial fashion parallel to the photoreceptors. Their single or multiple dendrites pass outwards to synapse principally with photoreceptors (but also with horizontal cells), while their single axon passes inwards and synapses with ganglion and amacrine cells. In the foveal region of the central retina the ratio of cones : bipolar cells : ganglion cells can be 1 : 1 : 1, whereas in the peripheral retina one bipolar cell receives stimuli from up to 50–100 rods. In intervening regions the ratio corresponds to the decreasing visual acuity present in the peripheral retina. This summation of stimuli is a crucial factor in the sensitivity of the rod system to low levels of illumination. Bipolar cells have been subdivided in humans into nine morphological subtypes (Figs 1.26B and 1.28A), one rod bipolar type and eight types of cone bipolars. The latter group can be subdivided into five types of diffuse cone bipolars and three types of midget bipolars.

Rod bipolar cells

Rod bipolar cells have a receptive field or dendritic tree, which is small in the central retina (15 µm wide, 10–20 rods) and larger in the peripheral retina (30 µm and 30–50 rods). These represent 20% of all bipolar cells and are most dense around the fovea. In the periphery they contact up to 50 rods and synapse with AII amacrine cells; only rarely do they synapse directly with diffuse ganglion cells.

Diffuse cone bipolar cells

Diffuse cone bipolar cells are concerned with converging information from many cones. Their dendrites fan out (up to 70–100 µm) to end in clusters of between five and seven cone pedicles (can be as high as 15–20). The overlap of adjacent cells of this type is extensive in the perifoveal region.

Midget bipolar cells

Invaginating midget bipolar cells are the smallest of the bipolar cells whose dendrites penetrate the base of a single cone pedicle (occasionally two) to form a central element in triads. The near 1 : 1 ratio of midget bipolar cells to cones decreases peripherally. Their dendrites may synapse with amacrine cells and midget ganglion cells.

Flat midget bipolar cells connect single cones with single midget ganglion cells or more rarely may connect several cones. They are similar to invaginating midget bipolar cells except their dendrites do not invaginate deeply into the cone pedicle. Potentially, therefore, most cones can be in contact with these two types of midget bipolar cells (flat and invaginating midget) as well as the diffuse type.

Blue cone-specific bipolar cells (blue S-cone) have been described in primates and humans (Kolb et al., 1992) and appear to make invaginating contact with only a limited number of cones in their territory, the suggestion being that these are specifically blue cones.

Ganglion cells

The cell bodies of most ganglion cells are located in the innermost nucleated layer of the retina (ganglion cell layer) situated between the nerve fibre layer and the inner plexiform layer (Figs 1.23 and 1.26); however, 'displaced' ganglion cells have been identified in the inner nuclear layer. Ganglion cells are the last neuronal link in the retinal component of the visual pathway (Fig. 1.26B). Their axons form the nerve fibre layer on the innermost surface of the retina and synapse with cells in the lateral geniculate nucleus of the thalamus. The axons form bundles separated and ensheathed by glial cells (Fig. 1.28E). The bundles leave the eye to form the optic nerve. Upon exiting through the *lamina cribrosa*, the axons become myelinated with oligodendrocytes. There are up to seven layers of ganglion cell bodies in the central retina or fovea (ganglion cell layer is 60–

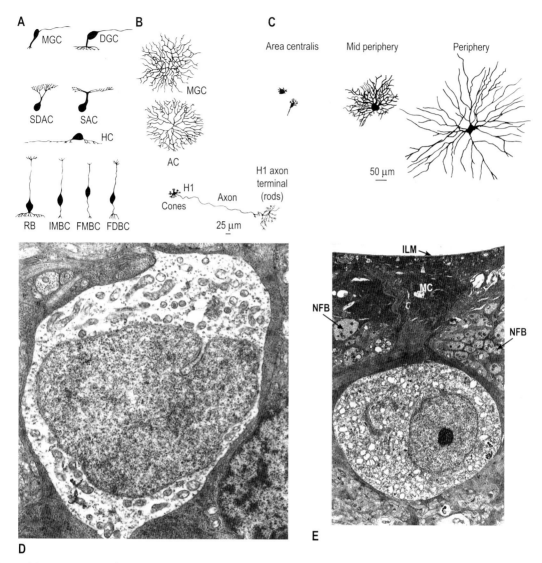

Fig. 1.28 **(A)** Diagram showing the arrangement and location of major neuronal cell types as seen in Golgi-stained preparations in relation to their position in the layers of the retina: DGC, diffuse ganglion cell; FDBC, flat diffuse bipolar cell; FMBC, flat midget bipolar cell: HC, horizontal cell; IMBC, invaginating midget bipolar cell; MGC, midget ganglion cell; RB, rod bipolar; SAC, stratified amacrine cell; SDAC, small diffuse amacrine cell. **(B)** Shape of dendritic fields of midget ganglion cell (MGC), amacrine cell (AC) and H1 horizontal cell (HC) as seen in Golgi preparations or single cell injections in retinal wholemounts. **(C)** Cat ganglion cells increasing in dendritic tree span with increasing eccentricity from the fovea. (Parts B and C, after Kolb et al., 1992, 1994.) **(D)** Electron micrograph of amacrine cell. **(E)** Ganglion cell body and adjacent nerve fibre bundles (NFB): ILM, inner limiting membrane; MC, Müller cell. Original magnifications: **D**, ×7100, **E**, × 4200.

80 μm thick) and as few as one cell layer in the peripheral retina (10–20 μm thick). There are approximately 1.2 million of these cells per retina, thus theoretically there are approximately 100 rods and four to six cones per ganglion cell. While they are functionally diverse, ganglion cells are characterized morphologically by a large cell body, abundant Nissl substance (arrays of rough endoplasmic reticu-

lum), and a large Golgi apparatus (Fig. 1.28E). They are classified into different types on the basis of cell body size, dendritic tree spread, branching pattern and branching level in the five strata of the inner plexiform layer (Fig. 1.26B). Some ganglion cells in the macular area may contain yellow (xanthophyll carotenoid) pigment in the cytoplasm, although the cone axons and Müller cells are thought to also

49

contain these pigments in the macular region (Yemelyanov et al., 2001). Impulses are received primarily from bipolar cells and amacrine cells via axodendritic and axosomatic synapses, the former occurring predominantly in the inner plexiform layer (Fig. 1.26B) where their dendrites repeatedly branch to form the 'dendritic tree', whose form and size varies considerably and may be correlated with location in the retina and therefore function (receptive field size) (Fig. 1.28B,C). The morphological diversity of ganglion cells (up to 25 types in mammalian and 18 types in human retinas) has prompted classification of these cells into categories, α, β and γ, or X, Y and W types, predominantly based on research in the cat (Rowe, 1991; Kolb et al., 1992).

Recently a non-rod, non-cone photoreceptive pathway, arising from a population of retinal ganglion cells, was discovered first in nocturnal rodents and then in primates. These ganglion cells express the putative photopigment melanopsin and by signalling gross changes in light intensity serve the subconscious, 'non-image-forming' functions of circadian photoentrainment and pupil constriction. The primate retina, in addition to being intrinsically photosensitive, is strongly activated by rods and cones to signal irradiance over the full dynamic range of human vision. Thus, in the diurnal trichromatic primate, 'non-image-forming' and conventional 'image-forming' retinal pathways are merged, and the melanopsin-based signal might contribute to conscious visual perception (Dacey et al., 2005)

Midget ganglion cells

These cells synapse exclusively with amacrine cells and one midget bipolar cell (and thus usually one cone) (Fig. 1.26B). Dendritic spread is around 5–10 μm in diameter in the central retina; however, this increases 10-fold in a zone of 2–6 mm eccentricity and attains a maximum of over 100 μm (Fig. 1.28C). Neighbouring midget ganglion cell dendritic fields do not overlap but form mosaics. In humans they are also known as P-cells because they project to the parvocellular layer of the lateral geniculate nucleus (LGN).

Diffuse (parasol) ganglion cells

These comprise a large synaptic field with all types of bipolar cells except midget bipolar cells. They occur in the central retina and their cell bodies (soma) are 8–16 μm in diameter with 30–70 μm dendritic fields, these being smaller nearer the fovea than the periphery. They are also known as M-cells because they project to the magnocellular layer of the LGN.

The finding that midget ganglion cells synapse exclusively with the midget bipolar cells, and that both are common near the fovea, provides the anatomical basis for the observation of small receptive fields and high visual acuity in this region. There are five types of diffuse ganglion cell, classified on the basis of morphology (Kolb et al, 1992; http://webvision.med.watch.utah.edu). The anatomical basis of antagonistic fields surrounding receptive fields is complex, although they do not appear to vary much in size from within an 8-mm radius of the fovea. The basis of the antagonist field may be the lateral extensions of the amacrine cell, with its extensive interconnections with ganglion cell dendrites and bipolar cells as well as fellow amacrine cells.

Association neurones (amacrine and horizontal cells) (Figs 1.26B and 1.28A,B)

Horizontal cells

These cells derive their name from the extensive horizontal extensions of their cell processes. There are two distinct morphological varieties in the retina of most species of which the cat is the most extensively studied: type A is a large sturdy axonless cell with stout dendrites that contact only cones; type B has a smaller bushier dendritic tree that contacts cones exclusively but, in addition, has an axon up to 300 μm in length that ends in extensive arborization that is postsynaptic only to rods (Figs 1.26B and 1.28B). Type A cells have much larger receptive fields than type B. In primates it appears that the two types of horizontal cell, HI (approximates to type B) and HII (approximates to type A), both possess axons. A third type (HIII) has been described in the human retina (Kolb et al., 1994). Each rod has connections with at least two horizontal cells and each cone with three or four horizontal cells of each type. In primates the stout dendrites of HI cell soma processes contact around seven cones near the fovea (dendritic tree covering 15 μm); this number increases to as many as 18 further from the fovea (dendritic tree covering 80–100 μm). The axon from HI cells passes laterally and terminates up to 1 mm away in a thickened axon terminal bearing a fan-shaped protrusion of lollipop-like endings in rod spherules (up to 100) (Fig. 1.28B). HII dendritic trees are more spidery and contact about twice as many cones. Their axons are generally shorter (100–200 μm) and contact cone pedicles by small wispy terminals. The manner of their insertion is depicted in Figure 1.26B. Their cell bodies are located primarily in the outer part of the inner nuclear layer. They have few distinctive cytoplasmic organelles except the crystalloids, a series of densely stacked tubules with associated ribosomes. Their processes ramify in the outer plexiform layer close to the cone pedicles. The overlap between horizontal cells is considerable and any one area of retina may be served by up to 20 horizontal cells. Horizontal cells have an integrative role in retinal processing and release inhibitory neurotransmitters, mainly γ-aminobutyric acid (GABA). Recent evidence suggests that there is some colour-specific wiring for the three types of horizontal cells in the human retina (see Ahnelt and Kolb, 1994, for details).

Amacrine cells (Figs 1.26B and 1.28D)

These association neurones were thought to lack axons; however, recent studies have shown that some do indeed possess an axon. They are located in the vitread or inner aspect of the inner nuclear layer (bipolar cell layer) and are distinguishable as a result of their larger size (12 μm) and oval shape. They display a remarkable degree of morphological (and pharmacological) diversity. There are at least 25 different types in the monkey and human retina. Their cell body is usually flask-shaped and the numerous dendritic processes of these cells ramify and terminate predominantly in the synaptic complexes formed by the bipolar and ganglion cell processes, namely the inner plexiform layer. The shape of their dendritic fields is highly variable and a few examples are shown in Figure 1.28A,B. They can be divided into subtypes on several criteria such as the stratification of their dendrites in the inner plexiform layer (Mariani, 1990) or their shape (see Rowe, 1991); for example, diffuse, starburst and stratified. Diffuse types can cover narrow fields (approximately 25 μm wide), their fibres being cone-shaped. Other types may spread their axon-like processes several millimetres. They may also be classified on the basis of their neurotransmitters. Amacrine cells may be GABAergic and dopaminergic or can release acetylcholine indicating, together with their morphology, that these cells play a role in modulation (most probably inhibitory) of signals reaching ganglion cells. A sub-class of amacrine cells are also thought to be the principle source of the peptide somatostatin, an important neuroactive peptide, in the retina. It may function as a neurotransmitter, neuromodulator or trophic factor (Thermos, 2003).

Retinal neuroglia

Astrocytes

Astrocytes are not the principal or predominant glial cell in the retina. This role is fulfilled by Müller cells, which are analogous to central nervous system oligodendrocytes. Astrocytes are predominantly located in the nerve fibre layer, ganglion cell layer, inner plexiform layer (site of cell bodies), and their outer limit is the vitread aspect of the inner nuclear layer in humans. They form an irregular honeycomb scaffold between vessels and neurones (Chan-Ling, 1994) perpendicular to the Müller cells. They may occur as fibrous (elongated) or protoplasmic (rounded) astrocytes. They both contain abundant cytoplasmic structural fibrils (10 nm in diameter) consisting of glial fibrillary acid protein (GFAP) (Fig. 1.29B). Astrocytes are often oriented perpendicular to the direction of the neurone cell bodies or processes, such as in the nerve fibre layer (Fig. 1.29). It seems their role may be to isolate the receptive surfaces of neurones in the retina, thus preventing unwanted signals or effects in neighbouring neurones. They have abundant intracytoplasmic glycogen and form 'gap junctions' with neighbouring astrocytes. Their pedicles or foot processes were once believed to constitute an important functional component of the blood–retinal barrier (see below).

Proliferative vitreal retinopathy

When injured, the retina frequently responds by forming astroglial scars. Indeed, normal age-related degenerative processes in the peripheral retina are accompanied by astrocyte proliferation. Disruption of the inner limiting membrane can lead to astrocyte proliferation in the subhyaloid space and in the vitreous itself.

Müller cells

Müller cells (Fig. 1.30A,B) are the principal supporting glial cells of the retina and are considered analogous to central nervous system radial glial or ependymal cells. They have a radial orientation and extend through the depths of the retina from the inner surface, where their expanded 'foot process' lies adjacent to the inner limiting membrane, to their outer limit where they have adherens junctions with photoreceptor inner segments to form the external limiting membrane. They envelop blood vessels, neuronal cell bodies and processes, creating glial 'tunnels' via a series of cytoplasmic processes, as shown in Figure 1.30A,B. Müller cells in humans contain little glycogen, in contrast to species with avascular retinae. Their cytoplasm contains abundant endoplasmic reticulum and microtubules, reflecting their role in protein synthesis, intracellular transport and secretion (Fig. 1.30C). These cells may help to nourish and maintain the outer retina, which lacks a direct blood supply.

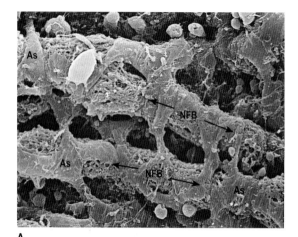

A

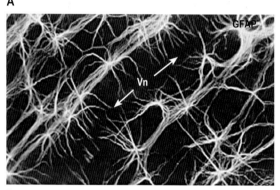

B

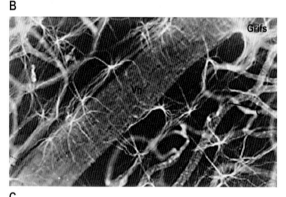

C

Fig. 1.29 (**A**) Scanning electron micrograph (viewed from the vitreous aspect) of astrocytes (As) surrounding nerve fibre bundles (NFB) in the inner retina (the inner limiting membrane has been removed to expose the underlying nerve fibre layer). (**B** and **C**) Double-colour immunofluorescence illustrating the relations of astrocytes shown with an antibody to glial acidic fibrillary acidic protein (GFAP) conjugated to Texas red (**B**) and the *Griffonia simplicifolia* (Grifs) lectin conjugated to fluorescein isothiocyanate (**C**) which binds to blood vessels. Vn, retinal vein; C, capillaries. Original magnifications: **A**, × 1500, **B**, × 150; **C**, × 150. (Parts B and C courtesy of Dr T. Chan-Ling, 1994.)

While there is extensive coupling between astrocytes and Müller cells, which allows the exchange of tracer molecules, recent studies have demonstrated an absence of significant spread of spatial buffer current between retinal glial cells. Both astrocytes and Müller cells have high K^+ membrane conductances, and most spatial buffer current will flow out through these conductances rather than spreading into neighbouring glial cells through gap junctions. In contrast to electrical coupling, chemical coupling between astrocytes is sufficiently strong to mediate propagation of intercellular signals such as the spread of metabolites and ions between glial cells. Coupling between glial cells, therefore, could serve to enhance the transport of key metabolites, such as glutamate, glutamine and lactate, both into and out of glial cells, by allowing them to diffuse between neighbouring cells in the glial syncytium (Ceelen et al., 2001). Clearly the underlying arrangement of both astrocytes and Müller cells reflects this function.

Microglia

Microglia (Fig. 1.30D) are a highly specialized subpopulation of the mononuclear phagocyte system that reside in the central nervous system (McMenamin and Forrester, 1999). These bone-marrow-derived cells are characterized by an extremely arborized morphology and an immuno-phenotype of resting macrophage. The cell bodies

---

Fig. 1.30 (**A**) Micrograph of a horseradish peroxidase (HRP) filled Müller cell in the rabbit retina. The dark band at the top of the micrograph is composed of Müller cell endfeet and the labelled axons of ganglion cells in the nerve fibre layer. The Müller cells possess side-processes that form different strata in the inner plexiform and they send numerous processes to wrap around the somata of photoreceptors: NFL, nerve fibre layer; GCL, ganglion cell layer; IPL, inner plexiform layer; INL, inner nuclear layer; OPL, outer plexiform layer; ONL, outer nuclear layer; IS, inner segments. (**B**) Diagram of the shape and position of a Müller cell: RPE, retinal pigment epithelium. (**C**) Morphology of a Müller cell (MC) within the outer nuclear layer. Note the intracytoplasmic microfilaments. (**D**) Microglial cells (specialized macrophages) in a retinal wholemount from a transgenic mouse in which eGFP is expressed alongside the locus for the chemokine receptor CX_3CR1. All microglia in these animals express CX_3CR1 and thus appear fluorescent green in confocal microscopy. Original magnifications: **A**, bar 10 mm; **B**, × 4400, **C**, × 200. (Part A courtesy of Dr. S. Robinson, from Robinson and Dreher, 1990.

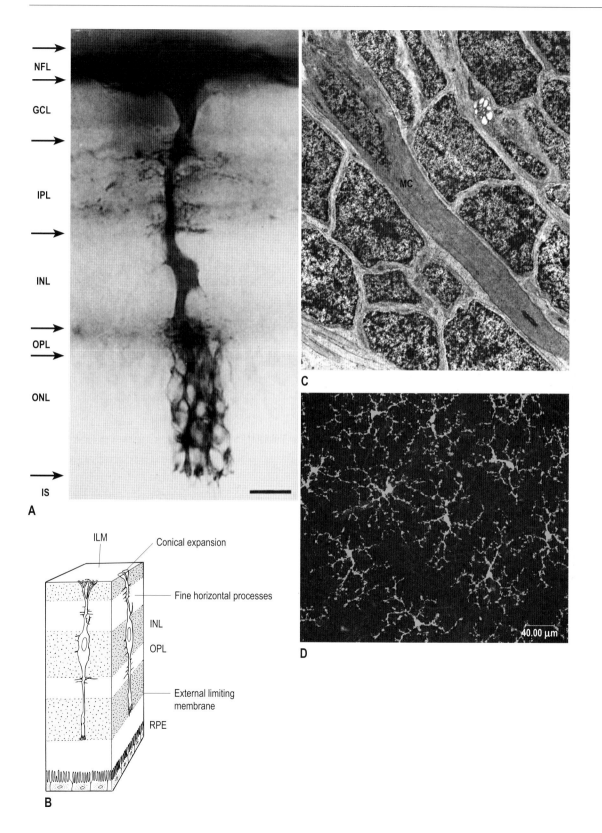

NFL

GCL

IPL

INL

OPL

ONL

IS

A

C

B

ILM

Conical expansion

Fine horizontal processes

INL

OPL

External limiting membrane

RPE

D

40.00 μm

are located largely in two strata, one at the nerve fibre layer–ganglion cell layer interface, the other at the inner nuclear layer–outer plexiform layer. Their processes form a three-dimensional net within the retina extending only as far as the outer limiting membrane. Although generally evenly distributed throughout the retina, they are absent from the foveal pit and may be more numerous in the peripheral retina (Diaz-Araya et al., 1995). Less arborized subtypes, sometimes referred to as perivascular macrophages, which closely resemble homologous cells in the parenchyma of the brain, are associated with the perivascular space of retinal capillaries (Fig. 1.32) although they are less numerous than brain perivasular macrophages. Retinal microglia share many properties with brain microglia including tissue homeostasis and host defence. Their highly arborized processes are constantly on the move sampling their immediate microenvironment (Nimmerjahn et al., 2005). Upon injury to the retina these cells become activated and assume the role of wandering phagocytes. Activated microglia play a role as immune effectors, via the release of chemokines and cytokines, however their role as potential antigen-presenting cells (they are predominantly MHC class II⁻), or indeed as immunomodulators limiting leucocyte infiltration of the retina, is controversial (see Dick et al., 2003).

Blood supply of the retina
(Figs 1.24A and 1.31)
The retina is an extremely metabolically active sheet of neural tissue with the highest oxygen consump-

tion (per weight) of any human tissue. Like the brain, the retina has a highly selective blood–tissue barrier, which serves primarily to regulate the optimal extracellular environment to facilitate neural transmission (Rowland, 1985). It also regulates the passage of pathogens and intravascular leucocytes, thus partly protecting the neural environment from 'surveillance' by immune cells (McMenamin and Forrester, 1999). In humans, the retina has a dual blood supply, the inner two-thirds being nourished by branches from the central retinal vessels, while the outer one-third is nourished by the choroidal circulation (see below). The choroidal circulation has a high flow rate (150 mm/s), low oxygen exchange and a fenestrated capillary bed; the retinal circulation has a low flow rate (25mm/s) and high oxygen exchange. The blood–retinal barrier is defined by two sets of characteristics. The first is the structural character of the endothelial and RPE cells located at the endothelial and RPE tight junctions, and the second is the membrane-associated transport characteristics.

Central retinal artery and branches
(Figs 1.24A, 1.31 and 1.32)
This vessel (0.3 mm in diameter) arises from the ophthalmic artery either in the optic canal or close to the optic foramen where the ophthalmic artery lies bound to the dural covering of the nerve (see p. 71). The central retinal artery then travels forward on the undersurface of the nerve within its dural covering. About 1–1.5 cm behind the eye it pierces the inferomedial aspect of the remainder of

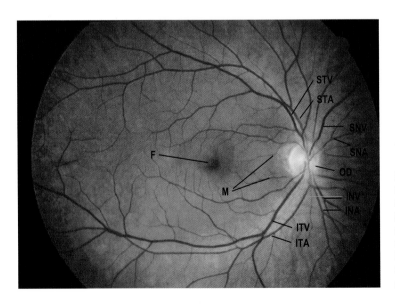

Fig. 1.31 Wide-field photograph of the normal human fundus: F, fovea; OD, optic disk; M, macular vessels; STV and STA, superior temporal vein and artery; ITV and ITA, inferior temporal vein and artery; INV and INA, inferior nasal vein and artery; SNV and SNA, superior nasal vein and artery. (Courtesy of C. Barry.)

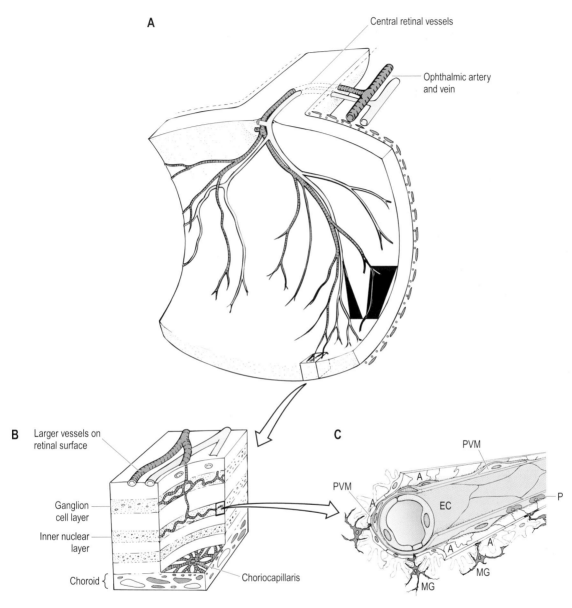

Fig. 1.32 Diagrams of the retinal blood supply. (**A**) The diagram illustrates the manner in which the central retinal artery obtains access to the optic nerve after branching from the ophthalmic artery. (**B**) The levels of the retinal capillary networks. (**C**) High-power diagram illustrating the components of a retinal (or brain) vessel wall that contribute to the blood–retinal (or blood–brain) barrier. From the lumen outwards these are the vascular endothelial cells (EC, pale orange), basal lamina (green) and the glia limitans composed of astrocyte foot processes (A). Note the position of the perivascular microglia (MG), perivascular macrophages (PVM) and pericytes (P). (From McMenamin and Forrester, 1999.)

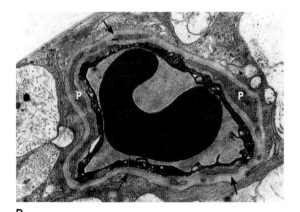

D

Fig. 1.32 *Continued* **(D)** Electron micrograph of a retinal capillary. Note the thickened basal lamina (arrows) and pericyte processes (P) surrounding the endothelial cell. Original magnification: × 6000.

meningeal coverings to pass through the subarachnoid and then pierces the nerve. As it passes forward in the centre of the optic nerve, the artery is accompanied by the central retinal vein and some sympathetic fibres. It resembles other muscular arteries and indeed is affected by conditions such as atheroma and giant cell arteritis. It pierces the papilla centrally, having passed through a constriction or gap in the lamina cribrosa (Fig. 1.12E). This is a potential site for partial or complete occlusive disease. It branches into superior and inferior branches, which subdivide into nasal and temporal arteries, a pattern best appreciated and investigated clinically by fluorescein angiography. A small vessel, the cilioretinal artery, may be present near the optic nerve head and provide a small anastomotic connection between the choroidal and retinal circulations. The central retinal artery diameter decreases to 100 μm upon emerging from the disk. The large retinal arterial branches travel in the nerve fibre layer beneath the inner limiting membrane. These vessels have no internal elastic lamina (which is lost at the optic disk) and are thus not affected in temporal arteritis. They possess a well-developed muscularis, and numerous pericytes lie within the endothelial basal lamina. Each of its four major branches (Figs 1.24A and 1.31) supplies a sector of the retina between which there is no overlap, i.e. they are *functional end-arteries*. The superior and inferior temporal arteries curve above and below the macula and foveal region. Arteries pass over veins and may in some pathological situations cause 'nipping' or narrowing of the veins. There are two

main levels of capillary networks, which spread like a vast cobweb throughout the retina (Fig. 1.32B). The inner plexus is situated at the level of the ganglion cell layer and the outer plexus at the level of the inner nuclear layer. The concept of these two laminae is not universally accepted, although patterns of vascular disease support the concept (see Ch. 9). There may be up to four layers of capillaries in the peripapillary zone, and single layers in the perifoveal region and at the ora serrata.

A further lamina of capillaries fans out over the nerve fibre layer in the peripapillary region. This unique radial capillary network may be more vulnerable to raised intraocular pressure in glaucoma because of its long course (over 1000 μm), infrequent arterial input and lack of anastomoses. Flame-shaped haemorrhages (due to hypertension or papilloedema) or cotton-wool spots (in ischaemic disease) occur predominantly in this unusual capillary network.

In the human, retinal capillaries pass only as far as the sclerad margin of the inner nuclear layer, the outer retina being normally avascular. Capillaries are most dense in the macula but are absent from the fovea itself (capillary-free zone 500 μm in diameter), which is dependent on the choriocapillaris for nutritional support. Larger arterioles are also surrounded by a capillary-free zone. Capillary network density decreases towards the peripheral retina.

Retinal capillaries are characterized by complete circumferentially oriented endothelial cells joined by non-leaky tight junctions (zonulae occludentes); however, the high number of endocytotic vesicles suggests that they are more permeable than brain capillaries (Fig. 1.32C,D). They are surrounded by a thick basal lamina, pericytes and astrocyte foot processes (Fig. 1.32C), which are four times more numerous around retinal vessels than brain capillaries and may act as a second front in the blood–retinal barrier and thus compensate for the more permeable nature of retinal vascular endothelium (Stewart and Tuor, 1994).

Pericytes

The numbers of these supportive cells decrease in diabetes, macroglobulinemia and other ischaemic diseases (see pp. 480 and 481).

The luminal diameter of retinal capillaries (3.5–6 μm) is somewhat smaller than that of conventional capillaries. There is very little extravascular connective tissue around retinal vessels. Mast cells, a common perivascular element in other tissues, including the choroid, are absent in the retina, which has a high threshold of tolerance to histamine. There are *no lymphatic* vessels in the retina.

Central retinal artery occlusion

This condition is a vivid reminder of the 'functional end-artery' status of the retinal blood supply. In complete central retinal artery occlusion, irreversible changes occur after 1–2 hours and the inner retina becomes white and oedematous except at the fovea, which survives owing to the underlying choroidal circulation, which shows through as a round red patch.

THE CHOROID

The choroid (Fig. 1.33A–G) is the posterior portion of the middle vascular coat of the eye, the *uveal tract*. It is homologous to the pia–arachnoid of the brain. The choroid is a thin, highly pigmented, vascular, loose connective tissue situated between the sclera and the retina, whose principal function is to nourish the outer layers of the retina. It also acts as a conduit for vessels travelling to other parts of the eye and may also have a thermoregulatory role. Furthermore, absorption of light by choroidal pigment aids vision by preventing unwanted light from reflecting back through the retina as occurs in some nocturnal species that possess a tapetum. The regulation of blood flow in the choroid may also influence intraocular pressure by affecting perfusion rates of the ciliary processes.

Tapetum

Many mammalian (carnivores, ruminants, cetaceans, seals) and non-mammalian (fish, crocodiles) species possess a reflective tapetum that may serve to increase photoreception in low light conditions. This may be located in the choroid or the RPE. The choroidal tapetum may be cellular or fibrous and may occupy only part, usually the upper portion, of the globe. In carnivores it generally consists of several layers of flattened cells containing reflective material (e.g. guanine, zinc cysteine). In ruminants (e.g. cows, sheep) and cetaceans (dolphins) it is fibrous (tapetum fibrosum) and consists of fine regularly arranged collagen bundles which cause diffractive patterns depending on their orientation. A retinal tapetum generally consists of lipid (e.g. opossum) or guanine (fish, crocodiles) deposits within the RPE.

The choroid extends from the optic nerve margins to the ciliary body and, although its thickness is probably dependent on blood flow dynamics, it is quoted as being approximately 220 μm at the posterior pole and 100 μm anteriorly. Its inner surface is smooth and forms part of Bruch's membrane beneath the RPE. The outer surface, the suprachoroid, is irregular and firmly attached to the lamina fusca of the sclera. Histologically the human choroid consists of five layers: Bruch's membrane, the choriocapillaris, two vessel layers [large vessels (Haller's layer) and medium-sized vessels (Sattler's layer)], and the suprachoroid (Fig. 1.33E).

Bruch's membrane (lamina vitrea)

This modified connective tissue layer is 2–4 μm thick and histologically appears as an acellular glassy membrane beneath the RPE (Figs 1.25A,B and 1.33F,G). Bruch's membrane comprises five layers: the RPE basal lamina (0.3 μm thick) (not truly part of the choroid); an inner collagenous zone; a middle elastic layer (incomplete interwoven bands or perforated sheets of elastic 'fibres'); an outer collagenous zone (which blends with the stroma between the choriocapillaris); and the basement membrane of the endothelial cells in the choriocapillaris. Age-related changes in Bruch's membrane lead to areas of diffuse or discrete thickening known as drusen (see Ch. 9, p. 493).

Choriocapillaris

This is an extraordinarily rich bed of wide-bore fenestrated capillaries that extends only as far anteriorly as the ora serrata and functions to provide nutritional support for the outer retina, especially the photoreceptors. The capillary 'network', when studied by resin-casting methods, is observed to be more of a perforated vascular 'net' than a network of capillaries (Fig. 1.33B–D).

Resin vascular casting

This experimental method has been used extensively to investigate the detailed microvasculature of the eye and other organs. It involves perfusing an experimental subject with acrylic resin via a major vessel. When the resin has polymerized, the tissues are digested with warm potassium hydroxide to expose the hardened cast of the vascular system. The three-dimensional configuration of the microvessels is best viewed by scanning electron microscopy (Fig. 1.33C,D).

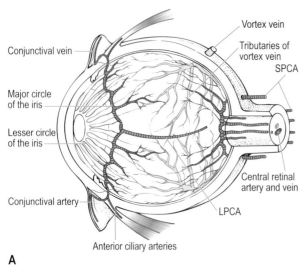

- Conjunctival vein
- Major circle of the iris
- Lesser circle of the iris
- Conjunctival artery
- Vortex vein
- Tributaries of vortex vein
- SPCA
- Central retinal artery and vein
- LPCA
- Anterior ciliary arteries

A

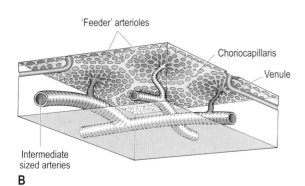

- 'Feeder' arterioles
- Choriocapillaris
- Venule
- Intermediate sized arteries

B

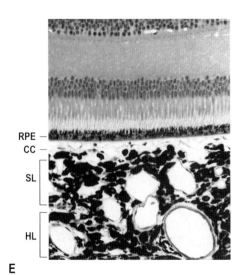

- RPE
- CC
- SL
- HL

E

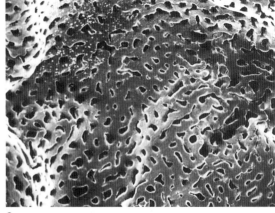

C

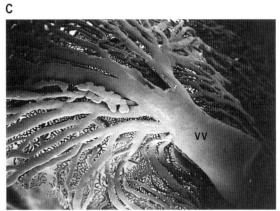

VV

D

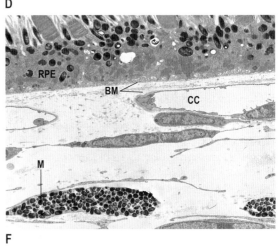

- RPE
- BM
- CC
- M

F

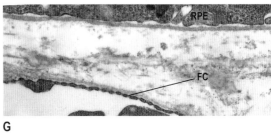

- RPE
- FC

G

The bore of the capillaries (20–40 μm) and the density of the 'net' (Fig. 1.33C) are greatest near the macula. The capillaries are fenestrated (75–85 nm diameter) on their retinal aspect (Fig. 1.33F,G) and these fenestrae occur at a density of approximately 46 per μm^2 (Guymer et al., 2005). Smooth muscle cells are not usually present in this layer. This sheet or net of capillaries is fed from arterioles, from the layer composed of arterioles and venules (Sattler's) in the manner depicted in Figure 1.33B, i.e. hexagonal patches or 'lobules' of choriocapillaris are fed by a central precapillary arteriole that runs perpendicular to the flat choriocapillaris. This lobular pattern is clinically significant because choroidal ischaemia often occurs as pale hexagonal patches (mosaic pattern). The venous channels drain the periphery of these lobules (Fig. 1.33B).

Vascular layer

This layer (Fig. 1.33E) lies beneath the choriocapillaris and can be subdivided into an outer component (major arteries and veins, Haller's layer) and an inner layer of intermediate-sized vessels (arterioles and venules, Sattler's layer). The blood supply of the choroid is chiefly from the long and short posterior ciliary arteries, although recurrent branches from the anterior ciliary arteries anastomose with anterior choroidal vessels (Fig. 1.33A). Venous drainage occurs via a series of large vortex veins (venae vorticosae), of which there are usually four (up to six), each draining a sector of the choroid. These large veins pierce the sclera through emissary canals (Figs 1.12A and 1.33A,D) and drain into the superior and inferior ophthalmic veins in the orbit.

The choroidal stroma consists of randomly arranged collagen fibres (type I), flattened ribbon-like elastic fibres, fibrocytes and numerous melanocytes (Fig. 1.33F). The extent of choroidal pigmentation influences the appearance of the fundus, with the highly pigmented choroid of black people showing through more than in the fundus of a white person, in which the red–orange reflex is primarily the result of the choroidal vasculature. The choroid, being a connective tissue, contains resident populations of immunocompetent cells including occasional plasma cells and lymphocytes, numerous perivascular mast cells (Fig. 1.34A–C) and networks of resident tissue macrophages and dendritic cells (Fig. 1.35; Butler and McMenamin, 1996). Recent studies of mice deficient in monocyte chemotactic protein-1 (MCP-1 or Ccl2), a chemoattractant for macrophages, revealed evidence of degenerative changes in the choroid, retinal pigment epithelium and retina which bear striking resemblance to those seen in age-related macular degeneration. The deposition of complement and immunoglobulin G that accompanies the senescent changes in this model and the impaired macrophage recruitment and/or decreased homeostatic scavenging by the resident macrophages and dendritic cells may contribute to the accumulation of debris and the formation of drusen and to the eventual choroidal neovascularization (Ambati et al., 2003; Forrester, 2003).

Suprachoroid

This is a 30-μm thick transition zone between the choroid and the sclera. It consists of thin interconnected lamellae of melanocytes, fibroblasts and connective tissue fibres separated by a thin 'potential' (supra- or perichoroidal) space, which in pathological conditions may become separated by fluid and blood. It is frequently artefactually enlarged in histological preparations. It is an avascular layer, the only vessels being those that traverse the suprachoroid entering or leaving the choroid. The lamellae blend with the choroid and the lamina fusca of the sclera. The suprachoroidal space is continuous with the supraciliary space anteriorly. Recent research has unveiled a previously unrecognized, highly organized network of non-vascular smooth muscle cells in the suprachoroid. These networks were particularly evident behind the fovea, around the entry points of the posterior ciliary arteries and nerves and in bundles running parallel to vessels traveling ante-

Fig. 1.33 (A) Diagram of the uveal tract blood supply. (B) Schematic representation of the hexagonal units in the choricapillaris fed by small arterioles. (C) Resin vascular cast of the choriocapillaris viewed from the retinal aspect. (D) Resin vascular cast of a quadrant of the choroid viewed from the external aspect showing a large vortex vein (VV). (E) Semi-thin resin section of the outer retina and choroid in the primate eye. Note the heavy degree of pigmentation and the layers of the choroids. (F) Low-power electron micrograph of the retinal pigment epithelium, Bruch's membrane (BM) and the closely related choriocapillaris in a primate eye. (G) Higher power electron micrograph of the basal aspect of the RPE with its basal lamina forming part of Bruch's membrane. Note the fenestrated capillaries (FC) in the endothelial lining of the choriocapillaris. Note the capillary endothelial cells are characterized by fenestrae (FC) on the retinal aspect adjacent to Bruch's membrane. RPE, retinal pigment epithelium; CC, choriocapillaris; HL, Haller's layer; SL, Sattler's layer; M, melanocyte; SPCA, short posterior ciliary arteries; LPCA, long posterior ciliary arteries. Original magnifications: C, × 350; D, × 35; E, × 120; F, × 2400; G, × 14 000.

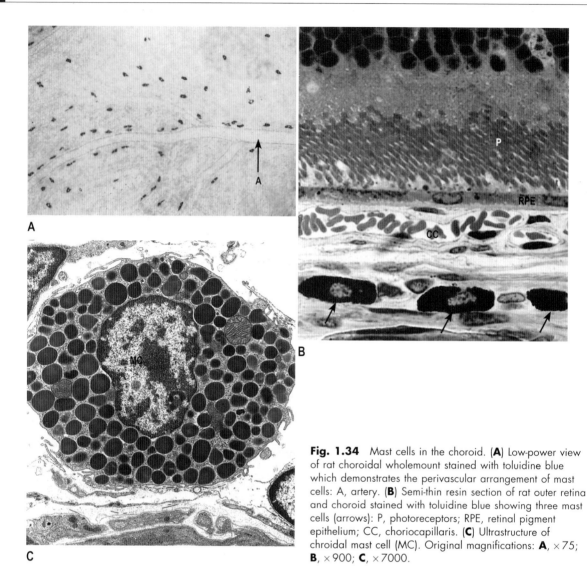

Fig. 1.34 Mast cells in the choroid. (**A**) Low-power view of rat choroidal wholemount stained with toluidine blue which demonstrates the perivascular arrangement of mast cells: A, artery. (**B**) Semi-thin resin section of rat outer retina and choroid stained with toluidine blue showing three mast cells (arrows): P, photoreceptors; RPE, retinal pigment epithelium; CC, choriocapillaris. (**C**) Ultrastructure of chroidal mast cell (MC). Original magnifications: **A**, ×75; **B**, ×900; **C**, ×7000.

riorly from the posterior pole as far as the exit points of the vortex veins. The function of this network of smooth muscle cells in the human choroid remains speculative.

Choroidal infarctions

These appear on angiograms to take the form of triangular areas near the equator, with the apex pointing towards the optic disk. There is probably less functional anastomosis between choriocapillaris lobules than was once suspected; however, some degree of anastomosis in the subcapillary arterioles exists. Peripheral retinal cobble or paving-stone degeneration represents chronic focal ischaemic changes in the anterior choroid.

Nerve supply of the choroid

The choroid is innervated by the *long and short ciliary nerves*. The long ciliary nerves (from the nasociliary branch of V_1) pass through the choroid and transmit sensory fibres to the cornea, iris and ciliary body. Sympathetic fibres are also carried in these nerves to the dilator pupillae (see p. 32). The *short ciliary nerves* arise from the ciliary ganglion and carry sensory (from nasociliary), sympathetic and parasympathetic fibres (derived predominantly from nerve III, but also from VII). The latter have already synapsed in the pterygopalatine ganglion (Ruskell, 1971a). Both long and short ciliary nerves pierce the sclera in the form of a ring 2–3 mm anterior to the optic nerve sheath, along with the long and short

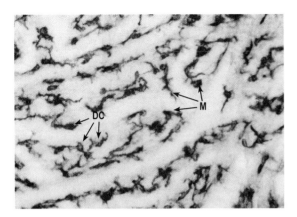

Fig. 1.35 Double-colour immunohistochemistry of rat choroidal wholemount stained with monoclonal antibodies specific for macrophages (M; blue) and major histocompatibility class II-positive dendritic cells (DC; red). This method of examining stained tissue provides a 'plan view' that clearly demonstrates the distinct networks of both these cell types in the choroid. Original magnification: × 600.

OPTIC NERVE

The optic nerve (Fig. 1.36) is unique anatomically as it is the only tract in the central nervous system to leave the cranial cavity. Furthermore, it is subdivided into fascicles by connective tissue and glial septae and is surrounded by cerebrospinal fluid. It is also unique in that it is the only central nervous system tract that can be visualized directly by the clinician.

The optic nerve is formed by convergence of ganglion cell axons at the optic disk, the commencement of the nerve. Foveal/macula fibres constitute around 90% of all axons leaving the eye and form the distinct *maculopapillary bundle*. From the disk, the axons extend along the nerve through the orbit to traverse the optic canal in the sphenoid bone.

The optic nerve can be divided into four main portions: *intraocular* (1 mm in length), *orbital* (25–30 mm), *intracanalicular* (4–10 mm) and *intracranial* (10 mm). The latter portion is discussed on p. 95 in the context of the visual pathways.

Intraocular portion

The *intraocular portion* (Fig. 1.36A) extends from the surface of the optic disk to the posterior margins of the sclera. The nerve fibres are not myelinated in this portion. It can be further subdivided into three regions: the retinal (pars retinalis), choroidal (pars choroidalis) and scleral (pars scleralis) portions. Myelination commences approximately level with the termination of the subarachnoid space at the posterior limits of the lamina cribrosa. As the fascicles of nerve fibres pass posteriorly from the optic disk into the intraocular portion, the glial cells become more common; columns of glial cell nuclei are especially prominent in the scleral portion, where they account for up to 40% of the tissue mass (Fig. 1.36A). The commencement of the optic nerve, the *optic disk*, is approximately 1.5 mm in diameter. The layers of the retina and the choroid terminate at the edge of the disk as specialized regions of glial tissue, the intermediary tissue (of Kuhnt), and marginal border tissue (of Elschnig). The absence of retinal tissue in this region explains the 'blind spot' phenomenon. As the 1.2 million ganglion cell axons in the nerve fibre layer become crowded towards the disk, they create a raised area or *papilla*, which is thickest on the lateral aspect owing to the large number of fibres in the *maculopapillary bundle*. The raised margin of the optic disk surrounds an indentation, the *physiological cup*. As the fibres pass posteriorly, they pierce the sieve-like connective tissue

posterior ciliary arteries. The nerve terminals branch extensively and form plexi of unmyelinated fibres in the choroid and suprachoroid adjacent to vascular smooth muscle cells; however, they do not extend into the choriocapillaris. Fibres containing vasoactive intestinal peptide (VIP) and neuropeptide Y have been identified in the choroid and probably act as vasodilator and vasoconstrictor agents respectively. Multipolar and bipolar ganglion cell bodies immunoreactive for nitric oxide synthase (NOS) and VIP have been recently identified in the choroid and their axons may supply the choroidal vasculature (vasodilatory) or non-vascular smooth muscle cells. Their structure and immunohistochemical charateristics suggest that they may have a mechanosensory role (May et al, 2004).

Physiological notes

1 Blood flow through the choroidal capillaries is one of the highest in the body (800–1200 ml per 100 g tissue/min).
2 85% of blood flow to the eye goes to the choroid and only 4% to the retina.
3 Blood flow in the choroid is little affected by high intraocular pressure.
4 The oxygen tension of venous blood is closer to that of arterial blood than in most tissues of the body.

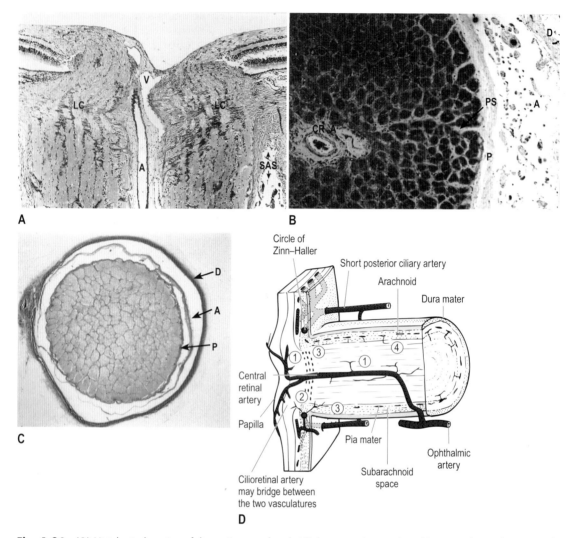

Fig. 1.36 (**A**) Histological section of the optic nerve head: LC, lamina cribrosa; A and V, central retinal artery and vein; SAS, subarachnoid space. (**B**) Transverse section (Loyez stain) of the orbital portion of the optic nerve revealing the arrangement of the myelinated nerve fascicles (darkly stained) separated by pial septae (PS) which penetrate as far as the central retinal artery (CRA) in the middle of the nerve. The three layers of meninges surrounding the nerve (D, dura; A, arachnoid; and P, pia mater) are clearly visible here and in C. (**C**) Cross-section (trichrome stain) of an entire optic nerve and surrounding meninges posterior to the entry of the central retinal artery. (**D**) Blood supply of the optic nerve. The four sources of vessels supplying the optic nerve include: 1, branches from the central retinal artery or its branches; 2, branches from the circle of Zinn–Haller; 3, choroidal branches; 4, pial branches. Original magnifications: **A**, × 60; **B**, × 290; **C**, × 40. (Part A reproduced courtesy of W.R. Lee and Springer-Verlag.)

mesh, the *lamina cribrosa*, which fills the posterior scleral foramen. The lamina cribrosa is formed by irregular collagen fibre bundles continuous with the sclera (Fig. 1.12E). These bundles are arranged in the form of circles or a figure of eight (Thale and Tillman, 1993). Elastic tissue from the choroid and Bruch's membrane is continuous with and 'anchored'

to the adventitia surrounding the central retinal artery and vein. The collagenous bundles in the lamina cribrosa are separated from the axons by a covering of glial tissue, which may protect the nerve fibres as they pierce the irregular openings. The *scleral canal* is some 0.5 mm long and may vary in shape from cone-like (narrowest portion nearest the disk) to double cone or funnel-like. Posterior to the pars scleralis, the nerve fibres become myelinated by *oligodendrocytes* (Fig. 1.36B), causing a doubling of the thickness of the optic nerve.

> The fact that the optic nerve is myelinated by central nervous system-type glial cells (oligodendrocytes), and not peripheral nervous system glia (Schwann cells), partly explains the lack of regenerative capacity of this nerve.

Glaucoma

> The intraocular portion is that part of the optic nerve damaged in glaucoma because of raised intraocular pressure. Axonal damage may be a consequence of either interference with blood flow or interruption of axonal transport. No single hypothesis has been proposed that adequately explains why specific regions of the nerve are more likely to be damaged than others, resulting in the characteristic visual field defects or *scotoma*.

Orbital portion

The *orbital portion* of the optic nerve (Fig. 1.36C,D) extends backwards and medially from the back of the eye to the optic canal in the sphenoid at the apex of the orbit. It is covered by three layers of meninges: pia, arachnoid and dura. The dura and arachnoid blend with the sclera, and the subarachnoid space around the nerve terminates at the posterior surface of the sclera in the form of a fluid-filled ring (Fig. 1.36A).

> The central retinal vessels must cross the subarachnoid space and are therefore vulnerable, particularly the vein, in cases of raised intracranial pressure.

The majority of the axons in the nerve are 1 μm in diameter and approximately 10% are between 2 and 10 μm. The glial septae between fascicles present in the intraocular portions extend into the orbital portion but become less distinct as the orbital apex is approached. The orbital portion of the optic nerve has a slight S-shaped bend, which allows a full range of ocular movement without stretching the nerve. As the optic nerve approaches the orbital apex it is surrounded by the tendinous annulus, which gives origin to the rectus muscles.

Intracanalicular portion

The *intracanalicular portion* of the optic nerve passes through the optic canal (foramen), accompanied by the ophthalmic artery and sympathetic nerves. The dura surrounding the nerve splits at the orbital opening, the majority continuing as the dural sheath of the nerve inside the canal and a thinner portion blending with the periorbita (Fig. 1.37).

Blood supply

The optic nerve has a complex blood supply, which has been extensively investigated because of its importance in the pathogenesis of glaucoma (see Ch. 9). The intraocular portion is supplied by branches from four sources: central retinal vessels and their branches, scleral vessels (the circle of Zinn–Haller), choroidal vessels and pial vessels (see Fig. 1.36D). The first three are derived from the ophthalmic or central retinal artery, and pial vessels from the adjacent branches of the internal carotid artery. The majority of capillaries pierce the nerve and course longitudinally within the nerve via the glial septae.

Papilloedema

> The swelling of the papillary fibres, which appears as a raised white disk margin, is partly the result of the lack of Müller cells in this region. These cells serve to bind the nerve fibres together in the remainder of the retina.

Meningitis

> The continuation of the subarachnoid space from the cranial cavity along the nerve may facilitate the spread of infection or tumours from the orbit to the cranium and vice versa.

Streaks

> The occurrence of white streaks at the optic disk is the result of aberrant myelination of ganglion cell axons in the retina (medullated nerve fibre layer). Interestingly, the myelination is still interrupted at the intraocular portion of the nerve fibres.

ORBITAL CONTENTS

GENERAL ARRANGEMENT

The orbits are a pair of bone sockets that, for descriptive purposes, can be divided into an *intraconal space* (within the cone of rectus muscles) and an

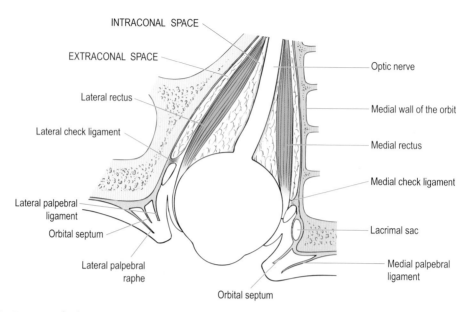

Fig. 1.37 Diagram of a horizontal section through the orbit illustrating the formation of an intra- and extraconal space by the four rectus muscles (only medial and lateral rectus shown in this section).

extraconal space (outside the muscle cone) (Figs 1.37 and 1.38). The orbital cavity has a volume of about 30 cm³.

The topographic anatomy of the orbit is summarized in a series of annotated diagrams and dissections (Figs 1.39–1.41). The lacrimal gland is discussed on p. 92. The course and function of nerves supplying the eye and orbit are discussed separately on pp. 72–82, and extraocular muscles are described on pp. 69–71.

PERIORBITA AND ORBITAL FIBROADIPOSE TISSUE
(Figs 1.37 and 1.38)

The orbital contents are bound together and supported by fibroadipose tissue. This connective tissue has classically been divided into separate components.

- *Periorbita* or periosteum of the orbit. This layer of connective tissue is frequently described as having a dense outer layer and a looser inner layer, which invests orbital nerves and the lacrimal gland. It is not very tightly bound to the bone except at the sutures, fissures and foraminae in the orbital walls, and also to the posterior lacrimal crest where it covers the lacrimal sac and is continuous

with the fibrous lining of the nasolacrimal duct. It forms a dense membrane over the inferior and superior orbital fissures with sufficient gaps for transmission of nerves and vessels. It is continuous with the periosteum lining the optic foramen and with the sheath of the optic nerve, itself an extension of dura mater of the brain. The periorbita is firmly attached at the orbital margins anteriorly where it becomes continuous with the orbital septum (palpebral fascia) in the eyelids (see p. 87).
- *Bulbar fascia (Tenon's capsule)*, a thick fibrous sheath enclosing the globe but separated from it by a layer of loose connective tissue.
- Muscular fascial sheaths that surround the extraocular muscles and blend with the bulbar fascia.
- *Medial and lateral check ligaments.*
- *Suspensory ligament (of Lockwood).*

The stereotypical structure and organization of the orbital connective tissue described by Koornneef (1982) and several others (see review Demer, 2004) based on serial sections of large numbers of intact human orbits (Fig 1.38), besides confirming the presence of those features detailed above also demonstrated that the arrangement of the orbital fibroadipose tissues is bilaterally symmetric and consistent between individuals. Furthermore, a fibrous intermuscular membrane was observed to

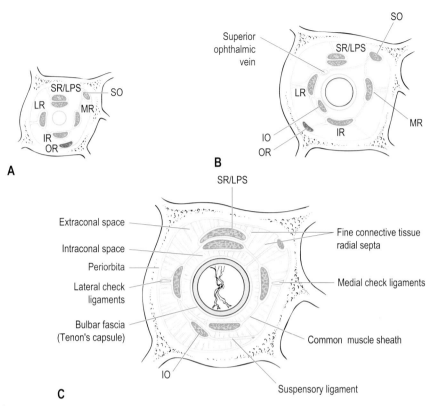

Fig. 1.38 Schematic diagrams of the connective tissue septae associated with each extraocular muscle at three levels in the orbit: (**A**) near orbital apex; (**B**) posterior part of the globe; (**C**) close to the equator of the globe. SO, superior oblique; MR, medial rectus; LR, lateral rectus; IR, inferior rectus; SR, superior rectus; LPS, levator palpebrae superioris; IO, inferior oblique; OR, orbitalis. (Modified from Koornneef, 1982.)

connect the four rectus muscles, thus helping create the intraconal space (best developed in the anterior part of the orbit; incomplete behind the globe). This connective tissue is continuous with the perimysium around each muscle and anteriorly with the bulbar fascia or Tenon's capsule around the globe (Fig. 1.38B,C). These studies also showed that each extraocular muscle has its own characteristic connective tissue system. Specific attachments via fibrous bands to the orbital walls throughout their course (Fig. 1.38A–C). A theoretical framework, known as the 'active pulley hypothesis', has recently been proposed (see review Demer, 2004) that postulates a crucial role for these connective tissue bands, known as 'pulley suspensions' in understanding the kinematics of extraocular muscle action. These suspensions pass between the orbital wall and the 'pulley sleeve' of each muscle, which is described as a ring-like extension of the connective tissue from Tenon's capsule posteriorly around the muscle. The tone of the pulleys is possibly under neuronal control because of the presence of smooth muscle fibres, which have been identified to varying extents by numerous investigators (Koornneef, 1982; Demer et al., 1997; Ruskell et al., 2005). The 'active pulley hypothesis' proposes that the rectus muscles have a so-called 'orbital layer' of fibres that are continuous with (or 'blend with' or 'insert into') these sleeves (and thus also into the pulley suspensions), in essence one part of a bifid insertion. The inner half or 'global layer' of the rectus muscle continues through the sleeve and bulbar fascia to insert directly into the sclera. The newly postulated function for orbital connective tissue in the 'active pulley hypothesis', which states in effect that this dual insertion allows the pulleys to act as a second 'origin' and thus influence the direction of pull of the extraocular muscles, has gained wide acceptance but some investigators have questioned the anatomical evidence of orbital muscle fibres terminating in

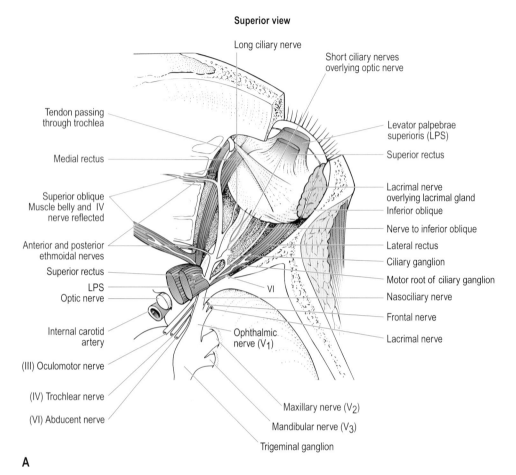

Superior view

Long ciliary nerve

Short ciliary nerves
overlying optic nerve

Tendon passing
through trochlea

Levator palpebrae
superioris (LPS)

Medial rectus

Superior rectus

Lacrimal nerve
overlying lacrimal gland

Superior oblique
Muscle belly and IV
nerve reflected

Inferior oblique

Nerve to inferior oblique

Anterior and posterior
ethmoidal nerves

Lateral rectus

Superior rectus

Ciliary ganglion

LPS

Motor root of ciliary ganglion

Optic nerve

VI

Nasociliary nerve

Internal carotid
artery

Ophthalmic
nerve (V₁)

Frontal nerve

Lacrimal nerve

(III) Oculomotor nerve

(IV) Trochlear nerve

Maxillary nerve (V₂)

(VI) Abducent nerve

Mandibular nerve (V₃)

Trigeminal ganglion

A

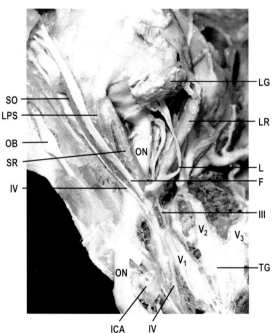

SO
LPS

LG

OB

LR

SR

IV

L
F

ON

III

V₂

V₃

V₁

TG

ON

ICA   IV

B

Fig. 1.39 Diagram (**A**) and prosected specimen (**B**) of the orbit viewed from above, revealing the relations of the orbital nerves and extraocular muscles. Orbital fat and vessels have been excluded for the purposes of clarity.

- The roof of the orbit and superior orbital fissure have been removed and the periorbita divided.
- In (**A**) the lacrimal (L), frontal (F) and trochlear (IV) nerves have been cut. In (**B**) these nerves are intact as they pass external to the tendinous ring or annulus.
- In (**A**) only one long ciliary nerve is shown arising from the nasociliary nerve.
- The sensory root of the ciliary ganglion emerges from the nasociliary. The motor root (parasympathetic fibres) arises from the branch of the oculomotor supplying inferior oblique.
- In (**A**) and (**B**) the lateral dural covering of the cavernous sinus has been removed to expose the cranial nerves before they pass through the superior orbital fissure: TG, trigeminal ganglion; V₁, V₂, V₃, divisions of the trigeminal nerve; OB, olfactory bulb; ICA, internal carotid artery; III, oculomotor nerve; VI, abducens nerve; SO, superior oblique; LR, lateral rectus; LG, lacrimal gland; LPS, levator palpebrae superioris; SR, superior rectus; ON, optic nerve.
- The optic canal has not been opened.

Lateral view

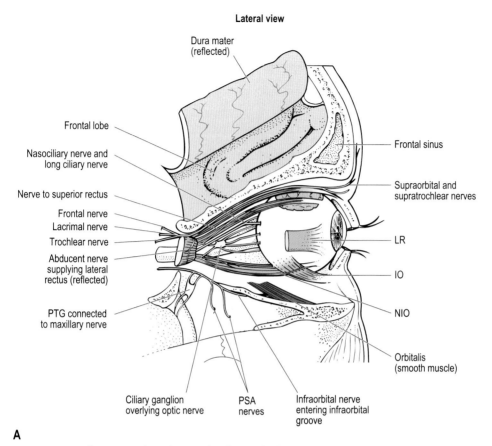

A

Fig. 1.40 (**A**) Diagram illustrating a lateral view of a dissected orbit revealing the relations of the orbital nerves and extraocular muscles (vessels have been excluded for the purposes of clarity).

- The lateral wall has been removed and the infratemporal fossa has been dissected to expose the pterygomaxillary fissure and pterygopalatine fossa.
- The cranial cavity has been opened to reveal the dura (reflected) covering the frontal lobe.
- The lateral rectus has been divided and reflected to expose the optic nerve and other cranial nerves entering the orbit through the tendinous ring. Note the abducent nerve entering its bulbar surface.
- The ciliary ganglion lies between the lateral rectus and the optic nerve. Note the motor root and sensory root as seen in the superior view. The nerve to inferior oblique (NIO) is a useful landmark for finding the ciliary ganglion. The short ciliary nerves emerge from the ganglion and enter the globe around the optic nerve.
- Note the three nerves which enter the orbit outside the tendinous ring–lacrimal, frontal and trochlear.
- The nerve to superior rectus (branch of superior division of III nerve) pierces the muscle and enters the levator palpebrae superioris, which it supplies, from below.
- Branches of the pterygopalatine ganglion enter the orbit through the inferior orbital fissure and contribute to the formation of the retrobulbar plexus (not shown).
- Inferior oblique passes backwards, laterally and superiorly beneath the inferior rectus.
- Orbitalis (Müller's muscle), a band of smooth muscle, covers the inferior orbital fissure.

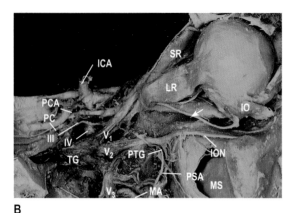

B

Fig. 1.40 *Continued* **(B)** Dissection of the orbit similar to the diagram above except that lateral rectus has not been cut and the course of the orbital nerves within the cavernous sinus is also shown (by removal of the lateral dural wall). ICA, internal carotid artery; PCA, posterior communicating artery; PC, posterior cerebral artery; MA, maxillary artery; TG, trigeminal ganglion; V_1, V_2, V_3, divisions of the trigeminal nerve; PTG, pterygopalatine ganglion; PSA, posterior superior alveolar nerves; ION, infraorbital nerve; IO, inferior oblique; LR, lateral rectus; SR, superior rectus; arrow, nerve to superior oblique branch of oculomotor nerve (III); IV, trochlear nerve; MS, maxillary sinus.

connective tissue other than the sclera (McClung et al., 2005; Ruskell et al., 2005).

An intricate system of fine radial connective tissue septae subdivides the orbit. Fat locules are interposed between the septae (Fig. 1.38C). Other less distinct septae lie parallel to and surround the globe. There are well-recognized but variable amounts of smooth muscle within the orbital connective tissue, including the sleeves of some of the recti muscles, whose functions (besides the superior and inferior palpebral muscles) are presently unclear. It has been suggested that like the smooth muscle covering the inferior orbital fissure (orbitalis or Müller's muscle) they may represent a redundant evolutionary remnant (see Ruskell et al., 2005 for discussion).

Veins passing through the orbit are supported by connective tissue septae (Fig. 1.38B), although arteries do not demonstrate this arrangement and instead travel among the fat locules and frequently pierce the septae. A thickened band of orbital fibrous tissue connects the superior rectus and the levator palpebrae superioris. This aids in coordinating lifting of the eyelid when the eye is directed upwards by the superior rectus.

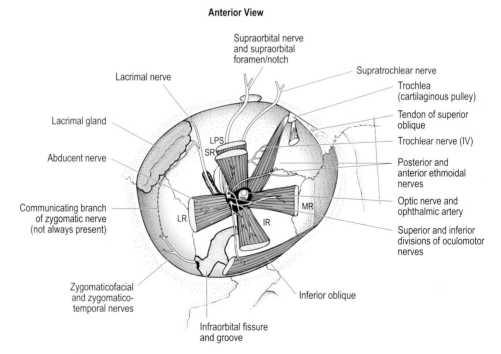

Fig. 1.41 The orbit from in front with the globe removed to show the origins of the extraocular muscles and the orbital nerves (vessels and fat are not included in this diagram).

The complex and interlinked nature of the fibroadipose system of connective tissue septae may explain why patients with orbital floor 'blow-out' fractures display vertical ocular mobility problems. It is not necessary to invoke the incarceration of the inferior rectus and inferior oblique muscles in the fracture to explain the symptoms.

EXTRAOCULAR MUSCLES

There are six true extraocular muscles responsible for movements of the globe. In addition there is one further 'orbital' muscle, the levator palpebrae superioris, which originates at the orbital apex and inserts into the tarsal plate and upper eyelid (see p. 85).

The true extraocular muscles comprise *four rectus muscles*, which arise from the tendinous ring at the apex of the orbit and insert into the sclera about 4–8 mm behind the limbus, and *two oblique muscles* (superior and inferior) whose tendons approach the globe from in front and insert into the posterior aspect of the sclera (Figs 1.39 and 1.42). Details of the six true extraocular muscles, including their innervation, origin, insertion, tendon length (important in the surgical management of strabismus), length of muscle belly, the angle subtended by the muscle axis to the vertical, and the size of the motor units, are provided in Table 1.2. The origins of the muscles are shown in Figure 1.41 and the pattern of insertion into the sclera is shown in Figure 1.42. The collagen bundles of the tendons blend with the scleral collagen as shown in Figure 1.12C. The relations of the orbital muscles to each other and to the orbital nerves are summarized diagrammatically in Figures 1.39 and 1.40. Movements are discussed in Chapter 5 (p. 310).

Microscopic anatomy of extraocular muscle

Histologically, extraocular muscle differs from skeletal muscle in the following respects (compare Fig. 1.43A with Fig. 1.43B).

- The epimysium or muscle sheath of extraocular muscle is generally very thin by comparison with other muscles.
- The fibres are not tightly packed but are separated by unusually large amounts of connective tissue (perimysium) rich in reticulin and elastic fibres.
- The muscle fibres are rounded or oval in shape with small fibres (5–15 μm) around the periphery of the muscle and larger fibres (10–40 μm) in the centre.

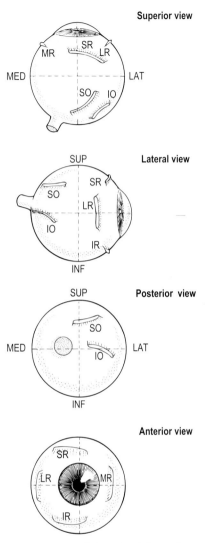

Fig. 1.42 Four views of the right globe to demonstrate the insertions of the extraocular muscles.

- Extraocular muscle is the most vascular in the body, next to myocardium. The most vascularized region is the orbital aspect.

> The extraocular muscles are supplied by muscular branches arising directly from the ophthalmic artery or indirectly from its branches.

- In normal extraocular muscle there often appear to be histopathological or ultrastructural changes normally associated with myopathy, i.e. mild mononuclear cellular infiltrate, centrally placed nuclei, disorganization of the sarcolemma,

Table 1.2 Summary of anatomical features of human extraocular muscles

Muscle	Innervation	Origin	Insertion (mm from cornea)	Tendon length (mm)	Length of muscle belly (mm)	Size of motor unit	Comment
Medial rectus	III (inf)	Tendinous ring	5.6	3.6	40	1:1.7–1:4	Largest of the ocular muscles
Inferior rectus	III (inf)	Tendinous ring	6.6	5	40	1:2–1:6	
Lateral rectus	VI	Tendinous ring via two heads	7.0	8.4	40	1:3–1:6	Opening between the two heads bridging the medial end of superior orbital fissure
Superior rectus	III (sup)	Tendinous ring	7.8	5.4	41	1:4	Lies beneath levator palpebrae superioris
Superior oblique	IV	Superomedial to optic canal	Lateral aspect of posterosuperior quadrant	Tendon forms 10 mm before winding around trochlea	32	1:5–1:6	The only extraocular muscle with a fusiform shape. IV nerve enters the muscle on its upper border
Inferior oblique	III (inf)	Behind orbital margin lateral to nasolacrimal canal	Posterolateral quadrant, mostly below horizontal	Very short tendon; muscle fibres almost reach the sclera	34	1:7	The only extraocular muscle not to originate at apex of orbit. Passes between the eye and lateral rectus

Values are approximate means based on several studies; for full details and ranges see Eggers (1982). III (inf), inferior division of oculomotor nerve; III (sup), superior division of oculomotor nerve.

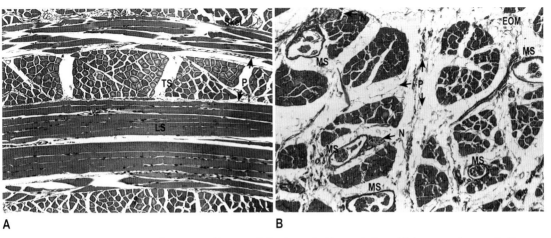

A   B

Fig. 1.43 Histological section of (**A**) normal human skeletal muscle fibres (Skel) and (**B**) extraocular muscle fibres (EOM): LS, longitudinal section of fibres; TS, fibres in transverse section; P, perimysium; MS, muscle spindles; N, nerve. Original magnifications: **A** and **B**, × 100.

Table 1.3 **Classification of mammalian extraocular muscle fibres**		
Type A	Type B	Type C
Large diameter	Intermediate diameter	Small diameter
Single end-plate	Multiple end-plates	Small *en grappe* plates
Fast twitch	Slow twitch	Tonic contractions
Required for saccadic movements	Needed for smooth pursuit movements	Function to align both visual axes, i.e. fine local contractions

disruption of the Z lines, and mitochondrial clumping.

- Extraocular muscle contains large numbers of specialized sensory or proprioreceptive endings, including large muscle spindles up to 1 mm long (nuclear bag fibres, nuclear chain fibres and annular nerve terminals). Golgi tendon organs are also numerous and are generally found within the tendons of extraocular muscles in greater numbers than in skeletal muscle (Fig. 1.43). The afferent fibres from extraocular muscles are transmitted initially for part of their course in the respective cranial nerve innervating the muscle (either III, IV or VI); however, they leave these nerves and join the ophthalmic division of the trigeminal, either in the cavernous sinus or in the brainstem. Their cell bodies are situated in the mesencephalic nucleus, although some muscle afferents have been traced to Purkinje cells in the cerebellum, and play an important role in positional sense and control of ocular movements (both saccadic and tracking).

The structural differences between extraocular and skeletal muscle outlined above are not surprising in light of the fundamental differences in function, namely the constancy of activity (even during sleeping) and the rapidity and fine gradation of contraction of extraocular muscle required to fixate subjects of interest, thus ensuring the image falls on the fovea. Since both eyes must move together, both sets of six muscles must be highly coordinated and move simultaneously (see Ch. 5). Up to six types of muscle fibre have been identified morphologically, but functionally there appear to be three main types (Table 1.3).

BLOOD VESSELS OF THE ORBIT
(Fig. 1.44)

The orbital contents are supplied chiefly by the ophthalmic artery, which usually arises from the internal carotid artery shortly after it emerges from the roof of the cavernous sinus. It commences its course beneath the optic nerve, closely bound to the dura

71

while in the optic canal, then winds around its lateral aspect, and finally passes above the nerve. It then proceeds forward above the medial rectus and under the superior oblique. It ends its tortuous course by dividing into dorsal nasal and supratrochlear branches. The branches are summarized in Figure 1.44. There are several important points of anasto-

Blood supply of the orbit

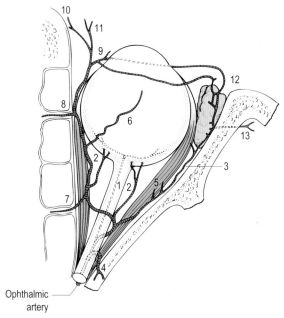

Ophthalmic artery

Fig. 1.44 Diagram summarizing the blood supply of the orbit as seen in a superior view. 1, central retinal artery; 2, posterior ciliary arteries [usually emerge as two trunks that divide into the short posterior ciliary arteries (seven or more) and the long posterior ciliary arteries (usually two, medial and lateral)]; 3, lacrimal artery; 4, recurrent branches (to meninges); 5, muscular branches (give rise to anterior ciliary arteries); 6, supraorbital artery; 7, posterior ethmoidal artery; 8, anterior ethmoidal artery; 9, superior and inferior medial palpebral arteries; 10, dorsalis nasi; 11, supratrochlear; 12, superior and inferior lateral palpebral arteries; 13, zygomatic branches of the lacrimal artery.

mosis between arteries derived from the internal carotid and the external carotid arteries (Table 1.4).

These anastomoses may be important during occlusive vascular disease of the ophthalmic artery by serving as alternative routes of blood supply to the eye and orbit. The veins that accompany the above arteries, in common with most veins of the head and neck, lack valves and thus there are several sites of communication between veins on the upper face and lids with intraorbital veins (superior and inferior ophthalmic veins) which drain posteriorly into the cavernous sinuses. The inferior ophthalmic vein may drain via the inferior orbital fissure into the pterygoid venous plexus. These communications are important clinically as they act as potential routes for the spread of infection from the face around the nose and eye to the cavernous sinuses and the cranial cavity (see p. 11).

CRANIAL NERVES ASSOCIATED WITH THE EYE AND ORBIT

GENERAL FUNCTIONAL ARRANGEMENT

Cranial nerves contain a diversity of functional components. Besides those found in spinal nerves (somatic efferents, somatic afferents, general visceral efferents, general visceral afferents), cranial nerves also contain additional functional categories including special visceral efferents (branchiomotor), special somatic afferents (special senses, hearing and balance), and special visceral afferents (taste and smell). The functional classification of cranial nerve components and their target organs and tissues are summarized in Table 1.5. The sites of origin of the cranial nerves from the brainstem are illustrated in Figure 1.45A,B.

OCULOMOTOR NERVE (CRANIAL NERVE III) (Fig. 1.46)

This is the largest of the extraocular nerves and supplies all the extraocular muscles except the lateral rectus and superior oblique.

Table 1.4 Sites of anastomosis between branches of the internal and external carotid arteries		
External carotid branch	Internal carotid branch	Region of anastomosis
Angular artery (facial)	Dorsalis nasi (ophthalmic)	Medial palpebral margin
Transverse facial artery (superficial temporal)	Lacrimal artery (ophthalmic)	Lateral palpebral margin
Middle meningeal artery and deep temporal artery	Lacrimal artery (ophthalmic)	Orbit

Table 1.5 Functional analysis of cranial nerve components

Functional classification	Modality/target (*ontogeny/phylogeny*)	Present in cranial nerves
Somatic efferent (general motor)	Supplies skeletal muscle of somatic origin (*preotic somites – extraocular muscles; occipital somites – tongue musculature*)	III, IV, and VI XII
Somatic afferent (general sensory)	Pain, temperature and touch. Supplies skin and mucous membranes of the head and neck	Predominantly in V but several minor elements in VII, IX and X
General visceral efferents* (parasympathetic)	Supplies smooth muscle (viscera), cardiac muscle, glands, blood vessels and intrinsic eye muscles (ciliary muscle and sphincter pupillae)	III, VII, IX, X and XI. X (vagus) is largest parasympathetic nerve in the body
General visceral afferents	Pain and sensibility of viscera	VII, IX and X
Special visceral efferents (branchiomotor)	Skeletal muscles of mastication and facial expression (*i.e. pharyngeal arch or visceral evolutionary orgin*)	V, VII, IX, X and XI
Special somatic afferent (special senses concerned with body position, excluding vision)	Maintenance of balance and reception of sound (vestibulocochlear organ)	VII
Special visceral afferent (special visceral senses, taste and smell)	Olfactory epithelium in nasal cavity and taste receptors in tongue and palate	Olfaction (smell) in I; taste in VII, IX and X

*Sympathetic nerve fibres, originating from upper thoracic segments of the spinal cord and synapsing in cervical ganglia may 'hitchhike' with various cranial nerves and/or blood vessels to reach ocular and obital structures, e.g. dilator pupillae muscle and tarsal muscle (see pp. 32, 94; Fig. 1.58).

Origin

The oculomotor nerve nuclei consist of two main types:

1. a complex of five individual motor (*somatic efferent*) nuclei containing the cell bodies of the multipolar motor neurones whose axons directly innervate their respective extraocular muscles;
2. a *general visceral efferent* nucleus, the Edinger–Westphal nucleus, containing small spindle-shaped preganglionic (first-order) *parasympathetic* neurones.

The oculomotor nuclei lie at the level of the superior colliculus in the ventral region of the periaqueductal grey matter and extend cranially for a short distance into the floor of the third ventricle. The *medial longitudinal fasciculus* lies lateral to the nucleus and contains the axons of internuclear neurones that pass vertically between the brainstem nuclei of the III, IV and VI nerves. The fibres emerge from the oculomotor nuclei, pass anteriorly through the tegmentum of the midbrain and red nucleus, and emerge medial to the cerebral peduncle at the upper border of the pons (Figs 1.45 and 1.46).

Intracranial and intracavernous course

The nerve passes forward, laterally and slightly downward in the interpeduncular fossa (one of the enlargements of the subarachnoid space or cisterns) lateral to the posterior communicating artery (Fig. 1.46). It passes between the posterior cerebral artery (above) and the superior cerebellar artery (below). It grooves the posterior clinoid process and courses forward before it passes through the dural roof of the cavernous sinus (Fig. 1.40B). The nerve runs forward in the upper part of the lateral wall of the cavernous sinus (Fig. 1.8D,E) and enters the intra-

---

Intracavernous lesions

The oculomotor, like other cranial nerves coursing through the cavernous sinus, can become involved in pathological processes such as venous thrombosis or aneurysms of the internal artery. Pituitary enlargements more commonly affect the oculomotor and trochlear nerves than the abducent, which is protected by the internal carotid artery. Meningioma or expanding lesions in the region of the superior orbital fissure can also compress the nerve.

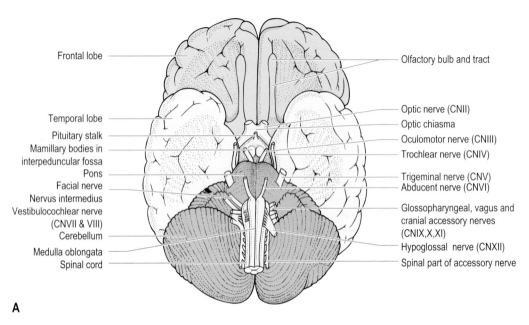

Frontal lobe

Olfactory bulb and tract

Temporal lobe

Optic nerve (CNII)
Optic chiasma

Pituitary stalk
Mamillary bodies in
interpeduncular fossa
Pons
Facial nerve
Nervus intermedius
Vestibulocochlear nerve
(CNVII & VIII)
Cerebellum
Medulla oblongata
Spinal cord

Oculomotor nerve (CNIII)
Trochlear nerve (CNIV)

Trigeminal nerve (CNV)
Abducent nerve (CNVI)

Glossopharyngeal, vagus and
cranial accessory nerves
(CNIX,X,XI)
Hypoglossal nerve (CNXII)
Spinal part of accessory nerve

A

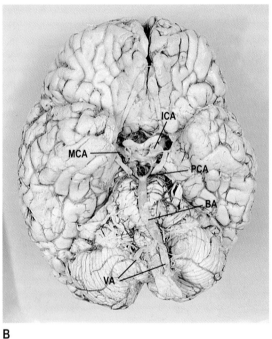

B

Fig. 1.45 Ventral views of the brain to demonstrate the origin of the cranial nerves: (**A**) diagram without vessels; (**B**) photograph of a whole brain with vessels. ICA, internal carotid artery; MCA, middle cerebral artery; PCA, posterior cerebral artery; BA, basilar artery; VA, vertebral artery.

conal space of the orbit through the superior orbital fissure within the tendinous ring (Fig. 1.5), where it divides into superior and inferior divisions.

Intraorbital course
In the orbit the nasociliary nerve is interposed between the two divisions of the oculomotor nerve.

The superior supplies the superior rectus, which it pierces to reach levator palpebrae superioris. The inferior division splits into several branches which supply the medial rectus and inferior rectus, and a long branch passes forward on the lateral aspect of inferior rectus to reach inferior oblique (Fig. 1.40B). It is from this latter branch that the stout motor root

Oculomotor nerve

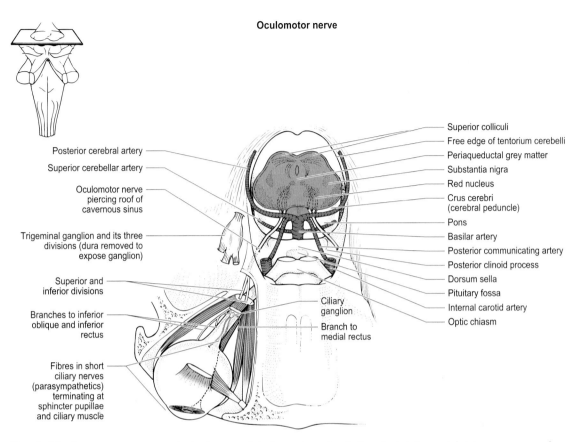

Fig. 1.46 Diagram summarizing the brainstem origin (inset shows level of section), intracranial, intracavernous and intraorbital course of the oculomotor nerve.

(preganglionic parasympathetic fibres) passes to the ciliary ganglion, the site of postganglionic parasympathetic (second-order) neurones (Fig. 1.39A). Axons from the postganglionic neurones travel in the short ciliary nerves to supply the choroid, sphincter pupillae of the iris, and the ciliary muscle (Fig. 1.46).

The nerves that supply extraocular muscles generally pierce the muscle one-third of the way along the muscle belly on the bulbar aspect.

Nerve lesions

Complete lesions of the oculomotor nerve (e.g. trauma) result in:

- inability to look upwards, downwards or medially
- lateral or *external strabismus* because of unopposed action of lateral rectus
- diplopia
- complete ptosis (paralysis of levator palpebrae superioris and unopposed orbicularis oculi)

- dilated non-reactive pupils (unopposed dilator pupillae)
- lack of accommodation.

Incomplete lesions – some of the symptoms above may be present.

Internal ophthalmoplegia – loss of parasympathetic components only. This may be the first sign of nerve palsy as the parasympathetic fibres are located superficially in the nerve and they may be damaged first in intracranial lesions; thus pupil dilation is a crucial sign of compression within the cranial cavity following head injury.

External ophthalmoplegia – the loss of extraocular muscle supply.

Intracranial lesions affecting the oculomotor nerve – aneurysms of adjacent arteries around the brainstem may cause compression of the nearby nerve. Meningitis can involve the nerve along its course in the subarachnoid space.

TROCHLEAR NERVE (CRANIAL NERVE IV) (Fig. 1.47)

This is the only somatic efferent nerve to emerge from the posterior aspect of the central nervous system. It is also unusual in that it decussates before leaving the brainstem. It supplies only one extraocular muscle, the *superior oblique.*

Origin

The nucleus lies in the anterior part of the periaqueductal grey matter at the level of the inferior colliculus (caudal to III nerve nucleus) in line with the other oculomotor nuclei. The fibres first pass anteriorly and laterally towards the tegmentum before turning and passing posteriorly around the periaqueductal grey matter and into the superior medullary velum (part of the roof of the fourth ventricle)

where they decussate before emerging from the posterior surface of the brainstem in the posterior cranial fossa (Fig. 1.45B).

Intracranial and intracavernous course

The trochlear nerve winds around the crus of the midbrain (cerebral peduncles) above the superior cerebellar artery and the pons and below the posterior cerebral artery. It continues anteriorly immediately beneath the free edge of the tentorium cerebelli. It pierces this dura and enters the lateral wall of the cavernous sinus beneath the oculomotor nerve (Figs 1.8D,E; 1.39B and 1.40B). The trochlear nerve then passes upwards, thus coming to lie above the oculomotor nerve before entering the orbit outside the tendinous ring in the lateral part of the superior orbital fissure.

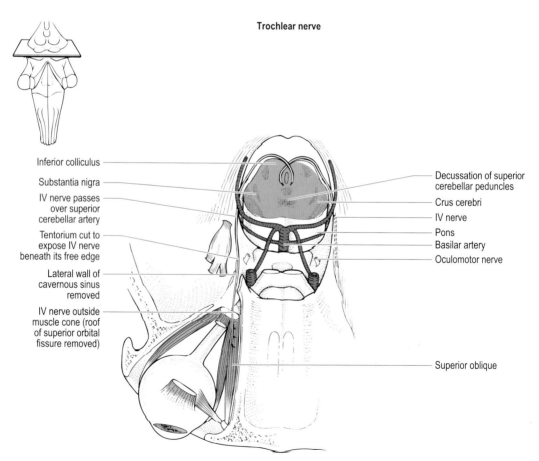

Fig. 1.47 Diagram summarizing the brainstem origin (inset shows level of section), intracranial, intracavernous and intraorbital course of the trochlear nerve.

Intraorbital course

It passes forward above the origin of levator palpebrae superioris close to the bone, to enter the upper free edge of the superior oblique (Figs 1.39A,B; 1.41 and 1.47).

Intracranial lesions affecting the trochlear nerve

The trochlear nerve is rarely paralysed alone, although it is particularly vulnerable at its posterior exit from the brainstem and as it winds round the midbrain. Lesions causing compression on the undersurface of the tentorium may affect the trochlear nerve. It may also be involved in pathological processes in the cavernous sinus (see p. 14). Patients suffering paralysis of the superior oblique because of trochlear nerve lesions suffer diplopia when looking down and have difficulty in looking down when the eye is adducted because the superior oblique is the only depressor in the adducted state. Patients characteristically carry the head tilted to the non-affected side with the chin lowered to compensate for the overaction of the inferior oblique producing unopposed torsion on the eye.

ABDUCENT NERVE (CRANIAL NERVE VI) (Fig. 1.48)

The abducens nucleus lies in the midpons beneath the floor of the upper part of the fourth ventricle, close to the midline beneath the facial colliculus. The fibres pass anteriorly to emerge on the lower border of the pons above the medulla near the midline (Fig. 1.45).

Intracranial and intracavernous course

The abducent nerve has the longest intracranial course of any cranial nerve. It courses upwards in the pontine cistern between the brainstem and the clivus, either side of the basilar artery. It is crossed or 'bound down' to the brainstem close to its origin by the anterior inferior cerebellar artery. It may pierce the dura early in its upward course upon the clivus close to the inferior petrosal sinus (2 cm below the posterior clinoid process). On reaching the upper border of the apex of the petrous temporal bone, it crosses the inferior petrosal sinus from medial to lateral and changes direction sharply from a vertical to a horizontal course and runs forward beneath the *petrosphenoidal ligament (of Gruber)* and *superior petrosal sinus*. The abducent nerve passes forward *within the cavernous sinus*, surrounded by venous spaces and suspended by fine connective tissue tra-

beculae. It lies *lateral* to the ascending portion of the internal carotid artery and then inferolateral to its horizontal portion (Fig. 1.8D,E). The abducent nerve enters the intraconal space of the orbit by passing within the tendinous ring (Fig. 1.5).

Intracranial lesions affecting the abducent nerve

The abducent nerve is considered the 'weakling of the cranial contents'. It is very susceptible to damage in head injuries, such as fractures to the base of the skull or any type of expanding cerebral lesion, owing to its long intracranial course. If the brainstem is displaced downward (due to raised intracranial pressure) the nerve may be compressed against the inferior cerebellar artery or severed where it bends sharply over the apex or crest of the petrous temporal bone. Within the *cavernous sinus* the nerve is more susceptible than the other intracavernous nerves, not being protected by the dura of the lateral wall (see p. 14). For example, atheromatous changes in the internal carotid artery may compress the abducent nerve. Lesions of the abducent nerve result in paralysis of lateral rectus; thus the patient is unable to abduct the eye and suffers esotropia (*internal strabismus*) as a result of the unopposed action of the medial rectus.

Intraorbital course

The abducent nerve has a short intraorbital course. It enters the bulbar surface of the lateral rectus one-third of the way from its origin. This is the only muscle supplied by the abducent nerve.

Brainstem lesions

There are a number of oculomotor palsies associated with lesions in the brainstem such as vascular disturbances. These may be associated with palsies of other cranial nerves, such as the association of VI and VII nerve palsies owing to their close relation in the floor of the fourth ventricle. Readers should consult specialist neurological or neuroanatomical texts for full consideration of the range of these disorders.

Sensory endings in oculomotor nerves

The cell bodies of proprioreceptive fibres in the extraocular muscles are located in the mesencephalic nucleus of the trigeminal nerve (see p. 69). The mesencephalic nucleus also receives proprioreceptive terminals from neck and face musculature.

Abducent nerve

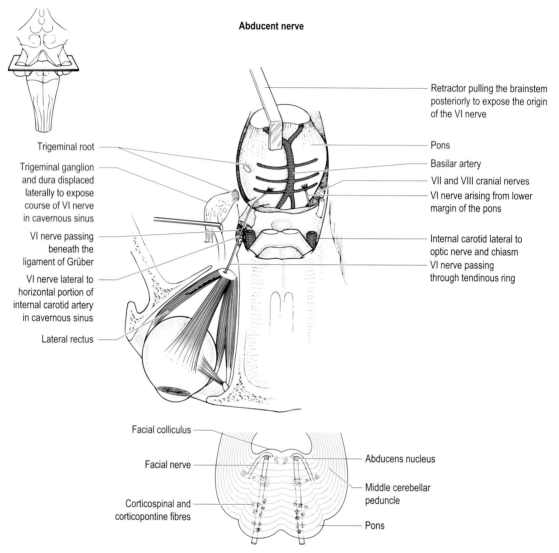

Retractor pulling the brainstem posteriorly to expose the origin of the VI nerve

Trigeminal root

Trigeminal ganglion and dura displaced laterally to expose course of VI nerve in cavernous sinus

VI nerve passing beneath the ligament of Grüber

VI nerve lateral to horizontal portion of internal carotid artery in cavernous sinus

Lateral rectus

Pons

Basilar artery

VII and VIII cranial nerves

VI nerve arising from lower margin of the pons

Internal carotid lateral to optic nerve and chiasm

VI nerve passing through tendinous ring

Facial colliculus

Facial nerve

Corticospinal and corticopontine fibres

Abducens nucleus

Middle cerebellar peduncle

Pons

Fig. 1.48 Main diagram summarizes the intracranial, intracavernous and intraorbital course of the abducent nerve. The smaller lower diagram shows the neurohistological features at the level of the abducens nuclei (level of mid-pons on brainstem).

The coordination of simultaneous movements of the head and eyes is dependent on conjugation of sensory (proprioceptive) information from the musculature of the neck and eyes, and input from cerebellar oculomotor centres (see Ch. 5).

TRIGEMINAL NERVE (CRANIAL NERVE V) (Fig. 1.49)

The trigeminal is the largest of the cranial nerves. It is the main sensory nerve of the head supplying the mucous membranes of the oronasal cavities, middle ear, paranasal sinuses, skin of the face, the teeth, the cornea, the temporomandibular joint, and the dura of the anterior and middle cranial fossae (Fig. 1.49A,B). Its embryological origin is complex (see Ch. 2). Briefly, the ophthalmic division represents the nerve to the frontonasal swelling; the maxillary and mandibular divisions are the nerves of the superior and inferior components of the first pharyngeal arch respectively. The dermatomes corresponding to its three major subdivisions and the cutaneous branches of the ophthalmic and maxillary nerves are shown in Figure 1.49A.

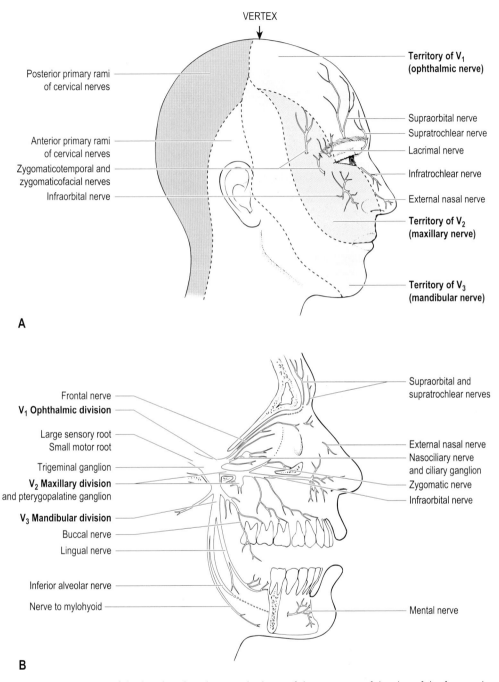

Fig. 1.49 (**A**) Sensory 'map' of the head and neck. Note the limits of the territories of the skin of the face and scalp supplied by the three divisions of the trigeminal nerve (ophthalmic, maxillary and mandibular). (**B**) Stylized diagram showing the origin of the motor and sensory roots of the trigeminal, the position of the pterygopalatine and ciliary ganglia, and the territories of some of the major branches of the three divisions.

There is less overlap between these dermatomes than is characteristically associated with spinal nerves; thus lesions of one or more divisions will present clinically as areas of paraesthesia whose distribution closely matches the territory shown in Figure 1.49A.

The mandibular division, besides its sensory component, supplies motor fibres to the muscles of mastication and also receives proprioceptive fibres from these muscles, together with the muscles of facial expression.

The trigeminal nerve arises from the brainstem in the posterior cranial fossa as a large *sensory root* and a small *motor root*. The sensory root consists of the central processes of pseudounipolar sensory neurones whose cell bodies lie in the large *trigeminal ganglion* located in the cavum trigeminale, a bony depression near the apex of the petrous temporal bone lined by evaginating dura mater from the edge of the tentorium cerebelli and roofed over by dura of the middle cranial fossa. The ganglion is partly surrounded by cerebrospinal fluid, which is continuous with the subarachnoid space of the posterior cranial fossa. The ganglion is homologous to a dorsal root or sensory ganglion of a spinal nerve. It is from the anterolateral convex surface of this flattened ganglion that the three named branches emerge, the ophthalmic (V_1), maxillary (V_2) and mandibular (V_3) (Fig. 1.49B).

The *ophthalmic division* or nerve (Fig. 1.50A) splits in the anterolateral portion of the cavernous sinus into three main branches: the *lacrimal, frontal* and *nasociliary*. The pathway and termination of these nerves are summarized in Figures 1.39–1.41, 1.49B and 1.50A.

The *maxillary nerve* (Figs 1.49B and 1.50B) passes through the *foramen rotundum* and spans the *pterygopalatine fossa* before entering the orbit through the *inferior orbital fissure* as the *infraorbital nerve*. It lies beneath the periorbita and is thus not truly an orbital content. The nerve passes forward from the inferior orbital fissure to the *infraorbital groove*, which becomes the *infraorbital canal*, the nerve eventually emerging through the *infraorbital foramen*. Here it radiates out as a number of cutaneous branches supplying the lower eyelid, the nose, upper lip and cheek (Fig. 1.49A). The *zygomatic nerve*, a branch of the infraorbital, runs along in the inferior orbital fissure, beneath the periorbita, to the lateral wall of the orbit where it pierces the zygomatic bone as two branches, the *zygomaticotemporal* and *zygomaticofacial* nerves (both cutaneous). Traditionally, a communicating branch is described as passing up the lateral wall of the orbit to join the lacrimal nerve; however, the presence or importance of this nerve has been disputed (Ruskell, 1971b). Other branches of the maxillary nerve, which pass through the *pterygopalatine ganglion* (without synapsing), supply the nasal cavity, upper alveolar arch and hard and soft palate (Fig. 1.49B). More details of these branches and those of the mandibular division are provided in standard anatomical texts.

The four parasympathetic ganglia of the head and neck (ciliary, pterygopalatine, otic and submandibular) are associated with the branches of the

Fig. 1.50 Diagram summarizing the origin, intracranial, intracavernous and intraorbital course of the ophthalmic nerve and its three main branches.

- The *frontal nerve* passes obliquely above the levator palpebrae superioris and divides into the supraorbital nerve and the supratrochlear nerve.
- The supraorbital nerve passes through the supraorbital notch or foramen and ascends in the subcutaneous tissue of the forehead to supply the skin.
- The supratrochlear nerve passes along the medial wall of the orbit to pass above the trochlea and supply the skin at the root of the nose, upper eyelid and the medial part of the forehead.
- The *lacrimal nerve* travels forward along the upper border of the lateral rectus and sends fibres to the gland before ending as *lateral palpebral branches* to the conjunctiva and skin of this region.
- Branches of the *nasociliary nerve* include the *sensory root* to the ciliary ganglion (from which the short ciliary nerves emerge), *long ciliary nerves, posterior ethmoidal nerve* (supplies ethmoidal and sphenoidal sinuses), the *anterior ethmoidal nerve* and *infratrochlear nerves*.
- The anterior ethmoidal briefly re-enters the cranial cavity at the cribriform plate (beneath the dura) before piercing the bone to exit the cavity to terminate as the *medial* and *lateral internal nasal branches* (supply the nasal cavity), the latter of which ends as the *external nasal branch* which supplies the skin on the lower half of the nose.
- The infratrochlear nerve runs along close to the medial orbital wall, passes beneath the trochlea and supplies the skin at the angle of the eye and upper part of the skin of the nose.

(B) Diagram of the orbital floor and the course of the maxillary and infraorbital nerves.

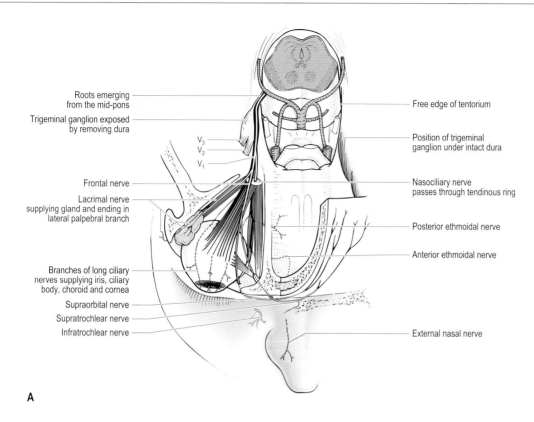

Roots emerging from the mid-pons

Trigeminal ganglion exposed by removing dura

V₃
V₂
V₁

Frontal nerve

Lacrimal nerve supplying gland and ending in lateral palpebral branch

Branches of long ciliary nerves supplying iris, ciliary body, choroid and cornea

Supraorbital nerve

Supratrochlear nerve

Infratrochlear nerve

Free edge of tentorium

Position of trigeminal ganglion under intact dura

Nasociliary nerve passes through tendinous ring

Posterior ethmoidal nerve

Anterior ethmoidal nerve

External nasal nerve

A

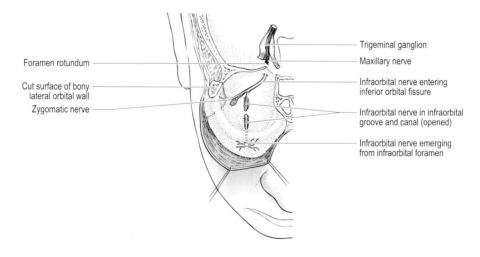

Foramen rotundum

Cut surface of bony lateral orbital wall

Zygomatic nerve

Trigeminal ganglion

Maxillary nerve

Infraorbital nerve entering inferior orbital fissure

Infraorbital nerve in infraorbital groove and canal (opened)

Infraorbital nerve emerging from infraorbital foramen

B

trigeminal (Fig. 1.49B). They are generally connected by short stalks containing pre- and postganglionic fibres, and the terminal fibres are distributed with the branches of the trigeminal – they may share the same perineural sheath for part of their course ('hitch-hikers'). Sympathetics may also hitch-hike with branches of the trigeminal for part of their course and be distributed to the territories of this large nerve.

Sensory nuclei of the trigeminal nerve

There are three sensory nuclei in the brainstem associated with the trigeminal nerve:

- *Mesencephalic nucleus* The only central nervous system nucleus containing unipolar neurones, it receives sensory (proprioceptive) information from muscles of mastication, muscles of facial expression (including orbicularis oculi) and extraocular muscles. The peripheral processes are distributed with all three divisions of the trigeminal.
- *Pontine nucleus* Concerned with discriminative tactile information from the face. Fibres from all three divisions enter this nucleus.
- *Spinal nucleus* Continuous with the substantia gelatinosa of the posterior grey horn of the spinal cord. Concerned with tactile, nociceptive and thermal information from the territories of the three divisions.

The afferent fibres terminating in the last two nuclei are the central processes of sensory neurones whose cell bodies are located in the trigeminal (Gasserian) ganglion. The peripheral processes terminate in appropriate sensory receptors in the territories of the three divisions.

Trigeminal neuralgia (tic douloureux)

This is a condition characterized by excruciating pain in the territory of one or more of the divisions of the trigeminal nerve. Thus, the clinician should be familiar with structures supplied by each division. Many causes have been suggested including osteitis of the petrous temporal bone or compression of the root or ganglion in the cavum trigeminale by enlarged or engorged vessels; however, in many cases the aetiology is unknown. The territory of the maxillary nerve is most frequently involved, then the mandibular, and less commonly the ophthalmic nerve. Three commonly performed surgeries include glycerol rhizotomy, stereotactic radiosurgery and microvascular decompression with a more recent trend towards endoscopic vascular decompression (Kabil et al., 2005).

FACIAL NERVE (CRANIAL NERVE VII)

The facial nerve is the nerve of the second pharyngeal (hyoid) arch. It contains a number of functional components (Table 1.5). The *facial nerve proper* (containing *branchiomotor* or *special visceral efferents*) supplies the muscles of facial expression (including the orbicularis oculi and other muscles around the orbit) (Fig. 1.51) (see p. 84), in addition to the stapedius (small muscle in middle ear), stylohyoid, and the posterior belly of the digastric. The second component, the *nervus intermedius*, contains secretomotor or *parasympathetic* fibres (*general visceral efferent*), which synapse in the pterygopalatine ganglion and supply the lacrimal gland and choroid in addition to other glands in and around the nose and mouth. The nerve also contains taste fibres (*special visceral afferents*) from the anterior two-thirds of the tongue. The extracranial branch of cranial nerve VII exits the skull through the *stylomastoid foramen* and pierces the parotid gland to emerge at the anterior border of that gland (Fig. 1.51). The facial nerve is important to the eye and orbit primarily because of its parasympathetic supply to the lacrimal gland (and some intraocular branches) and its motor supply to the periorbital facial muscles (especially orbicularis oculi). It is the most frequently paralysed of all peripheral nerves.

Lesions of the facial nerve

Supranuclear lesions – caused by vascular stroke in which descending corticonuclear and corticospinal fibres are damaged in the internal capsule. The upper facial motor nucleus (supplying upper half of facial muscles) receives input from 'face' areas of both the ipsilateral and contralateral motor cortices. The lower part of the facial nucleus has only contralateral input. The effect of a stroke, therefore, is to cause contralateral paralysis or weakness of the limbs and lower face. The upper face survives because of the bilateral supranuclear supply to the upper part of the facial nucleus.

Nuclear lesions – direct damage to the facial nucleus, such as thrombosis of the pontine branches of the basilar artery, results in complete paralysis of structures supplied by the facial nerve (and abducent nerve; see Fig. 1.48) together with motor weakness of the limbs on the opposite side (owing to pyramidal decussation occurring below this level).

Infranuclear lesions – Bell's palsy involves direct neuritis of the facial nerve in the bony canal within the temporal bone and results usually in complete facial paralysis.

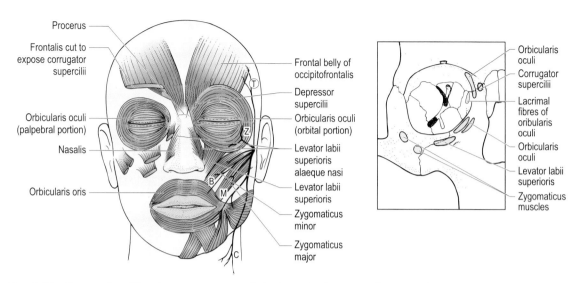

Fig. 1.51 The muscles of facial expression, particularly those of relevance to the eye and orbit. Inset shows the bony origins of some of these muscles around the orbit. Some of orbicularis oculi and frontalis muscle fibres have been removed on the right side of the face to display underlying musculature. The extracranial motor branches of the facial nerve that supply the muscles are shown on the right: T, temporal or frontal branches; Z, zygomatic branches; B, buccal branches; M, marginal mandibular branch; C, cervical branches.

Table 1.6	Reflexes involving the facial nerve		
	Corneal reflex	Blinking to light or fast approaching object	Blinking to noise
Receptor	Sensory ending in corneal epithelium	Retina	Cochlea
Afferent pathway	Long ciliary nerves, nasociliary nerve, ophthalmic nerve	Optic nerve	Vestibulocochlear nerve
First synapse	Spinal nucleus of trigeminal	Superior colliculus	Inferior colliculus
Second synapse	Facial nucleus	Facial nucleus	Facial nucleus
Efferent pathway	Temporal and zygomatic branches of facial nerve	Temporal and zygomatic branches of facial nerve	Temporal and zygomatic branches of facial nerve
Effector muscle	Orbicularis oculi	Orbicularis oculi	Orbicularis oculi

The patient is unable to move the lips (saliva and food drools from the corner of the mouth), eyebrows or close the eyelids (lids may be lax, causing epiphora), and suffers hyperacusis (due to paralysis of the stapedius). Some patients may also have reduced lacrimal and salivatory secretions and loss of taste to the anterior two-thirds of the tongue. Other causes of infranuclear lesions include multiple sclerosis, tumours of the cerebellopontine angle (acoustic neuromas), middle ear disease and tumours of the parotid gland.

There are three reflex arcs in the brainstem involving the facial nerve, of which the corneal reflex is an important clinical test (Table 1.6).

The autonomic innervation of smooth muscle and glands associated with the eye, eyelids and orbit has been described under the relevant sections. A general account of the *autonomic nervous system* can be found in any anatomy or neuroanatomy textbook.

OCULAR APPENDAGES (ADNEXA)

MUSCLES OF THE EYELIDS AND ADJACENT FACE

The muscles that are primarily responsible for movement of each eyelid include the *orbicularis oculi* (a muscle of facial expression), which is responsible for lid closure, and the *levator palpebrae superioris* (an extraocular muscle), which raises the lid.

The *muscles of facial expression* derive their motor innervation from the facial nerve (VII) (see Ch. 2). The muscles of facial expression (Fig. 1.51) of primary interest around the eye and eyelids are the *orbicularis oculi*, *corrugator supercilii* and *occipitofrontalis*.

Other small facial muscles that arise near the orbit but that may be concerned with the shape of the nasal apparatus or mouth are also of some interest because they may be used in reparative or reconstructive surgery of the eyelid region. They include *procerus*, *nasalis*, *levator labii superioris alaeque nasii*, *levator labii superioris* and *zygomaticus major* and *minor* (Fig. 1.51).

Orbicularis oculi (Fig. 1.51)

Shape: The orbicularis oculi muscle is a broad, flat, sheet of skeletal muscle with orbital, palpebral and lacrimal portions. The circular orientation of the fibres is a reflection of the sphincter-like function of this muscle. The *orbital portion* arises from the medial palpebral ligament and the adjacent orbital margin (Fig. 1.51, inset). Its fibres run circumferentially in an elliptical fashion around and beyond the orbital margin. Most pass round the lateral orbital margin without interruption, although some fibres (known as *depressor supercilii*) are inserted into the skin and connective tissue of the eyebrow. The *palpebral part* is an extremely thin muscle that originates from the *medial palpebral ligament*. Its fibres pass laterally within the eyelid anterior to the orbital septum and tarsal plate (see below), and interlace to form the *lateral palpebral raphe*. The small *lacrimal component* of the muscle passes deep to the medial palpebral ligament and is attached to the posterior lacrimal crest (behind the lacrimal sac) as two muscle slips (upper and lower). These fibres are inserted laterally into the tarsi close to the lacrimal canaliculi; they help draw the eyelids and lacrimal papillae medially and in addition dilate the lacrimal sac during blinking. This helps to suck tears into the lacrimal punctum from the lacus lacrimalis (see p. 94).

Nerve supply Temporal and zygomatic branches of the facial nerve.

Action The *orbital* portion, owing to its elliptical form and medial attachments, acts like a pursestring, drawing the skin of the forehead, temple, cheek and orbital margin towards the medial angle of the orbit, firmly closing the lids (for example, when in very bright light). The *palpebral* portion of orbicularis oculi can act under both voluntary and involuntary control to close the eyelids during normal blinking (and sleeping). This blinking reflex (Table 1.6) is essential to the integrity of the ocular tear film and function of the cornea.

Excess use of this muscle leads to permanent prominent skin folds ('crows' feet') along the lateral orbital margin. Vertical folds may also develop at this site owing to loss of muscle tone with age.

Corrugator supercilii

This is a small pyramidal muscle at the medial aspect of the eyebrow (Fig. 1.51), beneath the occipitofrontalis and orbicularis oculi. It draws the eyebrow downwards and medially (frowning), producing vertical skin furrows on the forehead. It assists in protecting the eyes in bright light. It is supplied by small subdivisions of the temporal branch of the facial nerve.

Occipitofrontalis

This fibromuscular layer covers the dome of the skull from the eyebrows to the nuchal lines. It consists of two occipital bellies posteriorly attached via a thick fibrous layer, the *galea aponeurotica*, to the two frontal bellies. Only the frontal part is of relevance to the eye and orbit. Its fibres form a thin quadrangular sheet that is attached to the superficial fascia above the eyebrows. The medial fibres are continuous with procerus (Fig. 1.51), the intermediate fibres with corrugator supercilii and orbicularis oculi, and the lateral fibres with the lateral fibres of the orbicularis oculi. The frontal belly is supplied by the temporal branches of the facial nerve. Upon contraction it draws the scalp backwards and elevates the eyebrows, causing transverse wrinkles on the scalp as in expressions of surprise, horror, fright, or when glancing upwards.

Levator palpebrae superioris

This muscle lies within the orbit and is responsible for opening the eyelids and, upon relaxation, allows lid closure due to gravity. The muscle has its origin from the lesser wing of sphenoid, above and in front of the optic foramen, blending with the origin of superior rectus. The muscle belly passes horizontally forward above superior rectus, close to the orbital roof. Behind the orbital margin it curves downwards into the lid where it becomes aponeurotic. The aponeurosis fans out, on either side, to form medial and lateral horns, which extend the whole width of the eyelid. The levator palpebrae superioris inserts into the skin of the upper lid (causing the horizontal palpebral sulcus or furrow) and the anterior surface of the tarsal plate. The lateral horn of the aponeurosis forms the *lateral palpebral ligament*, which inserts into the lateral orbital tubercle, and the medial horn forms the *medial palpebral ligament*, which inserts into the frontolacrimal suture. The levator palpebrae superioris is supplied by the superior division of the oculomotor nerve (see p. 73 and Fig. 1.46). Upon contraction it elevates the upper lid, thereby opening the palpebral fissure. On the inferior aspect of the levator palpebrae superioris is a small band of smooth muscle, the *superior tarsal* or *Müller's muscle*. It is attached anteriorly to the upper surface of the tarsal plate and conjunctival fornix. It has a sympathetic innervation and upon contraction assists the levator in elevating the eyelid. While there is no equivalent muscle to the levator in the lower lid, there is a small group of smooth muscle fibres (inferior tarsal muscle) that originate from the fascial sheath of the inferior rectus and insert into the lower tarsus (Ruskell et al., 2005).

THE EYELIDS

The eyelids are thin curtains of skin, muscle, fibrous tissue, and mucous membrane that serve to protect the eyes from injury and excessive light and also to distribute tears over the ocular surface during blinking. The upper lid, when open, normally just overlaps the corneoscleral junction, and it is this lid that undergoes most displacement during eyelid closure, the lower lid moving only minimally during normal blinking.

On external examination (Fig. 1.52) each lid is seen to be divided into *orbital* and *tarsal portions* by a horizontal *palpebral sulcus*, which is most evident on the upper lid. The upper lid is limited superiorly by the eyebrow, whereas the lower lid blends with the skin of the cheek. The upper and lower lids meet at

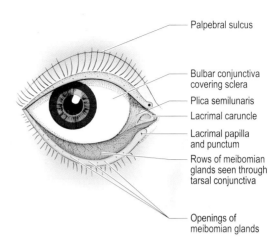

the *medial* and *lateral canthi* or angles, and are separated from one another by an elliptical opening – the *palpebral fissure*. The lateral canthus is an acute angle (60°) and lies close to the eyeball; the medial canthus is rounded, elongated medially, and lies 6 mm from the eyeball. It is separated from the eye by a triangular zone, the *lacus lacrimalis* (lake of tears), in which a small raised red swelling, the *curuncula lacrimalis*, is situated. There are obvious racial differences in the shape and form of the eyelids and canthi, the most conspicuous being the vertical *epicanthal fold* in Oriental and Asian races.

The *eyelid margins* (Figs 1.52 and 1.53) are approximately 30 mm in length, 2 mm in thickness, and relatively square in profile along most of their length, except the medial one-sixth, which is rounded and lacks eyelashes. Eyelashes are modified, thick, stiff hairs that occur as double or triple rows close to the anterior lid margin. They curl away from the lashes of the opposite lid. Notable features on the lid margins include:

- *Lacrimal puncta* located at the medial ends of the upper and lower lids. These drain tears from the lacus lacrimalis. The puncta are more easily identified if tension is placed on the lids causing the papillae to blanch.
- Openings of *tarsal (meibomian) glands* are visible to the naked eye as a row of minute openings on the lid margin posterior to the eyelash follicles. There are around 30 in the upper lid and slightly fewer in the lower lid.

Fig. 1.52 Surface anatomy of the eye and eyelids. The bottom lid has been slightly everted to reveal the inner surface of the lid, lacrimal papillae and puncta and the openings of the meibomian glands along the lid margin.

85

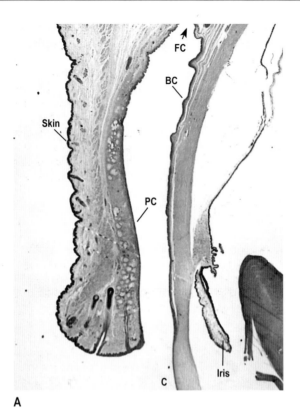

A

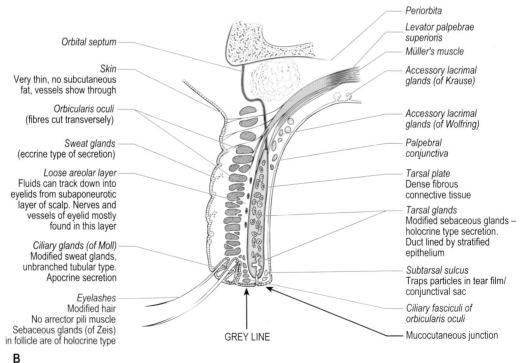

Orbital septum

Skin
Very thin, no subcutaneous
fat, vessels show through

Orbicularis oculi
(fibres cut transversely)

Sweat glands
(eccrine type of secretion)

Loose areolar layer
Fluids can track down into
eyelids from subaponeurotic
layer of scalp. Nerves and
vessels of eyelid mostly
found in this layer

Ciliary glands (of Moll)
Modified sweat glands,
unbranched tubular type.
Apocrine secretion

Eyelashes
Modified hair
No arrector pili muscle
Sebaceous glands (of Zeis)
in follicle are of holocrine type

GREY LINE

Periorbita

Levator palpebrae
superioris

Müller's muscle

Accessory lacrimal
glands (of Krause)

Accessory lacrimal
glands (of Wolfring)

Palpebral
conjunctiva

Tarsal plate
Dense fibrous
connective tissue

Tarsal glands
Modified sebaceous glands –
holocrine type secretion.
Duct lined by stratified
epithelium

Subtarsal sulcus
Traps particles in tear film/
conjunctival sac

Ciliary fasciculi of
orbicularis oculi

Mucocutaneous junction

B

Fig. 1.53 (**A**) Histological preparation of the upper eyelid, conjunctiva and anterior segment: PC, palpebral conjunctiva; FC, forniceal conjunctiva; BC, bulbar conjunctiva; C, cornea. (**B**) Schematic diagram of the upper eyelid in longitudinal section (sagittal plane). Original magnification: **A**, × 15. (Part A courtesy of W.R. Lee and Springer-Verlag.)

- The *skin/conjunctival transition zone* mucocutaneous junction occurs at the level of the opening of the tarsal glands.
- The *grey line* marks the anterior boundary of the tarsal plate and is a useful landmark for surgical incisions.

The histological structure of the eyelid is summarized in Figures 1.53 and 1.55. Note that the fibrous framework of the lids is formed by the *orbital septum* arising from the orbital margin (Fig. 1.37) and the *tarsal plates*. The *tarsal plates* are modified regional thickenings of the orbital septum that provide rigidity to the upper and lower lids and separate the orbit and its contents from the lids.

Herniation of orbital fat through weakened regions of the septum occurs in the elderly, producing bulging, sagging lids (blepharochalasis).

The tarsal plates consist of dense fibrous connective tissue and are approximately 25–30 mm from the medial to lateral borders. They are 1 mm thick and the upper plate is greater in height (10–12 mm) than the lower plate (5 mm). They are attached at either end via their continuations, the *medial* and *lateral palpebral ligaments*. Skin moves freely over their anterior surface, although the conjunctiva is tightly bound to the posterior surface. External examination of an everted eyelid reveals vertical rows of yellowish tarsal glands. They are embedded in the matrix of the tarsal plate and consist of modified sebaceous glands. Histologically the acinar cells are replete with lipid droplets that are secreted in a holocrine manner on to the eyelid margin, which functions to retain tears in the conjunctival sac and contributes to the lipid layer of the precorneal tear film.

Chalazion Localized, painless swelling in the lid due to obstruction and chronic inflammation of a tarsal gland.

Hordeolum (sty) Can be either an acute infection of an eyelash follicle or its sebaceous gland, infection of a ciliary sweat gland (external hordeolum), or acute infection of a tarsal gland (internal hordeolum).

Ectropion Drooping of lower lid owing to paralysis of orbicularis oculi. Because of paralysis of the fibres of orbicularis that enclose the lacrimal sac, the puncta no longer suck up tears, which may thus pass over the lid margin (*epiphora*).

The blood supply and nerve supply of the lids and surrounding areas are summarized in Figure 1.54. Lymphatics drain to the superficial parotid or submandibular lymph nodes. The pretarsal portion derives its arterial supply from the superficial temporal and facial arteries (branches of the external carotid), while the posttarsal portion is supplied by branches of the ophthalmic artery (branch of internal carotid artery) (see Fig. 1.44). Venous drainage follows a similar pattern to the arterial supply (see p. 72 for consideration of anastomoses between the internal and external carotid arteries). The posttarsal venous drainage is via the ophthalmic veins to the cavernous sinus.

Movements of the eyelids

The eyelids close as a result of the action of the palpebral fibres of the orbicularis oculi and relaxation of the levator palpebrae superioris. Opening of the lids occurs via the pull of levator palpebrae superioris on the skin, tarsal plate and forniceal conjunctiva. The nerve supply to these muscles is from three sources: orbicularis oculi – the facial nerve (VII); levator palpebrae superioris – the oculomotor nerve (III); while its smooth muscle component, superior tarsal (Müller's) muscle, is supplied by sympathetic nerves. The latter is important in times of fear or excitement when the width of the palpebral fissure is further increased.

Horner syndrome

Because of the complex neuroanatomy of the sympathetic nervous system, Horner syndrome, which is characterized by classical symptoms of unilateral ptosis, miosis and dry facial skin (anhidrosis) and blushing on the affected side, may result from a wide variety of lesions in the central and peripheral nervous system. These include iatrogenic interruption of the sympathetic chain in the neck, dissection of the internal carotid artery, cervical disc dislocation and the lysis of the first rib affecting the stellate ganglion associated with Pancoast tumour. Other symptoms may include heterochromia and enophthalmos, although the latter is debatable in humans.

THE CONJUNCTIVA

The conjunctiva (Figs 1.53A,B and 1.55) is a thin translucent mucous membrane that derives its name from the fact that it attaches the eyeball to the lids. It consists of a superficial conjunctival epithelium overlying a loose connective tissue stroma. The epithelium is continuous with the corneal

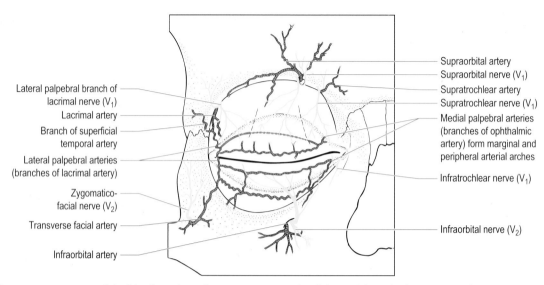

Lateral palpebral branch of lacrimal nerve (V₁)
Lacrimal artery
Branch of superficial temporal artery
Lateral palpebral arteries (branches of lacrimal artery)
Zygomatico-facial nerve (V₂)
Transverse facial artery
Infraorbital artery

Supraorbital artery
Supraorbital nerve (V₁)
Supratrochlear artery
Supratrochlear nerve (V₁)
Medial palpebral arteries (branches of ophthalmic artery) form marginal and peripheral arterial arches
Infratrochlear nerve (V₁)
Infraorbital nerve (V₂)

Fig. 1.54 Summary of the blood supply and sensory nerve supply of the eyelids and adjacent areas from cutaneous branches of the ophthalmic (V₁) and maxillary (V₂) divisions of the trigeminal nerve.

epithelium at the limbus and with the skin at the mucocutaneous junction on the lid margin. The conjunctiva is reflected from the anterior portion of the sclera at the superior and inferior fornices onto the tarsal surface of the eyelids. Thus, when the lids are closed a potential sac, the *conjunctival sac* is formed. The volume of this sac is approximately 7 μl, which explains the tendency for eye drops from commercial dispensers (volume 50–70 ml) to over-flow unless the lower lid is held away from the globe. The conjunctiva is responsible for the production of the mucous component of the tear film and, in common with other mucous membranes, has a variety of immunological defence mechanisms that protect the ocular surface from infection (Knop and Knop, 2005; see p. 429). For descriptive purposes the conjunctiva can be divided into three main regions.

Palpebral conjunctiva (Fig. 1.53A,B)
This part lines the inner surfaces of the eyelids. It is tightly bound to the tarsal plate, the subepithelial connective tissue stroma being thin in this region. The lacrimal puncta open onto the palpebral con-junctiva; thus the conjunctival epithelium is contin-uous with the lining of the inferior meatus of the nasal cavity, which explains the manner in which infection spreads between these two sites. A small

Fig. 1.55 Histology of the conjunctiva. (**A**) Low-power light micrograph of human conjunctiva [periodic acid–Schiff (PAS) stain] showing the irregular nature and goblet cell content (purple and red PAS⁺ profiles) of the epithelium (compare to corneal epithelium; Fig. 1.11). Note the accumulations of lymphoid cells in the highly vascular connective tissue stroma, a common feature in eyes of elderly patients. CT, subepithelial connective tissue or connective tissue stroma. (**B**) Electron micrograph of goblet cells (GC) in the conjunctival epithelium: Ep, epithelium. (**C**) 'Plan view' of MHC class II⁺ intraepithelial cells [red; sometimes called Langerhans' cells (LC)] in the limbal/conjunctival epithelium in mouse wholemount preparation (blue – DAPI-stained nuclei). (**D**) Toluidine-blue-stained conjunctival wholemount illustrating the orientation and distribution of mast cells around limbal vessels (V) and in the bulbar conjunctiva (Conj) where they are more rounded. (**E**) Toluidine-blue-stained semi-thin resin section of the limbal region showing a mast cell (MC) adjacent to a large venule (V). (**F**) Primate conjunctiva (histological preparation, H & E) showing melanocytes in the basal layer of the conjunctival/limbal epithelium. Note the intraepithelial melanin granules throughout the conjunctival epithelial layers. (**G**) Melanocytes as seen in a limbal wholemount preparation. Note their highly dendriform shape (arrows) and how they form a halo (dotted lines) of melanin granules within the adjacent epithelial cells ('epithelial-melanin unit'). Original magnifications: **A**, × 150, **B**, × 3000, **C**, × 200, **D**, × 100, **E**, × 650, **F**, × 150; **G**, × 160. (Part B courtesy of Prof: W. R. Lee.)

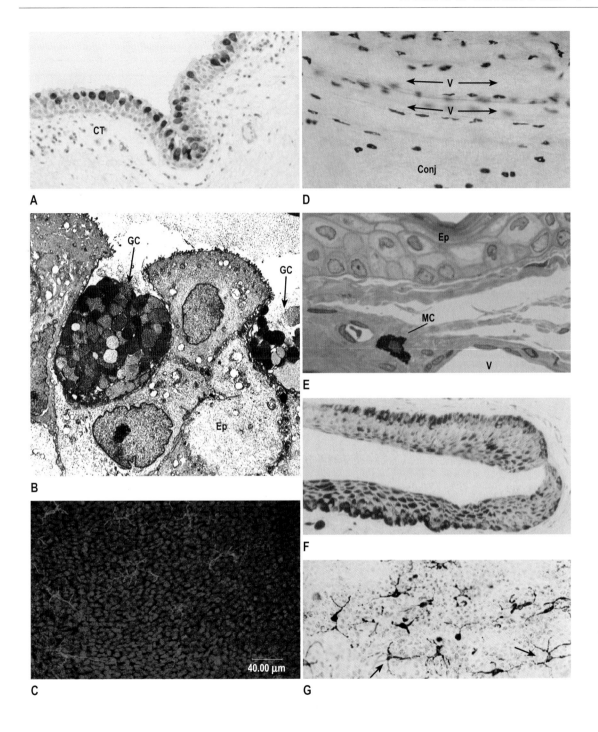

A

CT

B

GC

GC

Ep

C

40.00 μm

D

V

V

Conj

E

Ep

MC

V

F

G

subtarsal sulcus, close to the lid margin, is important in trapping and removing foreign particles and debris on the ocular surface.

Clinical examination of the everted lid for signs of ocular allergy and infection is a common procedure. Two major types of abnormal accumulations of immune cells may occur: *follicles*, which are similar to mucosal-associated lymphoid follicles elsewhere and consist primarily of lymphocytes; and *papillae*, which are focal aggregates of chronic inflammatory cellular infiltrates and accompanying vascular changes. These are usually associated with allergic conditions and irritation of the ocular surface, such as in contact lens wear.

Forniceal conjunctiva (Fig. 1.53A)

The superior and inferior fornices are continuous at the medial and lateral canthi, thus forming a circular *cul de sac*. It is into the superolateral fornix that the ducts of the main lacrimal gland and the bulk of accessory lacrimal glands empty. The forniceal conjunctiva is loosely attached to the fascial sheaths of levator palpebrae superioris and the rectus muscles, and thus moves slightly with the eye during contraction of these muscles.

Bulbar conjunctiva

The white sclera is visible through the normal translucent bulbar conjunctiva (see Figs 1.15A and 1.52). It clothes the anterior part of the eyeball including the extraocular muscle insertions and Tenon's capsule. Near the limbus the conjunctiva is tightly bound to the globe, but further from the limbus there is a loose episcleral tissue layer (Fig. 1.55A) within which lies the pericorneal vascular plexus (Fig. 1.55D). These vessels can become dilated and conspicuous as a result of physical and inflammatory stimuli.

There are two specializations of the conjunctiva in the medial fornix. First, the semilunar fold (*plica semilunaris*) which is probably homologous to the nictitating membrane of lower mammals and many non-mammalian vertebrates. It is highly vascular and rich in goblet cells and interstitial immunocompetent cells. The function of this loose fold may be to facilitate lateral movement of the eye. Second, the *caruncle* (*caruncula lacrimalis*) is a highly vascular nodule of modified skin in the medial corner of the eye containing large nests of accessory lacrimal and sebaceous glandular tissue.

The conjunctiva may manifest signs of several important systemic diseases: pathognomonic signs are present in sickle cell anaemia, jaundice [scleral icterus (yellowing)] and vitamin A deficiency (Bitot's spots).

Structure of the conjunctiva

Histologically the conjunctival epithelium varies in structure, depending on location, from a stratified squamous non-keratinizing epithelium (close to the lid margin) to a stratified columnar epithelium (bulbar). In general it consists of between two and seven layers of epithelial cells that are organized into three main types: basal, intermediate and superficial. There is no 'prickle' layer as found in corneal epithelium, indicating that there are fewer desmosomes between the conjunctival epithelial cells. There are numerous other cell types resident within the epithelium, reflecting its protective function, including the following.

- *Goblet cells* (Fig. 1.55A,B) – unicellular mucus-secreting cells that vary in density in different regions of the conjunctiva, being most numerous in the fornices and plica semilunaris. They are responsible for the secretion of the majority of conjunctival mucins.
- *Melanocytes* (Fig. 1.55F,G) – degree of melanization varies dependent on race, although melanocytes are present in all eyes. Melanosomes are synthesized within the melanocyte before exocytosis and subsequent uptake by surrounding epithelial cells as occurs in the epidermis.
- *Intraepithelial MHC class II-positive bone marrow-derived dendritic cells* (sometimes referred to as Langerhans' cells because of their similar morphology to analogous dendritic cell populations in the epidermis of the skin) (Fig. 1.55C) – function as 'sentinels' on the ocular surface and are responsible for trapping and internalizing antigens and transporting these signals to either local lymph nodes (such as the preauricular nodes) or conjunctival associated lymphoid tissue (CALT) or follicles, where they are capable of presenting antigens to naive T cells and inducing primary immune responses or driving antigen-specific B-cell maturation and immunoglobulin production (see Ch. 7). The latter role may be important in relation to CALT because there is no clear evidence of the specialized antigen-transporting intraepithelial M cells that are typically found in

other mucosal associated lymphoid tissues (MALT) such as Peyer's patches or tonsils (Gebert and Pabst, 1999; Knop and Knop, 2005). Conjunctival epithelial dendritic cells are continuous with and phenotypically identical to the dendritic cell populations of the limbal epithelium and peripheral corneal epithelium (Fig. 1.55C).

- *Intraepithelial lymphocytes* – a feature of normal conjunctiva, but increased numbers occur in inflammatory conditions and close to subepithelial lymphoid accumulations. These are predominantly CD3$^+$ T cells although occasional B cells are present (Hingorani et al., 1997; Knop and Knop, 2005).

The epithelium has an irregular basal aspect adjacent to the underlying connective tissue which is sometimes described as having a looser lymphoid layer and a deeper fibrous layer. Distinct papillae, finger-like protrusions of connective tissue stroma that project into the epithelium, are found only near the limbus. The subepithelial connective tissue contains numerous immunocompetent cells such as mast cells (Fig. 1.55D, E), eosinophils, plasma cells and lymphocytes scattered among the matrix (Hingorani et al., 1997; Knop and Knop, 2005). In some eyes, particularly of older individuals (Wotherspoon et al., 1994), these may form diffuse or discrete aggregates. Knop and Knop (2005) have postulated that the follicles, some of which contain pale germinal centres, represent the afferent arm of a generalized eye-associated mucosal immune system. The diffuse subepithelial aggregates along with intraepithelial lymphocytes form the efferent arm of this system and aid in immunological protection of the ocular surface. The topographical distribution of the small (~ 0.3 mm) lenticular lymphoid follicles and epithelial crypts in the tarso-orbital conjunctiva suggests that they may approximate to the cornea during eye closure and thus function as an 'immunological cushion' (Knop and Knop, 2005)

The loose connective tissue stroma contains a rich vascular network, whose branches are similar to those of the eyelids. In addition it also receives blood from the anterior ciliary arteries (see Fig. 1.44).

The sensory nerve supply of the palpebral conjunctiva is almost entirely from branches of the ophthalmic division of the trigeminal (supraorbital, supratrochlear and lacrimal nerves). These contain the neurotransmittors substance P, calcitonin-gene-related peptide (CGRP) and gallanin. Only the medial portion of the inferior forniceal and palpebral conjunctiva derives its nerve supply from the maxillary division (infraorbital nerve) (see Fig. 1.54). The long ciliary nerves supply the bulbar conjunctiva. Parasympathetic nerves from the pterygopalatine ganglion (containing the neurotransmittors acetylcholine and VIP) and sympathetics (containing norepinephrine and neuropetide Y) travelling with branches of the ophthalmic artery are also present in the conjunctiva. Both parasympathetics and sympathetics have been identified around goblet cells whereas the sensory nerve endings were identified only among the stratified squamous epithelial cells (see review, Dartt, 2002).

Glands in the conjunctiva

Besides the unicellular mucous glands (goblet cells) distributed throughout the conjunctiva, there are several small collections of named glands, some of which are accessory lacrimal glands (glands of Krause in the upper fornices, glands of Wolfring in the upper border of the tarsus); others secrete mucus (glands of Henle). The accessory lacrimal glands are under sympathetic stimulation and are responsible for baseline tear production.

LACRIMAL APPARATUS (Fig. 1.56)

The lacrimal apparatus consists of the *lacrimal gland, lacrimal puncta, lacrimal canaliculi, lacrimal sac* and *nasolacrimal duct*. The lacrimal apparatus functions to produce tears that moisten the ocular surface, thus preventing desiccation of delicate ocular cells and tissues, and facilitating non-friction-bearing movements of the lids on the globe. Tears are thus essential in maintaining the functional integrity of the eye.

Tear film

The tear film (7–9μm) is composed of three layers: an outer oily or lipid layer (from meibomian and Zeis glands), a middle aqueous layer containing protein, electrolytes and water (mainly from lacrimal glands but also small contributions from conjunctival epithelia and cornea), and a deep hydrophilic mucin layer (from goblet cells and conjunctival epithelial cells and some from the corneal epithelium) associated with the microplicae-rich surface of the conjunctival epithelium (Fig. 1.55B).

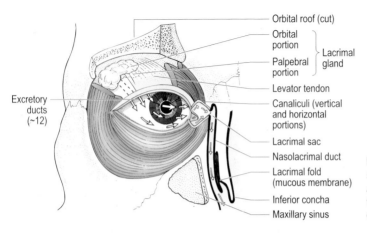

Fig. 1.56 Schematic diagram summarizing the entire lacrimal apparatus. Arrows indicate the direction of tears from the site of production to the site of drainage.

Lacrimal gland

The lacrimal gland measures approximately $20 \times 12 \times 5$ mm and weighs 78 mg. It is divided by the lateral horn of the aponeurosis of the levator palpebrae superioris into a large *orbital* and small *palpebral portion*, which are continuous via a small isthmus around the lateral border of the aponeurosis. The orbital portion is shaped like an almond with a convex outer surface that is lodged in the *lacrimal fossa* (easily felt in a dried skull with the pulp of the little finger – in the superolateral corner just behind the orbital margin; see p. 5 and Fig. 1.41). The concave inferior surface is moulded around the tendons of levator palpebrae superioris and lateral rectus (Fig. 1.56). The palpebral portion of the gland is approximately one-quarter of the total gland and its inferior surface lies close to the eye; indeed the gland can usually be seen when the upper lid is everted. In the orbital portion, fine interlobular ducts unite to form three to five main excretory ducts which then traverse the palpebral portion joining a further five to seven from this part of the gland before entering the superotemporal conjunctival fornix. As a result of this arrangement, removal of the palpebral portion renders the entire gland non-functional.

Histological structure (Fig. 1.57A–C)

The lacrimal gland is a branched tubuloacinar gland of the serous type. It is composed of many lobules separated by interstitial fibrovascular septae that are continuous with the poorly developed capsule. On section, each lobule contains numerous acini separated by abundant loose intralobular connective and adipose tissue. Histologically the acini resemble those of the parotid gland and appear as a series of rounded profiles in cross-section (Fig. 1.57A,B). Each acinus or tubuloacinar unit consists of a single layer of cuboidal or columnar cells whose apices are directed towards a central lumen (Fig. 1.57B–D). A layer of stellate-shaped myoepithelial cells surrounds each acinus. The central lumen of several acini unite to form intralobular ducts (Fig. 1.57A), which eventually form larger interlobular ducts that unite to form the main excretory duct system. The glandular epithelial cells have the characteristic histological and ultrastructural appearance of serous cells, namely basophilic cytoplasm, owing to large numbers of round or oval secretory ('zymogen') granules. The epithelial cells have been subdivided into various subtypes depending on the size and electron density of these granules; however, there is still debate as to whether these are functional subtypes or different stages in the life cycle of one cell type. The presence of true intracellular canaliculi (Fig. 1.57C), as observed in salivary glands, is also still controversial. The secretion of the gland is primarily proteinaceous, although some have shown that many of the granules contain mucopolysaccharides. The secretion also contains lysozymes, lactoferrin, B-lysin and immunoglobulin A (IgA), which are important in defence of the ocular surface against microbial infection (see p. 201). The IgA is derived from numerous plasma cells, present along with other immunocompetent cells such as lymphocytes and mast cells, in the intralobular connective tissue (Fig. 1.57B). The numbers of these cells increase with age concomitant with increased fibrosis and fatty infiltration and a decrease in the acinar elements especially in the orbital lobe (Obata et al., 1995).

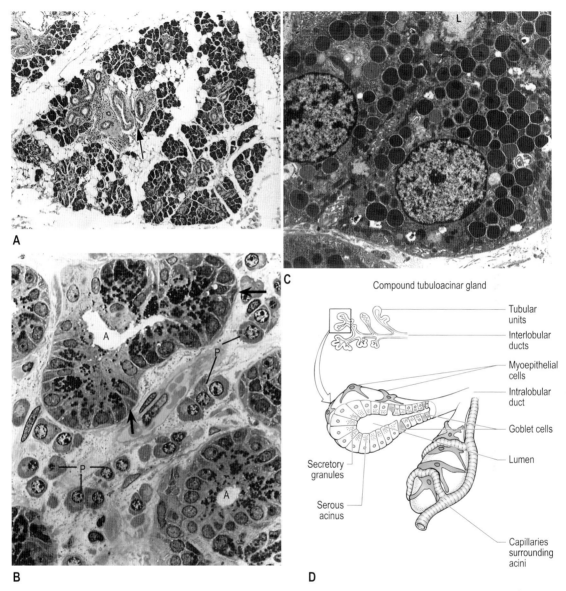

Fig. 1.57 Histology of the lacrimal gland. (**A**) Low-power micrograph of an entire lobule containing a series of large intralobular ducts (arrow). (**B**) Semi-thin section illustrating the arrangement of the glandular epithelial cells, containing numerous secretory granules, in acinar units (A). The vascular intralobular connective tissue is extremely rich in mature plasma cells (P). Arrows, myoepithelial cells. (**C**) Electron micrograph revealing the ultrastructure of a few pyramidal-shaped acinar cells whose apices are directed toward the central lumen (L). Note the numerous electron-dense zymogenic granules in the apical portion of the cells. An intracellular canaliculus is indicated (arrow): N, nucleus. (**D**) Three-dimensional diagram summarizing the arrangement of the epithelial cells, myoepithelial cells and capillaries in the lacrimal gland. Original magnifications: **A**, × 40, **B**, × 630, **C**, × 4400. (Part B courtesy of W.R. Lee.)

> Lacrimal gland tumours appear to arise from duct epithelial cells rather than acinar cells.

Nerve supply

The nerve supply of the lacrimal gland is summarized in Figure 1.58. The lacrimatory nucleus of the facial nerve lies at the rostral end of the general visceral efferent column of cell bodies in the brainstem, which include the superior and inferior salivatory nuclei. The cells are under the influence of the hypothalamus via descending autonomic pathways, thus explaining the neuronal pathways involved in excess lacrimation, which accompanies various emotional states. Reflex excess lacrimation occurs following irritation of the cornea, conjunctiva and nasal epithelia (afferent pathways in ophthalmic and maxillary divisions of the trigeminal). Interneurones connect the trigeminal sensory nuclei with the lacrimatory nucleus.

The course of secretomotor fibres from their origin in the facial nerve to the lacrimal gland via the pterygopalatine ganglion, rami orbitales, retro-orbital plexus and rami lacrimales has been reviewed recently by Ruskell (2004), who also points out that a previously unknown group of fibres may also arise from the otic ganglion. He also reinforces the point, made many years previously, that the traditional assumption that secretomotor fibres reach the gland via the zygomatic and lacrimal nerves is unlikely.

Blood supply

The lacrimal gland derives its blood supply principally from the lacrimal artery, an early branch of the ophthalmic artery, although a variable branch from the infraorbital artery (originating indirectly from the external carotid) may also aid in its supply. Venous blood drains posteriorly into the ophthalmic veins in the orbit and lymph drains to the preauricular node.

Collecting portion of the lacrimal apparatus (Fig. 1.57)

The collecting system serves to drain normal tears that have not evaporated (normally only a very small quantity) and those produced in times of increased lacrimation. Excess tears are drained from the medial aspect of the conjunctival sac via the canaliculi into the lacrimal sac and nasolacrimal duct, to empty into the inferior meatus of the nasal cavity (Fig. 1.56).

The *puncta* are small openings (visible to the naked eye on the medial margin of each lid) at the summit of small swellings, the *papillae lacrimalis* (see Fig. 1.52). Tears that enter the puncta from the *lacus lacrimalis* during blinking pass into the *lacrimal canaliculi* situated in the upper and lower lid behind the medial palpebral ligament. Each canaliculus is about 10 mm long (0.5 mm in diameter) and has vertical and horizontal components (Fig. 1.56) that may unite to form a common canaliculus before entering the *lacrimal sac*. The canaliculi are lined by stratified squamous non-keratinizing cells. They

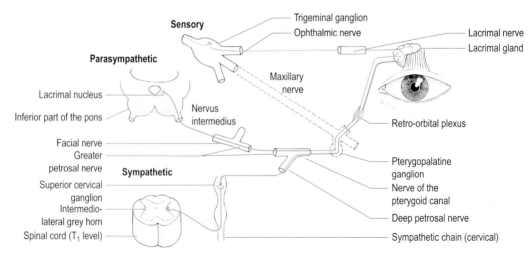

Fig. 1.58 Diagram summarizing the sensory (trigeminal nerve – green), secretomotor (facial nerve – red) and sympathetic (blue) innervation of the lacrimal gland.

enter the lacrimal sac by piercing the fascial covering. This sac is 12 mm long and in its upper portion the walls are usually in apposition. It lies in the lacrimal fossa (see p. 5; Fig. 1.5B), protected by the medial palpebral ligament anteriorly and the lacrimal fibres of orbicularis oculi posteriorly. It is related medially to the ethmoidal air cells and the middle meatus of the nasal cavity. The walls of the lacrimal sac consist of fibroelastic tissue and are lined by a mucous membrane consisting of stratified cuboidal/columnar epithelium containing goblet cells. This epithelium is continuous with that lining the canaliculi and the nasolacrimal duct inferiorly.

The nasoclacrimal duct empties into the anterior part of the inferior meatus of the nasal cavity, the opening being protected by a flap of mucous membrane, which prevents air and debris passing up the duct during nose 'blowing'. The duct lies in a bony nasolacrimal canal formed by the maxilla, the lacrimal bone and the inferior nasal concha. The duct is lined by a stratified columnar ciliated epithelium, which rests upon a vascular substantia propria. Knowledge of the position of a variety of constrictions and mucous membrane folds or 'valves' along the course of the canal is important during reconstruction of congenitally malformed lacrimal drainage systems.

ANATOMY OF THE VISUAL PATHWAY

The visual pathway is made up of the *retina, optic nerves, optic chiasma, optic tracts, lateral geniculate bodies, optic radiations* and *visual cortex* (summarized in Fig. 1.59). There are other areas of the cortex also associated with vision such as the frontal eye fields (see below). The visual pathway is effectively a tract within the central nervous system because the retinae develop as evaginations of the diencephalon (see Ch. 2) and, as discussed above (see p. 62), the optic nerves are covered by layers of meninges; even the corneoscleral envelope and uveal tract of the eye itself can be considered as homologous to the dura mater and pia–arachnoid respectively.

The retina has been described on p. 46. The intraocular, orbital, and intracanalicular portions of the optic nerve were described on p. 61. Description of the visual pathway will commence at the intracranial portion of the optic nerve.

INTRACRANIAL PORTION OF THE OPTIC NERVE (Figs 1.45 and 1.59)

The optic nerves leave the cranial end of the optic canal and pass medially, backwards, and slightly upwards within the subarachnoid space of the middle cranial fossa. They end by forming the optic chiasma in the floor of the third ventricle. Important relations include the olfactory tracts, frontal lobe (gyrus rectus) and the anterior cerebral arteries above. Each internal carotid artery as it emerges from the roof of the cavernous sinus lies lateral to the junction of the optic nerve and chiasma. Below the optic nerves lies the jugum of the sphenoid and the sulcus chiasmatis or optic groove.

OPTIC CHIASMA

The optic chiasma (Figs 1.59 and 1.60) is situated at the junction of the anterior wall and the floor or the third ventricle, approximately 5–10 mm above the diaphragma sella and the hypophysis cerebri. It is a flattened quadrangular bundle of nerves measuring 12×8 mm whose anterolateral angles are continuous with the optic nerves, and its posterolateral angles form the optic tracts. It usually lies just behind the optic groove or sulcus chiasmatis, but may rarely lie partly within the sulcus. The tuber cinereum (a sheet of grey matter that forms a median eminence around the base of the pituitary stalk or infundibulum) lies behind and below the chiasma between the mamillary bodies. The anterior perforated substance is an important lateral relation. The anterior communicating artery passes between the two anterior cerebral arteries, and lies above the chiasma. The partial crossing of optic nerve fibres in the optic chiasma is an essential requirement for binocular vision. The fibres from the nasal hemiretina of each eye cross the midline to enter the contralateral optic tract after taking a short loop in the ipsilateral tract or into the contralateral optic nerve. Nerve fibres from the temporal hemiretina do not cross at the chiasma (Fig. 1.59).

OPTIC TRACTS

The optic tracts (Figs 1.59 and 1.60) wind round the cerebral peduncles of the rostral midbrain and each divides into a large *lateral root*, which terminates posteriorly in the lateral geniculate body and is concerned with conscious visual sensation, and a smaller *medial root*. The medial root is connected both to the *pretectal area* and *superior colliculus* by the superior brachium and carries around 10% of tract fibres,

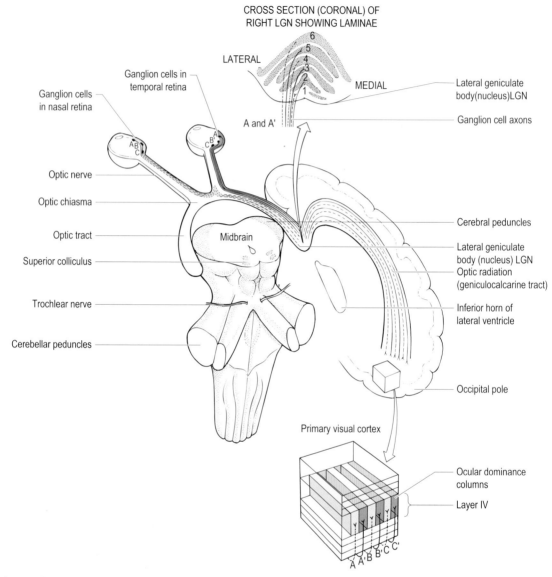

CROSS SECTION (CORONAL) OF
RIGHT LGN SHOWING LAMINAE

6
5
4
3
2
1

LATERAL

MEDIAL

Ganglion cells in
temporal retina

Ganglion cells
in nasal retina

A and A'

Lateral geniculate
body(nucleus)LGN

Ganglion cell axons

Optic nerve

Optic chiasma

Optic tract

Superior colliculus

Midbrain

Cerebral peduncles

Lateral geniculate
body (nucleus) LGN
Optic radiation
(geniculocalcarine tract)

Trochlear nerve

Inferior horn of
lateral ventricle

Cerebellar peduncles

Occipital pole

Primary visual cortex

Ocular dominance
columns

Layer IV

Fig. 1.59 Diagram summarizing the visual pathways. The manner of retinotopic projection to the lateral geniculate nucleus (LGN) and the ocular dominance columns in the primary visual cortex from left and right eyes are illustrated by three imaginary points or images (A, B, C) from the left visual field (not shown) falling on the right half of each retina (A, B, C in left eye and A', B', C' in right eye).

which functionally are not concerned with conscious vision. They contain six groups of fibres, three of which target the superior colliculus (involved in the visual grasp reflex, automatic scanning of images and visual association pathways); the remaining three enter either the pretectal nucleus (serve the pupillary light reflex), the parvocellular reticular formation (arousal function), or the retinohypothalamic tract, which terminates in the suprachiasmatic nucleus of the hypothalamus (possibly involved in photoperiod regulation and has been invoked to account for the beneficial effect of bright artificial light or sunshine on mood).

The *lateral root of the optic tract* passes backwards, a little upwards, and terminates in the lateral geniculate nucleus (LGN), part of the thalamus (a relay station for ascending sensory information). The

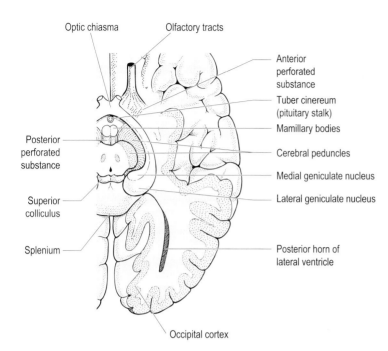

Fig. 1.60 The base of the brain with the brainstem and cerebellum removed to expose the optic nerves, optic chiasma, optic tracts and lateral geniculate nucleus and their relations.

lateral root does not lie completely free because its medial aspect is attached to the outer wall of the third ventricle by a narrow band of tissue. It rotates slightly on its own axis (90° inward twist) as it passes round the cerebral peduncles. It runs above the dorsum sella and crosses the third nerve from medial to lateral. Below and parallel to the optic tract runs the posterior cerebral artery (Figs 1.46 and 1.70). The middle portion of the tract is overlapped by the uncus and parahippocampal gyrus.

> The *superior colliculi* are two small rounded elevations located on the dorsal surface of the midbrain above the inferior colliculi, visible on external examination of the brainstem. The pineal body lies between and above the superior colliculi. The two pairs of colliculi are referred to collectively as the *tectum*. The mesencephalic or tectal termination of optic tract fibres is phylogenetically older than the forebrain termination (visual cortex).

LATERAL GENICULATE BODIES

Each lateral geniculate body (Figs 1.59 and 1.60) is distinguishable on the surface of the brain as an ovoid projection on the posteroinferior aspect of the thalamus, partly obscured by the overhanging temporal lobe (Fig. 1.60). It consists of a body, head, spur and hilum. The hilum is continuous with the groove between the medial and lateral root of the optic tract, which enters its anterior aspect. It lies at the anterior aspect of the pulvinar, which also partly surrounds it, particularly from above. The LGN in which the great majority of the optic tract fibres terminate consists of six laminae or cell layers (numbered 1 to 6 beginning at the hilum), oriented in a dome-shaped mound similar to a stack of hats (Fig. 1.59). On coronal section, the layers of cell nuclei (approximately one million) are separated by white matter (optic tract fibres). Nerve fibres derived from the contralateral eye (crossed fibres from the nasal half of the retina) terminate on cell bodies in layers 1, 4 and 6. Those of the ipsilateral eye (uncrossed) terminate in layers 2, 3 and 5. Thus each LGN receives information from both retinae. Each retinal ganglion cell axon may terminate on up to six geniculate cells; however, these are located in one lamina. Fibres from the upper quadrants of peripheral retinae synapse on the medial aspect of the LGN and those of the lower quadrant on the lateral aspect. The *macula* projects to a disproportionately large central wedge of the LGN. The posterior aspect of the LGN is dome-shaped, and it is from here that the geniculate cell axons that form the optic radiation emerge. The bulk of the LGN sends its fibres

97

via the optic radiation to the visual cortex (area 17). The LGN has input from areas 17, 18, 19, oculomotor centres and the reticular formation.

OPTIC RADIATIONS (GENICULOCALCARINE TRACTS)

These tracts (Fig. 1.59) consist of nerve fibre bundles whose cell bodies lie in the LGN. Their axons terminate in the visual (striate) cortex. The fibres form a wide forward and inferiorly directed fan-shaped loop (of Meyer), firstly into the retrolenticular portion of the internal capsule (posterior to sensory fibres and medial to auditory fibres). The fibres then pass into the temporal lobe around the inferior horn of the lateral ventricle (Fig. 1.61). Each tract then passes posteriorly along the lateral aspect of the posterior horn of the lateral ventricle before turning medially to enter the visual cortex. The optic radiations are of major clinical importance as they are frequently involved in cerebrovascular disturbance or tumours. Not all fibres loop to the same degree (Fig. 1.61). Those destined for the lower half of the visual cortex take a wider sweep into the loop around the tip of the inferior horn of the lateral ventricle than those designed for the upper half of the visual cortex. The fibres that swing furthest into the loop are associated with peripheral retina; those that pass more directly posteriorly originate closer to or within the macula region of the retina.

General comments on cerebral topography

On gross examination of the human brain the surfaces of the two cerebral hemispheres are characterized by conspicuous furrows known as *sulci* separated by raised ridges called *gyri*. The *lateral sulcus* and *central sulcus* together with imaginary lines serve to divide each hemisphere into four lobes (Fig. 1.62A), called frontal, parietal, occipital and temporal after the respective cranial bones to which they are related.

While the primary (area 17) and secondary (areas 18 and 19) visual areas of the cortex are located in the occipital lobe (Fig. 1.62B), other areas of the cerebral cortex outside the occipital lobe are associated with vision, for example the frontal eye field and secondary speech area (of Wernicke) (Fig. 1.62C).

PRIMARY VISUAL CORTEX (AREA 17)

The myelinated fibres of the geniculocalcarine tract (containing fibres from both eyes) enter the primary visual cortex, which lies within the depths of the calcarine sulcus and extends both above and below its margins on the medial surface of the occipital cortex extending as far posteriorly as the occipital pole (Fig. 1.62B) and as far anteriorly as the parieto-occipital sulcus. The area above the fissure is known as the *cuneus gyrus* and below is the *lingual gyrus*.

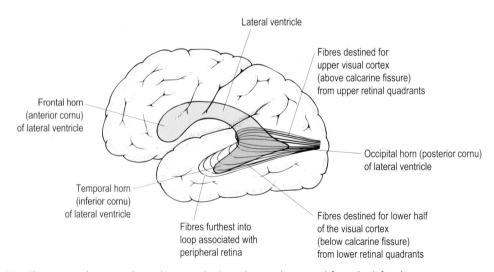

Fig. 1.61 The optic radiation and its relation to the lateral ventricle, viewed from the left side.

LATERAL VIEW

MEDIAL SURFACE

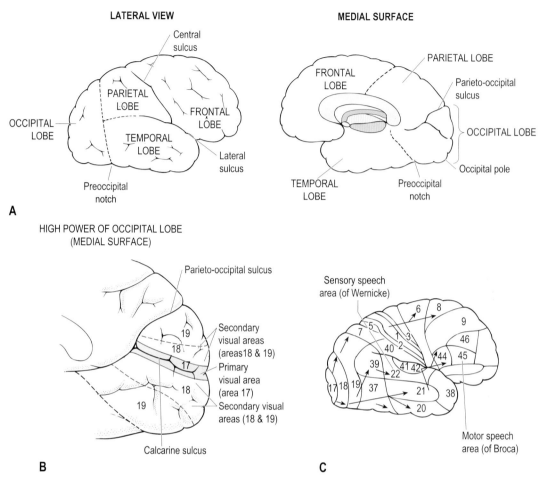

HIGH POWER OF OCCIPITAL LOBE
(MEDIAL SURFACE)

B

C

Fig. 1.62 **(A)** Simplified diagrams showing the boundaries of the lobes of the brain as viewed from the lateral and medial aspects. **(B)** The medial surface of the right occipital lobe indicating the sites of the primary and secondary visual areas. **(C)** The cytoarchitectural areas of the cortex as described by Brodmann. Higher visual projections are from area 17 of the left hemisphere. Those to and from area 20/21 are concerned with detail and colour. Projections to and from area 7 are associated with stereopsis and movement, while those to and from area 39 are concerned with recognition of letters and numbers.

Fibres from the superior retinal quadrants (representing the inferior visual field) pass to the upper lip of the calcarine sulcus. The fibres representing the macula account for one-third of the visual cortex (posterior portion of area 17). The myelinated fibres of the geniculocalcarine tract entering this area of cortex create the conspicuous white line or stria (of Gennari). This represents layer IV in the cortex (Fig. 1.63). The six basic layers of the primary visual cortex are shown in Figure 1.63. This region of cortex, although thinner (1.5 mm), is more cellular than other areas of cortex, the predominant cell type

not being pyramidal but small stellate cells. Alternating *ocular dominance columns* of these cells receive input from right and left eyes (Fig. 1.59). The geniculocalcarine projection is ordered in a manner whereby matching points from the retinae of both eyes are registered side by side in contiguous columns (see Ch. 5 for a discussion of binocular vision, colour vision, etc.). The cells in laminae II and III project to the secondary visual cortex (areas 18 and 19; Fig. 1.62B,C). Those in lamina V project to the superior colliculus, and those of VI to the LGN.

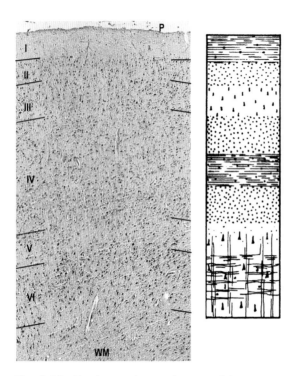

Fig. 1.63 Histology and cytoarchitecture of the primary visual cortex. Layers I–VI are indicated on the micrograph and adjacent diagram: P, pia; WM, white matter. Original magnification: ×35.

SECONDARY VISUAL ASSOCIATION AREAS (AREAS 18 AND 19)

These association areas (Fig. 1.62B,C), which lack the characteristic 'extra' stria found in the primary visual cortex, lie above and below area 17 and extend onto the lateral surfaces of the cerebral hemispheres. They possess the usual six layers, although layer IV is less extensive. Areas 18 and 19 receive afferent input fibres from area 17, the thalamus and pulvinar, together with other regions of the cerebral cortex. The connections of areas 18 and 19 mainly follow dorsal and ventral pathways (Fig. 1.62C). Outputs to area 7 in the parietal cortex are mainly involved in stereopsis and movement. Ventral

outputs to the inferotemporal cortex are concerned with analysis of colour and form, and connections to area 37 are associated with recognition of faces. Area 18 is also likely to be involved in sensory–motor eye coordination, as this is known to be linked to the frontal eye fields and oculomotor nuclei via descending pathways. This area also integrates information from two halves of the visual field via commissural fibres crossing the midline in the splenium of the corpus collosum (Fig. 1.60).

FRONTAL EYE FIELD

This frontal area (Fig. 1.62) corresponds to Brodmann's areas 6, 8 and 9, and is concerned with voluntary control of eye movements (saccades). Fibres pass from here to the superior colliculus, and in turn are connected to the 'extraocular' cranial nerve nuclei (III, IV and VI) and anterior horn cells (motor neurones) in cervical spinal cord segments, thus allowing coordination of head and neck movements with eye movements.

RETINOTOPIC ORGANIZATION OF THE VISUAL PATHWAY AND VISUAL PATHWAY DISTURBANCES
(Figs 1.64–1.70)

A large amount of neurobiological research in primates and non-primates, together with observations of visual dysfunction or abnormalities in human subjects by neuro-ophthalmologists, has led to a considerable body of knowledge regarding the position along the visual pathway of fibres originating from various points on the retina. This information has been crucial to our understanding of the physiology of vision (see Ch. 5), but in addition helps to explain the specific patterns of visual field disturbances following localized lesions in the pathway. Examples of these lesions and the resultant visual field loss are provided in Figures 1.65–1.70.

BLOOD SUPPLY OF THE VISUAL PATHWAY

The blood supply of the visual pathways is summarized in Figure 1.64.

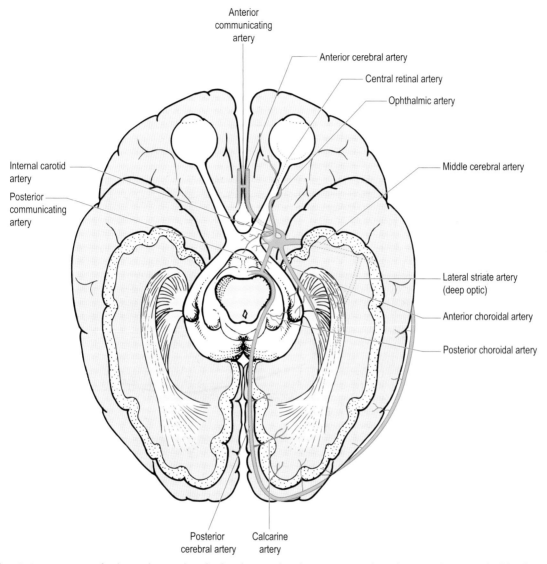

Fig. 1.64 Diagram of a brain dissected to display the visual pathways as seen from the ventral aspect. The blood supply to the various parts of the visual pathways is shown in red on the right-hand side of the diagram (corresponding to the *left side of the brain*). Note the blood supply to the following areas:

- Intracranial optic nerve: ophthalmic artery (an important inferior relation) and pial branches of the hypophyseal artery.
- Optic chiasma: adjacent related vessels including the superior hypophysial, internal carotid, posterior communicating, anterior cerebral and anterior communicating artery.
- Lateral root of the optic tract: anterior choroidal artery.
- Lateral geniculate body: anterior choroidal artery and branches of posterior cerebral artery.
- Commencement of the optic radiation (geniculocalcarine tract): anterior choroidal artery.
- Posteriorly directed fibres: lateral striate (deep optic) branch of the middle cerebral artery.
- Termination of geniculocalcarine tract and visual cortex: perforating branches of cortical arteries, principally the calcarine branch of the posterior cerebral although the middle cerebral may anastomose and aid in the supply of the cortex at the anterior end of the calcarine sulcus and at the posterior pole.

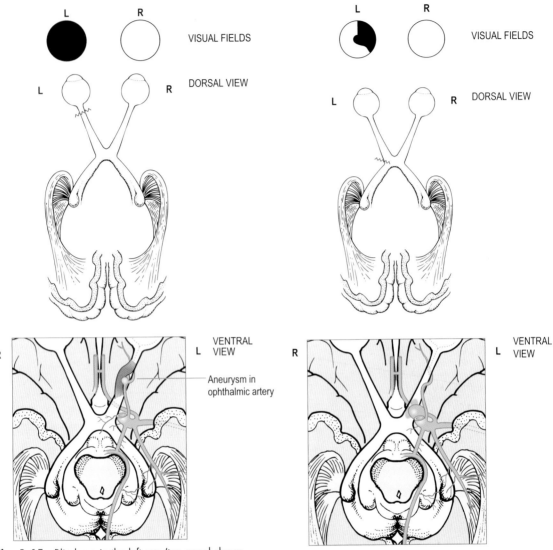

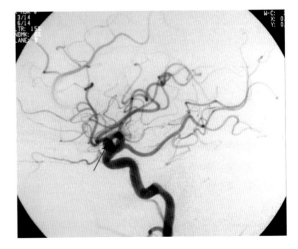

Fig. 1.65 Blindness in the left eye (top panel shows visual field deficit) caused by a lesion in the left optic nerve (middle panel). An example of such a lesion, an aneurysm in the ophthalmic artery, is illustrated (bottom panel: ventral view of the brain).

Fig. 1.66 (see right) Incongruous ipsilateral nasal hemianopia (top panel) caused by a lesion on the left side of the optic chiasma (middle panel). An example of such a lesion is an aneurysm of the terminal portion of the internal carotid artery (bottom panel). The radiographic image shows the digitally subtracted arterial phase of a carotid arteriogram of a 48-year-old patient suffering incongruous ipsilateral nasal hemianopia due to such an aneurysm (arrow). (Radiographic image courtesy of Prof. T. Chakera, Royal Perth Hospital.)

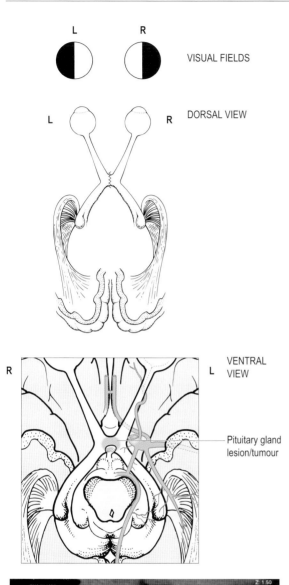

VISUAL FIELDS

DORSAL VIEW

VENTRAL VIEW

Pituitary gland lesion/tumour

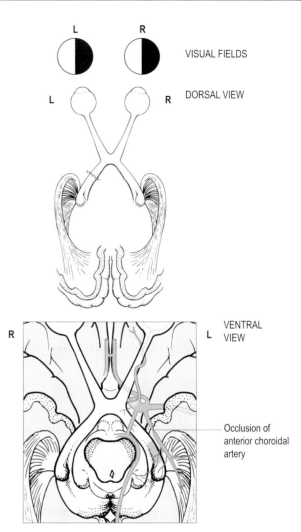

L R

VISUAL FIELDS

DORSAL VIEW

VENTRAL VIEW

Occlusion of anterior choroidal artery

Fig. 1.68 Contralateral homonymous hemianopia (top panel) caused by a lesion in the left optic tract (middle panel). Such a lesion would damage uncrossed fibres from the temporal retina of the left eye and crossed fibres from the nasal retina of the right eye and therefore cause disturbances in the right visual field. Causes of this type of deficit may include vascular disturbances such as occlusion of the anterior choroidal artery (bottom panel).

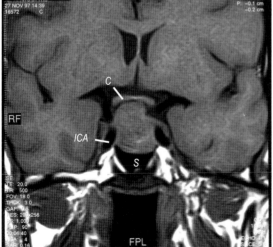

Fig. 1.67 (see left) Contralateral bitemporal homonymous hemianopia (top panel) caused by interruption or damage to the nasal retinal fibres decussating in the optic chiasma (middle panel). A common cause of such deficits is pituitary tumours (bottom panel). Radiograph: coronal MR image of the sellar region in a 31-year-old patient who presented with bitemporal hemianopia. A large pituitary tumour can be seen compressing the optic chiasma (C). S, sphenoid sinus; ICA, internal carotid artery. (Radiographic image courtesy of Prof. T. Chakera, Royal Perth Hospital.)

103

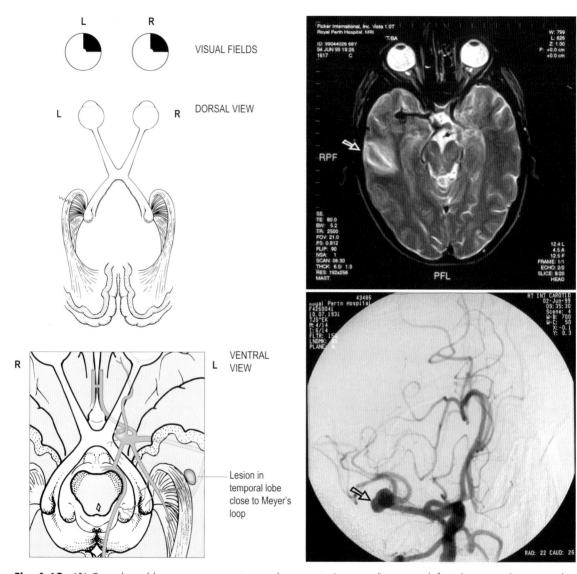

Fig. 1.69 (**A**) Contralateral homonymous superior quadrantanopia (top panel) may result from lesions in the temporal lobe affecting the fibres furthest into the optic radiation (middle panel) (see Fig. 1.61), which are derived from the inferior retinal quadrants and therefore cause deficits in the superior visual field. (**B**) Radiographic image of the brain of a 68-year-old patient with a stroke in the right middle cerebral artery (MCA) territory. Axial MR scan (diffusion weighted) shows the size and limits of the right temporoparietal infarct (arrow). (**C**) The digital subtraction carotid arteriogram (anteroposterior projection) shows the aneurysm (arrowhead) at the bifurcation of the right MCA. The extent of the ischaemic changes in the temporal lobe (involving the optic radiation) are consistent with the patient's loss of the left visual field causing him to bump into objects. (Radiographic images courtesy of Prof. T. Chakera, Royal Perth Hospital.)

L R

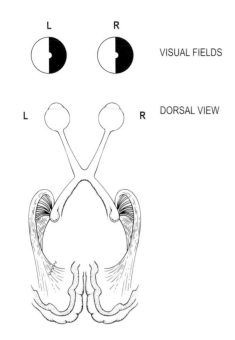

VISUAL FIELDS

DORSAL VIEW

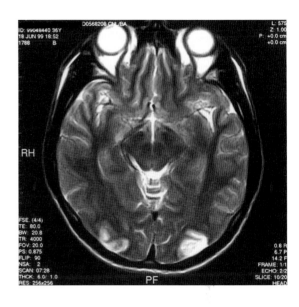

VENTRAL VIEW

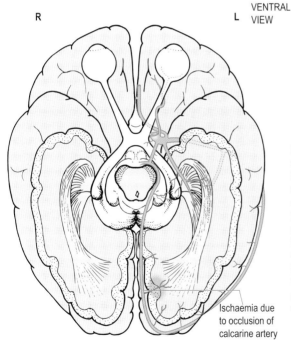

Ischaemia due to occlusion of calcarine artery

Fig. 1.70 Contralateral homonymous hemianopia with macular sparing (top left panel). This may be the result of lesions affecting portions of the occipital cortex, such as tumours or infarcts (bottom panel). Lesions affecting the entire occipital cortex can cause complete blindness. One such case is shown: MR scan of the brain in a 36-year-old intravenous drug user who presented with occipital headaches after injecting speed (amphetamine sulphate) with a dirty needle and waking 2 days later with total blindness and occipital headaches. Early CT scan (not shown) showed no sign of infarction but MR scan and diffusion-weighted imaging (not shown) clearly show bilateral occipital lobe infarcts which would explain the bilateral cortical blindness in this subject. (Radiographic image courtesy of Prof. T. Chakera, Royal Perth Hospital.)

FURTHER READING

Ahnelt P, Kolb H. Horizontal cells and cone photoreceptors in human retina: a Golgi-electron microscopic study of spectral connectivity. J Comp Neurol 1994; 343:406–427.

Ambati J, Anand A, Fernandez S, Sakurai E, Lynn BC, Kuziel WA, Rollins BJ, Ambati BK. An animal model of age-related macular degeneration in senescent Ccl-2- or Ccr-2-deficient mice. Nat Med 2003; 9(11):1390–1397.

Balazs EA. Functional anatomy of the vitreous. In: Jakobiec FA, ed. Ocular anatomy, embryology and teratology. Philadelphia: Harper and Row; 1982:425–440.

Bishop PN. Structural macromolecules and supramolecular organisation of the vitreous gel. Prog Retin Eye Res 2000; 19:323–344.

Bishop PN, Takanosu M, Le Goff M, Mayne R. The role of the posterior ciliary body in the biosynthesis of vitreous humour. Eye 2002; 16(4):454–460.

Butler TL, McMenamin PG. Resident and infiltrating immune cells in the uveal tract in the early and late stages of experimental autoimmune uveoretinitis. Invest Ophthalmol Vis Sci 1996; 37:2195–2210.

Ceelen PW, Lockridge A, Newman EA. Electrical coupling between glial cells in the rat retina. GLIA 2001; 35:1–13.

Chan-Ling T. Glial, neuronal and vascular interactions in the mammalian retina. Prog Ret Eye Res 1994; 13:357–389.

Chinnery HR, Ruitenberg MJ, Plant GW, Pearlman E, Jung S, McMenamin PG. The chemokine receptor CX3CR1 mediates homing of MHC class II-positive cells to the normal mouse corneal epithelium. Invest Ophthalmol Vis Sci 2007; 48:1568–1574.

Christensen AM. Assessing the variation in individual frontal sinus outlines. Am J Phys Anthropol 2004; 127: 291–295.

Dacey DM, Liao HW, Peterson BB, Robinson FR, Smith VC, Pokorny J, Yau KW, Gamlin PD. Melanopsin-expressing ganglion cells in primate retina signal colour and irradiance and project to the LGN. Nature 2005; 17(433):749–754.

Dartt DA. Regulation of mucin and fluid secretion by conjunctival epithelial cells. Prog Ret Eye Res 2002; 21:555–576.

Demer JL. Pivotal role of orbital connective tissue in binocular alignment and strabismus. Invest Ophthalmol Vis Sci 2004; 45:729–738.

Demer JL, Poukens V, Miller JM, Micevych P. Innervation of extraocular pulley smooth muscle in monkeys and humans. Invest Ophthalmol Vis Sci 1997; 38:1774–1785.

Diaz-Araya CM, Provis JM, Penfold PL, Billson FA. Development of microglial topography in human retina. J Comp Neurol 1995; 363:53–68.

Dick AD, Carter D, Robertson M, Broderick C, Hughes E, Forrester JV, Liversidge J. Control of myeloid activity during retinal inflammation. J Leuk Biol 2003; 74(2):161–166.

Eggers HM. Functional anatomy of the extraocular muscles. In Jakobiec FA, ed. Ocular anatomy, embryology and teratology. Philadelphia: Harper and Row; 1982:783–834.

Eisner G. Clinical anatomy of the vitreous. In Jakobiec FA, ed. Ocular anatomy, embryology and teratology. Philadelphia: Harper and Row; 1982:391–424.

Ertrurk M, Kayalioglu G, Govsa F, Varol T, Ozgur T. The cranio-orbital foramen, the groove on the lateral wall of the human orbit, and the orbital branch of the middle meningeal artery. Clin Anat 2005; 18:10–14

Fitzgerald MJF. Neuroanatomy. Basic and clinical, 2nd edn. London: Baillière Tindall; 1992.

Forrester JV. Macrophages eyed in macular degeneration. Nat Med 2003; 9:1350–1351.

Gausas RE. Advances in applied anatomy of the eyelid and orbit. Curr Opin Ophthalmol 2004; 15:422–425.

Gebert A, Pabst R. M cells at locations outside the gut. Semin Immunol 1999; 11:165–170.

Guymer RH, Bird A, Hageman G. Cytoarchitecture of choroid capillary endothelial cells. Invest Ophthalmol Vis Sci 2005; 45:1660–1666.

Halfter W, Dong S, Schurer B, Ring C, Cole GJ, Eller A. Embryonic synthesis of the inner limiting membrane and vitreous body. Invest Ophthalmol Vis Sci 2005; 46(6):2202–2209.

Hamrah P, Zhang Q, Liu Y, Dana MR. Novel characterization of MHC class II-negative population of resident corneal Langerhans cell-type dendritic cells. Invest Ophthalmol Vis Sci 2002; 43:639–646.

Hingorani M, Metz D, Lightman SL. Characterisation of the normal conjunctival leukocyte population. Exp Eye Res 1997; 64:905–912.

Ihanamaki T, Pelliniemi LJ, Vuorio E. Collagens and collagen-related matrix components in the human and mouse eye. Prog Ret Eye Res 2004; 23:403–434.

Jakobiec FA. Ocular anatomy, embryology and teratology. Philadelphia: Harper and Row; 1982.

Kabil MS, Eby JB, Shahinian HK. Endoscopic vascular decompression versus microvascular decompression of the trigeminal nerve. Minimally Invasive Neurosurgery 2005; 48(4):207–212.

Knop E, Knop N. The role of eye-associated lymphoid tissue in corneal immune protection. J Anat 2005; 206: 271–285.

Kolb H, Linberg KA, Fisher SK. Neurons of the human retina: a Golgi study. J Comp Neurol 1992; 31:147–187.

Kolb H, Fernandez E, Schouten J, Ahnelt P, Linberg KA and Fisher SK. Are there three types of horizontal cell in the human retina? J Comp Neurol 1992; 343: 370–386.

Koornneef L. Orbital connective tissue. In: Jakobiec FA, ed. Ocular anatomy, embryology and teratology. Philadelphia: Harper and Row.1982:835–857.

Last RJ. Wolff's anatomy of the eye and orbit. London: Lewis; 1968.

Lockwood C. The anatomy of the muscles, ligaments, fascia of the orbit etc. J Anat Physiol 1886; 20:1.

Lütjen-Drecoll E. Functional morphology of the trabecular meshwork in primate eyes. Prog Retin Eye Res 1998; 18:91–119.

Mariani AP. Amacrine cells of the rhesus monkey retina. J Comp Neurol 1990; 301:382–400.

May CA. Non-vascular smooth muscle cells in the human choroid: distribution, development and further characterization. J Anat 2005; 207:381–390.

May CA, Neuhuber W, Lutjen-Drecoll E. Immunohistochemical classification and functional morphology of human choroidal ganglion cells. Invest Ophthalmol Vis Sci 2004; 45:361–367.

McClung JR, Allman BL, Dimitrova DM, Goldberg SJ. Extraocular connective tissues: a role in human eye movements? Invest Ophthalmol Vis Sci 2006; 47:202–205.

McMenamin PG, Lee WR, Aitken DAN. Age-related changes in the human outflow apparatus. Ophthalmology 1986; 93: 194–208.

McMenamin PG, Forrester JV. Dendritic cells in the central nervous system and eye and their associated supporting tissues. In Lotze MT, Thomson AW, eds. Dendritic cells: biology and applications. San Diego: Academic Press; 1999:205–248.

Muller LJ, Pels L, Vrensen FJM. Novel aspects of the organisation of human corneal keratocytes. Invest Ophthalmol Vis Sci 1995; 36:2557–2567.

Muller LJ, Marfurt CF, Kruse F, Tervo TMT. Corneal nerves: structure, contents and function. Exp Eye Res 2003; 76:521–542.

Nimmerjahn A, Kirchhoff F, Helmchen F. Resting microglial cells are highly dynamic surveillants of brain parenchyma in vivo. Science 2005; 308(5726):1314–1318.

Obata H, Yamamoto S, Horiuchi H, Machinami R. Histopathologic study of human lacrimal gland. Ophthalmology 1995; 102:678–686.

Penfold PL, Madigan MC, Provis JM. Antibodies to human leucocyte antigens indicate subpopulations of microglia in human retina. Vis Neurosci 1991; 7:383–388.

Qiao H, Hisatomi T, Sonoda KH, Kura S, Sassa Y, Kinoshita S, Nakamura T, Sakamoto T, Ishibashi T. The characterisation of hyalocytes: the origin, phenotype, and turnover. Br J Ophthalmol 2005; 89(4):513–517.

Rada JA, Shelton S, Norton TT. The sclera and myopia. Exp Eye Res 2006; 82:185–200.

Raviola G. The structural basis of the blood–ocular barriers. Exp Eye Res (suppl.) 1977; 25:27–63.

Robinson S, Dreher Z. Müller cells in the adult rabbit retinae: morphology, distribution and implications for function and development. J Comp Neurol 1990; 292:178–192.

Rohen J. Ciliarkörper. In: von Möllendoff W, ed. Das Auge und seine Hilfsorgane. Ergänzung zu Band 111/2. Haut und Sinnesorgane. 4 Teil. Handbuch der mikroskopischen Anatomie des Menschen. Berlin: Springer; 1964:189–238.

Rowe MH. Functional organisation of the retina. In: Dreker B, Robinson SR, eds. Neuroanatomy of the visual pathways and their development. Vision and visual dysfunction (Cronly-Dillon J, general ed.), Vol. 3. Basingstoke: Macmillan UK; 1991:1–68.

Rowland LP. Blood–brain barrier, cerebrospinal fluid, brain edema, and hydrocephalus. In: Kandel ER, Schwartz JH, eds. Principles of neuroscience. New York: Elsevier; 1985:837–844.

Ruskell GL. Facial parasympathetic innervation of the choroidal blood vessels in the monkey. Exp Eye Res 1971a; 12:166–172.

Ruskell GL. The distribution of autonomic postganglionic nerve fibres to the lacrimal gland in monkeys. J Anat 1971b; 109:229–242.

Ruskell GL. Distribution of pterygopalatine ganglion efferents to the lacrimal gland in man. Exp Eye Res 2004; 78:329–335.

Ruskell GL, Kjellevold Haugen IB, Bruenech JR, van der Werf F. Double insertions of extraocular rectus muscles in humans and the pulley theory. J Anat 2005; 206:295–306.

Sebag J. Seeing the invisible: the challenge of imaging vitreous. J Biomed Optics 2004; 9(1):38–46.

Snell RS, Lemp MA. Clinical Anatomy of the Eye. Boston: Blackwell Scientific; 1989.

Stewart PA, Tuor UI. Blood–eye barriers in the rat: correlation of ultrastructure with function. J Comp Neurol 1994; 340:566–576.

Stiemke MM, Watsky MA, Kangas TA, Edelhauser HF. The establishment and maintenance of corneal transparency. Prog Ret Eye Res 1995; 14(1):109–140.

Summers Rada JA, Shelton S, Norton TT. The sclera and myopia. Exp Eye Res epub (in press)

Thale A, Tillman B. The collagen architecture of the sclera: SEM and immunohistochemical studies. Ann Anat 1993; 175:215–220.

Thermos K. Functional mapping of somatostatin receptors in the retina: a review. Vision Res 2003; 43(17):1805–1815.

Van Buskirk EM. The anatomy of the limbus. Eye 1989; 3:101–108.

Waring GO, Bourne WM, Edelhaauser HF, Kenyon KR. The corneal endothelium. Normal and pathologic structure and function. Ophthalmology 1982; 89:531–590.

Watson PG, Young RD. Scleral structure, organisation and disease. A review. Exp Eye Res 2004; 78:609–623.

Williams PL, Warwick R. Gray's Anatomy, 36th edn. Edinburgh: Churchill Livingstone; 1980.

Wotherspoon AC, Hardman-Lea S, Isaccson PG. Mucosa-associated lymphoid tissue (MALT) in the human conjunctiva. J Pathol 1994; 174:33–37.

Yemelyanov AY, Katz NB, Bernstein PS. Ligand-binding characterization of xanthophyll carotenoids to solubilized membrane proteins derived from human retina. Exp Eye Res 2001; 72(4):381–392.

Young RW. The renewal of photoreceptor cell outer segments. J Cell Biol 1967; 33:61–72.

Zhang HR. Scanning electron-microscopic study of corrosion casts on retinal and choroidal angioarchitecture in man and animals. Prog Ret Eye Res 1994; 13:243–270.

Zhivov A, Stave J, Vollmar B, Guthoff R. In vivo confocal microscopic evaluation of Langerhans cell density and distribution in the normal human corneal epithelium. Graefes Arch Clin Exp Ophthalmol 2005; 243(10):1056–1061.

2 EMBRYOLOGY AND EARLY DEVELOPMENT OF THE EYE AND ADNEXA

INTRODUCTION

This chapter aims to provide an embryological basis for understanding the anatomy of the eye and adnexa. Basic embryological events from the earliest formation of diverticula in the forebrain at the beginning of the fourth week to the maturation of the various components of the eye late in development are described. The contribution of the neural ectoderm or neuroepithelium, surface ectoderm, mesoderm, and neural crest to the final configuration of the adult eye and surrounding tissues of the head is emphasized. Disturbances in these embryological events and the interactive processes between the various embryonic tissue and cell types are the basis of congenital abnormalities, of which some examples are given. New data on the genetic basis for embryological events are briefly described.

GENERAL EMBRYOLOGY

Before considering eye development, which commences in the fourth week, it may be useful for some readers to review the embryological events of the first 3 weeks following fertilization (Fig. 2.1).

The male and female *gametes* unite at fertilization, which generally occurs within the oviduct or uterine tube, to form the *zygote*. The newly formed diploid cell undergoes *cleavage* as it travels towards the uterus. Within the solid mass of cells (30-cell stage) or *morula*, the *blastocyst cavity* appears. The earliest *differentiation* of the embryo occurs around this stage

109

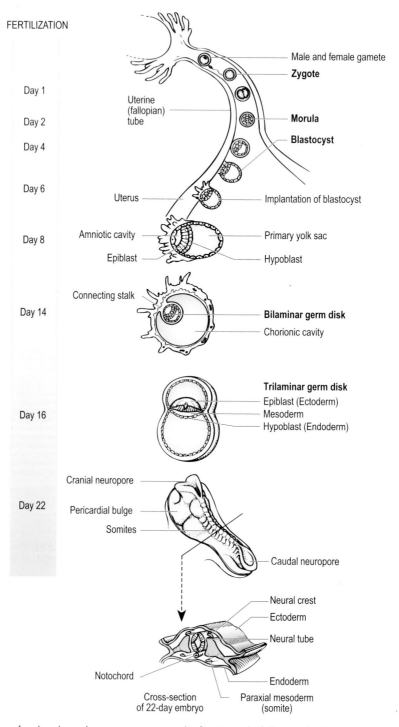

FERTILIZATION

Day 1

Day 2

Day 4

Day 6

Day 8

Day 14

Day 16

Day 22

Male and female gamete

Zygote

Uterine (fallopian) tube

Morula

Blastocyst

Uterus

Implantation of blastocyst

Amniotic cavity

Primary yolk sac

Epiblast

Hypoblast

Connecting stalk

Bilaminar germ disk

Chorionic cavity

Trilaminar germ disk
Epiblast (Ectoderm)
Mesoderm
Hypoblast (Endoderm)

Cranial neuropore

Pericardial bulge

Somites

Caudal neuropore

Neural crest
Ectoderm
Neural tube

Notochord

Endoderm

Cross-section of 22-day embryo

Paraxial mesoderm (somite)

Fig. 2.1 Summary of embryological events occurring in the first 3 weeks following fertilization.

when two groups of cells are formed: a peripheral *outer cell mass* or trophoblast and a central *inner cell mass* or embryoblast. The *embryoblast* will give rise to the embryo proper and some of its attached membranes. By day 5 or 6 the embryo is a hollow spheroid of around 100 cells, known as the *blastocyst*. The *embryoblast* is evident as a heterogeneous collection of cells at one pole of the blastocyst; the remainder forms the *trophoblast*. This differentiates into the syncytiotrophoblast and the cytotrophoblast, which contribute to the fetal component of the placenta. Around this time the blastocyst enters the uterus and commences implantation into its rich endometrial lining.

At the beginning of the second week two cavities appear within the embryoblast. One forms the *amniotic cavity*, lined by epiblast cells, while the other forms the *yolk sac*, lined by cells derived from the hypoblast. Where the two cavities impinge there is a double discoid layer of cells, the *epiblast* or *primary ectoderm* and the *hypoblast* or *primary endoderm*. These two flat disks of cells constitute the *bilaminar germ disk*, which will develop into the embryo proper.

The third week of development commences with formation of the *primitive streak* and *primitive knot* or node at the caudal (tail) end of the epiblast. It is here that epiblast cells detach and migrate laterally and cranially into the potential space between the epiblast and the hypoblast to form the *intraembryonic mesoderm* or third germ layer. Some of the epiblast cells also replace the original hypoblast to form the *definitive* or *secondary hypoblast*. The epiblast is now known as the *ectoderm*. Formation of the primitive streak establishes the craniocaudal axis and bilateral symmetry of the future embryo. The formation of the *notochord* by budding from the primitive knot induces the formation of the *neural plate*. A series of *paraxial mesodermal* condensations or *somites* form along each side of the neural plate as it folds to form the *neural tube*, the precursor of the central nervous system. A special group of cells, the *neural crest* cells, detach or delaminate from the margins of the neural folds and undergo extensive migration throughout the embryo where they differentiate into a remarkable variety of cells and tissues (Fig. 2.2). Derivatives of trunk neural crest cells are shown in Fig 2.2. Derivatives in the head are more extensive (see p. 118).

Anatomically, the human embryo is described as being in the prone (face-down) position. The terms dorsal and ventral correspond to posterior and

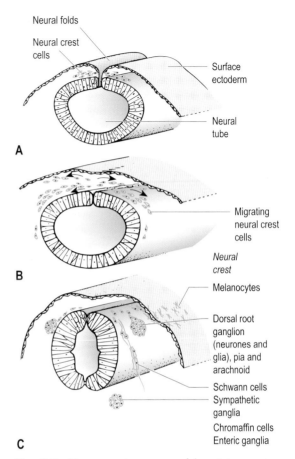

Fig. 2.2 Diagrammatic summary of the origin (**A**), migratory pathway (**B**), and derivatives (**C**) of neural crest cells in the trunk.

anterior in the adult. The terms rostral and caudal correspond to superior (head end) and inferior (tail end).

OCULAR EMBRYOLOGY: GENERAL INTRODUCTION

Eye development can be considered to commence around day 22 when the embryo has eight pairs of somites and is around 2 mm in length. The neural folds have commenced fusion to form the neural tube but before they have completed their closure rostrally and caudally the *optic sulci* (optic primordium) appear as shallow grooves or pits in the inner aspect of the neural plate or neural folds (Fig. 2.3A). The folds in this area fuse shortly afterwards and give rise to the future *diencephalon* region of the

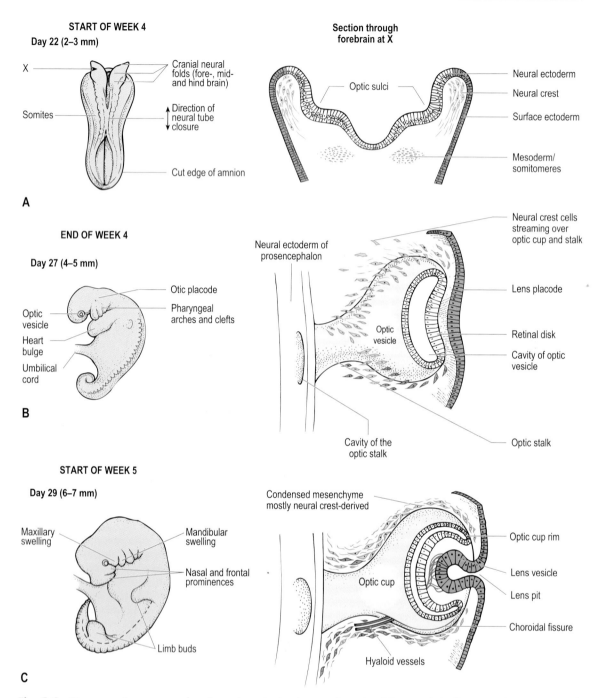

START OF WEEK 4

Day 22 (2–3 mm)

X — Cranial neural folds (fore-, mid- and hind brain)

Somites —

↕ Direction of neural tube closure

Cut edge of amnion

A

Section through forebrain at X

Optic sulci

Neural ectoderm

Neural crest

Surface ectoderm

Mesoderm/ somitomeres

END OF WEEK 4

Day 27 (4–5 mm)

Otic placode

Optic vesicle

Pharyngeal arches and clefts

Heart bulge

Umbilical cord

B

Neural ectoderm of prosencephalon

Neural crest cells streaming over optic cup and stalk

Lens placode

Optic vesicle

Retinal disk

Cavity of optic vesicle

Cavity of the optic stalk

Optic stalk

START OF WEEK 5

Day 29 (6–7 mm)

Maxillary swelling

Mandibular swelling

Nasal and frontal prominences

Limb buds

C

Condensed mesenchyme mostly neural crest-derived

Optic cup rim

Optic cup

Lens vesicle

Lens pit

Choroidal fissure

Hyaloid vessels

Fig. 2.3 Diagrammatic summary of ocular embryonic development from day 22 to week 8. The external appearance of the whole embryo at the equivalent period is shown on the left. The various 'germ layers' are colour-coded to illustrate their origin and final contribution to the eye and periocular tissues.

START OF WEEK 6

Day 37 (8–11 mm)

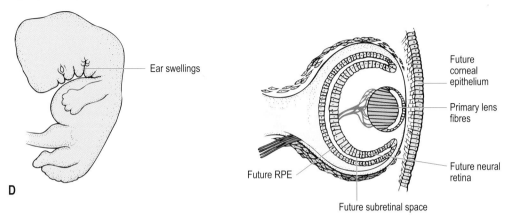

Ear swellings

Future corneal epithelium

Primary lens fibres

Future neural retina

Future RPE

Future subretinal space

D

START OF WEEK 7

Day 44 (13–17 mm)

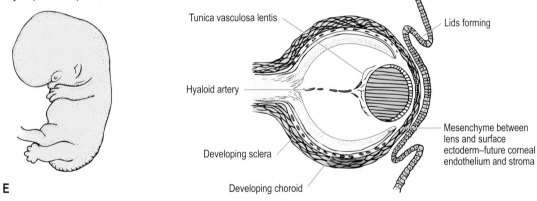

Tunica vasculosa lentis

Lids forming

Hyaloid artery

Mesenchyme between lens and surface ectoderm–future corneal endothelium and stroma

Developing sclera

Developing choroid

E

WEEK 8 (20–30 mm)

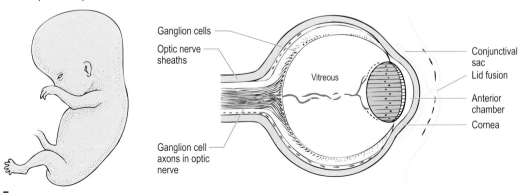

Ganglion cells

Optic nerve sheaths

Vitreous

Conjunctival sac

Lid fusion

Anterior chamber

Cornea

Ganglion cell axons in optic nerve

F

Fig. 2.3 *Continued*

prosencephalic (forebrain) vesicle. The optic sulci evaginate to form hollow diverticulae – the *optic vesicles* (Fig. 2.3B).

By about day 25 (20-somite stage) the hollow optic vesicles enlarge and become ensheathed by mesenchymal cells, except at the apex of the vesicle, which is closely apposed between the *surface ectoderm* on the lateral aspect of the developing head. This mesenchyme may be derived from cephalic neural crest and indeed from crest cells detaching from the outer surface of the optic vesicle itself (see below for full discussion).

Mesenchyme

This is a term used to describe the tissue occupying the embryo between the surface ectoderm (and derivatives such as neuroectoderm) and the endoderm-derived epithelial layers. It is a loose tissue consisting of stellate, amoeboid mesenchymal cells embedded in a matrix rich in glycosaminoglycans. Mesenchymal cells may be derived from several sources, namely mesoderm (dermatome or sclerotome component of the somites or lateral plate mesoderm) or neural crest. Thus this descriptive term 'mesenchyme' does not imply an origin from any particular embryonic germ layer.

A disk-shaped thickening of the neural ectoderm, the *retinal disk* (future neural retina), lies beneath a localized thickening of the surface ectoderm, which on day 27 is recognizable as the *lens placode* (Fig. 2.3B). Formation of the lens placode directly adjacent to the underlying neural ectoderm was considered, until recently, as one of the best examples of *induction* in developmental biology. However, experimental data (Saha et al., 1989; Sullivan et al., 2004) suggest lens placode formation may be the result of a complex series of interactions with other tissues including foregut endoderm, neuroectoderm and heart mesoderm.

Lens placode formation coincides with the formation of a constriction in the optic vesicle at its attachment to the wall of the forebrain to form the *optic stalk*. The *cavity of the optic vesicle* or *optic ventricle* (future subretinal space) is continuous, via the lumen in the optic stalk, with the future third ventricle (Figs 2.3B and 2.4A).

The single-layered spheroidal *optic vesicle* undergoes active invagination to become a goblet-shaped *optic cup*. The thickened retinal disk at the tip of the vesicle (Fig. 2.3B,C) and the ectoderm-derived lens

placode invaginate via a combination of differential growth (cell elongation and mitosis) and buckling to form the dorsal hemisphere of the optic cup and the lens vesicle. This combined invagination may also be aided by temporary fine cellular bridges between the lens placode and the retinal disk. The active growth of the optic cup is not uniform around the circumference, which leads to the development of a groove at the distal and ventral aspect where the margins form the *choroidal* or *optic fissure*. By day 29 invagination of the retinal disk and lens placode is almost complete (Figs 2.3C and 2.4A). A small *lens pit* can be identified just before the surface ectoderm seals over the site of lens placode invagination. By the start of day 36 the *lens vesicle* separates from the surface ectoderm. The lens epithelial cells enclose the *lens cavity* and are surrounded externally by a basal lamina which will form the future *lens capsule*. The longitudinal groove of the optic fissure which extends into the optic stalk, acts as a temporary deficiency in the expanding and invaginating cup through which vascular mesenchyme and a branch of the ophthalmic artery, the *hyaloid artery*, become incorporated into the fissure and thus gain access to the lentoretinal space. By the end of the sixth week the growing edges of the choroidal or optic fissure meet and fuse; thus the hyaloid vessels and associated mesenchyme become situated in the centre of the optic stalk and form the future central retinal artery and vein (Fig. 2.3D, E). The fusion or closure of the optic fissure commences at the mid-portion of the optic stalk and continues both proximally and distally. It is completed distally at the margins of the optic cup that will eventually form the pupil.

Coloboma

The word coloboma simply means 'a mutilation', but in clinical practice the term is used to describe a defect in the inferonasal quadrant in the iris, ciliary body or choroid. Colobomas are usually sporadic and bilateral and do not lead to significant complications. They are the result of a failure of closure of the (inferonasal) optic fissure. The consequence is an interference with the normal induction and formation of uveal tissues.

- A coloboma of the iris appears as an *inferonasal defect* in the stroma, the smooth muscle and the pigment epithelium.
- A ciliary body coloboma is characterized by absence of ciliary processes and presence of a diminutive muscle. The adjacent lens is indented, owing to a failure of formation of the zonular fibres.

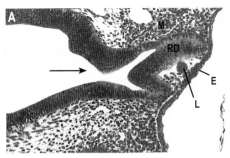

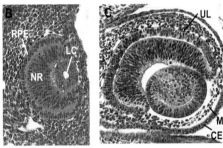

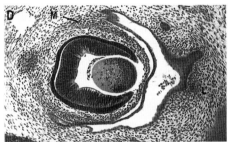

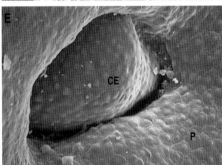

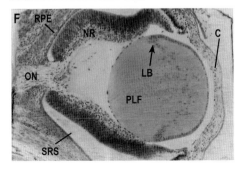

- In the colobomas associated with complex malformations and abnormalities (e.g. trisomy) there may be an ingrowth of mesodermal tissue into the retrolental space with formation of fat and cartilage.
- Colobomas involving the retina may be large and may extend to the disk. In the retina adjacent to the coloboma, proliferation of neuroblastic tissue leads to the formation of rosettes. The absence of induction by the retinal pigment epithelium in the region of the coloboma means that there is an absence of Bruch's membrane and choroidal tissue, although the underlying sclera is normal. In many cases of retinal coloboma there is glial and vascular ingrowth from the retina across the bed of the coloboma. Colobomas have been described in association with mutations in the *CHD7* gene (see Table 2.1).

In the CHARGE syndrome (*Coloboma, Heart disease, Atresia choanae, Retardation of growth and/or development; Genital hypoplasia, Ear malformation) the coloboma is posterior and inferonasal.

Fig. 2.4 Histological and scanning electron micrographs of early mammalian eye development (chronological sequence A–F). (**A**) The cavity of the optic vesicle is clearly in continuity via the cavity of the optic stalk with the forebrain ventricle (arrow) M, mesenchyme condensation; E, surface ectoderm/periderm; L, lens vesicle; RD retinal disk. (**B**) The lens vesicle, containing a distinct lens cavity (LC), fills the optic cup, which consists of two layers, an outer retinal pigment epithelium (RPE) and neural retina (NR). (**C**) Mesenchyme has condensed around the optic cup and migrated over the cup margin to form the future corneal endothelium/stroma (M) beneath the surface ectoderm-derived corneal epithelium (CE). Beneath the RPE the vascular mesenchyme has already formed a distinct row of vessels, the uveocapillary lamina (UL) or presumptive choroid. (**D**) Pigment is identifiable in the RPE layer. The lentoretinal space contains vascular mesenchyme. The mesenchyme (M) around the developing eye has now formed two layers, an outer dense avascular layer (future sclera) and an inner vascular layer (future choroid). Beneath the newly formed lids (L) lies the conjunctival sac. (**E**) Scanning electron micrograph of the embryonic corneal epithelial surface (CE) and periderm (P) just before lid closure. (**F**) Late embryonic eye with well-developed cornea (C), large lens consisting of primary lens fibres (PLF) whose nuclei form the lens bow (LB). The neural retina (NR) is artefactually detached from the RPE, producing a large subretinal space (SRS). Axons have commenced migration along the optic nerve (ON). (From McMenamin and Krause, 1993, with permission.) Original magnifications: (**A**) × 120; (**B**) × 180; (**C**) × 160; (**D**) × 55; (**E**) × 100; (**F**) × 65. (From McMenamin and Krause 1993, with permission.)

Following separation of the lens vesicle from the surface ectoderm this layer regenerates and forms the future corneal epithelium (Fig. 2.4E). Around this time (day 39) a 'wave' of mesenchyme passes over the rim of the optic cup, directly beneath the surface ectoderm (Figs 2.3D,E and 2.4C,D). The cells in the first of the three waves of mesenchyme, which lie posteriorly closest to the lens, become flattened and form apicolateral contacts. These contacts become continuous bands of junctional complexes and thus form an endothelium. The other waves of mesenchyme will form much of the cornea (except the epithelium), iris stroma and iridocorneal angle mesenchyme (Cvekl and Tamm, 2004; Creuzet et al., 2005).

By the end of the embryonic period (defined as the end of week 8) the retina can be clearly differentiated into a thin outer layer, which will form the *retinal pigment epithelium* (RPE) and a much thicker inner *neural retina* (Figs 2.3F and 2.4F). These two layers are separated by a narrow *intraretinal or subretinal space*, the remains of the almost obliterated ventricular cavity of the optic vesicle. Melanin first appears in the RPE around 5 weeks (Fig. 2.4C,D) and is visible on external examination of embryos of this gestational age. The neural retina commences its centrifugal differentiation into an *inner* and *outer neuroblastic layer* near its continuity with the optic stalk. The lens cavity disappears as the posterior cells elongate to form the *primary lens fibres* (Fig. 2.3D and 2.4D). Mesenchyme, mostly derived from neural crest cells, condenses around the external surface of the optic cup. The innermost layer of this mesenchyme is loose and highly vascular and will form the *choroid* (uveocapillary lamina) (Fig. 2.4C,D). It lies adjacent to a distinct basement membrane formed by the RPE, which is continuous with a similar membrane around the forebrain. Indeed, the choroid is homologous in its embryonic origin with the *pia mater* and *arachnoid* investing the brain. A series of genes regulate the molecular events that control migration and differentiation of ocular neural crest cells (Table 2.1); however, the molecular mechanisms remain unclear (Cvekl and Tamm, 2004).

The outer layer of the condensed mesenchyme will form the *sclera*, which is homologous to, and indeed continuous with, the dura mater around the optic nerve and brain posteriorly.

In the eighth and last week of the embryonic period (Figs 2.3F and 2.4F), ganglion cell axons grow from the inner retina towards the optic stalk. The axons travel within the stalk towards the brain, thus forming the optic nerve. Other major landmarks in development occurring in the eighth week include formation of secondary lens fibres, lens sutures and the secondary vitreous (see pp. 127 and 129).

In summary, by the end of the embryonic period the eye comprises a double-layered neural ectoderm-derived optic cup containing a surface ectoderm-derived lens, both enveloped by condensed mesenchyme comprising a dense outer layer (the bulk of the future cornea and sclera) and an inner vascular layer which will form the choroid and stroma of the iris and ciliary body. At this stage the human embryo is 30 mm in length (crown–rump length) and the developing eye is 1.5–2.0 mm in diameter (Figs 2.3F and 2.4F).

Malformations of the neural tube and optic vesicle

These occur in the first month of embryonic life and include:

- *Anophthalmia* Extremely rare and the result of a failure of formation of the optic vesicle. The orbits do not contain ocular tissue, but the extraocular muscles (mesoderm) and lacrimal gland (ectoderm) are present. Mutations in the *RX* (*RAX*) and *SOX2* genes have been associated with anophthalmia (Table 2.1).
- *Nanophthalmia and microphthalmia* Formation of the optic vesicle without proper subsequent development produces a rudimentary eye in the orbit – nanophthalmia (or dwarf eye). In microphthalmia there is a small but recognizable eye that contains recognizable elements, e.g. lens, choroid and retina.
- *Synophthalmia* Fusion of the two eyes may result from a malformation of the mesenchymal tissue between the optic vesicles or faulty inductive processes. Only rarely is a single eye (cyclops) formed by this mechanism and in most cases there are two recognizable corneas and lenses, and identifiable parts of the iris and ciliary body. The midline sclera and uveal tissue may be absent and the optic nerve may be single or duplicate. This malformation may be associated with a deletion of chromosome 18.
- *Congenital cystic eye* A disorganized cystic structure may arise owing to disturbances in the process of invagination of the retinal disk.

It is now clear that *epigenetic development*, the process by which organisms develop their definitive characteristics through the gradual alteration of simpler precursors, in vertebrates and non-vertebrates, is regulated by *cascades of gene expression*. Namely, early acting regulatory genes initiate developmental processes and induce the expression of 'downstream' genes, which may subsequently lead to expression of

Table 2.1 Critical genes in ocular development

Mouse gene	Human gene	Expression pattern	Ocular defects in mouse mutants	Ocular defects in humans with known mutations in related gene
Pax-6	PAX6	Anterior neural plate, optic sulcus/cup and stalk. Surface ectoderm (future lens and corneal/conjunctival epithelium). Weakly expressed in mesenchymal cells	Micro-ophthalmia, cataract, hypoplastic iris, incomplete separation of cornea and iris, corneal defects	Anophthalmia, anterior segment dysgenesis, congenital glaucoma, Peter's anomaly, Axenfeld–Rieger syndrome (aniridia)
Pitx3	PITX3	Developing lens vesicle	Persistent lens stalk, malformed lens	Congenital cataract, leucoma, Peter's anomaly
Chd7	CHD7	Neuroectoderm, lens vesicle	CHARGE-like features, keratoconjunctivitis sicca	CHARGE syndrome (see box, p. 115)
Maf	MAF	Lens placode, lens vesicle, primary lens fibres (transcription factors for alpha crytallin gene along with Sox1)	Failure of lens fibres to elongate, lens vesicle fails to separate from surface ectoderm	Defects in lens, cornea and iris (coloboma), Peter's anomaly
Foxe3	FOXE3	Lens placode	Failure of lens to separate from surface ectoderm	Peter's anomaly, posterior embryotoxon, cataract
Pitx2 Fox1	PITX2 FOXC1	Periocular mesenchyme (presumptive cornea, eyelids, trabecular meshwork, extraocular muscle)	Anterior segment abnormalities	Iridogoniodysgenesis, Axenfeld–Rieger syndrome, 50% develop juvenile glaucoma
Sox1, Sox2, Sox3	SOX1, SOX2, SOX3	Central nervous system, sensory placodes, Sox2 in lens placode	Micro-ophthalmia, cataract	Anophthalmia without cataract
Rx	RX	Anterior neural plate, optic vesicle, developing retina, photoreceptors	Eyeless	Anophthalmia
Crya, Cryb, Cryg	CRYA, CRYB, CRYG	Lens	Various forms of cataract	Various forms of cataract

further genes and so on until genes encoding actual structural and functional characteristics of specific cells and tissues are activated (Larsen, 1997). There is overwhelming evidence that these cascades have been conserved throughout evolution from insects to fish to mammals. The *Drosophila*, or fruit fly, zebra fish and mouse are the most intensively studied experimental species in each respective group and recent research has shed light on some of the critical genes in ocular development, some of which have been remarkably conserved in evolution. Table 2.1 is a summary of some of the genes influencing early eye development and readers interested in 'EVO–DEVO' models of eye development are directed to a special edition of *International Journal of Developmental Biology* 2004; 48(8/9).

The basic body plan of all animal embryos is initially established by a class of regulatory genes called *selector* or *switch genes* which, like the *maternal effect genes* of the fruit fly, establish longitudinal or anteroposterior (head–tail), dorsoventral and left–right axes. A further class of genes, the *zygotic genes*, which includes *segmentation genes*, is switched on later, after the maternal effect genes. The changes induced by the segmentation genes cause the expression of another class of selector genes, the *homeotic genes*, which encode a region of DNA called a *homeobox* (termed *Hox* genes). These subsequently regulate many downstream genes and thus act as *master control genes*.

Hox gene activation plays a critical role in the differentiation of what initially appear as identical segments in the embryo (induced by earlier expression of segmentation genes) into, for example, cervical, thoracic, abdominal and sacral regions as well as the segmentation of the head and neck, particularly the pharyngeal arches and subdivision of the brain.

Paired-box (Pax) genes encode transcription factors involved in the regulation of several aspects of vertebrate and non-vertebrate early development and as such are also considered as 'master control genes'. In vertebrates two *Pax* genes, *Pax-6* and *Pax-2*, are important to early eye differentiation.

Pax-6 is expressed in the anterior neuroepithelium and lens placode-forming epithelium. Thus it appears that the gene defines a field of cells *competent to differentiate into eye tissues* (neural retina, retinal pigment epithelium, iris epithelium, ciliary body epithelium, lens and corneal epithelium). It also appears to be required to *maintain growth and proliferation* of cells in the optic vesicle (and other regions of the central nervous system). *Pax-6* is only weakly expressed on the optic stalks, whereas *Pax-2* expression is, by comparison, largely restricted to this area where it appears to be necessary for successful closure of the *choroid fissure*.

NEURAL CREST-DERIVED PERIOCULAR MESENCHYME

For many years it was widely held that the middle germ layer, the *mesoderm*, gave rise to most of the mesenchyme and its derivatives in the head and neck region in a similar manner to the pattern of differentiation in the trunk. A large body of experimental evidence from avian and mammalian studies has now shown that mesenchyme in the head region is derived from two sources, neural crest (*mesectoderm*) and mesoderm.

The limited fate of neural crest cells in the trunk (Fig. 2.2) contrasts with their diverse role in head and neck development. Neural crest cells originate at the neuroectoderm–surface ectoderm junction of the fore-, mid- and hindbrain regions before fusion of the neural folds. They migrate ventrally into the pharyngeal arches and rostrally around the forebrain and developing optic cup and into the facial region in a highly ordered manner, guided in their migration by components of the extracellular matrix, e.g. fibronectin and glycosaminoglycans (Fig. 2.5). The pattern of appearance and migration of cranial neural crest is closely associated with the expression products of the Homeobox (*Hox*) gene family within the rhombomeres of the hindbrain (see Hunt et al., 1991; Noden, 1991; Gilland and Baker, 1993; Mendelson et al., 1994). In the face region, neural crest cells contribute significantly to mesenchyme-derived tissues, such as bone, cartilage, connective tissues, meninges and ocular and periocular connective tissues (normally not associated with neural crest in the trunk), as well as giving rise to the usual crest derivatives – melanocytes, dorsal root ganglia equivalents (sensory ganglia of V, VII, IX and X) and parasympathetic ganglia (ciliary, otic, pterygopalatine and submandibular).

At the same time as cephalic neural crest cell migration commences, the optic stalks begin to constrict, thus creating a pathway between the stalk and surface ectoderm into which predominantly mesencephalic crest cells migrate (Fig. 2.5). The migration of these cells ceases when they reach the choroid fissure on the ventral aspect of the optic cup.

Neural crest cells also migrate directly from the optic vesicle in human and primate embryos (Bartelmez and Blount, 1954; Blankenship et al., 1996).

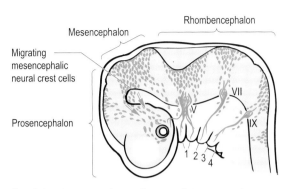

Fig. 2.5 Diagram of neural crest cell origins and migration pathways in the head region (based on avian studies of Noden). The bulk of the periocular neural crest is derived from mesencephalic neural crest. A large component of the sensory ganglia of cranial nerves V, VII and IX is also neural crest-derived. The pharyngeal arches are numbered in craniocaudal sequence. The neural crest associated with rhombomere 2 (R2) (not shown on diagram) migrates into and forms the basis for the first pharyngeal arch; R4 neural crest migrates into the second arch; R6 migrates into the third arch. Neural crest is not associated with R3 or R5.

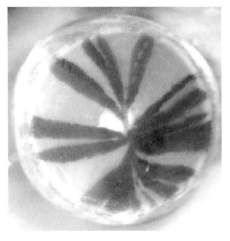

Fig. 2.6 Chimeric and mosaic analysis of growth and cell migration in the murine cornea. The radial stripes in the corneal epithelium of adult LacZ$^+$ – LacZ$^-$ chimeric mice stained with X-gal. Courtesy of Martin J. Collinson (University of Aberdeen) and John D. West (University of Edinburgh). (See Collinson et al., 2004 for discussion on the analysis of mouse eye development using chimeric and mosaic models).

Experimental methods of mapping neural crest cell migration and fate

The fate of neural crest cells from various regions of the neural plate has been mapped in birds (see reviews Noden, 1982, 1988; Creuzet et al., 2005) and also in mouse and rat embryos (Erickson et al, 1989; Fukisha and Morriss-Kay, 1992; Trainor and Tam, 1995). Avian experiments have used a variety of cell-tracing methods, including transplanted radiolabelled donor crest cells, chick–quail transplant chimeras and subsequent tracking of quail cells using natural nucleolus marker or anti-quail nuclear antigenic determinant (see review Creuzet et al., 2005).

Tracking the fate of neural crest cells in mammals has been aided by the production of mouse mutants with neural developmental anomalies and more recently by utilizing transgenic mice in which a transgene (bacterial *lac Z* 'reporter' gene which codes for β-galactosidase) is introduced into the mouse genome in a position where it will be coexpressed alongside proteins specific for the cell types under investigation, such as peripherin or retinoic acid receptor, which are expressed on neural crest cells during and after migration. The migration pathways of the cells carrying the transfected genome can thus be visualized with appropriate chemical substrates for bacterial β-galactosidase (Mendelson et al., 1994). Other techniques that are unveiling the destiny and diffentiation of various cell types in embryonic development include micromanipulative cell grafting and labelling using fluorescent cell markers (DiI and DiO), in-situ hybridization and chimeric and mosaic mouse models (Osumi-Yamishita et al., 1990; Trainor and Tam, 1995; Collinson et al., 2004) (Fig 2.6).

Paraxial mesoderm (somites and the less distinct rostrally situated *somitomeres*) forms most of the walls and floor of the brain case, all voluntary muscles of the craniofacial region (including extraocular muscles), all vascular endothelial cells, the dermis and connective tissues of the dorsal region of the head, and the meninges caudal to the prosencephalon. The seven rostrally situated somitomeres differentiate in a segmental manner within the pharyngeal arches (see p. 137) and they play an important role in eye development by influencing neural crest cell migration and differentiation and by directly contributing to the periocular mesenchyme. The spatial distribution of cranial paraxial mesoderm (somitomeres) and neural crest cells during craniofacial development in mouse embryos shows that paraxial mesoderm mixes extensively in the periocular, facial, periotic and cervical mesenchyme but appears to be segregated in the pharyngeal arches (Figs 2.7 and 2.8) (Trainor and Tam, 1995).

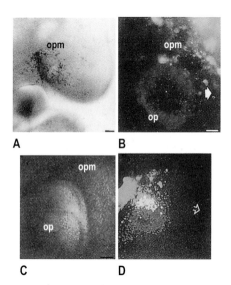

Fig. 2.7 Colonization of the periocular mesenchyme (opm) by cells derived from somitomere I in the mouse embryo. In (**A**) the cells have been labelled with X-gal (blue) and in (**B**) with DiO (green fluorescence). In (**B**) the red cells are DiI-labelled neural crest cells. (**C**) A bright field view of the same specimen showing the orientation of the optic vesicle (op) and periocular mesenchyme (opm). (**D**) A confocal image showing the codistribution of the two cell populations showing that neural crest cells are found in both the neural epithelium of the optic vesicle and in the surrounding mesenchyme where they share territory with somitomeric-derived mesenchyme (yellow indicates areas of overlapping distribution but not double-labelled cells). Arrow points rostrally. Bar, 500 μm. (Reproduced from Trainor and Tam, 1995, with permission.)

Thus mesodermally derived mesenchyme contributes more to the periocular connective tissues than experimental studies in birds had previously suggested.

DEVELOPMENT OF STRUCTURES DERIVED FROM NEUROEPITHELIUM: THE NEURAL RETINA AND RETINAL PIGMENT EPITHELIUM

The thickened portion of the optic vesicle that invaginates, the *retinal disk*, is destined to differentiate into the *neural retina*, while the thinner outermost layer of the optic vesicle is destined to form the RPE. These layers are continuous at the optic cup margin, where a sharp transition in morphology is evident (Figs 2.3B,C and 2.4A–D). The *optic cup margin* will later be the site from which the neuroepithelial

component of the iris and ciliary body will arise (see pp. 130–133) and ultimately form the *pupil margin*. Because of the invagination of the optic cup the apical aspect of the primitive neural retina comes to lie adjacent to the apical surface of the RPE, thereby obliterating the intraretinal space (Fig. 2.3C). As the ependymal cells that line the developing (and adult) ventricular spaces in the brain are ciliated, the apposing surfaces of the primitive neural retina and future RPE are also ciliated. The cilia of the neural retina are important later in development, in the formation of rods and cones. The cilia of the RPE degenerate.

RETINAL MORPHOGENESIS (Fig. 2.9)

The primitive neural retina consists of an *outer nuclear zone* and an *inner acellular* or *marginal zone*. The outer nuclear zone is homologous with the proliferative neuroepithelium of the neural tube. Both the inner and outer layers of the optic cup rest on their respective basal laminae: that of the inner layer becomes the *inner limiting membrane*, the outer is incorporated into *Bruch's membrane*. Differentiation of the retinal layers commences at the posterior pole and progresses in a centrifugal manner, thus a gradient of retinal differentiation can be seen within an individual eye. Miotic activity in the primitive neural retina is greatest in the outer part of the nuclear zone (Fig. 2.9A). Around 7 weeks of gestation (16–20 mm) newly formed cells migrate in a vitread direction into the marginal zone to form the *inner neuroblastic layer*. The outer nucleated zone is now referred to as the *outer neuroblastic layer* (Figs 2.9B and 2.10A). The two neuroblastic layers are separated by an acellular zone – the *transient layer of Chievitz*. The earliest differentiated cells, which form the inner neuroblastic layer, are future ganglion cells, Müller cells (radial glial) and amacrine cells. Elegant studies using chimeras and mosaic mouse models have revealed that clones of cells radiate in a vitread direction and as the retina begins to stratify, proliferation and differentiation cells that have arisen from these original 'clones' appear as columns. Subsequently some cells disperse laterally (Reese et al., 1999).

The nerve fibre layer becomes identifiable on the inner aspect of the inner neuroblastic layer owing to growth of ganglion cell axons that converge towards the optic stalk. A zone where the processes of cells from the inner neuroblastic layer intermingle (the *inner plexiform layer*), becomes identifiable at approximately 10.5 weeks gestation, thereby obliterating

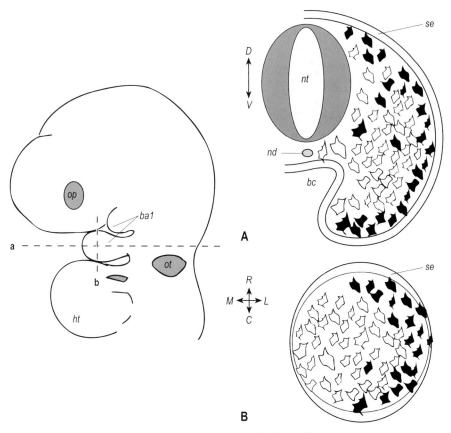

Fig. 2.8 Diagram summarizing the localization of neural crest cells (filled cells in diagram) and somitomeric mesoderm (open cells) in the facial mesenchyme and branchial arches (ba1) of the mouse embryo. The diagram on the left indicates two planes of section (a, transverse; b, coronal) as shown by the dotted lines. The neural crest cells are located around the periphery of the branchial arch in caudal, rostral and lateral aspects (C, R and L respectively) beneath the ectoderm and segregated from the somitomeric mesoderm. There is some intermingling of the two populations in the paraxial region. Abbreviations: bc, buccal cavity; ht, heart; nt, neural tube; op, optic vesicle; ot, otic vesicle; se, surface ectoderm. (Reproduced from Trainor and Tam, 1995, with permission).

the transient layer of Chievitz (Figs 2.9C and 2.10A). A new intermediate nucleated layer, the *inner nuclear layer*, becomes identifiable in the posterior pole retina and already contains the amacrine and Müller cell bodies, and shortly afterwards the bipolar and horizontal cells differentiate from the outer neuroblastic layer and migrate into this new nucleated layer (Fig. 2.9C). The remaining components of the outer neuroblastic layer will form the *outer nuclear layer* containing the cell bodies of the photoreceptors (rods and cones). The zone where fibres from this layer intermingle with those of the inner nuclear layer constitutes the new *outer plexiform layer* (Fig. 2.9D). The *external limiting membrane* (not a membrane *per se*) of the retina is identifiable in the

earliest stages as rows of tight junctions between adjacent neuroblasts (Fig. 2.11B).

Further important landmarks in retinal development include:

- synaptogenesis in cone pedicles at approximately 4 months, but not in rod spherules until 5 months,
- photoreceptor outer segment formation commences around the fifth month,
- horizontal cells become distinguishable around the fifth month,
- microglia (resident tissue macrophages) invade the retina via the retinal vasculature and peripheral subretinal space (10–12 weeks onwards),

121

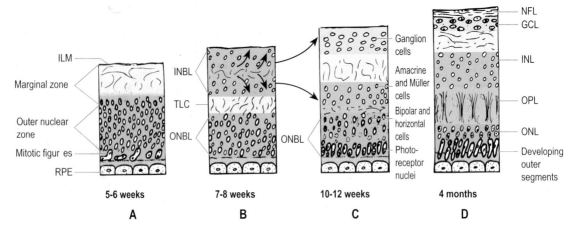

Fig. 2.9 (A–D) Summary of early retinal morphogenesis in the human eye. Arrows indicate major patterns of cell movements. ILM, inner limiting membrane; RPE, retinal pigment epithelium; INBL, inner neuroblastic layer; ONBL, outer neuroblastic layer; TLC, transient layer of Chievitz; NFL, nerve fibre layer; GCL; ganglion cell layer; INL, inner nuclear layer; OPL, outer plexiform layer; ONL; outer nuclear layer.

- the terminal expansions of the Müller cells beneath the inner limiting membrane mature around 4.5 months, at around the same time as their processes can be identified between the rods and cones.

Malformations of the retina

Failure of organization of the neuroblastic cells within the retina leads to thickening and distortion of normal architecture: 'retinal dysplasia,' is seen as nests of neuroblastic cells misplaced during differentiation, forming circular or oval structures, termed rosettes (see Ch. 9). More subtle abnormalities can occur in the formation of rods and cones which lead, for example, to defects in colour vision or poor visual acuity and congenital nystagmus.

MACULA AND FOVEAL DEVELOPMENT

Maculogenesis is first evident as a localized increase in ganglion cell density temporal to the optic disk at around 4.5 months. By 6 months, the ganglion cell layer may be eight or nine cells deep in this region. The thickened immature outer nuclear layer consists predominantly of immature cones. In the seventh month, there is a displacement of ganglion cells and formation of a *foveal depression*. There are approximately two layers of ganglion cells in the foveal region in the eighth month and at birth this is reduced to one. By 4 months postpartum the inner nuclear and ganglion cell layers have receded to the margins of the fovea, leaving only cone nuclei in the foveal region. Elongation of the inner and outer segments occurs over the next few months.

PERIPHERAL RETINA

Until approximately 10–12 weeks of gestation the periphery of the retina extends to within 50–100 μm of the optic cup margin (Fig. 2.4F). By 14 weeks the retina terminates immediately posterior to the newly formed ciliary folds, with minimal pars plana. However, a definite pars plana and a poorly formed ora serrata are present by 6 months (see p. 131). The pars plana and the region from the ora serrata to the equator of the eye continue to grow after birth with continued growth of the eyeball, which occurs up to 2 years of age. The area of the retina is approximately 600 mm^2 at birth and reaches 800 mm^2 by 2 years.

DEVELOPMENT OF RETINAL VASCULATURE

The vessel incorporated into the choroidal fissure is the *hyaloid artery*, a branch of the ophthalmic artery, itself a branch of the internal carotid artery (Fig. 2.12A). The hyaloid artery, upon emerging from the centre of the optic stalk, spreads between the lens surface and the marginal zone of the primitive neural retina (lentoretinal space). With growth of the optic cup and formation of the vitreous cavity,

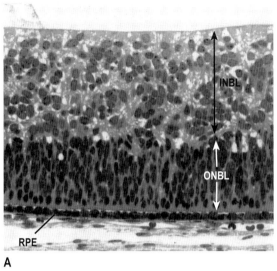

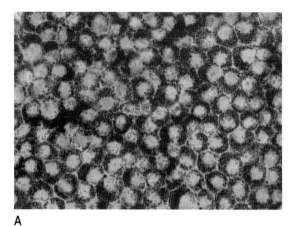

A

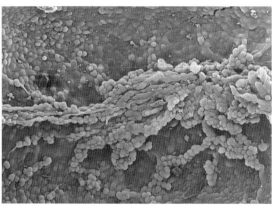

B

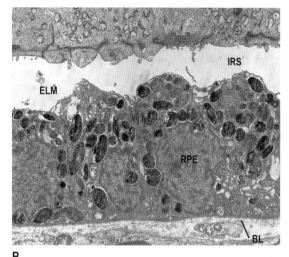

B

Fig. 2.10 (**A**) Human fetal retina (12–13 weeks) showing inner and outer neuroblastic layers (INBL, ONBL). The inner neuroblastic layer has commenced differentiation and the transient layer of Chievitz is obliterated. RPE, retinal pigment epithelium. Original magnification: × 115. (**B**) Scanning electron micrograph of 'cords' of endothelial and supporting cells (retinal vessel precursors) ramifying on the retinal surface. Original magnification: × 55.

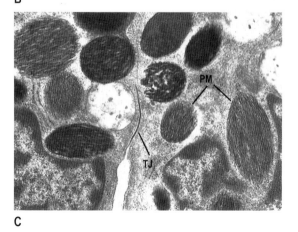

C

Fig. 2.11 (**A**) Human fetal RPE (15 weeks) viewed *en face* to demonstrate the regular hexagonal arrangement. Original magnification: × 100. (**B**) Transmission electron micrograph of human fetal RPE (12 weeks). ELM, external limiting membrane; IRS, intraretinal or subretinal space; BL, basal lamina. Original magnification: × 4100. (**C**) Premelanosomes (PM) and tight junctions (TJ) near apices of human fetal RPE (22 weeks). Original magnification: × 16000.

123

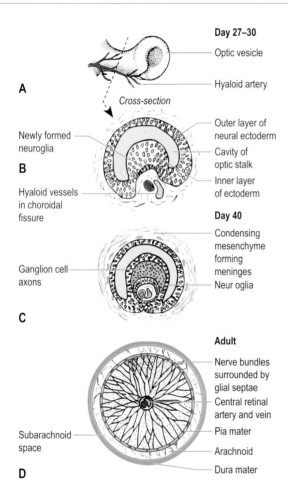

Day 27–30
- Optic vesicle
- Hyaloid artery

A

Cross-section

Newly formed neuroglia

B

- Outer layer of neural ectoderm
- Cavity of optic stalk
- Inner layer of ectoderm

Hyaloid vessels in choroidal fissure

Day 40
- Condensing mesenchyme forming meninges
- Neuroglia

Ganglion cell axons

C

Adult
- Nerve bundles surrounded by glial septae
- Central retinal artery and vein
- Pia mater

Subarachnoid space

- Arachnoid
- Dura mater

D

Fig. 2.12 Diagram summarizing the major events in the development of the optic stalk and optic nerve.

the hyaloid artery elongates and courses through the primitive vitreous, within the *hyaloid canal*, to reach the posterior lens surface.

Early in the fourth month of development, temporal clusters, or angiogenic buds, develop from the hyaloid vessels at the optic disk. These strands consist of endothelial cells, future glial cells and macrophages (Fig. 2.10B). The endothelial cells are canalized and form new vessels that course along the nerve fibre layer towards the peripheral retina at approximately 0.1 mm per day, to reach the ora serrata by the eighth month. At the same time, dividing vascular endothelial cells penetrate the depth of the neural retina to the outer border of the outer nuclear layer, a process not completed until the ninth month. Here they form a polygonal network of vessels, the outer retinal plexus (Chan-Ling, 1997).

The intraneural portion of the hyaloid vessels becomes the *central retinal artery*. Developing capillaries are united by immature punctate tight and gap junctions and their basal laminae are incomplete.

Retinopathy of prematurity

Altered oxygen tension has complex effects on the formation of capillary networks in the retina. Placing premature infants in high oxygen environments can result in a delay or reduction in retinal vascularization. Upon returning to normal oxygen tension, the retinal tissues experience hypoxia which induces the release of angiogenic factors, resulting in episodes of abnormal neovascularization within the retina and vitreous, known clinically as *retinopathy of prematurity* or *retrolental fibroplasia*. Now that the detrimental effects of high oxygen tension on the developing retina are better understood, this blinding condition is becoming less prevalent.

DEVELOPMENT OF THE RETINAL PIGMENT EPITHELIUM

One of the most dramatic events in eye development is the appearance of melanin in the embryonic RPE, which occurs as early as 28 days after fertilization (6–7 mm embryo). Initially the RPE comprises a mitotically active pseudostratified columnar ciliated epithelium. The cilia disappear as melanogenesis commences. The RPE cells are hexagonal in shape and homogeneous in size (Fig. 2.11A) and in section appear as simple cuboidal epithelium (Fig. 2.11B), although a columnar morphology is maintained in the peripheral retina for a longer period. By the fourth month the RPE has only minimal apical microvilli, few or no basal infoldings, primitive basolateral interdigitations (Fig. 2.11B), mature apical junction complexes, and intracytoplasmic premelanosomes (Fig. 2.11C). Mitotic activity appears to take place early in development and is reputed to have ceased by birth; therefore growth of the eye, and consequently of the RPE itself, is accommodated by hypertrophy or enlargement of the existing cells. A component of the future five-layered Bruch's membrane, the RPE basal lamina, is recognizable at the optic cup stage. Collagen fibrils are subsequently laid down beneath the basal lamina around 10 weeks; the first evidence of the elastic fibre layer can be detected around 3.5 months and by midterm the elastic layer forms a fenestrated sheet.

OPTIC NERVE AND DISK DEVELOPMENT

The hollow optic stalk forms a connection between the cavity of the forebrain (future third ventricle of the brain) and the cavity of the developing optic vesicles (Fig. 2.3B, 2.4A). It is formed by the constriction of the proximal portion of the vesicle, particularly on the dorsal aspect concurrent with the expansion of the distal part (Fig. 2.12A). At this stage of morphogenesis (26–28 days) the central hollow, fluid-filled stalk is lined by neuroectodermal cells. Invagination of the optic stalk at the 'choroidal' fissure, on the ventral aspect, which occurs simultaneously with invagination of the optic vesicle, results in a double layer of neuroectoderm with narrowing and eventual obliteration of the intervening fluid-filled cavity (Fig. 2.12B). The invagination process in the distal and ventral portions of the stalk leads to the incorporation of the hyaloid vessels and surrounding mesenchyme (Fig. 2.12B). The lips of the optic stalk start closing over the hyaloid vessels near the forebrain (5–6 weeks) and gradually extend distally. This fusion lags behind that of the cup. The stalks lie at approximately 65° to the mid-sagittal plane, compared with 40° in the adult.

Axons from developing retinal ganglion cells grow towards the optic stalk and upon reaching the optic disk, change direction and course towards the brain among the inner neuroectodermal cells of the developing optic nerve (Fig. 2.12B,C). The choroidal fissure closes soon after, and by 6 weeks the optic nerve contains numerous axons that surround the hyaloid artery and vein. The outer neuroectodermal layer of the stalk differentiates into the peripheral glial mantle and the glial component of the lamina cribrosa. A cone-like structure, Bergmeister's papilla, consisting of glial cells and the remnants of hyaloid vessels, may persist at the optic nerve head in some individuals. An outer layer of condensed mesenchyme forms the optic nerve dura, which blends with the sclera. The glial septae surrounding the nerve bundles are composed of astroglia that differentiate from the cells of the inner layer of the optic stalk. The latter also gives origin to the oligodendroglia that surround the individual axons and are myelinated as far as the posterior margin of the lamina cribrosa. The nerve is displaced nasally during the third month by enlargement of the temporal side of the eye.

Malformations of the optic nerve head

When there is a failure of closure of the posterior part of the optic fissure, the optic nerve head is deformed by a *coloboma*, located inferonasally and associated with bulging of the sclera (scleractasia). The coloboma may take the form of a small recess (*optic pit*) at the rim of the disk: this is a herniation of the retina into the meninges and adjacent optic nerve. The clinical importance of an optic pit lies in its association with visual loss as a result of leakage from the pit and exudation of fluid beneath the macula.

Axial coloboma or 'morning glory syndrome'
There are numerous names for a symmetrically enlarged and excavated optic disk – a condition that may be unilateral or bilateral. The most extreme axial malformation is the 'morning glory syndrome', so-called because of the similarity to the American flower of the same name. This malformation is complicated by severe visual dysfunction and characterized by retrodisplacement of the optic disk into the meninges of the optic nerve. The abnormality is the result of a defect in mesodermal organization in the disk; the lamina cribrosa is not formed and there is fat and smooth muscle in the meninges.

DEVELOPMENT OF THE FIBROUS COAT OF THE EYE

Around weeks 6 and 7, periocular mesenchyme, probably derived from the neural crest, begins to condense around the optic cup (Figs 2.3D,E and 2.4C,D). This mesenchyme can be differentiated into an *inner vascular layer* (uveocapillary lamina), which forms the stroma of the choroid, ciliary body and iris, and an *outer fibrous layer*, which will form the sclera and cornea.

DEVELOPMENT OF THE SCLERA

Mesenchymal condensation is most conspicuous at the future site of insertions of the extraocular muscles (limbal–equatorial region). In the third month, active fibroblasts are already embedded in an irregular matrix of collagen, elastic fibrils and glycosaminoglycans. By 12 weeks a well-formed fibrous coat envelops the eye posteriorly as far as the optic nerve where the connective tissue forms a perforated plate, the lamina cribrosa, through which glia-covered ganglion cell axons pass.

DEVELOPMENT OF THE CORNEA

The *surface ectoderm* that seals over the lens pit forms the future corneal epithelium. It is a stratified squamous epithelium of three or four layers, the basal layer of which rests on a thin basal lamina. The first 'wave' of mesenchymal cells that passes over the optic cup margin migrates centripetally in the space between the anterior surface of the lens and the surface ectoderm to form the *corneal endothelium* (around 33 days) (Fig. 2.4C). Around day 49 a *second 'wave' of mesenchyme* commences migration from the optic cup margin and penetrates the space between the basal surface of the corneal epithelium and endothelium to form the corneal stroma (Fig. 2.4D). Both waves of mesenchyme are derived from the neural crest (see review, Cvekl and Tamm, 2004). The epithelium, which is continuous with the surface ectoderm, becomes stratified (three or four layers) and over the next few weeks the eyelids form and fuse (week 9–10). Around 8 weeks the first evidence of loosely arranged collagen fibres can be detected amidst the actively synthetic fibroblasts, now known as *keratoblasts*. The endothelium, which until now has been a double layer, becomes initially a simple cuboidal and ultimately a simple squamous layer resting on a thick basal lamina – the precursor of *Desçemet's membrane* (Fig. 2.13B). Within the corneal epithelium an intermediate layer of wing cells does not appear until the fourth or fifth month (Fig. 2.13A). By this time all the corneal layers are present with the exception of *Bowman's membrane*, which becomes identifiable by 5 months as an acellular collagenous zone beneath the epithelium (Fig. 2.13A). The stromal collagen bundles become organized into highly oriented *lamellae*, and the keratoblasts mature into long flattened *keratocytes*. This maturation process commences first in the posterior or deeper layers of the cornea and progresses more anteriorly or superficially.

Corneal thickness and diameter continue to increase throughout development by both interstitial growth (thickening of lamellae) and appositional growth (addition of new lamellae). The glycosaminoglycan constituents are known to alter during development and are thought to underlie the initial swelling of the cornea (when lids are fused) and its subsequent thinning, which occurs during eyelid opening (24 weeks) (Zieske, 2004). Corneal transparency is gradually attained before birth owing to maturation of the superficial lamellae and the hydration activity of the endothelial cells. Innervation of the cornea commences at 3 months and reaches the epithelium at 5 months.

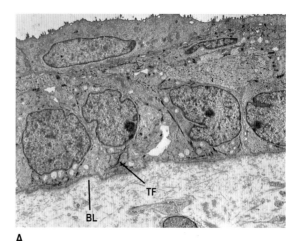

A

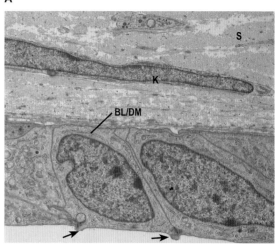

B

Fig. 2.13 Transmission electron micrographs of human fetal cornea (16 weeks). (**A**) Epithelium consists of three cell layers joined by desmosomes resting upon a thin basal lamina (BL). Note the electron-dense intracytoplasmic tonofilaments (TF). Original magnification: × 2300. (**B**) Developing endothelial cells. Note that the cells are cuboidal with apical junctional complexes (arrows) and rest on the basal lamina (BL/DM), which is already showing evidence of thickening to form the future Desçemet's membrane. K, keratoblast; S, collagenous stroma. Original magnification: × 5000.

In summary, the cornea develops from the interaction of a surface ectoderm-derived epithelium and neural crest-derived mesenchyme, which gives rise to the deeper layers including Bowman's layer, stroma, endothelium and its thick basal lamina, Desçemet's membrane.

Corneal malformation (corneal leucoma)

Corneal opacification may be the result of a failure of the keratocytes to produce collagen fibres arranged in a lamellar array: instead the pattern resembles sclera (scleralization of the cornea). *Peter's anomaly* is a term used to describe a posterior axial stromal defect associated with incarceration of the pupillary part of the iris at the edge of the defect. A mild form of malformation is the presence of thickening at the periphery of Desçemet's membrane (Schwalbe's line). When this is visible clinically (by gonioscopy) it takes the form of a bow, hence the term *embryotoxon* (Gk. *toxon* – a bow). Broad strands of tissue derived from the iris are sometimes seen in the chamber angle. In *Axenfeld's anomaly*, iridocorneal strands are localized to Schwalbe's line. When 'iris hypoplasia' is present, the malformation is known as *Rieger's (or Axenfeld–Rieger's) anomaly* (see Table 2.1 for mutations associated with these abnormalities).

DEVELOPMENT OF THE INTRAOCULAR CONTENTS

LENS DEVELOPMENT (Fig. 2.14)

The thickened disk of ectodermal cells that forms the *lens placode* can be identified at 27 days. Differential elongation of these cells and contraction of their apical terminal bar causes the placode to invaginate, producing a *lens vesicle* with a central depression, the *lens pit*, leading into a hollow *lens cavity* that is connected briefly to the amniotic cavity via the *lens pore* (Figs 2.3C and 2.4B). As the vesicle, surrounded by its basal lamina, detaches from the surface ectoderm (10 mm, 33 days) it sinks into the underlying rim of the optic cup (Figs 2.3D and 2.4B). Occasionally, degenerating cells (epitrichial or periderm cells) are seen within the lens cavity. It now appears that lens induction is a multi-stage process requiring signalling by bone morphogenetic protein (Bmp) and also probably fibroblast growth factor (Fgf) combined with the expression of a number of transcription factors, the most important of which appears to be *Pax-6* (Lang, 2004)

Under an inductive signal from developing neural retina, the posterior cells of the lens vesicle elongate to form the *primary lens fibres* (Fig. 2.14A) and commence synthesis of a new group of intracytoplasmic proteins known as *crystallins*. Fibroblast growth factor, as well as being an inductive signal, is likely to be involved in lens fibre differentiation (Schulz et al., 1993; McAvoy et al., 1999). The base of each elongating lens cell remains anchored to the basal lamina posteriorly and their apices grow towards the *anterior lens epithelium*, thereby obliterating the lens cavity (Figs 2.3D,E; 2.4C and 2.14B,C). The nuclei migrate forward within the elongated cell body to produce a *lens bow* with a conspicuous forward convexity (Figs 2.4F and 2.14C,G). Subsequent lens fibres arise from mitotic activity within the *anterior lens epithelium* at the equatorial zone and are known as *secondary lens fibres* (Fig. 2.14D,G). The tips of the secondary fibres extend around the primary fibres and meet at the Y-shaped anterior and posterior *lens sutures* (Fig. 2.14D). Every subsequent generation of fibres throughout embryonic, and indeed later, life is added superficial to the previous layer. Early in embryonic development the lens is nearly spherical or possibly longer in its anteroposterior axis; however, as secondary fibres are added at the equator the lens becomes more ellipsoid, a trend that continues till birth and into adulthood. Basal lamina material is continually deposited by the lens epithelium on its external aspect and encases the lens in a membranous non-cellular envelope, the *lens capsule*. During embryonic and fetal development the lens receives nourishment via an intricate vascular net, the *tunica vasculosa lentis* (Fig. 2.14E,F,G), which completely encompasses the lens by approximately 9 weeks.

Malformations of lens

The lens is particularly susceptible during its formation and early growth, to intrauterine toxic insults such as rubella (German measles). The disorganization that ensues causes degeneration in the fibres and visible opacities in the lens (congenital cataract). If the lens fibre cells recover, the opacities become buried in the inner part of the cortex by the newly formed lens fibres.

Small (microphakic) or round (spherophakic) lenses do not exhibit a strikingly abnormal histology. Axial bulges on the anterior and posterior surfaces of the lens are referred to respectively as anterior and posterior lentiglobus and are presumed to be the result of abnormalities in the lens epithelium and the lens capsule.

Lenticulocorneal fusion

Lenticulocorneal fusion occurs when a relatively normal lens is fused with the posterior surface of the cornea, possibly as a result of failure of the lens vesicle to separate from surface ectoderm. A number of mutations have been linked to disturbances in these early events (Table 2.1).

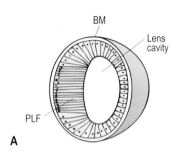

A

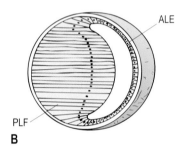

B

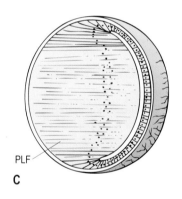

C

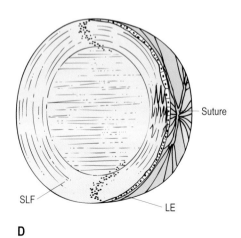

D

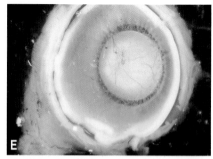

E

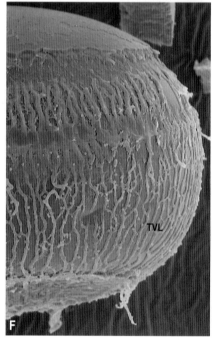

F

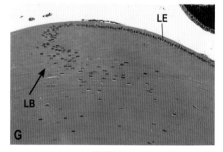

G

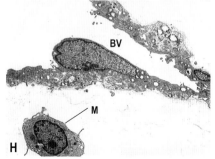

H

DEVELOPMENT OF THE VITREOUS AND HYALOID SYSTEM

At 5 weeks of gestation the lentoretinal space is narrow and occupied by the *primary vitreous* (Figs 2.3C,D, and 2.15A), which consists of the *hyaloid artery* and its branches, the *vasa hyaloidea propria*, namely vascular mesenchyme, which become incorporated into the optic cup through the choroidal fissure (see p. 114). Surface ectodermally derived elements that surrounded the lens during invagination are also thought to contribute to the primary vitreous. Thus the primary vitreous may be of mixed ectodermal and mesenchymal origin.

The *tunica vasculosa lentis* has two sources. The first (visible at around 5 weeks) is a series of capillaries that arise from the hyaloid vessels and form a palisade-like network of vessels, the *capsulopupillary vessels*, around the equator of the lens (Fig. 2.14F, 2.15B). This capillary network anastomoses with the anterior component of the tunica, the *pupillary membrane (lamina iridopupillaris)*, on the anterior lens surface (Fig. 2.15B). The pupillary membrane vessels are derived predominantly from branches of the long posterior ciliary arteries, which form an annular vessel close to the optic cup margin and whose branches pass over the rim of the optic cup to supply the anterior portion of the lens (Fig. 2.15B). The hyaloid system has no veins and venous drainage occurs anteriorly via the pupillary membrane and the uveal vessels. The expression of vascular endothelial growth factor by the lens is thought to be a critical molecular event in the formation of the hyaloid vascular system (Saint-Geniez and D'Amore, 2004).

An avascular *secondary (definitive) vitreous* composed of finely fibrillar material is deposited behind the primary vitreous between 5.5 and 12 weeks. The primitive hyalocytes appear around this time. These cells are now widely recognized as belonging to the

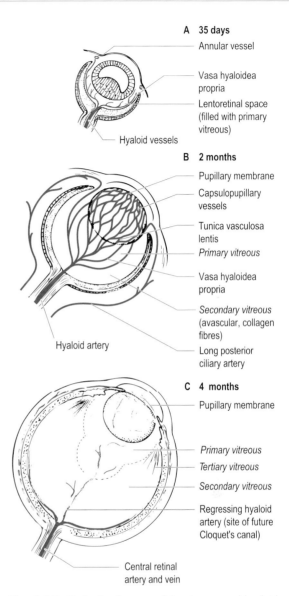

Fig. 2.15 Early development of the vitreous and hyaloid system.

Fig. 2.14 (A–D) Diagrammatic summary of lens morphogenesis. BM, basement membrane of lens cells; ALE, anterior lens epithelium; PLF, primary lens fibres; SLF, secondary lens fibres; LE, lens epithelium (former anterior lens epithelium). **(E)** Macroscopic view of human fetal eye (20 weeks) with posterior segment removed to reveal the hyaloid artery (HA) and tunica vasculosa lentis (TVL) around the lens. Original magnification: × 10. **(F)** Scanning electron micrographic view of a fetal rat lens surrounded by the fine vessels of the TVL. Note the small spherical macrophages associated with the vessels on the lens surface. Original magnification: × 95. **(G)** Fetal lens showing the lens bow (LB) arising from the equatorial region. LE, lens epithelium. Original magnification: × 90. **(H)** Electron micrograph of macrophage (M) associated with a blood vessel (BV) of the tunica vasculosa lentis. Original magnification: × 2800.

mononuclear phagocyte system, although it has been postulated that they may also synthesize hyaluronan in the secondary vitreous. Mesenchymal cells in the adventitia of vitreal vessels may also contribute to the vitreous matrix. Much of the hyaluronan and collagen (type II) in the vitreous gel is added after birth.

Around the end of the third month distinct condensations of secondary vitreous become evident in the space between the optic cup margin and the lens. The fibres, which are firmly attached to the inner limiting membrane of the retina in the developing pars plana region, are sometimes referred to as the *tertiary vitreous* and, when mature, will form the *vitreous base* (Fig. 2.15C). It seems likely that the non-pigmented ciliary epithelial cells in this region are responsible for synthesis of the tertiary vitreous and zonular fibres.

During the fourth month the remains of the primary vitreous, the hyaloid vessels and the vasa hyaloidea propria, together with the tunica vasculosa lentis, begin to atrophy (Fig. 2.15C). The regression occurs contemporaneously with the formation of the retinal vasculature (see review, Saint-Geniez and D'Amore, 2004). The course these vessels took through the vitreous is evident in the adult as a narrow fluid-filled central channel, Cloquet's canal. Macrophages play an important scavenging role in the regression of the hyaloid vessels (Fig. 2.14F,H) (Lang and Bishop, 1993; McMenamin et al., 2002) and may also be responsible for the induction of apoptosis of vascular endothelial cells. Small portions of the pupillary membrane may persist in otherwise normal eyes.

Malformations of the vitreous and hyaloid artery system

Normally, the hyaloid system of vessels vanishes completely but in some disorders regression does not occur.

Persistent tunica vasculosa lentis
Persistence of the anterior part of the tunica vasculosa lentis or the pupillary membrane causes deformation of the iris.

Persistent hyperplastic (anterior) primary vitreous
If the embryonic fibrovascular tissue in the anterior vitreous face persists, the ciliary processes are drawn internally, providing a valuable clinical diagnostic feature that is visible when the pupil is dilated. The lens is opaque in persistent hyperplastic anterior primary vitreous, because a retrolental fibrovascular mass erodes the posterior lens capsule and penetrates the lens cortex. The white retrolental mass (leucocoria) produced by this malformation can lead to a mistaken clinical diagnosis of retinoblastoma.

Persistent (posterior) hyperplastic primary vitreous
A persistent hyaloid artery and the condensed posterior primary vitreous project from the optic disk and the adjacent retina. Distortion of the disk by prepapillary and preretinal fibrous membranes is associated with radial or falciform folds in the retina.

DEVELOPMENT OF THE UVEAL TRACT

THE CHOROID

The choroid arises very early in development from the loose vascular layer of mesenchyme that surrounds the optic cup (Fig. 2.3C,D). A palisade layer of vessels lies immediately external to the RPE and forms the basis of the future choriocapillaris. Fenestrations in the endothelium become evident very early in development. This layer of vessels forms communications with the precursors of the posterior ciliary arteries at around 2 months. A second layer of vessels forms at around 4 months external to the future choriocapillaris and consists of thin-walled venous channels that will eventually unite to form rudimentary vortex veins and branches of the long and short posterior ciliary arteries. An intermediate or middle layer (future Sattler's layer) of mainly arterioles forms between the larger vessels (Haller's layer) and the choriocapillaris. The choroidal vessels are initially embedded in a loose collagenous stroma; however, elastic fibres form later in development in the outer choroid (future lamina suprachoroidea) and pigment-bearing melanocytes appear around the seventh to eighth month of gestation.

THE CILIARY BODY

The development of the ciliary body has similarities to iris development because it involves an interaction between mesenchyme and neuroectoderm. Ciliary body and iris development commence in the 11–12th week with indentation of the outer pigmented layer of the neuroectoderm (presumptive pigmented ciliary epithelium) near the optic cup rim by small capillaries in the inner vascular mesenchyme (Fig. 2.16A,B). Investigations of *Hox* gene

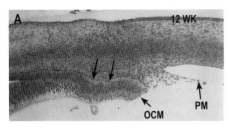

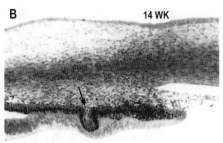

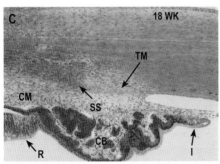

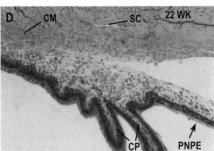

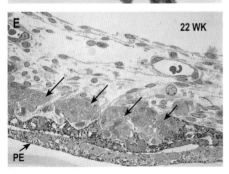

expression during early ocular development in the mouse revealed a highly restricted expression of *Hox 7.1* in the non-pigmented or inner neural epithelium just behind the optic cup margin at the site of the prospective ciliary body and iris (Monaghan et al., 1991). This gene is expressed 2 days before any morphological evidence of these structures is evident and thus it may be an early molecular marker for regional specialization and differentiation in the eye.

Initially, the inner non-pigmented ciliary epithelium is flat, but as the vascular sprouts enlarge they push inwards to form primitive radial folds. This arrangement of a vascular connective tissue core overlaid by a double layer of ciliary epithelial cells forms the basis of adult ciliary process anatomy (see Ch. 1). The 70–75 radial folds that develop in this manner appear initially as smooth undulations (Figs 2.16B and 2.17); however, between weeks 14 and 22 they increase in height and complexity (Fig. 2.16C,D). Early in development the primitive neural retina terminates immediately posterior to the ciliary folds (Fig. 2.16C), but later a smooth area, the future *pars plana*, separates the two regions and continues to expand during the remainder of gestation with continued growth of the eye. The ciliary epithelium may commence aqueous production as early as 20 weeks, coinciding with concomitant changes in the iridocorneal angle (see p. 133).

The ciliary muscle differentiates at around 15 weeks' gestation from the mesenchyme between the neuroectoderm and scleral condensation external to the early ciliary folds, namely the region that will form

Fig. 2.16 (A–D) Development of the ciliary body and iris in the human fetal eye from 12 to 22 weeks (the lens has been removed in all specimens). Note that the earliest evidence is the vascular mesenchyme indenting the outer neuroectoderm layer (arrows) near the optic cup margin (OCM) in 12- and 14-week specimens. PM, pupillary membrane; CM, ciliary muscle; SS, scleral spur; TM, trabecular meshwork anlage; I, iris; CB, ciliary body; R, retina; SC, Schlemm's canal; PNPE, posterior non-pigmented epithelium of the developing iris; CP, ciliary processes. **(E)** Electron micrograph of iris margin in a 22-week-old human fetal eye to illustrate sphincter pupillae smooth muscle bundles (arrows) differentiating from the anterior pigmented iris epithelium. Note that the posterior epithelium (PE) is showing early evidence of melanogenesis. Original magnifications: **A**, ×75; **B**, ×95; **C**, ×110; **D**, ×80; **E**, ×420.

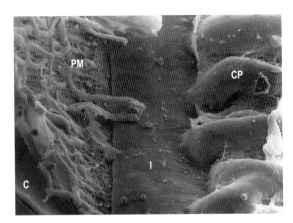

Fig. 2.17 Scanning electron micrograph of the developing human ciliary processes and iris (20-week fetus). Note the smooth outline of the ciliary processes (CP), the short iris (I), and vessels of the pupillary membrane (PM). C, cornea. Original magnification: × 120.

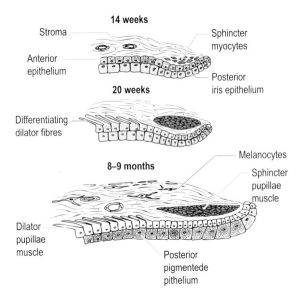

Fig. 2.18 Summary of human iris development showing the differentiation of the sphincter and dilator pupillae from the anterior iris epithelium (neuroectoderm).

the future ciliary body stroma. The longitudinally oriented smooth muscle fibres terminate in the region of the trabecular anlage during fetal development. Circular or radial ciliary muscle fibres do not differentiate until much later in development and indeed are not fully formed until about 1 year of age.

THE IRIS

Until 12–13 weeks of development there are no morphological signs of iris differentiation at the rim of the optic cup, and the cup margin lies posterior to the lateral recess of the anterior chamber (Fig. 2.16A). At around 14 weeks there is an expansion or growth of neuroepithelial cells at the cup margin anterior to the presumptive ciliary body (Fig. 2.16B,C). The optic cup neuroectoderm grows in a centripetal manner between the mesenchyme that has formed the cornea and the anterior lens surface. As it grows it incorporates some of the vessels of the lamina iridopupillaris or pupillary membrane, which lie on the anterior surface of the lens. This vascular mesenchyme is effectively split by the centrally growing neuroepithelial cells into vessels of the iridopupillary membrane, which now face the anterior chamber and form the future iris stroma (Fig. 2.16C,D), and deep to the epithelium the vessels of the capsulopupillaris.

The smooth muscles of the iris, the *sphincter* and *dilator pupillae muscles*, are unique in embryological

terms because they differentiate directly from neuroectoderm. The sphincter pupillae differentiation commences before that of the dilator pupillae. Around 13–14 weeks, anterior iris pigment epithelial cells delaminate, lose their melanin, develop intracytoplasmic microfilaments (actin) and dense bodies, and deposit a basal lamina. These are classic characteristics of smooth muscle cells. Cell-to-cell contact (gap junctions) among the smooth muscle cells in this circumferential muscle band is not fully established until 7 months (Fig. 2.16E), and the muscle becomes free in the stroma at around 8 months. The dilator pupillae muscle develops much later, around 6 months, as basal extensions of the anterior or pigmented epithelial layer of the iris (Fig. 2.18), and continues to develop even after birth. These basal extensions are arranged radial to the pupil. This muscle never becomes fully independent of the epithelium because, even in adulthood, it is composed of modified basal processes of the neuroepithelial cells (Fig. 2.18).

During development the posterior (inner) iris epithelium is largely amelanotic. It is continuous with the non-pigmented ciliary epithelium and thus the neural retina. Intracytoplasmic melanin increases in the fourth month, initially near the pupil margin (Fig. 2.16E), and by months 7–8 this layer is heavily pigmented (Fig. 2.18) and the anterior layer has lost its pigment.

Iris innervation, both adrenergic and cholinergic, is not established until late in development. In common with the choroid, pigment-bearing melanocytes are not identifiable in the iris stroma until late in development, around birth or later (Fig. 2.18). The thickness of the stroma and degree of melanogenesis are determining factors in eye colour at birth, and indeed full pigmentation and the pattern of the anterior surface are not complete until a few years postpartum. Blue irides are the result of interference and reflection of light from stromal collagen, whereas a thin stroma may allow the brownish colouration of the posterior epithelium to show through. Later in life brown irides are the result of heavily pigmented melanocytes within the stroma.

Aniridia

Aniridia is a rare autosomal dominant bilateral disease in which there is an apparent absence of the iris. The term is a misnomer because histologically the abnormal iris is seen as a stump of hypercellular stroma, often with an abnormal proliferation of the pigment epithelium. Malformation or hypoplasia of the outflow system occurs in aniridia, as do anterior and posterior cortical lens opacities. The lens may dislocate (ectopia lentis) and the optic nerve may be hypoplastic. It is now well known that aniridia is caused by mutations of the *Pax-6* gene. Other mutations have been identified in Peter's anomaly and corneal dystrophy, supporting the suggestion that this gene is a crucial transcription factor gene for ocular development (Lang, 2004). The murine Small eye (*Sey*) gene is homologous to the human *Pax-6* gene, and thus a common molecular mechanism involving the regulation of differentiation and growth of the neuroepithelium may underlie these genetic disorders.

DEVELOPMENT OF THE ANTERIOR CHAMBER ANGLE AND AQUEOUS OUTFLOW PATHWAYS

As early as the 12th week a roughly wedged-shaped distinctive mass of mesenchyme, the trabecular anlage, can be identified at the junction of the pupillary membrane and lateral margins of the cornea, namely the future anterior chamber angle (Figs 2.16A and 2.19A). The trabecular anlage consists of a dense collection of stellate mesenchymal cells (neural-crest-derived) and some loosely arranged extracellular matrix (Fig. 2.19A,D). The deep aspect of the wedge-shaped anlage is characterized by a row of small capillaries (Fig. 2.19A), which most probably have grown in from the capillary plexus on the external surface of the eye (future episcleral plexus) and are thus lined by mesoderm-derived vascular endothelial cells. By weeks 20–22 (fifth month) the connective tissue matrix of the trabecular anlage consists of flattened 'trabecular' endothelial-lined sheets and cords (early trabeculae) separated by intervening spaces (Fig. 2.19B,D). On the deep aspect of the fetal trabecular meshwork the collection of small capillaries fuses to form a single elongated slit-like vessel, the *canal of Schlemm*, lined by endothelial cells that are continuous with those of the collector channels and episcleral vessels. The characteristic 'giant vacuoles' (Fig. 2.19B) in the canal endothelium that are responsible for the passage of aqueous across the inner wall of the canal (see Ch. 1) appear at around 18–20 weeks of gestation. Chick–quail chimera studies have confirmed that vascular endothelial cells in the eye, including those lining Schlemm's canal, are not neural-crest-derived but are mesodermal in origin (Noden, 1988).

During the remainder of fetal development the meshwork becomes further specialized into cord-like inner uveal trabeculae, numerous intermediate layers of lamellar corneoscleral trabeculae, and a deep loosely arranged cribriform meshwork (Fig. 2.19B). The scleral spur is formed by month 4–5 (Fig. 2.16C). It has been thought for some time that during early angle development the inner surface of the meshwork is lined by a layer of uninterrupted cuboidal endothelial cells continuous with the corneal endothelium and that perforations between these cells appeared around the time of birth. However, scanning electron microscopy of the developing angle reveals that this layer is incomplete and numerous perforations allow communication between the anterior chamber and the spaces of the developing meshwork from 15 weeks onwards (Fig. 2.19C).

Congenital glaucoma

Theories on the aetiology of congenital glaucoma include:

- Persistence of a cellular or acellular membrane (Barkan's membrane) over the inner surface of the angle. This explanation is unlikely in light of the findings that such a cellular membrane never exists during normal development (McMenamin, 1991).

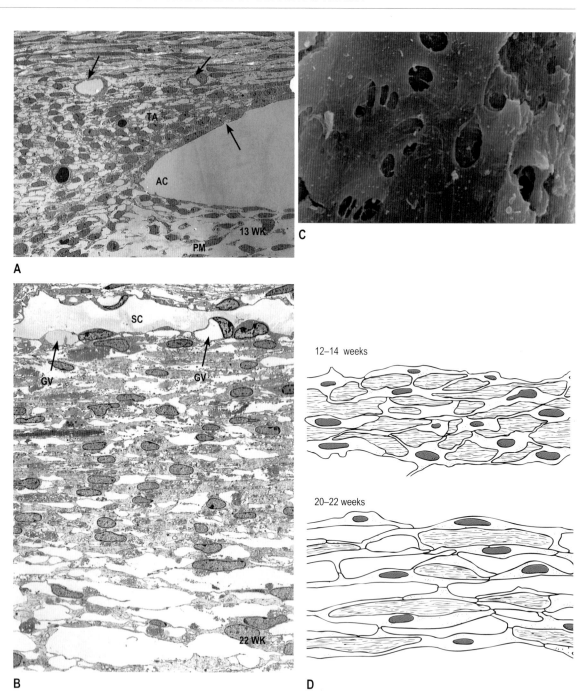

A

B

C

D

12–14 weeks

20–22 weeks

- Failure of cleavage. This theory has largely been discounted because the so-called cleavage is most likely a tissue-processing artefact.
- Failure of atrophy. Programmed cell death (apoptosis) has been observed only rarely during human angle development.
- Failure of differentiation or alterations in differential growth rates. This is a strong candidate because the few pathological accounts of congenital glaucoma describe the tissue as undifferentiated, or as lacking the typical organized trabeculae and intertrabecular spaces, especially in the outer or cribriform zone.

Chamber angle malformation (goniodysgenesis)

A failure of remodelling of the progenitor tissue in the angle leaves very obvious strands between the iris stroma and the trabecular meshwork, or between the iris and cornea. Abnormalities in the outflow system, 'goniodysgenesis', include hypoplasia of the scleral spur with extension of the ciliary muscle into the outer part of the trabecular meshwork and an excessive amount of trabecular tissue.

There are a number of more generalized abnormalities of the mesenchyme and mesoderm, which display altered iridocorneal angle structure and may manifest as *infantile glaucoma*. These include posterior embryotoxon, Axenfeld syndrome, Rieger's anomaly and Peter's anomaly. A number of mutations or deletions have been associated with iridogoniodysgenesis (Table 2.1; Cvekl and Tamm, 2004).

DEVELOPMENT OF THE EXTRAOCULAR MUSCLES

The extraocular muscles are some of the few periocular tissues that have been shown not to be of neural crest origin. They are thought to arise from presumptive myocytes in the *preotic region (paraxial mesoderm)* in the area of the prochordal plate (Fig. 2.20). They migrate ventrally and caudally around the developing eye. The presumptive myocytes concentrate particularly in the equatorial zone external to the mesenchymal condensation, which forms the sclera. Here they proliferate and differentiate, eventually fusing with the sclera anteriorly via flattened collagenous tendons.

Investigations of *MyoD* gene expression in transgenic mice (using the *LacZ* reporter gene) have shown evidence of myogenesis in situ around the developing eye as early as E10.5 (day 10.5 of embryogenesis), at about the time when myocytes are appearing in the hyoid arch mesenchyme (Patapoutian et al., 1993).

The extraocular muscles appear in approximately the following sequence: lateral rectus, superior rectus and levator palpebrae superioris (week 5), superior oblique and medial rectus (week 6), followed by inferior oblique and inferior rectus (common primordium).

The axons of the *general somatic efferent* neurones of cranial nerves III, IV and VI, which innervate these muscles, are 'dragged' behind the migrating myocytes from the site of their cell bodies in the developing brainstem to the periocular region.

Fig. 2.19 Development of the iridocorneal or chamber angle (see also Fig. 2.16). (**A**) Electron micrograph of the trabecular anlage (TA) in a 13-week-old human fetus. Note the two small capillaries (arrows) on the deep aspect of the anlage, the high density of trabecular cells, and the poorly developed extracellular matrix. AC, anterior chamber; PM, pupillary membrane (future iris stroma). Original magnification: × 500. (**B**) Electron micrograph of the trabecular meshwork in a 22-week-old human fetus. Note the enlarged intratrabecular spaces separated by well-formed connective tissue trabeculae and the size of Schlemm's canal (SC), which possesses giant vacuoles (GV) in its inner wall. Original magnification: × 100. (**C**) Scanning electron micrograph of the inner surface of the trabecular anlage in a 13-week-old human fetus revealing the incomplete nature of the endothelial cells facing the anterior chamber. These perforations most likely allow free passage of cells and fluids from the anterior chamber to the developing meshwork from this early stage onwards. Large arrow in (**A**) indicates the perspective from which the scanning micrograph was obtained. Original magnification: × 1600. (**D**) Summary of the morphogenetic changes that occur during remodelling of the loose mesenchyme of the trabecular anlage to form the trabecular meshwork. (Parts A–C from McMenamin, 1989, 1991; with permission.)

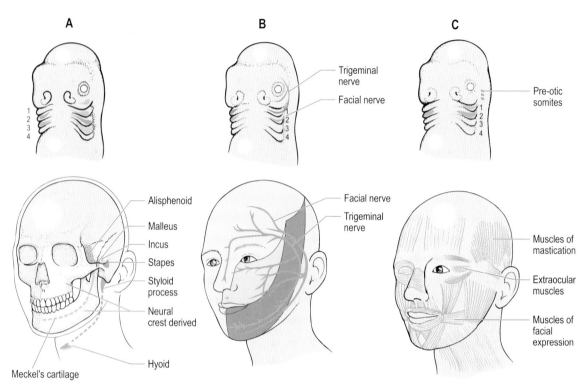

Fig. 2.20 Summary of the embryonic pharyngeal arches and their derivatives in the adult. (**A**) Arch cartilages (yellow shaded areas represent bones derived from the neural crest); (**B**) arch nerves and the sensory territories of the three divisions of the trigeminal nerve shaded green (V_1), blue (B_2) and grey (V_3) (see also Fig. 1.49); and (**C**) arch musculature.

DEVELOPMENT OF THE EYES AND SURROUNDING STRUCTURES IS INFLUENCED BY THE PATTERN OF DEVELOPMENT OF THE SKULL, PHARYNGEAL ARCHES AND FACE

DEVELOPMENT OF THE SKULL

The orbit lies at the junction of the neurocranium (skull vault) and viscerocranium (facial skeleton), and has also evolved partly from the primitive sensory capsules around the eyes. Therefore, to understand the embryology and development of the orbit, it is essential to appreciate that the entire craniofacial skeleton is formed by a combination of several components.

Chondrocranium

The *chondrocranium* forms the skull base initially as cartilaginous precursors that develop in a rostral to caudal sequence, namely the prechordal plate, hypophyseal and parachordal cartilages. These subsequently ossify to form the midline bones in the base of the skull from the interorbital region (body of the sphenoid) to the occipital region. The *sensory capsules* that evolved to support the olfactory organs, eyes and inner ear develop separately alongside this midline basal cartilage. These capsules develop initially as cartilage and in humans are represented by bones in the nasal cavity (ethmoid from prechordal cartilages), orbits (body of the sphenoid – hypophyseal cartilages, lesser wing, and medial part of the greater wing of the sphenoid) and part of the temporal bone.

Membranous bones

The *membranous bones*, evolved from 'dermal' bones like those seen in fossils of primitive placoderm fishes, ossify directly from mesenchyme ('in membrane'). They are derived from neural crest and parachordal (head) mesoderm and form the calvaria or cranial vault in the human skull. They are represented in the orbit by the orbital plate of the frontal bone.

Viscerocranium

The *viscerocranium* evolved to support the *branchial (gill) arches* in fish. In humans there are five pairs of *pharyngeal arches*, either side of the foregut tube, whose derivatives contribute to the viscerocranium (see below).

THE PHARYNGEAL ARCHES

The pharyngeal arches play an important role in the morphogenesis of the head and neck; the first and second arches in particular are important to the development of the periocular region. Pharyngeal arches form in a craniocaudal sequence and are not all at similar stages of development at any point in time. In humans, five arches develop that correspond to arches 1, 2, 3, 4 and 6 of their evolutionary precursors in fish. The first or mandibular arch has two components, one forming the upper jaw the other the lower jaw; the second or hyoid arch has evolved to support the jaw, tongue and larynx (Fig. 2.20). The third arch also contributes to the hyoid.

The fourth and sixth arches help form the larynx. Each arch has an inner covering of endoderm (separated by endodermal *pharyngeal pouches*) and an outer covering of ectoderm (separated by ectodermal *pharyngeal clefts*), a cartilaginous component (e.g. Meckel's cartilage), an arch nerve and an arch artery, together with a core of mesenchyme (Fig. 2.21). This mesenchyme is a mixture of somatic mesoderm and neural crest-derived mesectoderm [derived from rhombomere 2 (first arch), rhombomere 4 (second arch) and rhombomere 6 (third arch); (see Hunt et al., 1991; Noden, 1991; Maden et al., 1992; Hall, 2005)]. Table 2.2 and Figure 2.20 summarize the skeletal, neuronal and muscular derivatives from the pharyngeal arches. The migration of neural crest cells into each of the pharyngeal arches is like all axial organization (i.e. neural tube, somitic mesoderm and endoderm) controlled by the *Hox* code. Only a few elements of the viscerocranium, such as the medial part of the greater wing of the sphenoid (alisphenoid), incus, malleus and stapes, arise directly from the cartilaginous component (Fig.

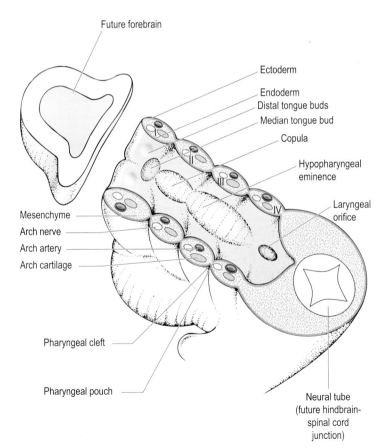

Future forebrain

Ectoderm
Endoderm
Distal tongue buds
Median tongue bud
Copula
Hypopharyngeal eminence
Laryngeal orifice

Mesenchyme
Arch nerve
Arch artery
Arch cartilage

Pharyngeal cleft

Pharyngeal pouch

Neural tube (future hindbrain–spinal cord junction)

Fig. 2.21 Schematic diagram of the floor of the embryonic mouth as viewed from above in a horizontal section of the head. Note the pharyngeal arches (I–IV) have been cut to expose their neural (yellow), arterial (red), cartilaginous (green) and mesenchymal (orange stipple) contents. The arches are lined externally by ectoderm (blue) and internally by endoderm (purple).

Table 2.2 Pharyngeal arch derivatives (arch arteries and their derivatives not included)

Pharyngeal arch	Pouch endoderm	Skeletal elements		Cranial nerve	Muscles
		Ossify in cartilage	Ossify in membrane		
1	Tympanic cavity Pharyngotympanic tube (Cleft ectoderm – external auditory meatus)	Arch cartilage – palatoquadrate bar: alisphenoid, incus Meckel's cartilage – malleus	Arch mesenchyme: upper part – maxilla, zygoma, squamous temporal bone lower part – mandible	Maxillary division of trigeminal (V) (upper part of arch 1) Mandibular division of trigeminal (V) (lower part of arch 1)	From cranial somitomere 4: Muscles of mastication (temporalis, masseter, pterygoids) plus mylohyoid, anterior belly of digastric, tensor tympani, tensor veli, palatini
2	Epithelial lining of tonsillar crypts and tonsillar fossa	Reichert's cartilage: stapes, stylohyoid ligament, upper part of hyoid		Facial nerve (VII)	From somitomere 6: Muscles of facial expression plus posterior belly of digastric, stylohyoid, stapedius
3	Dorsal wing – inferior parathyroid Ventral wing – epithelioid cells of thymus (Hassall's corpuscles and epithelial reticulum)	Lower part of hyoid		Glossopharyngeal nerve (IX)	From somitomere 7: Stylopharyngeus
4	Dorsal wing – superior parathyroid Ventral wing – ultimobranchial body: C cells in thyroid gland		Upper laryngeal cartilages (mesoderm)	Superior laryngeal branch of vagus nerve (X)	From occipital somites 2–4: Pharyngeal constrictors, cricothyroid, levator veli palatini
6			Lower laryngeal cartilages (mesodem)	Recurrent laryngeal nerve (X)	Intrinsic muscles of the larynx

The accessory nerve has all the hallmarks of a branchial arch nerve as its cell bodies in the brainstem and cervical spinal cord are in line with other branchial efferent cell bodies (branchial efferent column), however its evolutionary history, or more specifically the muscles it supplies (sternocleidomastoid and trapezius), is controversial as are many of the musculoskeletal elements of the neck and shoulder (Matsuoka et al., 2005).

2.20A); the majority of the cartilaginous elements of the pharyngeal arches regress and become encased within membrane bones that ossify directly from neural-crest-derived mesenchyme. Such membranous bones include the maxilla, zygoma, squamous temporal bone and dentary (described in most textbooks as the mandible) (Fig. 2.20A).

Some of the cranial nerve sensory neurones (part of V, VII, IX and X), like the dorsal root ganglia of the trunk, arise from the neural crest, as do the four parasympathetic ganglia of the head and neck.

Craniofacial abnormalities

Skeletal development can be considered to have three essential steps: (1) classic induction [as the result of mesenchyme–epithelium interactions mediated by highly conserved signalling molecules such as Bmp (bone morphogenetic protein) and Fgf (fibroblast growth factor)]; (2) condensation of mesenchyme; and (3) overt differentiation. Interestingly 65% of skeletal abnormalities of the head and neck are the result of defects in this first signalling step (Hall, 1998).

It is now recognized that a group of craniofacial abnormalities, the mandibulofacial dysostoses, including Treacher Collins and Hallerman–Streiff syndromes are caused by deficits in neural crest cell migration and differentiation in the first and second pharyngeal arches. These are manifest as abnormal ear development, hypoplasia of the maxilla and mandible, and lower lid defects. These and more generalized disturbances of neural crest migration, e.g. Rieger syndrome, Pierre Robin syndrome, and conditions affecting primarily the periocular region such as Peter's anomaly, are increasingly being classified as *neurocristopathies* because of their proposed link to disturbances in neural crest cell migration, proliferation and differentiation.

DEVELOPMENT OF THE FACE
(Fig. 2.22)

Development of the face commences around the fourth week and is largely complete by week 10. The basic arrangement of the face is the result of fusion of five swellings around the stomodeum (primitive mouth), nasal pits and eyes. There are paired maxillary and mandibular processes plus an unpaired frontonasal process (Fig. 2.22A). The mesenchyme of the frontonasal process, a conspicuous swelling over the developing forebrain vesicles, arises from the neural crest and does not appear to have any association with pharyngeal arch development. The frontonasal process is innervated by the ophthalmic division of the trigeminal nerve and forms the

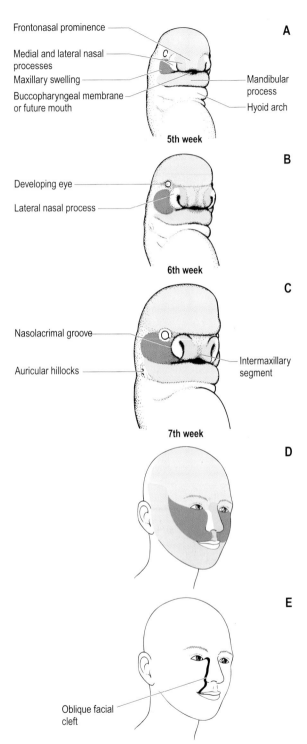

Fig. 2.22 Early development of the face (**A–C**), the adult form (**D**), and one of the many congenital abnormalities, oblique facial cleft (**E**), that results from incomplete fusion of the facial swellings.

tissues above the eye as far back as the vertex, thus explaining the sensory cutaneous distribution in the adult (see p. 79). The frontonasal process also gives rise to medial and lateral nasal swellings around the nasal pits (Fig. 2.22B). The maxillary processes grow medially beneath the developing eyes and form the lower eyelids. Concomitant with this growth, the eyes also move from their position on the lateral aspect of the embryonic head to the front of the face. The *nasolacrimal groove* on each side lies along the line of fusion of the maxillary process with the lateral nasal swelling (Fig. 2.22C). The ectoderm of the groove invaginates (10-mm stage) into the surrounding mesenchyme to form the *nasolacrimal duct*, which at this stage consists of a solid cord of ectodermal cells that grows upwards into the lids to form the canaliculi and downwards into the nose. Canaliculization of the solid columns of cells commences first in the vicinity of the lacrimal sac (3 months). Mesenchyme condenses and ossifies around this cord of cells to form the bony walls of the nasolacrimal canal.

The upper eyelid develops from the frontonasal process and both lids are visible early in the second month (Fig. 2.3E). The primitive lid folds fuse in weeks 9–10 of gestation, enclosing a surface ectoderm-lined cavity, the conjunctival sac (Fig. 2.4D). Myocytes differentiate in the mesenchyme of both lids and eventually form the orbicularis oculi muscle (second arch derived – nerve supply, facial nerve). Meibomian glands, sebaceous glands and eyelashes develop as invaginations of the conjunctival epithelium or epidermis and are therefore ectodermal derivatives. In the seventh week the future *lacrimal gland* arises as a bud of epithelial cells from the region of the upper temporal conjunctiva sac.

Developmental anomalies of the nasolacrimal duct

Disturbances in morphogenetic processes may lead to multiple canaliculi and punctae, abnormal diverticulae, and blockage of the nasolacrimal duct, possibly because of debris from the degenerating central cells producing a mucocoele (not uncommon in the first few weeks after birth).

There is a range of *congenital facial defects*, of which cleft lip and palate are the most common. These are a consequence of complete or partial failure of fusion of the various processes and swellings in the face. Oblique facial clefts occur along the course of the nasolacrimal duct (Fig. 2.22E). The aetiology of these conditions is multifactorial, although maternal exposure to anticonvulsant drugs (phenytoin) and vitamin A are known

---

teratogenic agents that produce these defects. The spatial and temporal expression of retinoic acid receptors during embryological development is currently the subject of much research. While details are still emerging, it is clear that the patterns of expression partially explain the effects of retinoic acid (a vitamin A derivative) as a potent morphogen. Retinoic acid appears sequentially to activate genes of the *Hox* cluster, thereby influencing the normal segmental pattern of hindbrain development (rhombomeres), neural crest migration pathways into pharyngeal arches, and development of the face (Maden et al., 1992).

At birth and in the infant, the eyes in humans are in a comparatively advanced state of development relative to the rest of the face; the orbits are therefore large, although the remainder of the facial skeleton is small by comparison with the adult. During infancy and childhood, as a consequence of the development of teeth and growth of the paranasal sinuses, the facial skeleton steadily increases in size relative to the neurocranium. With the exception of the frontal sinuses, the paranasal sinuses develop as diverticulae from the nasal passages around the fifth month of gestation and are rudimentary at birth. The frontal sinuses appear in the fifth to sixth postnatal year as evaginations from the ethmoid sinuses or middle meatus.

CONGENITAL MALFORMATIONS

Classification of congenital malformations or abnormalities is difficult for several reasons. First, the aetiology is often unknown and, even where a single genetic or environmental cause is suspected, it is often difficult to ascribe full responsibility to such agents or events because exposure to widely different teratogenic agents, such as drugs or trauma, can result in identical developmental defects. Second, defects may be strongly associated with chromosomal abnormality (e.g. trisomy 13).

Trisomy 13 (Patau syndrome)

The ocular pathology in trisomy 13 illustrates various forms of malformation. The cornea and chamber angle are malformed and persistent hyperplastic primary vitreous is common. An anterior coloboma is present and is characterized by a fibrous ingrowth that contains nodules of cartilage. Retinal dysplasia is extensive. Optic nerve malformation is limited to hypoplasia. The systemic malformations are not compatible with survival and are extreme forms of brain malformation (arrhinencephaly) with cardiac and renal malformation.

Trisomy 21 (Down syndrome)

The systemic disturbances in this disorder are well known. In ophthalmology the important components are a high incidence of keratoconus and cataract. Small nodules are formed by spindle cells on the iris (Brushfield's spots); myopia and the attendant complication of retinal detachment may require surgical intervention.

Furthermore, disturbances in basic cellular events such as neural tube closure may lead to multisystem pathologies. In common with more generalized developmental defects, the consequences of exposure to teratogenic agents are highly dependent on the timing of major embryonic or fetal developmental events occurring at the time of exposure: there are important known *periods of vulnerability*, or critical (sensitive) periods, during which morphogenesis of particular systems and organs may be at risk. In this respect the eye is highly vulnerable for a long period of embryonic and fetal development because there are crucial developmental landmarks from the point of formation of the optic pits (day 22) till late in gestation, with such events as retinal vascularization and pupillary membrane regression occurring close to birth.

Congenital malformations affecting ocular tissues may have the following causes.

GENETIC CAUSES

- *Chromosomal anomalies*: deletions (*cri-du-chat* syndrome, Turner syndrome), trisomies (trisomy 13 or Patau syndrome, Down syndrome, Klinefelter syndrome) and triploidy (see Table 2.1).
- *Hereditary*: either sporadic mutations (aniridia with Wilms' tumour) or dominant/recessive inheritance.

ENVIRONMENTAL CAUSES

- *Drugs*: alcohol, tobacco, anticonvulsants, thalidomide.
- *Vitamins and minerals*: excess (e.g. hypervitaminosis A) or deficiency (e.g. folic acid, zinc).
- *Infection*: e.g. rubella, syphilis, toxoplasmosis.
- *Radiation*: X-rays.

MATERNAL AGE

There is an increased incidence of genetic abnormalities in the oocyte with advancing maternal age.

FURTHER READING

Bartelmez GW, Blount MP. The formation of neural crest from the primary optic vesicle in man. Contr Embryol 1954; 35:55–71.

Blankenship T, Peterson PE, Hendricks AG. Emigration of neural crest cells from macaque optic vesicles is correlated with discontinuities in its basement membrane. J Anat 1996; 188:473–483.

Chan-Ling T. Glial, vascular, and neuronal cytogenesis in whole-mounted cat retina. Microsc Res Tech 1997; 36:1–16.

Collinson JM, Hill RE, West J. Analysis of mouse eye development with chimeras and mosaics. Int J Dev Biol 2004; 48:793–804.

Creuzet S, Vincent C, Couly G. Neural crest derivatives in ocular and periocular structures. Int J Dev Biol 2005; 49:161–171.

Cvekl A, Tamm ER. Anterior eye development and ocular mesenchyme: new insights from mouse models and human diseases. BioEssays 2004; 26:374–386.

Erickson CA, Loring JF, Lester SM. Migratory pathways of HNK-1-immunoreactive neural crest cells in the rat embryo. Dev Biol 1989; 134:112–118.

Fukisha Y, Morriss-Kay GM. Migration of neural crest cells to the pharyngeal arches and heart in rat embryos. Cell Tissue Res 1992; 268:1–8.

Gilland E, Baker R. Conservation of neuroepithelial and mesodermal segments in the embryonic vertebrate head. Acta Anat 1993; 148:110–123.

Hall BK. Evolutionary developmental biology. Dordrecht: Kluwer Academic Publishers; 1998.

Hall BK. Bones and cartilage: developmental and evolutionary skeletal biology. London: Elsevier Academic Press; 2005.

Hunt P, Wilkinson D, Krumlauf R. Patterning the vertebrate head: murine *Hox2* genes mark distinct subpopulations of premigratory and migratory cranial neural crest. Development 1991; 112:43–50.

Lang RA. Pathways regulating lens induction in the mouse. Int J Dev Biol 2004; 48:783–791.

Lang RA, Bishop JM. Macrophages are required for cell death and tissue remodelling in the developing mouse eye. Cell 1993; 74:453–462.

Larsen WJ. Human Embryology, 2nd edn. New York: Churchill Livingstone; 1997.

McAvoy JW, Chamberlain CG, de Jongh RU. Lens development. Eye 1999; 13:425–437.

McMenamin PG. The human foetal iridocorneal angle: a scanning electron microscopic study. Br J Ophthalmol 1989; 73:871–879.

McMenamin PG. A morphological study of the inner surface of the anterior chamber angle in pre- and post-natal human eyes. Curr Eye Res 1989; 8:727–739.

McMenamin PG. A quantitative study of the prenatal development of aqueous outflow system in the human eye. Exp Eye Res 1991; 53:507–517.

McMenamin PG, Krause W. Development of the eye in the North American opossum (*Didelphis virginiana*). J Anat 1993; 183:343–358.

McMenamin PG, Djano J, Wealthall R, Griffin BJ. Characterisation of the macrophages associated with the tunica vasculosa lentis of the rat eye. Invest Ophthalmol Vis Sci 2002; 43:2076–2082.

Maden M, Horton C, Graham A, Leonard L, Pizzey J, Siegenthaler G, Lumsden A, Eriksson U. Domains of cellular retinoic acid-binding protein I (CRABP I) expression in the hindbrain and neural crest of the mouse embryo. Mech Dev 1992; 37:13–23.

Mann I. The Development of the Human Eye, 3rd edn. New York: Grune and Stratton, 1964.

Matsuoka T, Ahlberg PE, Kessaris N, Iannarelli P, Dennehy U, Richardson WD, McMahon AP, Koentges G. Neural crest origins of the neck and shoulder. Nature 2005; 436:347–355.

Mendelson C, Larkin S, Mark M, LeMeur M, Clifford J, Zelent A, ChambonP. RARβ isoforms: distinct transcriptional control by retinoic acid and specific spatial patterns of promotor activity during mouse embryonic development. Mech Dev 1994; 45:227–241.

Monaghan AP, Davidson DR, Sime C. The *Msh*-like homeobox genes define domains in the developing vertebrate eye. Development 1991; 112:1053–1061.

Noden D. Periocular mesenchyme: neural crest and mesoderm interactions. In: Jakobiec FA, ed. Ocular anatomy, embryology and teratology. Philadelphia: Harper and Row; 1982:97–119.

Noden DM. Interactions and fate of avian craniofacial mesenchyme. Development 1988; 103 (suppl.):121–140.

Noden DM. Vertebrate craniofacial development: the relation between ontogenetic process and morphological outcome. Brain Behav Evol 1991; 38:190–225.

O'Rahilly R. The prenatal development of the human eye. Exp Eye Res 1966; 21:93–112.

Osumi-Yamashita NO, Noji S, Nohno T, Koyama E, Doi H, Eto K, Taniguchi S. Expression of retinoic acid receptor genes in neural crest-derived cells during mouse facial development. FEBS Lett 1990; 264:71–74.

Ozanics V, Jakobiec FA. Prenatal development of the eye and its adnexa. In: Jakobiec FA, ed. Ocular anatomy, embryology and teratology. Philadelphia: Harper and Row; 1982:11–96.

Patapoutian A, Miner J, Lyons GE, Wold B. Isolated sequences from the linked *Myf-5* and *MRF4* genes drive distinct patterns of muscle-specific expression in transgenic mice. Development 1993; 118:61–69.

Reese BE, Necessary BD, Tam PPL, Faulker-Jones B, Tan SS. Clonal expansion and cell dispersion in the developing mouse retina. Eur J Neurosci 1999; 11:2965–2978.

Robinson SR. Development of the mammalian retina. In: Dreher B, Robinson SR, eds. Neuroanatomy of the visual pathways and their development; Cronly-Dillon JR, series ed. Vision and visual dysfunction, Vol. 3. Basingstoke: Macmillan; 1991:69–128.

Saha MS, Spann C, Grainger RM. Embryonic lens induction: more than meets the optic vesicle. Cell Differ Dev 1989; 28:153–171.

Saint-Geniez M, D'Amore P. Development and pathology of the hyaloid, choroidal and retinal vasculature. Int J Dev Biol 2004; 48:1045–1058.

Schulz MW, Chamberlain CG, de Longh RU, McAvoy JW. Acidic and basic FGF in ocular media and lens: implications for lens polarity and growth patterns. Development 1993; 118:117–126.

Spaeth G, Nelson LB, Beaudoin AR. Ocular teratology. In: Jakobiec FA, ed. Ocular anatomy, embryology and teratology. Philadelphia: Harper and Row; 1982:955–1080.

Sullivan CH, Braunstein L. Hazard-Leonards RM, Holen AL, Samaha F, Stephens L, Grainger RM. A re-examination of lens induction in chicken embryos: in vitro studies of early tissue interactions. Int J Dev Biol 2004; 48:771–782

Trainor PA, Tam PPL. Cranial paraxial mesoderm and neural crest cells of the mouse embryo: co-distribution in the craniofacial mesenchyme but distinct segregation in the branchial arches. Development 1995; 121:2569–2582.

Zieske JD. Corneal development associated with eyelid opening. Int J Dev Biol 2004; 48:903–911.

3 GENETICS

- Chromosomes and cell division
- Molecular genetics (DNA and genes)
- Chromosome defects and gene mutations
- Clinical genetics
- Population genetics
- Understanding the human genome: DNA analysis
- Molecular biology and clinical medicine
- Molecular and cell biology: controlling cell destiny
- Molecular genetics and ophthalmology

Genetic disorders are often thought of as interesting but rare. However, in a population of 100 000, there will be 10 children born with a genetic disorder, a further 10 who will develop genetic disorders in later life, and 10% of adults will have a chronic illness with a strong genetic basis. The advances in medical and molecular genetics have increased our understanding of disease processes, which can be illustrated particularly with examples of inherited ophthalmic disorders.

CHROMOSOMES AND CELL DIVISION

CHROMOSOMES

Human cells contain 46 chromosomes (diploid), consisting of 22 almost identical pairs (homologous autosomes) and a pair of sex chromosomes, which constitute the karyotype of an individual. Chromosomes are numbered 1–22, as they decrease in size. The chromosome consists of two arms: the short arm is designated 'p' and the long arm 'q'. During somatic division, or mitosis, each chromosome, and therefore gene, replicates precisely. Gamete formation involves a special reduction division (meiosis), in which the homologous chromosomes separate from each other so that each cell contains 23 chromosomes (haploid). Since chance determines which chromosome of a pair ends up in a particular gamete, there is a possibility of 2^{23} combinations in the gametes. The different stages of the two forms of cell division are summarized below. The genes are located in a linear order along the chromosome, each gene having a precise location or *locus*. Each of a pair of chromosomes (homologous chromosomes) carries matching genetic information, i.e. they have the same sequence of gene loci. However, at any locus they may have slightly different forms, which are called *alleles*. Cytogenetic analysis of the

143

Box 3.1 Stages of mitosis

Interphase	Resting phase
Prophase	Chromosomes identifiable in nucleus
Metaphase	Chromosomes aligned in centre of nucleus
Anaphase	Centromere of chromosome divides with chromatid separation
Telophase	Daughter chromosomes separate

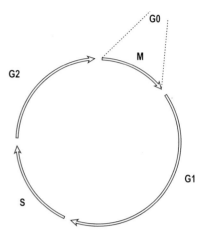

G0	Resting, quiescent
M	Mitosis and cytokinesis (division of cell cytoplasm)
G1 **G2** } Gap phases	– biosynthetic activity – preparation for division
S	Synthesis of DNA and chromosomal replication

Fig. 3.1 The cell cycle: S, synthesis of DNA; M, mitosis and cytokinesis; G₁ and G₂, gap phases.

chromosomes can be performed by looking at the banding pattern of individual chromosomes. Giemsa staining highlights the horizontal banding of the chromosome, by the characteristic pattern of light and dark staining (G-banding). More specific patterns of staining can be performed by looking at *high-resolution banding* with G-banding patterns at the early stages of mitosis (prophase; see below). *Fragile sites* are non-staining gaps that can be demonstrated only when the chromosomes are cultured in specific conditions (e.g. thymidine and folic acid deprivation) and then stained.

CELL DIVISION

Mitosis

During mitosis each chromosome, and with it every gene along its length, replicates to produce two identical daughter cells, so that every nucleated cell (except gametes) has 46 chromosomes (diploid). In culture, the cell cycle of most mammalian cells varies but is usually about 24 hours. Mitosis itself occupies approximately 1 hour of the total time, whereas the time taken to synthesize DNA required for replication is 6–8 hours (Fig. 3.1). The gap phases G_1, between mitosis and synthesis of DNA, and to a lesser extent G_2, between synthesis and mitosis, govern the turnover of the cells because some cells can rest in G_1 for days. It appears that late in G_1 the cell passes a *restriction point* after which it will proceed through the rest of the cell cycle at a standard rate. During the S phase each chromosome replicates, each with its own individual pattern, although homologous pairs of chromosomes replicate synchronously. During G_2, the cell gradually enlarges, doubling its total mass before the next mitosis. Some cells, however, do not divide once they are fully differentiated (e.g. neurones and erythrocytes) and are permanently arrested in a phase known as G_0.

Meiosis: formation of gametes

Meiosis takes place in two stages, both having the same stages as mitosis. In the first stage of meiosis there is a prolonged prophase, in which cell division of only the chromosomes occurs so that each subsequent daughter nucleus contains half the number of chromosomes (23), resembling mitosis but in the haploid state. The prophase of the first meiotic division is complex and may be divided into a further five stages:

- *Leptotene* Starts with the first appearance of the chromosome.
- *Zygotene* The homologous chromosomes pair and bind closely to form bivalents.
- *Pachytene* The main stage of chromosomal thickening; each chromosome consists of two chromatids and, because they are bivalent, has four strands. During this stage, chromatids of the chromosomes exchange material (crossovers), further ensuring a random assortment of paternal and maternal homologues.

- *Diplotene* The bivalents start to separate (the centromere of each remains intact).
- *Diakinesis* The bivalent chromosome formations separate and coil tightly.

The chromosomes then undergo *metaphase* and *anaphase*, where the bivalents disjoin, going to each equatorial plane of the cell, and as the cytoplasm divides each cell has 23 chromosomes, each with a pair of chromatids. The second meiotic division follows the first without an interphase and resembles mitosis. Thus meiosis gives rise to gametes that contain only one representative of each homologous pair of chromosomes and there is random selection of paternal and maternal homologues.

Box 3.2 Control of cell cycle

Cyclins are regulatory subunits within the cell that are periodically synthesized and degraded, regulating cyclin-dependent kinases (CDK) essential for cell cycle control.

Cyclins (of which to date there are nine; A–I) bind to CDKs, forming an active complex that in a controlled fashion drives the cell through its stages via phosphorylation of unique protein substrates, such as retinoblastoma protein, Rb, allowing progression into the next phase of the cycle. Interaction of cyclin–CDK complexes with the retinoblastoma (Rb) protein family (Rb, p107, p130) is regulated by proteins that block cyclin–CDK activity (e.g. p21). p53, a cell cycle regulator, leads to increased p21 expression.

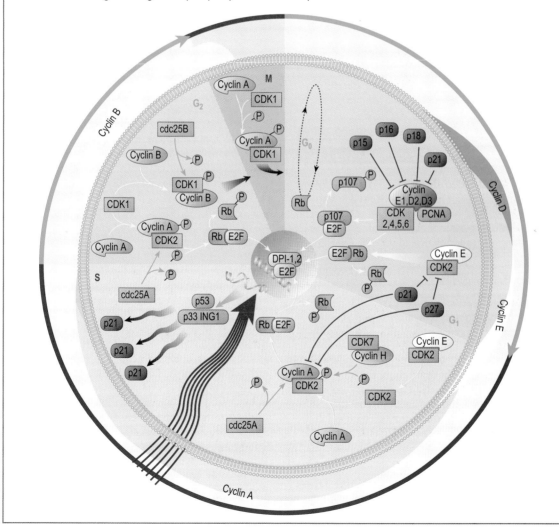

Genetic makeup

The genetic makeup of each individual or of a specific patient population is a result of mutations and natural selection in the past. During cell division, the division of chromosomes may be imperfect. A mutation is a sudden change in the gross or fine structure of DNA, such as might be caused by a replication error or a crossover defect between misaligned chromosomes at meiosis, giving rise to deletion or duplication of DNA. The mechanisms by which chromosomal abnormalities may occur are discussed below. A mutation may affect a specific gene and thus the protein structure it codes for. Equally, the mutation may alter the structure of the protein in such a way that the function of the protein is changed only slightly but the metabolism remains unaffected. If the gene is destroyed altogether, including the nucleotide sequence, which is critically important for the protein that it encodes, then the individual will be at an immediate disadvantage. It is therefore not surprising that it is genetic diseases that occur as a result of harmful mutations, as opposed to diseases with multifactorial inheritance patterns, which have a predictable mode of inheritance.

MOLECULAR GENETICS (DNA AND GENES)

The basis of inherited disease can be understood from information about chromosomal makeup, specific genes, and how proteins are encoded. The human haploid genome consists of 3×10^9 base pairs of double-stranded DNA (dsDNA). The genetic information that determines the sequence of amino acids in peptide chains is stored in the DNA by the order of the nucleotide bases: adenine (A), cytosine (C), guanine (G) and thymine (T). Three bases (a codon) code for a particular amino acid. A gene is part of the DNA that directs the sequencing of polypeptide chains. The gene itself consists of both coding regions (*exons*) and variable-length intervening regions (*introns*). There are also enhancer regions of the gene, which carry out regulatory activities, particularly the expression of genes in tissues. Similarly there is a family of regulatory molecules on the gene that activate or suppress both pairs of homologous genes (Fig. 3.2).

HOW GENES WORK: DECODING DNA

All proteins are encoded in DNA and, as mentioned above, each amino acid is represented by a triplet

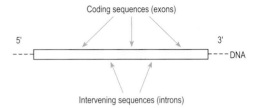

Fig. 3.2 Components of a gene.

code of bases (codon). Since the number of possible codons is greater than the number of amino acids, most amino acids, except methionine and tryptophan, may be encoded by more than one codon. The code AUG (methionine) acts as a starter signal for protein synthesis, and there are also codes that act as polypeptide chain terminators (stop codons).

Polypeptide chain synthesis occurs in two processes: *transcription* and *translation* (Fig. 3.3). During transcription one strand of DNA forms a template for the synthesis of messenger RNA (mRNA), catalysed by the enzyme RNA polymerase. RNA polymerase binds to a specific DNA sequence known as the *promoter*, which signals the unwinding of the DNA helix, which acts as a template for the complementary base pairs. The process moves along the DNA molecule, extending the RNA molecule in the 5′ to 3′ direction. This process continues until it meets the termination signal on the DNA molecule. The first transcript is an exact replica of the single strand of DNA. Before leaving the nucleus the introns are excised and the exons are spliced together. On leaving the nucleus the mRNA acts as a template on cytoplasmic ribosomes for protein synthesis. The mRNA 5′ end is blocked before the whole molecule is transcribed with 7-methylguanine joined 5′ to 5′ and a 3′ poly-A tail, which aids transport into the cytoplasm. The poly-A tail is added after transcription by *poly-A polymerase*. Translation of nucleotide sequences is performed by specific transfer RNA (tRNA): amino acids, each specific for three nucleotide bases, are attached before polymerization into polypeptide chains. They are attached by their C-terminal ends and are transformed into high-energy molecules, from which peptide bonds form to produce polypeptides. Each tRNA (anticodons) is linked with the appropriate codons on the mRNA. This process of translation is controlled by a set of enzymes called *aminoacyl-tRNA synthetases*, which couple each amino acid to the appropriate tRNA molecule. The mRNA sequence is read three nucleotides at a time from the 5′ to 3′ direction along the mRNA. The polypeptide chain is constructed from

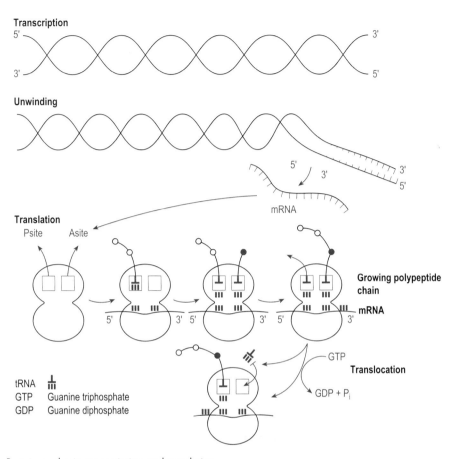

Fig. 3.3 Protein synthesis: transcription and translation.

its N-terminal end to its C-terminal end, and the growing C-terminal end of the protein remains activated by covalent attachment to the tRNA (peptidyl-tRNA molecule). The mRNA is coded with specific start and stop codons, which thus determine the length of the polypeptide chain. The initiation of polypeptide chain synthesis is under the control of initiation factor 2 (IF-2), which catalyses the reaction between a specific initiator tRNA molecule and the mRNA. The growing polypeptide chain must be exactly three nucleotides along the mRNA after the addition of each amino acid, which requires a multienzyme system incorporated within the ribosome. Ribosomes are half RNA by weight and have a groove that accommodates a growing polypeptide chain and a groove that accommodates each mRNA molecule. On the ribosome there are two different binding sites for tRNA. One site holds the tRNA and growing polypeptide chain, the peptidyl-tRNA binding site (P site), and the other site holds the incoming tRNA molecule, the aminoacyl-tRNA binding site (A site). The process of polypeptide chain elongation involves two steps. The first step involves an aminoacyl-tRNA molecule becoming bound to the A site adjacent to an occupied P site. The second step involves uncoupling the C-terminal end of the polypeptide chain from the tRNA in the P site and joining it to the tRNA molecule in the A site. The reaction is catalysed by *peptidyl transferase*, which is present on the ribosome. The new peptidyl-tRNA molecule is then transferred to the P site, releasing the now unoccupied tRNA molecule, and the whole process is repeated. The stop codon on the mRNA initiates a protein called *release factor* to bind to the A site, causing hydrolysation of the peptidyl-tRNA molecule on the P site and subsequent release of the polypeptide chain into the cell cytoplasm.

Genes are regulated by adjacent sequences on the genome. Upstream of the gene is the *promoter*,

147

Box 3.3 Summary of protein synthesis

Messenger RNA is produced from DNA transcription under control of the enzyme 5′–3′ RNA polymerase. Translation begins in the cell cytoplasm by the binding of mRNA to ribosomal subunits, to which an initiator tRNA molecule binds. Amino-acid-specific tRNAs have anticodons specific for a triplet of nucleotides (codon), forming the aminoacyl-tRNA molecule, which binds to the A site on the ribosome under the control of an enzyme, aminoacyl-tRNA synthetase. Each amino acid is added to the C-terminal of the growing polypeptide chain, progressing from codon to codon in the 5′ to 3′ direction of the mRNA. The length of the polypeptide chain is regulated by specific start and stop codons.

which is involved in the attachment of RNA polymerase to the DNA strand. Promoters have an element called a TATA box, which specifies the correct 5′ end of the RNA precursor. Several promoter-specific transcription factors have now been isolated, each specific for a gene promoter which, when bound, activates transcription. TATA binding protein is a general transcription factor for RNA polymerases I, II and III. *RNA polymerase III* is responsible for the synthesis of a variety of small RNA molecules including tRNA and small subunits of ribosomal RNA. *RNA polymerase II* carries out the transcription of genes, and *RNA polymerase I* synthesizes the large subunits of ribosomal RNA.

CHROMOSOME DEFECTS AND GENE MUTATIONS

During cell division the division of chromosomes may be imperfect. The extent, however, of genetically determined disease remains undetermined. The risk of genetic abnormality detectable at birth or in infancy is approximately 1 in 40. However, most fetuses with chromosomal aberrations are spontaneously aborted and it has been estimated that the frequency of genetic defects in live births is 0.6% and in stillbirths 5%. Chronic diseases with a significant genetic contribution occur in about 10% of the adult population. Abnormalities of the chromosomes are usually classified as numeric abnormalities, where somatic cells contain an abnormal number of normal chromosomes, or as structural abnormalities, where somatic cells contain one or more abnormal chromosomes, which in turn may affect either sex or autosomal chromosomes.

NUMERIC CHROMOSOMAL ABNORMALITIES

Aneuploidy arises from failure of paired chromosomes to disjoin or as a result of delayed movement during anaphase, thus producing an extra copy of the chromosome (trisomy) or a missing copy of the chromosome (monosomy). Meiotic aneuploidy can occur during either of the stages of meiosis. Polyploidy describes a complete extra set of chromosomes (69 in triploidy), which usually results from fertilization of the ovum by two sperm cells. This usually results in miscarriage.

Autosomal trisomies (Fig. 3.4)

Trisomy describes the individual chromosome that is somatically triplicated in the cell. Triplication of individual chromosomes gives rise to characteristic syndromes with multisystem disorders. Examples of

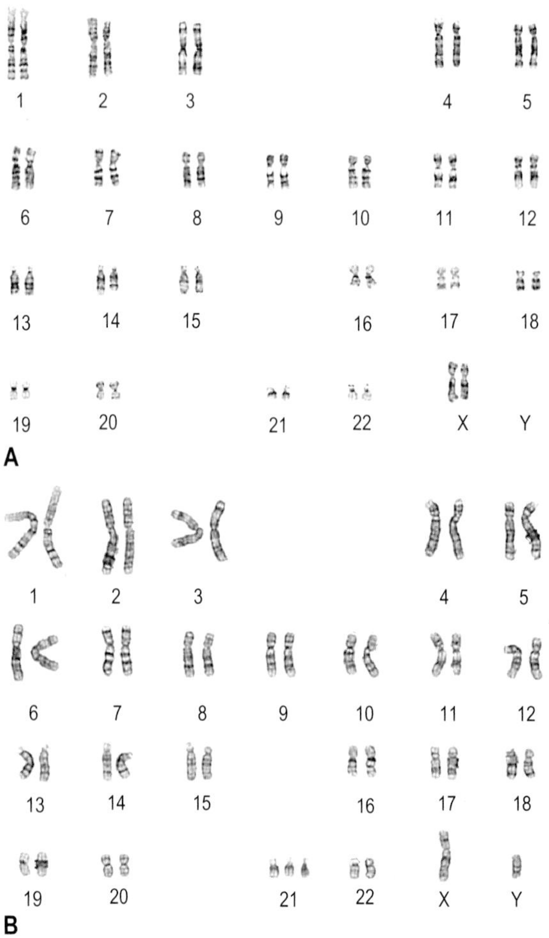

Fig. 3.4 (**A**) Normal human karyotype: 22 autosome pairs and sex chromosomes. (**B**) Trisomy of chromosome 21.

autosomal trisomies include trisomy of chromosome 21 (Down syndrome), chromosome 18 (Edwards syndrome) and chromosome 13 (Patau syndrome) (see Ch. 9). In each of the autosomal trisomies, mosaicisms (two or more cell lineages derived from a single zygote) may influence the clinical picture markedly, particularly when the normal cell line is present in a critical tissue. Trisomy, as mentioned above, may result from a failure of the separation of chromosome pairs during cell division (non-disjunction) or (in approximately 4% of cases) from translocation of one chromosome onto another inherited from one of the parents, thus giving the offspring a normal number of chromosomes but with a translocated copy of, for example, chromosome 21 (Robertsonian translocation) (see below).

Meiotic aneuploidy

Similar chromosomal anomalies exist with the sex chromosomes, whereby an extra X or Y chromosome gives rise to a phenotype not distinguished in the normal population. Loss of an X chromosome gives rise to Turner syndrome (45 X0), which again may not present with the characteristic phenotype because of the prevalence of mosaic forms and therefore normal sexual development may be present. This is also true for Klinefelter syndrome, in which there is an extra X chromosome (47 XXY).

STRUCTURAL CHROMOSOMAL ABNORMALITIES

Structural chromosomal abnormalities result from chromosomal breakage. Normally single breaks are repaired quickly, but if more than one break occurs repair mechanisms may cause random rejoining of the wrong ends. Spontaneous breakage increases with exposure to mutagenic chemicals and ionizing radiation. The following structural abnormalities may occur:

- Translocation – chromosomes break and exchange segments
- Inversion – segment of chromosome is inverted in sequence
- Deletion – section of chromosome is lost
- Mutation – point mutation occurs with a change in a single base of a triplet code of a gene.

Translocation usually results in no loss of DNA so that individuals may appear clinically normal. Translocation may be reciprocal if exchange of chro-

mosomal segments distal to the breaks occurs. *Robertsonian* translocation arises from breaks at or near the centromere in two acrocentric chromosomes (centromere near from one end of the chromosome). Translocation of segments on chromosomes 14 and 21 may occur and, during meiosis, a trivalent is formed which will then lead to a mosaic of normal and abnormal karyotype during anaphase. Insertional translocation requires the occurrence of three breaks in one or two chromosomes, resulting in deletion of one segment and insertion of another into the gap in the first chromosome. Inversions arise from two chromosomal breaks and the segment being inverted through 180°C between the breaks. Inversions interfere with the pairing of chromosomes during meoisis and crossovers are suppressed, generating unbalanced gametes. Deletion may also occur when only part of the chromosome is lost. This can occur between two breakpoints or as a result of breaks and loss of segments in both arms of the chromosome. Point mutations, on the other hand, occur when a single nucleotide base is replaced by another, which may in turn alter the amino acid coding for that protein.

GENE MUTATIONS

Many types of mutation may occur throughout the alleles at each locus. Within the normal population, and in examples of inherited disease, mutations can occur that range from a single base pair to deletion of large gene segments involving many millions of base pairs. The description of these mutations has led to increasing availability of diagnostic and screening tools for genetic disease. Box 3.4 details the diversity of gene mutations that occur within the human genome.

CLINICAL GENETICS

There are five main types of genetic disorders: chromosomal (see above), mitochondrial, multifactorial, somatic cell genetic and single gene (autosomal and X-linked inheritance) disorders.

AUTOSOMAL INHERITANCE

A trait that is determined by a gene on an autosome may be *dominant* or *recessive*. Heterozygotes are individuals with different alleles at the corresponding locus on the pair of homologous chromosomes. Homozygotes have the same allele. As such,

Box 3.4 Mutations within the human genome

Point mutation (nucleotide substitution)
A single nucleotide change in the transcribed codon leading to a different amino acid substitution in the polypeptide chain – *missense mutation*.

A single nucleotide change which results in a stop codon, giving rise to a shortened polypeptide chain, or vice versa resulting in an elongated polypeptide chain – *nonsense mutation*.

A single nucleotide base change which alters a critical splice junction and leads to abnormal RNA processing or a reduction in the normal gene product, or prevents the efficient addition of the poly-A chain for effective transcription – *splice site mutation*.

Deletions and insertions (frame shifts)
Deletion of one or two nucleotide bases leading to incorrect reading during translation and resulting in an inappropriate amino acid sequence and premature termination of the polypeptide chain.

Codon deletions and insertion (repeat expansions)
Insertion of a repeated codon (three nucleotide bases) that as a consequence interrupts the coding sequence. These mutations, known as *triplet repeats*, are found in myotonic dystrophy, the fragile X syndrome (X-linked mental retardation), Huntington's disease and spinocerebellar ataxia.

Box 3.5 Characteristics of Mendelian inheritance

Autosomal dominant
- Vertical transmission
- 50% of offspring affected
- Males and females affected equally
- Variable expressivity
- Unaffected persons do not pass on trait
- Homozygotes are more severely affected.

Autosomal recessive
- Recessive gene does not cause disease in heterozygote
- Disease expressed in homozygotes
- Males and females affected equally
- Constant expressivity
- Affected individuals have children who are carriers.

X-linked recessive
- Vertical transmission
- Usually only males are affected
- All daughters of affected males are carriers
- Heterozygous females may be affected because of 'lyonization'
- Variable expressivity.

case neither parent expresses the disease. Affected individuals have a 1 in 2 chance of passing it on to their child. This form of inheritance is not related to sex chromosomes and male-to-male transmission may occur. In contrast, X-linked disorders cannot be transmitted by males (see below). In clinical practice the detection of autosomal dominantly inherited disease is complicated by variation in expression of the gene and by new mutations. As such the clinical manifestation in an affected individual may not be apparent, giving rise to the view that the condition has skipped a generation. Most autosomal dominant disorders present clinically with features in later life, often after the carriers of the gene have completed their families. This raises difficulties in genetic

autosomal dominant refers to the situation where a monogenetic disorder manifests clinically in the heterozygous state, and inheritance is usually from one parent only.

Autosomal dominant disorders
The overall incidence of autosomal dominant inheritance (Fig. 3.5A) of disease in the UK is 7 per 1000 live births. Usually there is one affected parent, unless the trait occurs as a new mutation, in which

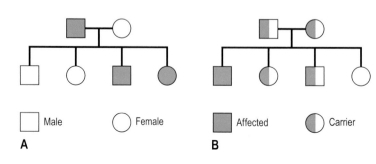

Male   Female   Affected   Carrier

Fig. 3.5 Pedigree of (**A**) autosomal dominant inheritance, (**B**) recessive inheritance.

A   B

counselling, and for this reason consideration is now being given to developing predictive tests based on gene tracking with DNA probes. The more severe the disorder the less likely the individual is to reproduce, so that the proportion of individuals affected as a result of new mutations will increase. Both new mutations and variable gene expression can combine to create difficult clinical decisions for the affected individuals as well as the clinical geneticist.

Autosomal recessive disorders

Autosomal recessive traits affect both sexes but the trait is manifest only if both abnormal genes are present (Fig. 3.5B), i.e. the patient has no normal allele at the affected locus. Usually both parents are heterozygous carriers of the gene in question and are clinically normal. Thus there is a 1 in 4 chance of any offspring being affected, a 1 in 2 chance of producing a heterozygous carrier, and a 1 in 4 chance of being normal. In rare recessive traits there is usually a strong family history of consanguinity between first cousins, who share 1 in 8 of their genes by virtue of their common ancestry. In practical terms the incidence of severe autosomal recessive disorders is low, making the risk to the sibling of first-cousin parents small. In the UK the overall incidence of autosomal recessive disorders is 2.5 per 1000 live births, the commonest being cystic fibrosis.

X-linked disorders

X-linked inheritance refers to the pattern of inheritance carried by the genes on the sex chromosomes. This inheritance therefore carries a characteristic family pedigree (Fig. 3.6). An X-linked recessive trait carried on the X chromosome is manifest only in females when the homozygous state exists, because in heterozygotes the normal dominant gene would be expressed. Such individuals may express disease traits. Traits are thus transmitted from healthy female carriers or affected males. An affected male would pass the trait to all his daughters, who would then be heterozygous carriers, but he would be unable to pass the disorder on to his sons, who receive only his Y chromosome. In some X-linked recessive disorders a proportion of female heterozygotes are affected more as a trait. The explanation lies in the fact that only one of the X chromosomes in a cell is active (Lyon hypothesis; see Box 3.6). This inactivation occurs early in ontogeny and thereafter the descendants of the cell have the same inactive X chromosome. By chance, therefore, females may inactivate the healthy chromosome and thus manifest the disease.

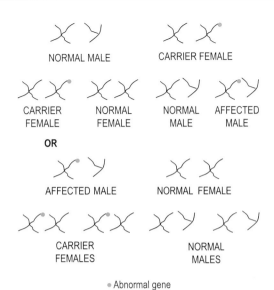

Fig. 3.6 Pedigree of X-linked recessive inheritance.

In the UK the incidence of X-linked inherited disorders is around 1 per 1000 live births. The term X-linked dominant has been used to describe X-linked inheritance where the heterozygous female is regularly affected. In these disorders males are frequently more severely affected and do not survive gestation (e.g. Aicardi syndrome: agenesis of the corpus callosum and chorioretinopathy). If the affected male does reproduce, none of the sons will be affected and all the daughters will be. Occasionally these pedigree patterns may be mimicked by autosomal traits that display sex limitation. If the affected males of an autosomal dominant trait with sex limitation are infertile, the pedigree pattern is identical to that of X-linked recessive traits, except that carrier females exhibit lyonization. The family pedigree will also show a smaller proportion of affected females than would be expected in X-linked dominant traits.

MITOCHONDRIAL INHERITANCE

Cells have multiple copies of an extranuclear chromosome, contained in mitochondria. The mitochondria contain about 10 single circular chromosomes, which replicate independently of the nuclear genome. Within their genome there are the genes for tRNA and ribosomal RNA necessary for mitochondrial protein synthesis and peptides involved in cellular oxidative phosphorylation. As the acrosome of the sperm is lost during fertilization, the inheritance of mitochondrial chromosomes

3 GENETICS

Box 3.6 Lyonization

Lyonization is the process of inactivation of one member of a pair of X chromosomes in every female somatic cell. The Barr body (densely stained mass of chromatin, which is the inactivated X chromosome) occurs in the trophoblast by day 12 after fertilization. Inactivation occurs only in somatic cells; it is random and then fixed for all subsequent generations of that cell line. The inactive X chromosome is not transcribed, except for a small region at the tip of the short arm. If loss of material occurs in one X chromosome, then the structurally abnormal chromosome is inactivated. About 30% of cells from buccal smears show a Barr body and 1–10% of female neutrophils will also show an inactivated X chromosome (Drumstick). Females have random expression of either paternal or maternal X chromosome, which clinically gives rise to patchy expression of mutant X-linked genes in carrier females (e.g. retinitis pigmentosa and choroidermia).

Table 3.1 HLA-linked disease associations

Disease	HLA allele	Relative risk
Ankylosing spondylitis	B27	90–100
Acute anterior uveitis	B25	8
Reiter syndrome	B27	40
Behçet syndrome	B51	4–10
Birdshot chorioretinopathy	A29	50–224
Intermediate uveitis	DR15	6
Sympathetic ophthalmia	DR4	14
Vogt-Koyanagi-Harada syndrome	DR4	12

is exclusively through the female ova, which gives rise to a characteristic form of cytoplasmic inheritance with the following features: there is no transmission from males to their offspring, although both males and females can receive the defective gene from their mother; if all the mitochondria carried the gene, then all offspring of the affected woman would also be affected. However, the precise pattern of the disease may not be recognized if only a proportion of the mitochondrial genes are affected.

MULTIFACTORIAL INHERITANCE

There are many conditions that have a familial incidence, yet the incidence of affected siblings is less than can be accounted for by unifactorial Mendelian inheritance. This is because the clinical presentation is influenced by several genes and by environmental factors. In multifactorial inheritance both genetic and environmental factors combine in varying proportions in different individuals to permit the disease to be manifest. Each trait is determined by the interaction of a number of genes at different loci. Multifactorial inheritance may be *continuous* or *discontinuous*. In discontinuous multifactorial traits the risk within affected families is raised above that in the general population, but is low compared with that of single-gene defects. In continuous traits there is a range of disease expression, with individuals falling between two extremes (for example, blood pressure).

Multifactorial discontinuous traits have an increased incidence in affected families compared with that in the general population. If multifactorial inheritance is suspected, twin concordance and family correlation studies are undertaken. For instance, in multifactorial inheritance the incidence of the trait in monozygotic twins will exceed that in dizygotic twins. Some discontinuous multifactorial traits will also show unequal sex distribution, indicating that for one of the sexes the threshold for disease penetrance is higher than for the other sex, i.e. a higher proportion of underactive genes is required before the disease is expressed.

DISEASE ASSOCIATIONS

One approach to identifying disease associations with a specific genotype is to examine major genetic polymorphisms in a population and search for associations. Strong associations have been obtained between ankylosing spondylitis and *HLA-B27*, and birdshot chorioretinopathy and *HLA-A29*. In practice it is perhaps the absence of such allelic correlations that is more useful in predicting disease occurrence. Disease associations can be expressed as relative risk by comparing the incidence of the allele within a control population with allelic expression in patients. Table 3.1 gives a list of some of the commoner associations. Currently, high-resolution typing that characterizes the nucleic acid sequence of major histocompatibility complex alleles has meant that, for example, classical DR4 associations are now further subtyped, e.g. the association of *DRB1 *0404* with sympathic ophthalmia and Vogt–Koyanagi–Harada syndrome.

Genetic polymorphisms

Within the human genome many gene loci possess commonly occurring alleles, which can be used to distinguish populations into discrete phenotypes. This was first described for components of human blood, particularly ABO and MNS phenotypes, where allelic differences in the former determine terminal sugar residues on membrane glycoproteins and those in the latter determine the amino acid sequence of membrane-bound glycoproteins. This is also true for the Rhesus system where polymorphisms exist for the Rhesus polypeptide on the red blood cell membrane. Genetic polymorphisms are defined as the occurrence of multiple alleles at a locus, where at least two alleles occur with a frequency greater than 1%. The existence of different versions of the same genetic material in different people has prompted their use as genetic markers. This is particularly the case for human enzymes and other proteins in which polymorphisms are detectable in population groups. The use of polymorphisms in genetics will be highlighted below when we discuss the types and uses of molecular polymorphisms. To summarize at this point, their practical use in medical genetics is seen for mapping genes to individual chromosomes by linkage analysis (see below), presymptomatic and prenatal diagnosis of genetic disease (see Box 3.9 on p. 109), evaluation of high-risk and low-risk persons with a predisposition to common adult disorders (e.g. diabetes mellitus), and tissue typing for both tissue and organ transplantation.

POPULATION GENETICS

Population genetics is the study of the distribution of genes within populations and how these gene frequencies are changed or maintained. This form of study is important for the understanding of *linkage analysis* (linked genes that have their loci within measurable distances of one another on the same chromosome) and *linkage disequilibrium* (the association of two linked alleles more frequently than would be expected by chance), which is described later.

GENE FREQUENCY

When contemplating the genetic makeup of whole populations, in particular when relating the frequency of people who are heterozygotes at a particular locus to the frequency of homozygotes, the *Hardy–Weinberg equilibrium* is employed. This calculation is based on the assumption that in a given population where random mating occurs, in the absence of mutation and selection, the genetic constitution remains the same from one generation to the next.

It is important to remember that genes are paired in alleles, so that within the Hardy–Weinberg equilibrium, p is the proportion of normal alleles and q is the proportion of abnormal alleles, so that $p + q = 1$. Since a pair of alleles occurs at each gene locus, the relative proportions of normal homozygotes, heterozygotes and abnormal homozygotes are given by the equation: $p^2 + 2pq + q^2 = 1$.

A few important points can be derived from this equation.

- Although the gene frequency determines the chance of any one chromosome carrying the abnormal allele, individuals have two alleles for each gene, which thus doubles the chance of having the abnormal allele on one or other chromosome.
- The heterozygote frequency is often twice the gene frequency.
- In autosomal recessive inherited disorders the gene frequency is the square root of the abnormal homozygote frequency.

It is also important to note that the Hardy–Weinberg equilibrium is concerned only with alleles at a single gene locus; in practical terms the relationship of gene loci to each other along the length of the chromosomes is of greater importance.

GENETIC LINKAGE AND LINKAGE ANALYSIS

Two genes may be transmitted more frequently than independent assortment would suggest.

During meiosis a crossing over between homologous chromosomes may occur at any point along the length of the chromosome. Therefore, the closer two genes are to each other, the more likely they are to be transmitted together. Gene loci on the same chromosome are therefore said to be linked when their alleles do not show independent segregation during meiosis (i.e. their loci are within measurable distance of one another on the same chromosome). Although genes may be mapped on the chromosome by techniques such as in-situ hybridization (see below), genetic linkage may also be shown by family studies, confirming a genetic background to the disorder. In a family linkage study two loci are

153

considered: one for the disease, the other for the trait.

One way of performing linkage analysis is to study family members who are heterozygous at each of the gene loci. One must first establish the linkage phase, determining which allele at locus 1 to be studied is on the same chromosome (of a pair) as a particular allele at locus 2 (marker locus). The family must of course be informative for the loci being considered (i.e. express the phenotype). The loci most informative for linkage analysis are those that are highly polymorphic and thus heterozygous in a large proportion of the population. The probability of meiotic crossing over between them is in effect a means of describing the distance between linked loci. Gene loci that are sufficiently well separated on the same chromosome will always have several crossovers between them and thus exhibit a 50% recombination rate (as if they were situated on different chromosomes and segregating independently). To establish the probability of two gene loci being linked, the number of opportunities for recombination and the proportion in which they have occurred is counted. This may be given as a ratio of the probability of observing the data in the sibship, based on the assumption that there is no linkage between the two loci. As large sibships are required to assess probability of linkage, it is calculated by computer and given as a logarithmic ratio, known as the Lod score (derived from log odds). In most situations there is significant linkage if the Lod score is greater than 3, and linkage can be ruled out if it reaches −2.

Linkage equilibrium and disequilibrium

Linkage equilibrium exists when, in the presence of random mating and given enough generations, the various combinations of alleles that could occur are expressed with equal proportion. *Linkage disequilibrium*, on the other hand, describes the association of two alleles more frequently than would occur by chance. This linkage may arise from mutation of one allele that has not yet established equilibrium because of a selective advantage or disadvantage. The same principles of equilibrium and disequilibrium can apply to alleles of any linked gene loci. At this point it should be emphasized that close linkage between a disease-specific gene locus and a gene showing considerable polymorphism does not necessarily mean association between the two particular alleles of the gene loci. The association between disease and human leucocyte antigens (HLA), for example, arises as a result of both genetic linkage

between *HLA* allele and the disease susceptibility gene, and linkage disequilibrium involving the particular allele at the *HLA* locus. Linkage disequilibrium is important clinically as a means of identifying disease-causing genes and identifying the origin and spread of mutations. As mentioned above, genetic polymorphism is the occurrence in the same population of two or more discontinuous traits at a frequency where the rarest trait would not be maintained by recurrent mutation alone. The most commonly accounted genetic polymorphisms exist within blood groups (ABO) and cell surface antigens (HLA) but more recently, with the advent of molecular biological techniques, DNA sequences of genes have shown that many are polymorphic (see below).

UNDERSTANDING THE HUMAN GENOME: DNA ANALYSIS

The advent of modern molecular biological techniques has benefited many branches of medicine, including ophthalmology. In particular the techniques described below have increased our fundamental understanding of such conditions as X-linked ophthalmic disorders, retinoblastoma and Leber's hereditary optic neuropathy. Some of the techniques used to examine genes and genetic linkage are shown, with examples of how this has helped in the identification and understanding of the molecular and genetic basis of ophthalmic diseases.

CLONING

Cloning (Fig. 3.7) is an *in vivo* technique that produces identical copies of DNA sequences, which can then be used as gene probes. Cloning is achieved by inserting the specific fragment of DNA to be studied into another DNA molecule, which can then be replicated quickly in bacteria (recombination). Fragments of DNA can consistently be obtained by cleaving the DNA with naturally occurring enzymes, known as *restriction endonucleases*. These restriction enzymes cut DNA at specific recognition sites, usually into lengths of four to six nucleotide base sequences. Reproducing large quantities of the same DNA fragment (i.e. cloning) can, however, be performed only by transferring the genetic material into a bacterium via a vector. The common vectors are bacteriophages or modified bacterial plasmids (extrachromosomal, self-replicating, circular DNA). The choice of vector is dependent on the size of DNA fragment to be cloned: bacteriophages have a capacity of 5–20 kilobases (kb) and plasmids a smaller

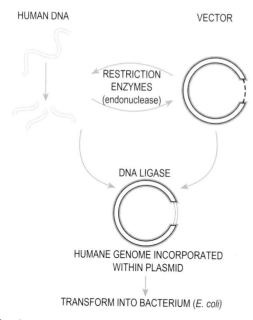

Fig. 3.7 Recombinant DNA technology: cloning.

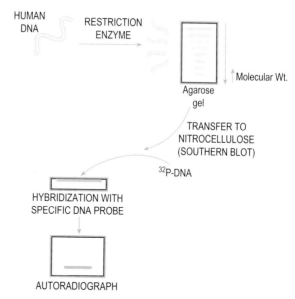

Fig. 3.8 Recombinant DNA technology: Southern blotting.

capacity of up to 10 kb. These vectors replicate their own DNA independently of the host DNA and also have single restriction enzyme sites, which allow insertion of recombinant molecules. After slicing the DNA molecule the recombinant DNA is prepared by incubation of the plasmid with the fragment in the presence of an enzyme, *DNA ligase*, which ligates or binds the DNA to the cut ends of the plasmid. To date, over 200 restriction enzyme sites have been recognized. Restriction enzymes are named according to the organism of origin, e.g. E-cor is derived from *Escherichia coli*.

MOLECULAR ANALYSIS OF HUMAN GENES AND MUTATIONS

Southern and Northern blotting

The total DNA from a sample of an individual's cells may be cut into fragments using restriction endonucleases. The fragments can then be analysed according to their molecular weight by electrophoresis. The DNA fragments are denatured into single-stranded DNA and blotted on to nitrocellulose. Single-strand copies of a segment of DNA that has been cloned and labelled with a radioisotope (^{32}P), known as a DNA probe, are then hybridized with the complementary nucleotide sequences by incubating the radioactive probe with the blotted DNA in the nitrocellulose membrane. The complementary sequences are revealed as bands, by autoradiography

(Southern blotting; Fig. 3.8). In a similar way, mRNA fragments can be detected by Northern blotting, in which labelled DNA probes are hybridized with electrophoresed and blotted mRNA fragments. Both the size and abundance of the mRNA from a specific gene in a sample of RNA can be determined.

DNA POLYMORPHISMS

Polymorphisms in DNA segments (genes) can be detected by many techniques, two of which are restriction fragment length polymorphism (RFLP) and variable number of tandem repeats (VNTR) polymorphism.

Restriction fragment length polymorphism

RFLP occurs because of point mutations in the human genome, which normally occur in the non-coding regions of the DNA molecule. As a result of these acquired polymorphisms, recognition sites for the restriction endonucleases are created or abolished. The consequence is that restriction enzymes will produce variable lengths of DNA fragments, which give characteristic banding on Southern blotting. If an individual is heterozygous for an RFLP, one restriction band on the electrophoretic gel corresponds to one chromosome and the other band to the other chromosome of the pair. This allows one to track the transmission of a single chromosome region through the family and perform classic linkage studies. The discovery of DNA polymorphisms has greatly increased the extent to which individual copies of particular genes are recognized as being truly unique. In fact, DNA polymorphisms are simply the molecular manifestations of variations in the genome, which have been recognized for a long time from studies of protein polymorphisms.

Variable number of tandem repeats polymorphism

Also within the genome are many tandem repeats of sequences that vary for each individual. The sequences act as spacers between restriction enzyme sites. VNTR polymorphisms are short sequences of DNA and the distance between the VNTR depends on the number of repeats. VNTR are heterozygous and can be detected using probes for the core sequence that gives rise to these repeats. VNTR are highly polymorphic and almost unique for each individual (genetic fingerprinting). VNTR markers are highly informative for genetic linkage analysis as well as for individual identification (paternity and forensic testing). Within the genome there are several classes of repetitive DNA, whose nucleotide sequence is repeated several hundred times within the genome. These tandem repeats are again highly polymorphic and can be used for genetic linkage studies.

POLYMERASE CHAIN REACTION

The polymerase chain reaction (PCR) is a technique that allows small amounts of DNA to be amplified for detection and analysis. PCR requires two flanking sequences to the sequence that is to be amplified. DNA primers are formed from short sequences of DNA with these flanking sequences. Amplification of the DNA sequence uses heat-resistant DNA polymerase to extend the short DNA primers of about 20 base pairs, which are hybridized at either end. Cycles of denaturation with heat and polymerization with cooling occur up to 50 times. As a result the target DNA is amplified 10^5–10^6 times. This process, which is largely automated, is proving a great asset in detecting specific DNA where the amount of starting material is very small, e.g. neonatal diagnosis and the identification of infective organisms in tissue samples, and as a research tool. However, quality control of false-positive rates must be established before its full clinical efficacy can be ascertained.

GENOMICS, TRANSCRIPTOMICS AND PROTEOMICS

The genome contains genes that, as we have already described in this chapter, are transcribed to produce RNA and ultimately generate proteins. What has been realized since the findings of the Human Genome Project is that there are very many more proteins in the *human proteome* than there are genes in the *human genome* (circa 400 000 proteins and 22 000 genes). The study of the *genome (Genomics)* has been made possible by the development of *gene arrays* (Fig. 3.9). Gene arrays are DNA microarrays (small solid platform devices with thousands of DNA sequences corresponding to genes, immobilized on a variety of surfaces – nylon membranes or glass) which give us the ability to look at many genes at one time. As such we can get a picture of the possible interactions among thousands of genes. The array is an orderly arrangement of gene-specific DNA that is hybridized to mixtures of labelled RNA in samples. Therefore, based on the amount of signal from successful hybridization, we can determine the relative expression of the corresponding gene. With such a capability we can now compare the extent of gene expression within a sample or of specific genes between samples (see Box 3.7).

However, the genome is only a source of information and the initial step to provide proteins involves the transcription to RNA, where the *transcriptome* is the complete set of RNA transcripts. *Transcriptomics* is the ability to study the dynamic *transcriptome*, which varies depending upon the cell, the stage of cellular development and activation and environmental influences. *Transcriptomics* allows us to investigate the control of RNA transcripts by activating or inactivating transcription factors that control RNA transcription, and this looking at gene expres-

---

Box 3.7 Gene arrays (Affymettrix GeneChips®)

- Isolate RNA from sample or samples to be compared
- Convert to DNA with reverse transcriptase – complementary or cDNA
- Hybridize the labelled cDNA (e.g. ^{32}P) to arrays with fixed DNA sequences (spot sizes on plate of 300 µm)
- Remove unhybridized cDNA
- Detect and quantify hybridized cDNA.

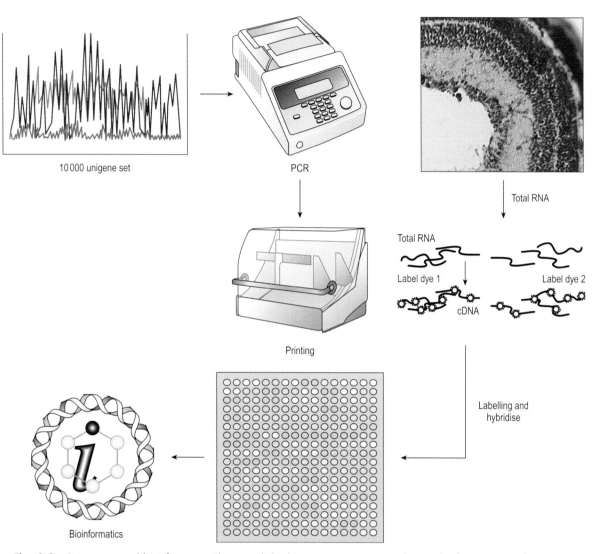

Fig. 3.9 Gene array and bioinformatics. The array hybridization generates many thousands of computational parameters describing upregulation and downregulation of genes that have been targeted and require quantification. (Courtesy of UOB Transcriptomics Facility and Dr Chungui Lu, School of Biological Sciences, University of Bristol.)

10 000 unigene set

PCR

Total RNA

Total RNA

Label dye 1

Label dye 2

cDNA

Printing

Labelling and hybridise

Bioinformatics

sion patterns under various conditions or comparing normal with pathology. The dynamics of the system are further exemplified by the fact that there are very many more proteins than genes. Also ultimately cell and tissue behaviour is defined by protein interactions both intracellularly and extracellularly. *Proteomics* studies these dynamic consequences of gene expression. The study relies on an ability to separate and identify proteins by, for example, mass spectrometry, gel quantification (two-dimensional electrophoresis) and protein sequence analysis. *Structural Proteomics* determines three-dimensional structure by X-ray crystallography and nuclear magnetic resonance spectroscopy. How proteins interact can be assessed by affinity chromatography and fluorescent resonance energy transfer (FRET). Finally, given the diversity of proteins observed but not accounted for at the gene level, their post-translational modifications can be studied by looking at the extent of phosphorylation or glycosylation.

157

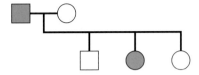

Fig. 3.10 Restriction endonuclease mapping. ■ and ● are affected individuals.

GENE MAPPING: TRACKING THE GENE THROUGH FAMILIES (Fig. 3.10)

The use of restriction endonuclease mapping (gene mapping) is now a well-established tool for analysing genetic disease. DNA obtained from tissues or cells (usually peripheral blood leucocytes) is treated with restriction enzymes and analysed by Southern blotting using a radioactively labelled gene probe. By using different restriction enzymes and orientation of the fragments, it is possible to build up restriction enzyme maps of sections of the human genome. Any normal or abnormal gene for which a specific probe has been generated can be analysed by this technique. Potential probes are chosen from a central library and screened for their ability to detect RFLPs by hybridizing them to Southern blots of DNA from a panel of unrelated individuals and by searching for restriction enzyme sites that give variable patterns. A disease gene can be mapped by collecting large pedigrees and comparing the segregation of the disease with the segregation of the RFLP. Once linkage has been clearly established, the probe is assumed to map to a chromosome region close to the disease gene and can be used to track the gene through families.

MOLECULAR BIOLOGY AND CLINICAL MEDICINE

GENE PROBES

Gene probes can be produced in several ways and fall broadly into three types: gene-specific probes, oligonucleotide probes, and polymorphic probes. Gene-specific probes are produced from specific mRNA by the enzyme reverse transcriptase, which synthesizes a complementary DNA copy (cDNA) from mRNA. If radioactive bases are added to the reaction mixture, the cDNA will be labelled and can thus be used as a hybridization probe to look for the complementary sequences. Probes can be used in *dot–blot hybridization*, where serial dilutions of DNA samples are held on DNA-binding membranes and

> **Box 3.8 Screening to identify candidate gene and mutation**
>
> Although the most sensitive method, sequencing is expensive, time-consuming and therefore limited to analysing only small areas of DNA at a time. Therefore, screening to identify positive samples to then sequence is performed by:
>
> - *Single strand conformation polymorphism analysis* (SSCP) – DNA is amplified by PCR and after denaturing the product one can electrophoretically identify two bands of DNA. Mutations will give rise to changes in electrophoretic mobility, producing four bands.
> - *Denaturing gradient gel electrophoresis* (DGGE) – fragments of DNA are incubated with cDNA and mutations are detected electrophoretically on a denaturing gradient gel because of abnormal band mobility. Radioactive cDNA probes (see below) will either bind as a *homoduplex* if no mutation or a *heteroduplex* if mutated, which can be detected following electrophoresis.
> - *Heteroduplex* – similar to SSCP because PCR products are used. Detection of mutations occurs as a consequence of the mutated product annealing with normal DNA and resulting in altered electrophoretic mobility.

the complementary radioactively labelled probes are hybridized *in vitro*, so that the amount of radioactive signal is proportional to the amount of target DNA present. The cDNA can also be cloned by synthesizing a second DNA strand from cDNA using a bacterial DNA polymerase, which is incorporated into a plasmid and grown in bacterial cells. These oligonucleotide probes recognize short sequences of DNA that correspond to the sequence known to occur in the gene. With a probe of this length, a single mismatched base pair is sufficient to impair hybridization and can be used to detect changes to a single base (point mutations). Similarly, probes can be developed that recognize the various DNA polymorphisms within the non-coding sequences, for example RFLP and VNTR. DNA probes can also be used to identify abnormal genes or gene products at the molecular level within cell cytoplasm or nucleus, by *in-situ hybridization*. This technique utilizes labelled DNA or mRNA probes which hybridize to the expressed genes in the cell in a manner similar to that used for immunohistochemistry. In-situ hybridization can thus establish whether the genomic material of interest is present in the DNA of the cell *in vitro*.

PRENATAL DIAGNOSIS

Prenatal diagnosis is possible in many genetic diseases and congenital or inherited malformations. Screening may be performed early in the second trimester with abdominal echography and estimation of serum α-fetoprotein (AFP) for the detection of neural tube defects, chromosomal abnormalities and other defects. The next most commonly used procedure, if required, is amniocentesis, performed at about 16 weeks' gestation. The cells in the amniotic fluid are fetal in origin, and cytogenetic, biochemical and cytological studies can be performed to identify genetic disease. A potentially important advance in prenatal diagnosis is that of chorionic villus sampling, usually at 9–12 weeks' gestation. The cells collected are particularly suitable for DNA diagnosis of inherited diseases (see Box 3.9). It is also possible to obtain samples of fetal blood at 18 weeks or more of gestation by ultrasonographically guided venepuncture of the umbilical cord. The lymphocytes can then be processed for DNA and chromosomal analysis. The process is currently indicated for rapid fetal chromosomal analysis in pregnancies at risk of the fragile X chromosome syndrome (mental retardation) or in those in which echography has revealed features suggestive of a chromosomal syndrome. It is also used for confirming equivocal chorionic villus sampling or amniocentesis results. Fetoscopy, which is more invasive, involves the insertion of a fetoscope through the abdominal wall into the amniotic sac. It is used for direct inspection of the fetus and for obtaining a pure sample of fetal blood, usually drawn from the umbilical cord close to its insertion into the placenta. This blood can be used for a variety of biochemical and cytogenetic investigations to help in the identification of genetic disease.

MOLECULAR AND CELL BIOLOGY: CONTROLLING CELL DESTINY

Cell death can occur by either necrosis (see Ch. 9) or apoptosis (programmed cell death). Apoptosis is a process whereby developmental or exogenous environmental signals trigger specific intracellular genes, which results in cell death. Ligation of cell surface receptors such as Fas-ligand (see Box 3.10), which is commonly associated with death domains that signal and stimulate caspases, disrupts mitochondrial membrane channel permeability. Apoptosis is essential for normal development and many of the genes that control apoptosis (see Box 3.10) have been highly conserved throughout evolution. Histologically, apoptosis is associated with chromatin condensation and nuclear DNA fragmentation. Only finally when caspase enzyme activation has occurred is membrane integrity affected and the cell eliminated via phagocytosis and the reticuloendothelial system without the secondary inflammatory response that occurs when cells undergo necrosis.

USING MOLECULAR BIOLOGICAL TECHNOLOGY TO DETECT APOPTOSIS

Observed, and therefore measurable, changes in apoptotic cells include intranucleosomal cleavage of DNA, which generates both monomers and multimers of DNA that can be detected by DNA electrophoresis (DNA laddering). Early changes can be detected by labelling DNA fragments at the 3′ OH ends with terminal deoxynucleotidyl transferase either immunohistochemically (TUNEL staining) or by flow cytometric analysis (see Ch. 9). Changes in apoptotic cell membranes can be detected by increased flip-flopping of the plasma membrane and exposure of

---

Box 3.9 Diagnoses made with chorionic villus sampling

Chromosomal abnormalities – trisomies including Down syndrome and translocation Down syndrome.

Enzymopathies – inherited metabolic disorders by enzyme assay. Assays can be performed on supernatants from amniocentesis samples and chorionic villus cell culture.

Single-gene mutations – single-gene defects by DNA analysis (haemoglobinaemias, cystic fibrosis, haemophilia).

Box 3.10 Gene regulation of apoptosis

- p53 – tumour suppressor protein which functions to activate DNA fragmentation and apoptosis, thus regulating tumour development
- Bcl-2 – gene for family of proteins which *inhibit* apoptosis
- BAX – gene for family of proteins which *activate* apoptosis
- Fas and TNFRI – death-domain-containing proteins which when cross-linked with ligand (Fas-ligand and tumour necrosis factor-α respectively) induce apoptosis.

3 GENETICS

Box 3.11   Ubiquitin (Ubq) – proteosome pathway maintains cellular homeostasis

Proteosomes are nuclear and cytosolic protease complexes that degrade proteins, which become covalently linked to Ubq via a cascade of enzymatic reactions (Ubq 1–3). Ubq is a highly conserved 76-amino-acid protein that has been implicated in the pathogenesis of genetic disease and malignancies. It is integral in the destruction of phosphorylated cyclins and cyclin inhibitors, such as p27 an inducible inhibitor of cyclin-dependent kinase activity (see Box 3.2, p. 145); transcriptional proteins such as STAT 1; and p53, a tumour suppressor gene product. Viruses (e.g. human papillomavirus) can upregulate p53 degradation in the Ubq–proteosome pathway, a process implicated in tumour formation. Proteosome inhibitors such as lactacystin can arrest cycle–cycle progression and therefore offer potential as chemotherapeutic agents.

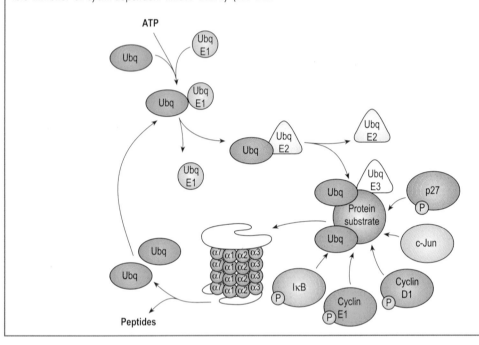

phosphatidylserine residues on its outer leaflet. Phosphatidylserine is detected by annexin V via either in-situ histochemistry or flow cytometry. Apoptosis ultimately increases intracellular caspase activity and cell lysates can be tested for levels of caspase enzymatic activity by simple fluorometric analysis.

GENE THERAPY

Gene therapy is the transfer of selected genes into a host with the intention of alleviating or curing disease. There are many gene therapy strategies that can be used; which one to choose depends upon the pathogenesis.

- *Gene augmentation therapy* For diseases caused by loss of gene function and which will supply more copies of normal gene in the hope of restoring normal phenotype, e.g cystic fibrosis,

haemophilia, severe combined immunodeficiency syndrome (SCID), retinitis pigmentosa.
- *Targeted killing of specific cells* Genes are directed to specific cell types and incorporated into the genome, expressed so that protein interferes with cell cycling and survival thus killing cells.
- *Targeted mutation correction* Can be performed using *ribozymes* (which cleave and repair mRNA), *triple helix oligonucleotides* (block gene transcription) and *anti-sense oligonucleotides* (that block mRNA translation).
- *Targeting inhibition of gene expression* When diseases display novel gene products or excessive expression of gene product then blocking at a single gene level (either DNA or RNA) or blocking protein can be possible to attain specific inhibition of expression.

Achieving gene therapy depends upon the size of the DNA fragments to be transferred (*transfection/*

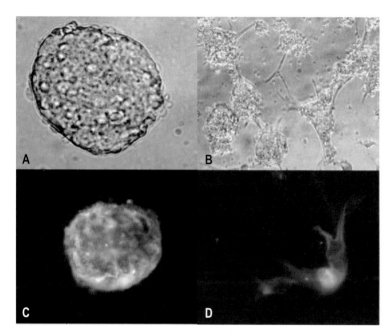

Fig. 3.11 Neurospheres generated from cell suspensions derived from the adult human retina and pars plana differentiate after dividing into neurones. Phase contrast photography showing (**A**) free-floating neurosphere at 3 weeks, which may attach to a fibronectin-coated coverslip (**B**). Neurospheres were generated at a rate of one neurosphere for every 200×10^4 vital cells in the retinal cell suspension. Neurospheres contained nestin-positive (red) cells, some of which colabelled with green GFAP (**C**). Primary and secondary (passaged) neurospheres were exposed to BrdU at 1 week. After dissociation, primary neurospheres incubated in the presence of BrdU (green nucleus) express neurofilament M (red) in monolayer cultures (**D**). (Courtesy of Dr Eric Mayer and Dr Debbie Carter, Academic Unit of Ophthalmology, University of Bristol.) GFAP, glial fibrillary acid protein; BrdU, bromodeoxyuridine.

Box 3.12 Vectors

Viral vectors
Retroviruses – e.g. lentiviruses (human immunodeficiency virus; simian immunodeficiency virus) Although RNA viruses, they possess reverse transcriptase so can generate complementary DNA.

Adenoviruses – have been engineered to remove replicatory ability and also antigenic coats, particularly to reduce the immune response to these vectors

Adeno-associated viruses (AAV) – a single strand of DNA virus without viral genes and therefore reduced immunogenicity. They only accommodate smaller DNA inserts but do establish long-term expression.

Non-viral vectors
Liposomes – spherical lipid bilayer vesicles. No limit to size of DNA to be carried but efficiency of transfer is low.

---

transduction). Techniques can include injection of naked DNA, which is not limited by size or number of genes but is inefficient (*gene gun*). Often therefore the gene to be transferred is not conventional and the coding DNA is engineered to be flanked by regulatory sequences to ensure high expression dependent upon the tissue. By whatever method, the aim is to insert the DNA into the chromosome of the cell. To assist entry of DNA into the cell, *vectors* are

used (see Box 3.12). These are currently attenuated viruses that have been engineered so that the replication and disease-causing components have been removed. Even with this manipulation they retain an efficient ability to enter cells – so called *transduction*.

NEURAL PROGENITOR CELLS

Stem cells have the capacity to self-renew, proliferate and have no limitation to their potential differentiation. Progenitor cells can divide but have restricted differentiation potential. In the adult vertebrate central nervous system, neural progenitor cells (NPC) have been identified and shown to generate neurones and glia. Both the developing and the postnatal vertebrate animal retina contain NPC, which divide, generate *neurospheres* and undergo neuronal and glial differentiation (Fig. 3.11). In humans, central nervous system-derived NPC have been successfully cultured from the adult brain and more recently adult retina and also NPC have been isolated from the human retina while it is still immature and undergoing development. One phenotypic marker of stem cells and NPC is nestin, which is an intermediate filament. The adult human retina contains nestin-positive neuronal and glial cells, as does epiretinal scar tissue. This evidence suggests that NPC exist throughout life in the human retina and, perhaps, are misdirected in retinal scarring disorders including proliferative vitreo-retinopathy, diabetes, retinal detachment and ocular inflammatory disorders. Human retinal NPC are currently under extensive investigation to look at their capacity to renew damaged retina via, for example, transplantation with potentially gene-modifying cells that have undergone gene therapy before administration.

MOLECULAR GENETICS AND OPHTHALMOLOGY

With the advent of modern molecular biological techniques, which have and will improve the understanding of the pathology of disease at both the cellular and molecular levels, considerable progress has been made, in particular in the study of X-linked disorders, several of which are of interest to the ophthalmologist.

The problem of how to find and identify an abnormal gene among the millions of genes in the human genome has already been discussed. To summarize briefly, the problem can be tackled principally by two approaches. The first is to find a gene marker in the human genome that is close to the causative gene defect. This approach, as described above, is the basis of genetic linkage and requires the analysis of DNA from affected families. Using the genetic marker, linkage analysis will locate the gene to loci on the same chromosome. Fragments of DNA from that region of the chromosome are cloned and sequenced to identify mutations in the gene.

The second approach is to identify candidate genes specifically expressed in the tissue, or which are known to code for proteins important in that tissue. Patients are then screened for mutation in these genes. By this method the discovery of mutant genes gives insight into the underlying pathophysiology of the condition, if the functions of the proteins from the genes studied are already known. This method of analysis is known as *candidate gene analysis*. Both of these methods have been used to study ophthalmic disorders.

THE X CHROMOSOME

Many molecular genetic studies have been based on an investigation of the X chromosome and of X-linked disorders. Mapping of disorders such as red–green colour blindness (Xq22–28), blue cone monochromacy (Xq28), and congenital stationary night blindness (Xp11) have come about with the

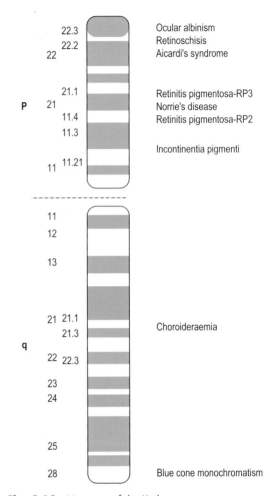

Fig. 3.12 Mapping of the X chromosome.

use of RFLP and recombinant DNA technology (see Ch. 5). Figure 3.12 demonstrates the approximate location on the X chromosome of the genes for various inherited ophthalmic X-linked disorders. Molecular biological techniques are more easily applied to the X chromosome than to autosomes, because the location of the genes in autosomal dominant or recessively inherited conditions is uncertain, and distances between genetic markers and the defective gene are appreciable, even if linkage has been established.

RETINITIS PIGMENTOSA (Fig. 3.13)

Retinitis pigmentosa is the term used to describe a heterogeneous group of rod–cone dystrophies that have a variety of clinical appearances by virtue of

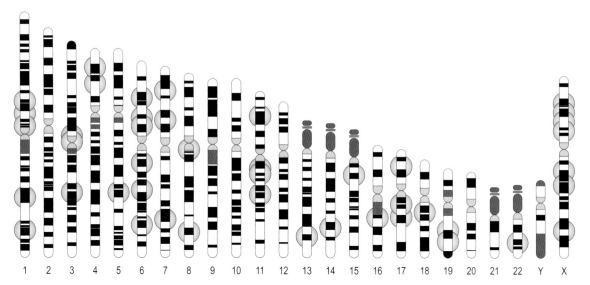

Fig. 3.13 A schematic representation of the human chromosomes, showing the various loci implicated in retinal disorders. (Courtesy of Dr Z. Mohamed, PhD thesis, University of Aberdeen.)

varying inheritance patterns. Studies have documented the frequencies of the various modes of inheritance. Approximately 43% are inherited by autosomal transmission, 20% by autosomal recessive transmission and between 8 and 25% by X-linked recessive transmission. Figures again vary, but approximately 20–25% of cases of retinitis pigmentosa appear to be isolated, or at least have unidentifiable patterns of inheritance. As the disease may be classified according to Mendelian inheritance patterns, the possibility of single-gene defects is high and this has prompted an energetic search for the isolation of such genes.

X-linked retinitis pigmentosa

Patients with this form of retinitis pigmentosa present with symptoms of night blindness from childhood; they have progressive constriction of visual fields and loss of vision in midlife, although the severity of the disease does vary. The gene for this condition has been mapped to Xp11.3 (short arm of the X chromosome). Further evidence also maps the X-linked gene to Xp21, particularly in families where the female carrier demonstrates the golden tapetoretinal reflex. Recently these gene loci have been designated *RP2* (Xp11.3) and *RP3* (Xp21.1). Currently, probes are available for identifying both loci and may be used for prenatal diagnosis and genetic counselling. However, to date, the function of these genes remains unknown.

Autosomal dominant retinitis pigmentosa

Several mutations have been found in candidate genes in up to 30% of patients with autosomal dominant retinitis pigmentosa. Mutations in two genes have been studied in particular. These include the rhodopsin gene on chromosome 3q (accounting for 20% of all cases) and the peripherin gene on chromosome 6p. The rhodopsin molecule, composed of 348 amino acids, exists as a seven-loop transmembrane protein in the rod outer segment (see Fig. 4.45). The C terminus of the protein is in the cytoplasm and the N terminus of rhodopsin is in the intradiscal space. Throughout the protein, several regions are affected by mutations, which fall into three main groups: (1) mutations affecting amino acids in the intradiscal space; (2) mutations affecting amino acids in the transmembrane domain; and (3) mutations affecting amino acids in the cytoplasm. Most of these mutations probably destroy the three-dimensional (tertiary) conformation of the protein and in some way affect protein function. To date, over 70 different mutations have been reported, the majority of which are point mutations, although deletions have also been discovered.

The peripherin gene codes for the retinal degeneration show (RDS) protein found in rats (see Ch. 5), which is a component of the rod outer segment disk membranes. More than 20 mutations have been discovered in this gene in association with autosomal dominant retinitis pigmentosa and other retinopathies, for example retinitis pigmentosa albescens and hereditary maculopathies. Recently, other genes have been identified in autosomal dominant retinitis pigmentosa, and these include one at the centromere of chromosome 8 and both the long and short arms of chromosome 7.

Autosomal recessive forms of retinitis pigmentosa have been less well studied; to date, only one gene mutation has been identified in a rhodopsin gene. Recently there has been a report that certain patients with autosomal dominant retinitis pigmentosa have defects in the gene coding for cyclic guanosine monophosphate phosphodiesterase (see Ch. 4).

CHOROIDERAEMIA

Choroideraemia presents in childhood with night blindness leading to eventual loss of vision in later life. Fundal changes show granular pigmentary changes early in the course of the disease and choroidal atrophy in the late stages. Like X-linked recessive retinitis pigmentosa with the *RP3* gene defect, carrier females also demonstrate patchy non-progressive equatorial pigmentary changes, as a consequence of lyonization. The gene locus for choroideraemia has been identified at the locus Xq21. Several point mutations, deletions and RFLPs resulting from aberrant splicing at the exon–intron junction have been associated with the locus.

NORRIE'S DISEASE

Norrie's disease affects males from birth. Features include bilateral congenital blindness secondary to retinal dysplasia and retinal vascular anomalies, impaired hearing, mental retardation, retinal detachment and cataract. This condition is similar to another congenital blinding condition, namely familial exudative vitreoretinopathy, which also shows abnormal vascular development, particularly of the retinal vessels. The gene locus for Norrie's disease has been identified as Xp11.1, Xp11.3. Similar gene loci have been suggested for familial exudative vitreoretinopathy, suggesting that these two disorders are related by expressing different mutations at the same gene loci, producing the two phenotypes. Mutations and deletions have been demonstrated at the gene loci for Norrie's disease. This locus codes for the cDNA of a protein that has no significant homology to known proteins. Also, cDNA that recognizes sequences coding for ornithine aminotransferase on the X chromosome was not expressed in affected males, which suggests that

these gene sequences could be used as DNA markers for the disease.

RETINOBLASTOMA

Retinoblastoma is a tumour of primitive photoreceptor cells. It is the commonest ocular malignancy of childhood with a prevalence of approximately 1 in 20 000, showing an equal sex distribution. Approximately 40% of cases are inherited. Unilateral tumour, however, is nearly always sporadic, with no family history. Bilateral cases usually have a strong family history of retinoblastoma and are inherited by autosomal transmission. These patients are also at greater risk in later life of developing osteosarcoma. It has been shown that retinoblastoma may be secondary to a deletion of 13q14 in about 4% of patients. The gene locus that encodes the enzyme d-esterase is also situated on chromosome 13, and patients with retinoblastoma show a much reduced level of this enzyme, indicating that the d-esterase and retinoblastoma loci are closely linked. Knudson proposed a hypothesis to explain the fact that inherited cases are usually bilateral, multifocal and of early onset, whereas sporadic cases are unilateral and solitary. The 'two-hit hypothesis' proposes two mutational events in inherited retinoblastoma. The first mutation is present in the germinal cell and would therefore be present in every cell. The second 'somatic' mutation must occur to induce tumour growth in cells with the initial mutation by releasing suppression or regulation of the retinoblast. Two somatic mutations to one retinoblast must occur in sporadic cases of retinoblastoma and are therefore likely to be solitary and unilateral. This retinoblastoma gene has therefore been proposed as a *tumour suppressor gene*, whose presence in normal retinoblasts prevents uncontrolled mitosis. The DNA sequence of the retinoblastoma gene has now been identified, and the surrounding complex gene locus identified as a *retinoblastoma predisposition gene*, which is structurally altered in patients with retinoblastoma, although its true function is unknown. As mentioned above, patients who survive retinoblastoma have an increased risk of developing osteosarcoma and, interestingly, in isolated patients with osteosarcoma the retinoblastoma gene has been found to be deleted.

ALBINISM

Albinism is a cause of poor visual acuity and nystagmus in children and is divided broadly into two groups: oculocutaneous and ocular albinism.

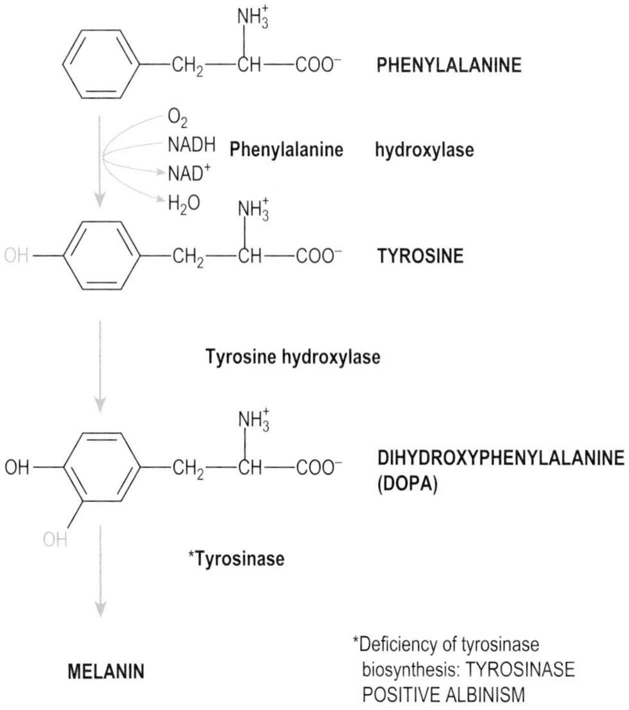

$$NH_3^+$$

$$\text{CH}_2-\text{CH}-\text{COO}^- \quad \textbf{PHENYLALANINE}$$

$$O_2$$
$$NADH \quad \text{Phenylalanine} \quad \text{hydroxylase}$$
$$\rightarrow NAD^+$$
$$H_2O \quad NH_3^+$$

$$\text{OH}-\text{CH}_2-\text{CH}-\text{COO}^- \quad \textbf{TYROSINE}$$

Tyrosine hydroxylase

$$NH_3^+$$

$$\text{OH}-\text{CH}_2-\text{CH}-\text{COO}^- \quad \textbf{DIHYDROXYPHENYLALANINE}$$
$$\text{(DOPA)}$$

OH

*Tyrosinase

MELANIN

*Deficiency of tyrosinase
biosynthesis: TYROSINASE
POSITIVE ALBINISM

Fig. 3.14 Enzyme defects in albinism.

Patients with oculocutaneous albinism may be further differentiated into tyrosinase-producing (tyrosinase-positive) and tyrosinase-non-producing (tyrosinase-negative) groups, shown in children over the age of 4 years by hair bulb incubation in tyrosinase solution (Fig. 3.14).

Oculocutaneous albinism

This form of albinism is inherited in an autosomal recessive Mendelian fashion and within the tyrosinase-negative group gives rise to severe disease with profound visual loss, photophobia, and nystagmus, as well as the classic features of iris transillumination, absent fundal pigmentation and absent foveal reflex. Most of the optic nerve fibres cross at the chiasma (90%), and further neuronal disorganization occurs within the lateral geniculate body.

Ocular albinism

Ocular albinism is present when most of the hypopigmentation (hypomelanosis) is confined to the ocular structures. Ocular albinism may be inherited in an autosomal recessive (Nettleship–Fells syndrome) or an X-linked recessive pattern. X-linked recessive ocular albinism gives rise to ocular disease of moderate severity, with a prevalence of approximately 1 in 50 000. Affected males have reduced

visual acuity, nystagmus, strabismus and iris translucency. Fundal examination shows classic hypopigmentation and foveal hypoplasia. In this condition giant melanosomes are present in the retinal pigment epithelium and are also found in skin biopsies; they are similar to the melanosome aggregates found in one of the albinoid syndromes, Chediak–Higashi syndrome (associated with phagocytic dysfunction). Carrier females, whose visual acuity is normal, also demonstrate iris transillumination, retinal pigment epithelial granularity and a preponderance of giant melanosomes in the skin. At-risk females, however, can pose a diagnostic problem, and accurate genetic counselling will be available only when future genetic diagnostic tests and techniques for identification of the candidate gene have been developed.

MYOTONIC DYSTROPHY

Myotonic dystrophy presents with progressive muscle weakness early in adult life. The condition is characterized by expressionless face, frontal balding, gonadal atrophy and myotonia when shaking hands. Patients often develop cataracts and may also develop a pigmentary retinopathy. Myotonic dystrophy is transmitted as an autosomal

Table 3.2 Summary of patterns of inheritance of ocular disease

Disease	Description
AUTOSOMAL DOMINANT	
Corneal dystrophies	
Meesmans	See Chapter 9
Reis–Buckler	See Chapter 9
Lattice	See Chapter 9
Granular	See Chapter 9
Posterior polymorphous	See Chapter 9
Syndromes affecting lens	
Marfan's	Mesodermal dysplasia syndrome with defects in collagen crosslinking. Gives rise to multiple ocular features including upward dislocation of lens and systemic features of aortic regurgitation, arachnodactyl, and arm span greater than height. Individuals have mutations in fibrillin-FBN1 gene
Ehlers-Danlos	Defect in type II collagen, which gives rise to ectopia lentis and systemic features of hyperextensible joints and skin. Spectrum of phenotype related to mutations in lysyl hydroxylase gene and COL1A1 and 2 genes
Aniridia	See Chapter 3
Congenital cataract	See Chapter 3
Myotonic dystrophy	See Chapter 3
Vitreoretinal disorders	
Macular coloboma	Failure of closure of optic fissure (see Ch. 2) affecting neural retina of macula
Myelinated nerve fibres	
Wagner's disease	Vitreous degeneration with peripheral retinal degeneration, myopia and retinal detachment
Stickler's syndrome	Arthro-ophthalmopathy syndrome, where patients have marfanoid habitus with vitreoretinal degeneration similar to Wagner's disease. Type 1 Stickler's phenotype have mutations in COL2A1 gene, whilst type 2 phenotype have mutations in COL11A1
Tritanopia colour blindness	See Chapter 5
Retinitis pigmentosa	See Chapters 3 and 9
Best's vitelliform dystrophy	See Chapter 9; mutation in VMD2 (encoding bestrophin)
Sorsby's fundus dystrophy	Subretinal neurovascularization and disciform macular degeneration. Mapped to 22q13 and TIMP-3 mutations
Primary congenital glaucoma	Associated with *CYP1B1* gene (2p21). Has been linked with mutations in myocilin gene (*MYOC*) and optineurin gene (*OPTIN*)
AUTOSOMAL RECESSIVE	
Corneal dystrophies	
Macular	See Chapter 9
Syndromes affecting lens	
Weil–Marchesani	Disorder of connective tissue metabolism giving rise to mental retardation, short stature, stubby fingers and spherophakia. Mapped to 19p13.3–p13.2 with reported cases of mutation with fibrillin-1 gene (15q21.1)
Homocystinuria	See Chapter 9
Sulphite oxidase deficiency	Enzyme involved in trace element metabolism which gives rise to ectopia lentis
Hyperlysinaemia	Deficiency in lysine dehydrogenase which leads to generalized psychomotor retardation and microspheropakia
Familial ectopia lentis	Isolated dislocated lens
Anterior lenticonus	Anterior aspect of the lens is conical with respect to the lens surface. This may be associated with Alport's syndrome (aminoacidura and nephritis), but may be present in isolation with cataract formation. Alport's is associated with mutations in the COL4A5 gene
Congenital cataract	

Table 3.2 Summary of patterns of inheritance of ocular disease (cont.)

Disease	Description
Vitreoretinal disorders	
Goldman–Favre disease	Syndrome of night blindness, foveal schisis, mental retardation and cataracts
Retinitis pigmentosa	See Chapters 3 and 9
Stargardt's disease	See Chapter 9; mutation in ABCA4 gene
Fundus flavimaculatus	See Chapter 9
Gyrate atrophy	Ornithine aminotransferase deficiency, which gives rise to progressive chorioretinopathy
Lysosomal storage diseases	
Sphingolipidoses	
Niemann–Pick	Sphingolipidosis secondary to sphingomyelinase deficiency. Later presentations may show a cherry-red spot at the macula. Type 1C is associated with mutations of NPC1 gene on chromosome 18
Metachromatic leukodystrophy	Secondary to sulphatase deficiency, which gives rise to optic atrophy, cherry-red spot at the macula; associated with dystonia and mental retardation
Tay–Sachs	Deficiency in hexaminidase, which catalyzes conversion of GM-2 ganglioside to GM-3 ganglioside. Known as infantile gangliosidosis. Neuronal cells of both central and autonomic nervous systems contain large amounts of GM-2, demonstrated by the presence of the classic cherry-red spot at the macula. A more severe form of gangliosidosis is Sandhoff's disease
Mucopolysaccharidoses	Group of conditions all secondary to inborn errors of metabolism in which activity of one of the exoglycosides is deficient. This gives rise to sulphated mucopolysaccharides in fibroblasts. Clinically there is optic atrophy, corneal clouding associated with mental retardation and physical deformity. Within this group of disorders are the conditions of Hurler's, Hunter's and Sanfilippo's syndromes
Mucolipidoses	Group of conditions where clinical features are a mixture of sphingolipidoses and mucopolysaccharidoses. Includes deficiency in neuraminadase, N-acetyl glucosamine phosphate transferase. Can give rise to corneal clouding
Batten's disease	Accumulation of autofluorescent lipopigments in neural tissue, which gives rise to pigmentary retinopathy, optic atrophy and psychomotor retardation
Refsum's syndrome	Heredopathia atactica polyneuritiformis. Otherwise known as phytanic acid storage disease, which is due to failure of α-hydroxylation of 3, 7, 11, 15-tetramethylhexadecanoic acid. Gives rise to a progressive polyneuropathy and ataxia with retinitis pigmentosa and cataracts. Individuals have defect in phytanol-CoA hydroxylase gene
X-LINKED RECESSIVE	
Norrie's disease	See Chapter 3
Incontinentia pigmenti	Gives rise to recurrent cutaneous bullous eruptions with pigmentation, and dysplastic retina with optic atrophy and cataract formation
Juvenile retinoschisis	Splitting of nerve fibre layer of the retina. Occurs in two forms involving either the fovea with a late onset of visual failure or peripheral involving predominantly inferotemporal quadrant of retina
Retinitis pigmentosa	See Chapters 3 and 9
Albinism	See Chapter 3
Choroideraemia	See Chapter 3

dominant trait with an incidence of 1 in 20 000. Gene loci for this disease have been localized with the use of RFLP and DNA probes to chromosome 19. However, because of the recent discovery of an unstable DNA mutation consisting of an increased number (more than 50) of a nucleotide triplet (CTG repeats), whose protein product is a member of the protein kinase family, family studies can confirm or exclude those at risk.

ANIRIDIA

Aniridia may be inherited in an autosomal dominant or, less commonly, an autosomal recessive pattern. It may also occur sporadically in association with Wilms' tumour. Most cases are associated with a deletion of a segment of chromosome 11p13, which includes a region coding for the enzyme lactate dehydrogenase (LDH-A gene). The level of this enzyme can thus be measured biochemically as part of the screening and diagnostic investigation of such patients. Clinical examination may reveal parents with a much less severe form of aniridia, who have no visual impairment because of the variable expression of the autosomal dominant form. The genetic basis for aniridia and Wilms' tumours may be similar to those of retinoblastoma, in that loss of a functional allele abrogates tumour suppressor gene function and allows uncontrolled cell proliferation.

MITOCHONDRIAL INHERITANCE

As has been stated above, mitochondria contain specific circular DNA that replicates separately from the nuclear DNA and is inherited solely from maternal mitochondria. Recently, some inherited disorders have been identified as having a mitochondrial mode of transmission, because they do not follow classic Mendelian patterns of inheritance.

Leber's hereditary optic neuropathy

This condition is characterized by rapid onset of visual failure particularly in boys, but it may affect either sex. The result of the initial hyperaemic disk swelling and peripapillary telangiectasia is optic atrophy and visual failure. Mothers characteristically pass the disease to their sons, but sons never transmit it (i.e. no male-to-male transmission). A characteristic point mutation causing histidine to be inserted instead of arginine at the 340th amino acid of NADH in complex I of the respiratory chain has been demonstrated in patients with this type of optic neuropathy. Other point mutations in mitochon-

drial DNA have also been documented. However, there has been no explanation as to why males are predominantly affected in this disorder, which cannot be explained purely on the basis of a single mitochodrial gene defect. With the advent of mitochondrial DNA analysis, investigation of patients with optic neuropathy of uncertain aetiology can be carried out to determine whether Leber's neuropathy is the cause. Also, recent studies have shown that the genotype of the condition is associated with a variable phenotype, in that some families with specific gene mutations demonstrate recovery of vision in up to 50% of patients. In addition, other gene mutations are linked to Leber's hereditary optic neuropathy and are associated with generalized neurological abnormalities.

Other mitochondrial disorders

Other mitochondrial inherited disorders also affect the eye. These include the mitochondrial myopathies, of which the most documented is Kearns–Sayre syndrome. This syndrome occurs secondary to multiple point mutations within the mitochondrial genome, which in turn lead to multiple deletions of varying size. The heterogeneity of the mutations accounts for the variance of the clinical signs encountered, which include a pigmentary retinopathy and progressive myopathy, involving cardiac and proximal limb muscles as well as a progressive external ophthalmoplegia.

FURTHER READING

Blau HM, Springer ML. Molecular medicine: gene therapy – a novel form of drug delivery. N Eng J Med 1995; 333:1204–1207.

Connor JM, Ferguson-Smith MA. Essential Medical Genetics, 5th edn. Oxford: Blackwell Scientific; 1997.

Gregory-Evans K. Molecular biology for ophthalmolgists. Eye News 1999; 5(5):6–12.

Grivell L. Mitochondrial DNA. Sci Am 1983; 248:78–89.

Humphries P. Hereditary retinopathies: insights into a complex genetic aetiology. Br J Ophthalmol 1993; 77(8):469–471.

Jay B, Jay M. Molecular aspects in clinical ophthalmology. Recent advances in ophthalmology, 8th edn. Edinburgh: Churchill Livingstone; 1992.

Lewis RA, Holcomb JD, Bromley WC, Wilson MC, Roderick TH, Hejtmancik JF. Mapping X-linked ophthalmic diseases III. Provisional assignment of the locus for blue cone monochromy to Xq28. Arch Ophthalmol 1987; 105:1055–1059.

Molday RS. Photoreceptor membrane proteins, phototransduction and retinal degenerative diseases.

The Friedenwald lecture. Invest Ophthalmol Vis Sci 1998; 39:2491–2513.

Mueller RF, Young ID. Emery's Elements of Medical Genetics, 10th edn. Edinburgh: Churchill Livingstone; 1998.

Reardon W, Macmillan JC, Myring J, Harley HG, Rundle SA, Beck L, Harper PS, Shaw DJ. Cataract and myotonic dystrophy: the role of molecular diagnosis. Br J Ophthalmol 1993; 77(9): 579–584.

Rigby P, Krumlauf R and Grosveld F. Transcriptional regulation in cell differentiation and development. J Cell Sci (Suppl.) 1992; **16**.

Rimoin DL, Connor JM, Korf B, Pyeritz RE, Emery AEH (eds) Priniciples and practice of medical genetics, 4th edn. New York: Churchill Livingstone; 1999.

Snead MP, Yates JR. Clinical and molecular genetics of Stickler syndrome. J Med Genet 1999; 36 (5):353–359.

Strachan T, Read AP. Human molecular genetics. Oxford: Bios Scientific Publishers Ltd; 1998.

Thompson MW, McInnes RR, Willard HF. Genetics in medicine, 5th edn. Philadelphia: WB Saunders; 1991.

Ulman S, Nelson LB, Jackson LG. Prenatal diagnostic techniques: chorionic villus sampling. Surv Ophthalmol 1985; 30:33.

4 BIOCHEMISTRY AND CELL BIOLOGY

INTRODUCTION

Almost all types of tissue cell are represented in the eye, including secretory cells, nerve cells, vascular cells, specialized fibroblasts and tissue macrophages, and supporting cells, while the matrices are composed of collagens, proteoglycans, glycoproteins, and basement membranes, as in any other tissue. The unique feature of cells and tissues in the eye, however, is that they are organized for the transmission, reception and conversion of light energy into cellular signals.

Cells respond to stimuli in a remarkably similar manner. What differentiates one cell from another are the stimuli each cell responds to and the mechanisms it uses to respond. In essence, cells possess specialized receptors in their cell membranes that respond to a specific stimulus by activating an intracellular second messenger system. This produces a programmed response in the cell, resulting in an effect, e.g. aqueous secretion from acinar lacrimal gland cells after stimulation by epinephrine, ocular muscle action potential after neurotransmitter release from nerve endings, or rhodopsin activation by a photon of light.

Cells are organized singly or in groups (tissues), to receive information from the environment (membrane receptors), to signal this information to the intracellular compartment (signalling networks), to convert the message into cellular responses (gene activation and protein transcription), and to relay this information to the outside world (e.g. changes in cell behaviour, tissue function, secretion, etc.). In recent years there has been a realization that many thousands of molecules and genes are involved in a single response by a cell through networks, in which thousands of molecular interactions may be connected through a system in which some molecules form many interactions with others ('hubs') while

171

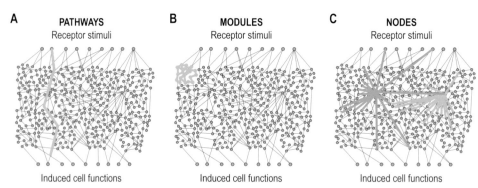

Fig. 4.1 Three concepts that are useful for describing signalling networks. Cell signalling is initiated by receptor stimuli. Each connection point reflects a signalling protein or second messenger, with lines indicating functional interactions. (**A**) Linear signalling pathways. (**B**) Modular structures within the network. (**C**) Nodes, which can be proteins or second messengers. Nodal points are regulated by many upstream events and/or regulate many downstream events. (From Meyer and Teruel 2003, with permission from Elsevier.)

other molecules make very few interactions and are on the periphery of the network (Fig. 4.1). These concepts have derived from the vast amount of information made available through full genetic analysis of various organisms (genomics) and the use of novel methods of investigation including microarray technology and informatics.

GENOMICS, PROTEOMICS AND THE EXPANDING CONCEPT OF '...OMICS'

Study of cellular function through the many thousands of molecules that may be affected in any single cellular activity is enshrined in one of the '...omics'. Genomics examines the many genes which may be involved by increased or decreased expression, transcriptomics studies the many transcription factors which may be activated or deactivated in any one cellular behaviour, such as cell division, and metabolomics investigates the many biochemical pathways which may be utilized, or not, in conversion of one molecular species to another. In these processes molecular networks are entrained, which in themselves reveal the extensive interdependence of molecular activities that one system has on another. In addition, the notion of central 'hub' molecular species without which the entire network would collapse allows a hierarchy of importance to be applied to molecules. This is demonstrated in the genetic mutagenesis studies in which certain molecules, such as transforming growth factor-β, are lethal to the embryo when deleted while others, such

as plasminogen activator inhibitor 1, barely alter the murine phenotype.

Signalling networks are a prime example of how cellular information is transmitted. It is now recognized that there are hundreds of signalling receptors in the cell membrane interacting with around 10 second messenger 'hubs' in large interacting intracellular networks of several thousand cellular proteins (Figure 4.1). Furthermore, 'hub' molecules are frequently transient in activity, one molecule acting as a hub during activation of one signalling pathway while the same molecule acts merely as a relay station during activity of another pathway. Information usually proceeds from 'outside in' to the cell, but on occasion information initiated outside the cell can be relayed back to extracellular targets (see Fig. 4.2). Many of the cellular proteins may not be directly involved in signalling but may act as adaptors or amplify/diminish the overall response. In addition, other proteins act as 'chaperones' to 'protect' proteins and signalling molecules for optimal function (see Box 4.1).

Typical general second messenger systems include:

- tyrosine-kinase-linked receptor systems
- ion channels and 'pumps'
- G-protein driven messengers.

Each of these may interact with other signalling systems and the signalling systems themselves may be 'customized' to respond selectively depending on the conditions (Fig. 4.3).

Box 4.1 Molecular chaperones in the regulation of signalling: a few recent advances

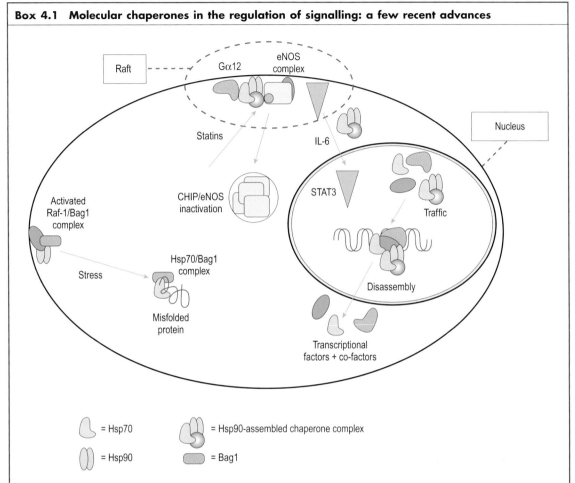

Chaperone proteins are everywhere in the cell, shepherding essential functional proteins such as enzymes and signalling molecules to ensure their proper functioning. Many different types of chaperone exist and some come into their own in certain circumstances such as heat-shock proteins (Hsp) while others are constitutively functioning such as lens crystallins (Fig 4.2). Chaperones play an essential role in the activation of protein kinases, for instance Bag1, the co-chaperone of Hsp70, which can activate the Hsp90-dependant process. Stress is known to inhibit cell prolifera-tion and sequestration of Bag1 may be how this occurs. Chaperones like Bag1 and Hsp70, play an essential role in the maturation and activation of hundreds of protein kinases regulating, for instance, cell proliferation in response to stress. Chaperones participate in raft-dependent signalling of molecules like eNOS, G-proteins and STATs. Chaperones also help the subnuclear trafficking and disassembly of transcriptional factors and related complexes. (From Söti et al. 2005, with permission from Elsevier.)

Signalling networks behave similarly to other biological networks, such as metabolic and gene transcriptional networks, and probably represent a basic biological organizing system. Three basic concepts underpin a signalling network: signalling pathways, signalling modules and signalling nodes (Fig. 4.1). Information is transmitted differently through each of these routes, for instance directly via linear signalling pathways or in a tightly regulated manner through nodes. Nodes themselves may be either protein sinks or second messengers. Modules may link scaffolding cytoskeletal proteins and signalling pathways.

Interaction with the extracellular matrix (inside-out signalling) is an important cell communication process (Fig 4.2). Examples include the interaction of endothelial cell surface integrin receptors with fibronectin and collagen to regulate angiogenesis, and the role of Bowman's layer in maintaining

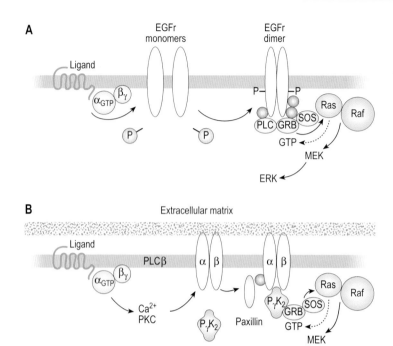

Fig. 4.2 Two models for cell activation using the MEK (MAPK–ERK: mitogen activated protein kinase–extracellular receptor kinase) system. (**A**) Soluble ligand binds to G protein-coupled receptor and activates tyrosine kinase-linked EGF receptor system. (**B**) Soluble ligand binds to G protein-coupled system and activates an ECM-αβ integrin-linked cascade to signal via MEK–ERK. EGF, epidermal growth factor; ECM, extracellular matrix.

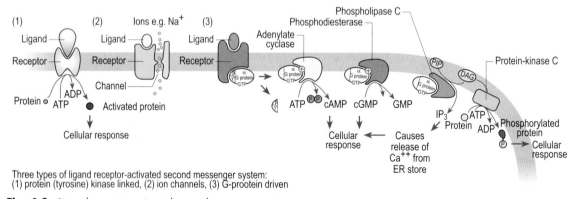

Three types of ligand receptor-activated second messenger system:
(1) protein (tyrosine) kinase linked, (2) ion channels, (3) G-prootein driven

Fig. 4.3 Ligand–receptor-activated second messenger systems.

integrity and non-keratinized status of the corneal epithelium.

CELLS AND TISSUES

THE CELL

General structure
The basic structure of the cell can be illustrated by the retinal pigmented epithelial (RPE) cell (Fig. 4.4)

as it contains most of the recognized cellular structures and intracellular organelles. While all cells have the potential and machinery for mitosis and motility, many adult tissue cells such as the RPE cell are considered terminally differentiated, non-motile cells, except under pathological conditions. The RPE cell is an example of a transporting epithelial cell with polarity, i.e. an apical surface with microvillous processes and a basal surface with numerous infoldings. The RPE cell is an example

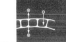

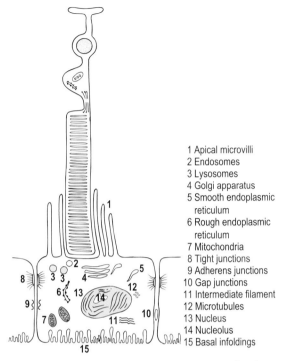

1 Apical microvilli
2 Endosomes
3 Lysosomes
4 Golgi apparatus
5 Smooth endoplasmic reticulum
6 Rough endoplasmic reticulum
7 Mitochondria
8 Tight junctions
9 Adherens junctions
10 Gap junctions
11 Intermediate filament
12 Microtubules
13 Nucleus
14 Nucleolus
15 Basal infoldings

Fig. 4.4 Diagram of RPE and photoreceptor cells. The photoreceptor outer segment lies in close apposition to the RPE cell, enclosed in a sheath of apical microvilli. The RPE cell is a terminally differentiated epithelial cell with several functions, one of which is to transport fluid across the cell towards the basal infoldings and into the choroid sink.

of how the basic structure of the cell has been modified extensively in several types of specialized cells in the eye.

The plasma membrane

The plasma membrane is a selective two-way barrier to passive diffusion, which also has active transport mechanisms subserved by specialized proteins (for instance ion channels, pumps and suspended transporters) floating in the lipid bilayer (Fig. 4.5A). Other proteins are also suspended in the plasma membrane, such as receptors for hormones, neurotransmitters, viruses and other cells. Many of these receptors have a three-part structure with an extracellular variably sized component, a transmembrane component, and a short intracellular section coupled to the second messenger system.

Previously held views that membrane proteins were present in low concentration have given way to the current concept of variably thick lipid bilayers 'crowded' with many membrane proteins (Fig. 4.5A).

The cell surface is irregularly pitted with invaginations and evaginations such as specialized structures for endocytosis (clathrin-coated pits), embedded in a glycoprotein-rich matrix (glycocalyx). Exocytosis occurs through vacuolar structures.

Recently it has been shown that the lipid bilayer itself not only varies in composition from cell to cell, e.g. in cholesterol content, but also may be inhomogeneous in lipid content in individual cells, thus possessing membrane microdomains (Fig. 4.5B). These may vary in size as well as lipid content and are specialized for discrete functions. Microdomains are frequently detergent-resistant and usually contain a specific protein such as caveolin in caveolae, or several proteins as occur in 'lipid rafts', areas specialized for specific functions such as the immunological synapse in antigen-presenting cells (see Chapter 7, Immunology). Other microdomains include tiny domains (nanodomains), which contain GTP-binding protein (inhibitory) (GPI)-anchored proteins (important in some types of signalling) and glycosphingolipids, transient confined zones of varying size, and small regions composed of more fluid lipids.

Many other specializations occur in the plasma membrane, depending on the cell type, such as junctional complexes, gap junctions, desmosomes, hemidesmosomes and contact sites with the basement membranes (see below). In the eye these membrane specializations are developed to a high level. For instance, the photoreceptor cell (Fig. 4.4) (see Ch. 1) is a highly polarized structure comprising a receptor component, a nucleus and a synapse. The rod photoreceptor (specialized for scotopic vision; see Ch. 5) develops as an evagination of the plasma membrane, which folds upon itself many times to form stacks of membranous disks by fusion of the peripheral disk membrane. The plasma membrane is typical of any cell, i.e. it comprises a lipid bilayer containing a high concentration of membrane proteins. The lipid bilayer is a self-assembling sheet of phospholipid that adopts the bilayer format because of the physicochemical properties of the polar phospholipids, ensuring that the polar groups are external and the hydrophobic groups form the inner layer of the leaflet (see Fig. 4.5). The photoreceptor can adopt this special arrangement because it has more cholesterol in its bilayer, not only making it less fluid but also preventing crystallization of the membrane by inhibiting possible phase transition of the hydrocarbons.

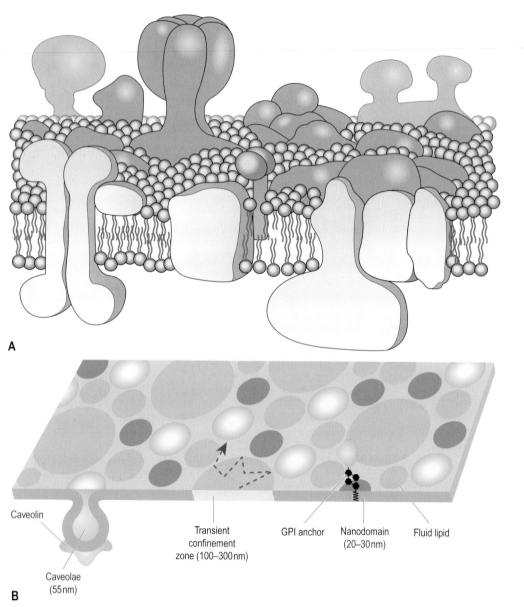

Fig. 4.5 (**A**) General models for membrane structure. The fluid mosaic model has been modified to the current view of a 'protein-crowded' membrane. From Engelman (2005). (**B**) Mosaic domain model of the plasma membrane. The plasma membrane is modelled as a mosaic of different lipid domains. These include caveolae, nanodomains enriched in GPI-anchored proteins and glycosphingolipids, transient confinement zones (TCZs) of various sizes and small regions enriched in fluid lipids. The relationships among these domains remain uncertain. For instance, the TCZs, caveolae and nanodomains may all be examples of detergent-resistant l_o domains. Nanodomains may exist within TCZs or be independent of them. Lipids and GPI-anchored protein are able to exchange in and out of these various domains. (From Maxfield 2002, with permission from Elsevier.)

Endoplasmic reticulum and Golgi apparatus

A wide variety of cell organelles are embedded in a cytoplasmic gel, which is traversed by a system of membranes, the endoplasmic reticulum (ER). The ER, a system of thin bilayered membranes, is a flowing dynamic system constantly forming and reforming. Cisternal, tubular and vesicular elements exist. The rough ER (RER) is distinguished from the smooth ER as a ribosome-studded structure that is highly developed in secretory cells such as the lacrimal gland acinar cell, and is specialized in other cells, e.g. the sarcoplasmic reticulum of striated (including extraocular) muscle. The RER is arranged *en face* in rows or rosettes of ribosomes (polysomes). Newly synthesized proteins come off the ribosomes and are threaded through the lipid bilayer into the interior of the ER where they are post-translationally folded, ready for secretion via the Golgi apparatus by vacuolar budding and fusion with the plasma membrane for exocytosis (see Boxes 4.2 and 4.3). The smooth ER is also the site of synthesis of molecules such as lipids, triglycerides and steroids, and is well demonstrated in cells such as the RPE and meibomian gland cells.

New evidence also indicates that the ER and the Golgi apparatus may be involved in signalling. The well-known series of signalling molecules, the small GTPases, as well as being activated through the plasma membrane have similar counterparts for signalling in the ER and Golgi body (see Box 4.3). In fact, small GTPases and other molecules, such as phosphoinositides, provide a signature for each organelle and are involved in the specific lipid membrane folding that characterizes each organelle (see Box 4.3).

The ER also forms the nuclear envelope during telophase, when a series of flat vesicles surround the chromosomes and fuse at their edges. The envelope contains many *nuclear pores*, which are composed of eight cylindrical filamentous structures in a highly organized arrangement. Pores act as molecular sieves, permitting rapid passage of small 4.5-nm (4.5 kDa) particles and slower passage of larger molecules (12–70 kDa). The outer aspect of the nuclear envelope in secretory cells is lined with ribosomes and polysomes, while the inner surface is in contact with a nuclear filamentous matrix.

Mitochondria

Mitochondria are small (2 mm) oval-shaped organelles comprising a two-membrane system of compartments the inner one of which is folded into cristae. The intermembrane space contains carrier proteins, which are responsible for the transport of metabolites between the two compartments and also between the cytosol and the outer compartment. Their transport systems include antiport, aspartate/glutamate, ornithine/citrulline, malate/citrate, symport, pyruvate/H^+, and urea and porphyrin synthesis. Mitochondria are the powerhouses of the cell and have several essential metabolic functions because they contain all the elements for the respiratory assembly, for the citric acid cycle and for fatty acid metabolism. Their main functions therefore are to act as the site of energy-rich adenosine triphosphate (ATP)/guanosine triphosphate (GTP) formation, to function as a calcium store mainly in the form of calcium phosphate, to engage in the uptake of energy-rich substances, and to facilitate the oxidative breakdown of ATP. In addition, recent studies have shown that mitochondria play an integral part in the process of apoptosis following activation of cytochrome C. Many other proteins (such as those shown in Box 4.4) have been implicated as 'death gene' products but studies in knockout mice have failed to confirm many of these. Even those known to be involved in cell death, such as the caspases, may also have a role in normal cell physiology. Mitochondria have their own complement of DNA but no histones, and ribosomal RNA/transfer RNA, and generate a series of mitochondrion-specific proteins associated with mutations and a number of discrete syndromes. Since mitochondria originate only from ova, transmission of these genetic defects is purely maternal.

The nucleus

Chromatin is a complex structure of highly extended DNA, RNA and protein in the interphase (non-dividing) cell, which becomes greatly condensed (by 400-fold) to form chromosomes during cell division. Packing of chromatin is effected by interaction between negatively charged DNA and certain basic proteins (histones) which carry a positive charge at the pH of the cell; euchromatin is less packed than heterochromatin, the proportion of which varies from nucleus to nucleus and may be characteristic of certain cell types, e.g. the 'clock-face' heterochromatin of plasma cells detectable in histological sections.

The nuclear membrane also contains receptors for ligands, which may be synthesized in the cytoplasm or may have been endocytosed through plasma membrane receptors. Typical nuclear membrane receptors include steroids, growth factors such as

Box 4.2 Endocytosis and exocytosis

Endocytosis is generally achieved via incorporation of ligand–receptor complexes in clathrin-coated vesicles. This applies to soluble proteins and to small and large particles such as viruses, which frequently use constitutive cell surface receptors to enter cells.

Clathrin-coated vesicles start as small pits on the cell surface. When the vesicle is fully intracellular it loses its clathrin coat and becomes an endosome, which fuses with primary lysosomes that have a high content of acid hydro-

lases and other proteases. These lead to degradation of the ingested material, and further processing depending on the cell type. Certain cell surface receptors are recycled to the cell membrane during this process to engage further extracellular ligand (**A**). Clathrin-coated pits are normally restricted to the region of the plasma membrane by the cortical cytoplasm actin organization. Relaxation of this actin assembly by proteins such as latrunculin B allows movement of the coated pits.

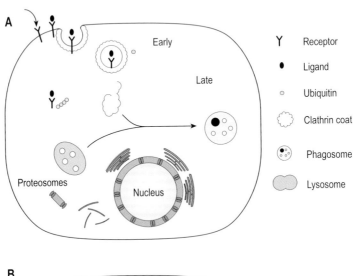

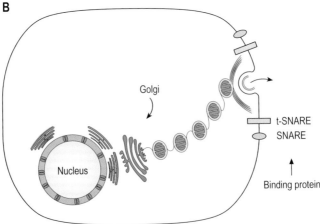

Exocytosis occurs by a similar process but in reverse. Cytoplasmic granules such as those in exocrine glands or in granulocytes are lipid vesicles containing material for extrusion. Secretory vesicles bud from the Golgi apparatus and are transported towards the plasma membrane by the cytoskeleton. There, they fuse in a lipid microdomain assisted by proteins such as SNARE and the SNARE-binding proteins in a 'targeting patch' (**B**). Fused secretory vesicle membranes act as targets for further secretory granule fusion in cells such as mast cells.

Box 4.3 Schematic representation of how mitogens activate cells

Ligand binding to the tyrosine kinase receptor (PKTR) activates the small GTPases, Ras, through a complex of signalling molecules (Grb2/SOS). Activated Ras on endosomes from the plasma membrane induces signalling in this organelle as well as in the Golgi apparatus (indirectly via phospholipase CgCa and another protein known as GRPI) while inhibition of the small Ras occurs in the endoplasmic reticulum via an inhibitor protein ERII. In this example of a signalling network, interstin and kinase suppressor of Ras serve as scaffold proteins while p14 acts as an adaptor protein in Ras-independent activation of the kinase, MEK-1 (mitogen-activated protein (extracellular signal regulated (ERR) kinase) kinase), by the endosome. The integration of organelles and signalling networks with cytosolic proteins is thus central to proper functioning of the cell in response to an external stimulus such as a mitogen.

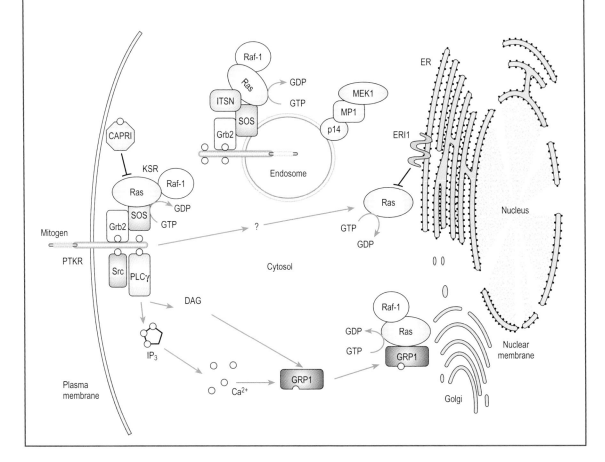

fibroblast growth factor and novel groups of proteins known as the peroxisome proliferator-activated receptors (PPARs), which are involved in many cell processes such as lipid and glucose homeostasis, wound healing and inflammation generally. PPARs are unique receptors that allow integration of signals mediated by lipophilic ligands with plasma membrane-derived signals (Fig. 4.6A,B). Nuclear membrane receptors may be organized for induction or suppression of genes in a co-ordinated fashion (Fig 4.6C).

The nucleolus is essentially composed of RNA and fibrillar material, and is the site of ribosomal RNA synthesis. It develops during the late stages of mitosis in association with specific regions on the chromosomes, the nucleolar organizer centre.

The intracellular matrix

The cytoplasm is a highly viscous aqueous medium that has deformability (elasticity). Physically, it exists at different times as a gel or as a sol. The cortical cytoplasm (ectoplasm) is more akin to a gel struc-

Box 4.4 Signalling pathways in apoptosis

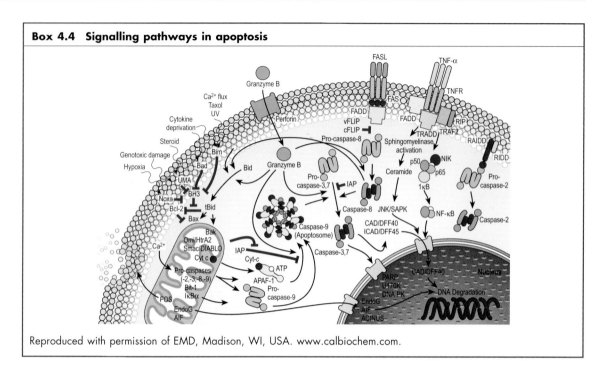

Reproduced with permission of EMD, Madison, WI, USA. www.calbiochem.com.

A Direct mechanisms

B Indirect mechanisms

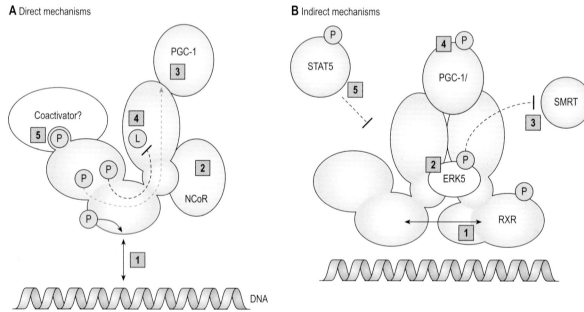

Fig. 4.6 (**A,B**) Mechanisms through which phosphorylation modulates PPAR activity. (**A**) Direct mechanisms. 1: Enhancement of DNA binding; 2: inhibition of NCoR association; 3: selective recruitment of PGC-1 by the E domain; 4: inhibition of the ligand binding; 5: putative recruitment of cofactors by the A/B domain. (From Laurent and Michalik 2005, with permission from Elsevier.) (**B**) Indirect mechanisms. 1: Allosteric control of PPAR through RXR and/or RXR-mediated recruitment of cofactors; 2: recruitment of phosphorylated ERK5; 3: inhibition of SMRT association; 4: modulation of cofactor acitivity; 5: inhibition by phosphorylated STAT5 (unknown mechanism). ERK, extracellular-signal-regulated kinase; NCoR, nuclear receptor co-repressor; RXR, retinoid X receptor; SMRT, silencing mediator for retinoid and thryoid hormone receptors. (From Stein *et al.* 2003, with permission from Elsevier.)

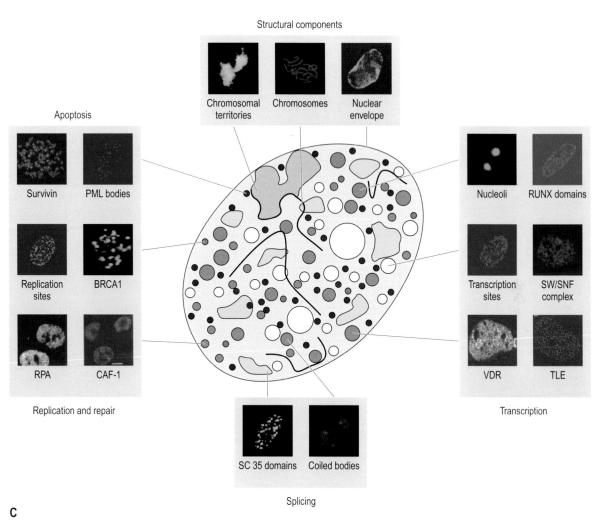

Fig. 4.6 *Continued* **(C)** The nuclear architecture is functionally linked to the organization and sorting of regulatory information. Immunofluorescence microscopy of the nucleus in situ has revealed the distinct non-overlapping subnuclear distribution of vital nuclear processes. (From Stein *et al.* 2003, with permission from Elsevier.)

ture, while the endoplasm is usually more fluid. Thus the cortical cytoplasm restricts movement of organelles such as coated vesicles (see Boxes 4.2 and 4.3). The gel-like properties of the cytoplasm are the result of the binding of 'structured' water molecules and Ca^{2+} ions to polymeric filaments, of which there are three types: microfilaments, intermediate filaments and group 3 cytoskeletal fibres.

Microfilaments

Microfilaments (5–7 nm), such as actin, tropomyosin and troponin, are universal constituents of cells and are involved in cell motility, contractility, and structural integrity, where they insert into cell junctional complexes (see Box 4.5). Actin bundles are brought to a highly developed level in muscle cells. Actin occurs in several forms within the cell, depending on its associated protein, e.g. as a fine lattice meshwork or as a sheaf of fibres (stress fibres).

The cellular distribution and, particularly, the degree of polymerization of microfilaments are determined by the nature of proteins that bind to them, i.e. the microfilament-associated proteins (Table 4.1). Monomeric soluble actin (G actin) is converted to gel-phase polymerized fibrils (F actin) by association

Table 4.1 Function of actin binding proteins

Function	Protein	Cell/structure
Gelation	Filamin	Smooth muscle/fibroblasts
Bundling	A actin Fimbrin Talin	Muscle Microvilli All cells
Severing	Gelsolin Villin B actinin	Macrophages Microvilli Skeletal muscle
Depolymerizing	Profilin Thymosin Actobinin	Lymphocytes All cells All cells
Membrane binding	Vinculin Spectrin	Adhesion sites Red cells, photoreceptors
Receptor transport	Capping proteins	Leucocytes
Junctional complex	Radixin	Liver cells

with certain proteins. In smooth muscle cells and fibroblasts, filamin assists polymerization; in contrast, in lymphocytes, profilin and thymosin maintain G actin in the depolymerized state, presumably to facilitate flexibility in cell shape during rapid migration within tissues. The specificity of these actin-binding proteins is remarkable; examples include the ankyrin–spectrin–actin combination, which effects the red cell biconcave shape, and the spectrin–peripherin–actin combination between rod outer segment disks and plasma membrane. Actin polymerization and depolymerization is a highly regulated process requiring addition of actin monomers to one end of the microfilament and removal at the opposite end, each of which has separate K_{on} and K_{off} constants. This process is under the control of actin-depolymerization factor/cofilins which alter these rate constants as necessary, leading to changes in the twist of the molecule and promoting severance of the actin filament.

Regulation of coordinated changes to the actin cytoskeleton is under the control of intracellular enzymes, particularly the Rho family of GTPases (this includes enzymes such as Rho, Rac and Cdc42, the last of which is a cell cycle-related protein). Certain kinases, known as the p-21 activated kinases (PAKs), are involved in regulating some of the diverse changes induced by Rac and Cdc42. PAKs may determine such cellular responses as polarity in epithelial cells and motility in fibroblasts. For example, coordinated functional regulation of the interaction between dynamin, cortactin, actin-binding protein 1, neuronal Wiskott–Aldrich syndrome protein 1 (N-Wasp-1), profilin and actin occurs during the pseudopodial extension of migrating fibroblasts (Fig. 4.7).

Several isoforms and at least three families of actin exist and some of these are located in specific parts of the cell, e.g. β-actin in the cell cortex.

Intermediate filaments

Intermediate filaments (10–12 nm) are coiled α-helices and act as stretchable components of the cytoskeleton scaffold. They occur in cell-, tissue- and differentiation-specific distribution (Fig. 4.8) in both cytoplasmic and nuclear compartments of the cell, and are classified into five groups depending on domain and sequence homology. Their major function is to protect cells from mechanical and non-mechanical damage, and gene mutations account for around 30 different diseases in man, mostly related to skin, muscle and nerve dysfunction. In general, intermediate filaments are important for the correct positioning and function of cell organelles such as mitochondria and ER. There are five classes of cytoplasmic intermediate filaments, often used to characterize cells in tissue culture or

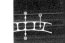

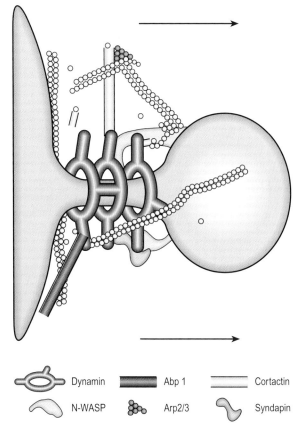

Dynamin   Abp 1   Cortactin

N-WASP   Arp2/3   Syndapin

Fig. 4.7 Dynamin-mediated tubulation and vesiculation of secretory and endocytic compartments. Model showing dynamin-mediated tubulation/vesiculation of membrane as it might occur at the plasma membrane. Dynamin, its binding protein and associated proteins are likely to function together during vesicle formation. The molecular 'pinchase' activity of dynamin, together with the enhanced actin filament nucleation at the membrane interface, results in the tubulation and severing of the membranous vesicle necks. (See text for details.) Large black arrows indicate the generation of force and the movement of nascent vesicles. (From Orth and McNiven 2003, with permission from Elsevier.)

tumours, and one class of nuclear intermediate filaments:

- *keratins* – found in epithelial cells; over 50 individual members grouped into two types, I and II, exist as heterodimers.
- *vimentin* – found in mesenchymal cells
- *desmin* – interconnects myofibrils of muscle cells, at site of Z disk and M line, thus maintaining their register
- *glial fibrillary acidic protein* (glia)

- *neurofilaments* – e.g. S100 protein in neuroectoderm; connect with microtubules via small projections
- *lamins* – line the inner surface of the nuclear envelope as a fibrous lattice (karyoskeleton); more than five types.

The function of intermediate filaments is to ensure normal cytoplasmic positioning and function of different organelles. Lamins undergo considerable molecular disruption during mitosis and may communicate with cytoplasmic intermediate filaments, but how this occurs is not clear. Others, such as keratins, provide mechanical strength to junctional structures such as desmosomes (see Box 4.6). They may also have a function in the positioning of the nucleus in the cell in a cage-like bundle of fibrils.

Considerable information is now available on the molecular organization of these junctions. For instance, while desmosomes and hemidesmosomes ('junctions' between the cell and basement membrane in epithelia) have some ultrastructural similarity, at the molecular level there are clear differences between the constituent proteins. Desmosomes are formed by a series of proteins spanning the cell membrane and the intercellular space (desmoglobin, desmoplakin, see Box 4.6), while hemidesmosomes contain other proteins such as the $\alpha_6\beta_4$ integrin receptor, which binds to laminin in the basement membrane, plus other proteins such as the bullous pemphigoid and the pemphigus antigens.

Interactions between intermediate filaments and microfilaments are mediated by plectin, a >500 kDa dumbbell-shaped protein that can self-associate and in addition can bind at both ends of the hemidesmosomal protein $\alpha_6\beta_4$ integrin and probably to other junctional proteins.

Group 3 cytoskeletal fibres

A third group of cytoskeletal fibrillar elements also exists but the fibres are less easy to categorize. Several thick filaments occur as part of the cytoskeleton, such as myosin (myosin comprises 25% of cytoplasmic protein in striated muscle) and microtubules. Microtubules are cylindrical structures about 24 nm wide, comprising 13 globular elements composed of the heterodimer ($\alpha\beta$) tubulin. Stable microtubules occur in flagellae and cilia, while labile microtubules are found in structures such as the muscle spindle. Microtubules are involved in movement and cell motility, including intracellular

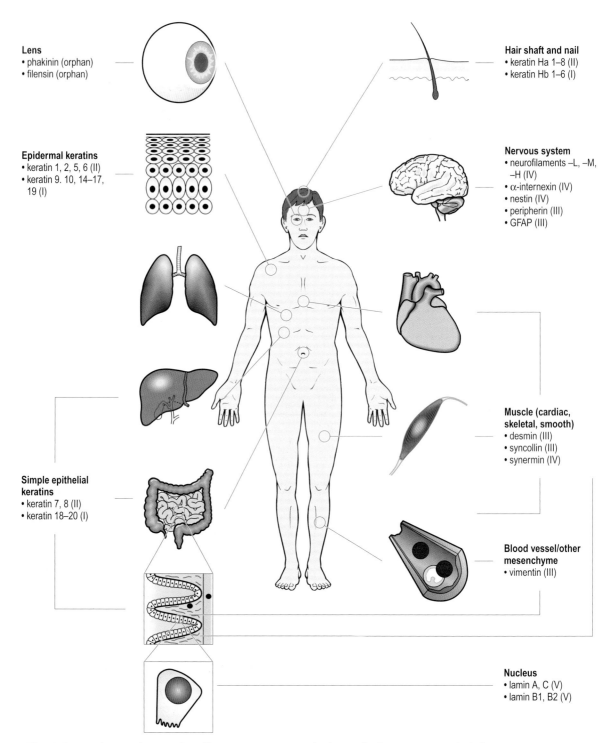

Lens
• phakinin (orphan)
• filensin (orphan)

Epidermal keratins
• keratin 1, 2, 5, 6 (II)
• keratin 9. 10, 14–17, 19 (I)

Simple epithelial keratins
• keratin 7, 8 (II)
• keratin 18–20 (I)

Hair shaft and nail
• keratin Ha 1–8 (II)
• keratin Hb 1–6 (I)

Nervous system
• neurofilaments –L, –M, –H (IV)
• α-internexin (IV)
• nestin (IV)
• peripherin (III)
• GFAP (III)

Muscle (cardiac, skeletal, smooth)
• desmin (III)
• syncollin (III)
• synermin (IV)

Blood vessel/other mesenchyme
• vimentin (III)

Nucleus
• lamin A, C (V)
• lamin B1, B2 (V)

Fig. 4.8 Distribution of intermediate filament (IF) proteins in the human body. IF proteins include five major types (I–V) and a separate 'orphan' category (IF type and category are listed in parentheses). Lamins (type V) are found in the nucleus of most mammalian cells whereas the remaining IFs (types I–IV) are cytoplasmic and expressed in a cell-tissue-selective manner. For each tissue, representative major IFs are listed for the principal cell type. (From Toivola *et al.* 2005, with permission from Elsevier.)

transport as in axoplasmic flow. Drugs such as colchicine (used in Behçet's disease) and taxol (proposed as prophylaxis for proliferative vitreoretinopathy) disrupt microtubule organization and inhibit cell motility.

With the recently identified superfine filaments, these elements combine to form an intracellular meshwork in which proteins do not exist in solution as previously surmised, but are attached to the filaments alongside other structures such as 'free' ribosomes and small vesicles (polysomes). This arrangement has special relevance to highly organized cells such as lens fibres.

Cell movement involves formation and release of focal contact sites in coordination with the actin cytoskeleton. However, contact sites are also implicated in signalling via the Rho family of small GTPases (see above), which in turn involve microtubules. Therefore this demonstrates the extensive interconnections between the three filamentous systems in at least one fundamental type of cell behaviour.

Certain discrete cellular structures are composed of microtubules, such as the centriole (the microtubular organizing centre, a cylindrical structure comprising nine groups of triplet microtubules) and the mitotic spindle. Cilia are remarkably constant structures in eukaryotic cells, composed of nine peripheral and two central bundles of three fused microtubules. Movement occurs by sliding of the outer arm of dynein along the core of tubulin.

The cytoplasm also contains several storage products such as glycogen granules, lipid droplets and melanin in melanosomes. With age, some cells, such as the RPE cell, accumulate lipofuscin granules as byproducts of undigested proteolipid (ethanolamine).

Intracellular signalling mechanisms

As stated above, cells respond to external stimuli by means of cell surface receptors, which convert the external stimulus to a series of intracellular signals (second messengers) directed towards specific cellular functions such as protein transcription for growth control or ion-channel gating in neural responses (see p. 174).

Second messenger systems are based on a network of reactions involving an agonist, a receptor and an interacting set of coupled proteins (see Fig. 4.1). Cyclic adenosine monophosphate (cAMP) is the archetypal second messenger, and the result of such a response is the phosphorylation of a regulatory intracellular protein via a kinase.

THE EXTRACELLULAR MATRIX

Cells exist within a structural framework, the extracellular matrix, which is secreted by the cells and consists of several classes of macromolecules, the most abundant of which is collagen (accounting for 30% of total protein in the organism) (Table 4.2).

Genetic and protein sequence analysis of extracellular proteins has shown that, despite the great variety of matrix molecules, extensive sequence homology exists between them with recurring structural motifs (see Box 4.6). Thus the 'epidermal growth factor' motif appears to be present in several apparently different extracellular matrix proteins.

Extracellular matrix proteins determine the structural nature of the tissue

Extracellular matrix proteins show modifications that are characteristic of the tissue in which they are found. Thus, the cornea contains type I collagen filaments, which do not form fibrils of diameter greater than 5 nm; this is important in corneal transparency. The vitreous contains an isoform of type IX collagen, which is different in certain characteristics from cartilage type IX collagen.

There are over 30 different types of collagen (Table 4.3), of which at least 22 have been detected in the developing and adult eye. The eye and cartilaginous tissues share six types of collagen not found very frequently in other tissues; indeed the collagen triple helix has been found as a domain of many proteins and it has been suggested that all such proteins should be included in the collagen family. Collagen types are determined by the combination of the three types of chain forming the α helix core. For instance, type I collagen triple helix is made up of two unique α_1 chains and a unique α_2 chain, coded

Table 4.2 Some extracellular matrix proteins	
Structural	Non-structural
Collagen	Fibronectin
Laminin	Thrombospondin
Elastin	Nidogen
Proteoglycan	Plasminogen activator inhibitor
Tenascin	α_2-macroglobulin

Box 4.5 Filaments and junctions

Intercellular connections or junctions are structures that make cells into tissues and tissues into organs. There are several types, each of which is composed of junction-specific proteins.

Tight junctions – have no detectable 'space' between the cell membranes. They are also known as zonulae occludens; they form a barrier to paracellular diffusion of all molecules, including water and ions. They are also involved in regulation of epithelial cell proliferation and differentiation. They occur at such sites as the blood–aqueous barrier of the ciliary body and the blood–retinal barrier at the apex of the RPE cell. They consist of a system of ridges and grooves, as seen by freeze–fracture studies. There are four major classes of tight junction proteins:

- transmembrane proteins – occludin, dandin
- adaptors – ZO-1, cingulin, MUPPI
- transcriptional and post-transcriptional regulators – AP-1
- signalling proteins – aPKC, CDK4.

Clandins have unique abilities to selectively permit transport of charged ions and vary from tissue to tissue (**A**).

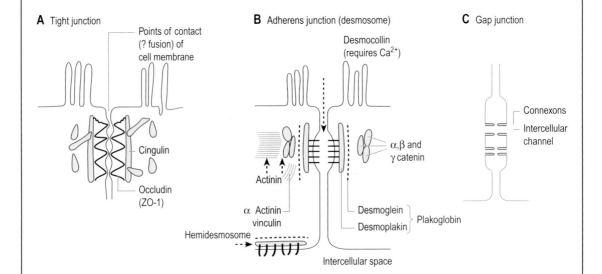

A Tight junction

Points of contact (? fusion) of cell membrane

Cingulin

Occludin (ZO-1)

B Adherens junction (desmosome)

Desmocollin (requires Ca^{2+})

Actinin

α,β and γ catenin

α Actinin vinculin

Desmoglein
Desmoplakin
Plakoglobin

Hemidesmosome

Intercellular space

C Gap junction

Connexons

Intercellular channel

Desmosomes – form specialized 'adherens' junctions of 20-nm width between cells. Two types are described: spot desmosomes (at single site) and belt desmosomes (as a ring round the apex of the cell). The latter are also known as zonulae adherens. Their probable role is mechanical adhesion: cytoplasmic filaments insert into spot (cytokeratin) and belt (actin) forms (**B**). Several proteins are involved in different regions of the desmosome, including desmocollin, desmoglein and desmoplakin, forming a subfamily of cadherins. The cadherins bind to β-catenin and then to actin-based cytoskeletal proteins such as vinculin and α-activin, ZO-1 and actin itself. The function of tight junctions (above) is dependent on the integrity of the adherens junctions. Hemidesmosomes have a similar plaque formed in this case by bullous pemphigoid antigen (BPAG1).

Gap junctions – so called because there is a 2-nm gap at this adhesion site between cells. Gap junctions occur in the basal regions of epithelial and other cells. They are a highly organized structure composed of 'connexons', plasma membrane domains containing connexins, which have a role in permitting the passage of larger ions such as Ca^{2+}, and other signalling molecules, so permitting a coordinated response by a group of cells, as in ocular or cardiac muscle (**C**).

Synapse – a specialized form of junction between nerves, or between nerves and muscles, and characterized by synaptic vesicles in the axon terminal and pre- and post-synaptic thickening of the plasma membrane (see Ch. 5).

Table 4.3 Some collagen types

Structural, fibrillar	Structural, non-fibrillar	Non-structural	Transmembrane
I	IV	IX	XIII
II	VI	XI	XVII
III	VIII	XII	XXIII
V	X		XXV
VII		XIV–XIX	

as $[\alpha_1(I)]_2 \, \alpha_2(I)$; type II collagen is composed of three identical unique α_1 chains, $[\alpha_1(II)]_3$. Each collagen therefore has a set of unique chains that make up the triple helix.

In certain collagens, particularly the non-fibrillar collagens such as types IV and IX, the protein is composed of short segments of triple helix (COL1, -2, -3, etc.) interspersed with sections of non-collagenous (NC1, NC2, etc.) protein. These are also sometimes referred to as FACII collagens (fibril-associated collagens) with interrupted triple helices. These proteins usually act as bridges or networks for binding other proteins and forming complex protein aggregates such as basement membranes. Collagens in essence are the structural components that hold organs and tissues together and the mechanism by which they form is interesting: the three polypeptide chains form a monomer by self-assembly from a small nucleus in a zipper-like fashion, much in the way that crystallization occurs, and the formation of fibrils from monomers is also entropy driven.

A subcategory of collagenous proteins is included as components of transmembrane proteins including types XIII, XVII, XXIII and XXV (Table 4.3) and remain following cleavage of the soluble fragment of the cytokine or adhesion molecule by enzymes known as 'sheddases'. They exist as homotrimers of a collagen-specific α-chain. Some transmembrane collagen-like molecules occur as specific receptors such as the macrophage scavenger receptors. Sheddases are of several types and include the ADAMTs (proteinases of the 'a disintegrin-and-metalloproteinase' family) which are involved for instance in the shedding of molecules such as soluble tumour necrosis factor-α-converting enzyme, TACE) from leucocytes (see Ch. 7). This general process is important in establishing the soluble regulatory constituents of particular extracellular matrices.

The transmembrane collagen XVII (originally described as bullous pemphigoid antigen 180, BP180) is important in cellular adhesion because it binds α_6 integrin and laminin 5 extracellularly and β_4 integrin, plectin and BP230 intracellularly. Degradation products of collagens, such as the non-fibrillar collagens XVIII and XV, which yield the anti-angiogenic products endostatin and restin after cleavage, have major roles in regulating cell function through inhibition of matrix metalloproteinases.

The eye contains a wide variety of different collagens (see Ch. 2). For instance, the cornea contains types I, V and VI in the stroma, while types IV and VII are present in the subepithelial layer. In addition, type XVI transmembrane linker collagen has been found in the basal epithelial cell matrix. The iris contains collagen types I, III and IV, while the zonule contains type IV. The lens contains only type IV, while the vitreous contains collagens II, IX and XI, complexed to the extracellular matrix protein fibrillin. This complex has an important role in vitreous matrix organization.

Certain types of collagen are unique to ocular tissue in that their structure has been modified. Examples include type VIII in Desçemet's membrane, types II and IX in vitreous (both similar but not identical to cartilage collagens) and type III in the distensible tissue of the choroid. Several of the newer collagens contain domains similar to type IX, and it has been suggested that these may represent a subfamily of type IX collagens (Table 4.3). The more recently described types XV, XVIII and XIX are located in basement membranes and may have a role in the formation of blood vessels.

Collagen and elastin are the major insoluble proteins of the extracellular matrix. While collagen occurs in all tissues, elastin is present only in

Box 4.6 Extracellular matrix proteins

Extracellular matrix proteins appear to be made up of building blocks ('structural motifs'), which are protein domains with extensive homology to existing protein structures. For instance, three fibronectin domains are reproduced in many other proteins; the epidermal growth factor-like domain also appears in modular form in proteins such as plasminogen; and the arginine–glycine–aspartate (RGD) cell adhesion site is present in many molecules (**A**).

Fibronectin is a dimer containing discrete domains for the attachment of other molecules (**A**). The modular structure of fibronectin shows that it consists of 12 type I modules (rectangles), two type II modules (violet ovals) and 15–17 type III modules (ovals). The alternatively spliced domains IIIB, IIIA and the V region are shown in yellow. Binding domains for fibrin, collagen, cells and heparin are indi-

cated; dimer forms via cysteine pair at the C-terminus (SS). From Mao and Schwarzbauer (2005)

Laminin is a cross-shaped trimer in which the B1, B2 and A chains form a triple helix in the stem of the cross. Laminin also has several discrete domains for attachment of various molecules. In addition, it contains a cryptic cell adhesion-binding site, which becomes exposed after partial proteolysis (**B**). Fibrillar collagen is organized in tissues by association with smaller non-fibrillar collagens, e.g. type I with type XII collagen, and type II with type IX collagen (**C**).

Part A from Yao and Schwarzbauer 2005, with permission from Elsevier. Parts B,C courtesy of S Miyayima and KM Yamada.)

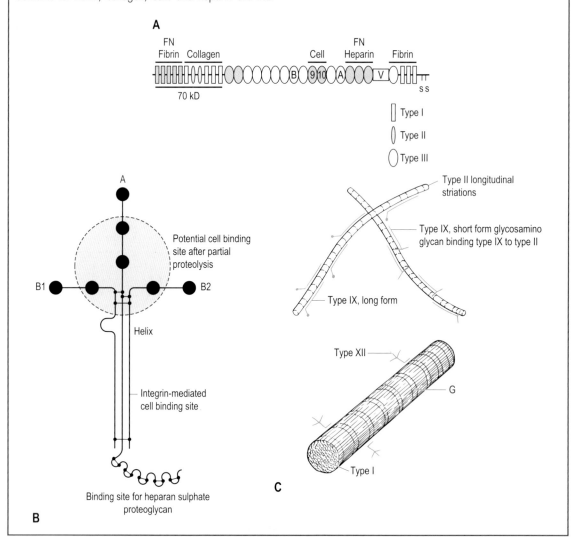

deformable tissues such as blood vessel walls, lung parenchyma and the zonule of the lens. Unlike collagen, elastin does not contain any methionine residues and is therefore separable from collagen after digestion with cyanogen bromide. Elastin is formed from soluble tropoelastin fibrils which crosslink at their lysine residues to form, via allysine intermediates, desmosine and isodesmosine crosslinks. Elastin has little order to its tertiary structure; instead it forms a random coil, which tends to become more ordered during deformation.

As for collagen, elastin degradation products have a role in regulating cell behaviour in the matrix, and under certain circumstances, may be pathogenic, e.g. in promoting tumour invasion and angiogenesis. Even smaller molecules derived from a range of matrix proteins (matrikines) have regulatory activity for connective tissue cells, for instance the tripeptide GHK which has stimulatory activity for several cell types and promotes collagen biosynthesis and wound healing overall.

Fibrillins are extracellular microfibrils that are responsible for the biomechanical properties of tissues. Cysteine-rich glycoproteins, composed of multiple repeats of a Ca^{2+}-binding epidermal growth factor-like domain, are secreted in a proform and polymerize extracellularly. They are present in vitreous (see above) and are an important component of the zonule. Fibrillins have a structural role in long-range elasticity of tissues. They also have a role in the fine tuning of growth factor signals such as those involving transforming growth factor-β (TGF-β) and particularly latent TGF-β-binding protein (PTBP) involved in morphogenesis.

Tenascins are extracellular matrix proteins that are functionally mysterious at present. Several forms are described (tenascin-C, -X, -W, etc.) and phenotypes in knockout mice are broadly normal although there may be some subtle defects in wound healing. Tenascin-Y appears to be restricted to neural tissue while mutations in Tenascin-X have been linked to Ehelrs–Danlos syndrome, in conjunction with known defects in pro-collagen and elastin biosynthesis. Tenascins are widely distributed and appear to have an anti-adhesive role particularly antagonizing the effects of fibronectin. Interestingly, fibronectin is found in the anterior lens capsule while tenascin is found in the posterior capsule.

Laminins are an integral part of basement membranes and have a characteristic cross-shaped structure composed of an A-coiled long chain and two B chains (B1 and B2) (see Box 4.6). There are several isoforms (at least 15) that are specific for different cell types (e.g. kalinin in epithelial cells) and that may reflect the different properties of each type of basement membrane.

Laminin 5 is specific for epithelial cells and binds to the $\alpha_3\beta_1$ and $\alpha_6\beta_4$ integrins (see above). Matrix metalloproteinases (MMP2 and MMP9 especially) are activated by laminin degradation products.

Laminin in the basement membrane is tightly bound to nidogen (entactin), a protein that mediates the binding of laminin to heparin-containing proteoglycans (heparin sulphate proteoglycan) such as perlecan and syndecan in the basement membrane matrix. The infrastructure of the basement membranes is composed of type IV collagen in a highly organized lattice network to which the complex of laminin–nidogen is also bound. The proteoglycan then acts as a space-filling molecule in the basement membrane (Fig. 4.9). Cells are bound to the basement membrane via anchoring fibrils containing type VII collagen and transmembrane proteins such as type XI collagen.

Non-structural proteins

Many other proteins are distributed throughout the extracellular matrix, which, although not having a direct structural role, have important functions in cell–matrix and cell–cell interactions. Probably the best known of these is fibronectin, a 250-kDa heterodimer that has multiple cell and molecule binding domains (see Box 4.6). One of the type III fibronectin domains contains the ubiquitous cell adhesion domain Arg-Gly-Asp-Ser (RGDS in single-letter amino acid nomenclature), found in many other proteins. Multiple forms of fibronectin occur by alternate splicing. Two major forms exist: plasma fibronectin, secreted by hepatocytes, and cellular fibronectin, secreted by fibroblasts and forming a fibrillar network on the cell surface. Fibronectin is not a constitutive component of basement membranes but may be present under certain circumstances. It may be involved in the initial stages of cell binding to the extracellular matrix, with a major role in the alignment of matrix proteins and the final organization of the basement membrane components. Fibronectin may be involved in integrin-mediated cell signalling and, through the actin-binding protein profilin, may regulate stress fibre formation in endothelial cells and fibroblasts. Fibronectin also has high-affinity binding sites for fibrin(ogen), thus promoting incorporation of fibrin into the extracellular matrix during wound healing. Fibrin binds growth factors such as fibroblast growth

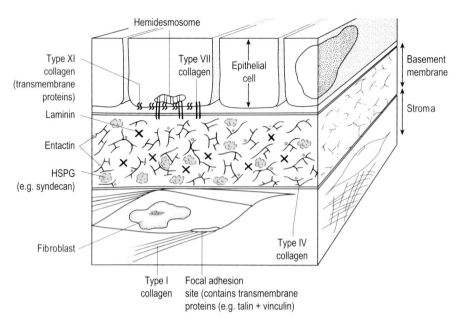

Fig. 4.9 Structure of basement membrane.

factor 2 and vascular endothelial cell growth factor, providing sources for angiogenic stimulation.

Thrombospondins are a group of extracellular matrix proteins that were first identified as platelet release proteins but that are now known to be secreted by endothelial cells and other cell types. Five forms of thrombospondin exist, two of which appear to be alternately spliced forms of the 'parent' molecule. Like extracellular matrix proteins, thrombospondins are composed of building blocks, each with specific cellular and molecular adhesive properties. Thrombospondins may be involved in the regulation of angiogenesis, which is of considerable importance in ocular disease (see Ch. 9). In this regard, they form complexes with a ubiquitous plasma protein, histidine-rich glycoprotein (HRG), which has many regulatory functions in wound healing, cell migration and immune cell function. In addition, thrombospondins are better regarded as matricellular proteins that regulate a variety of processes, including cell adhesion and collagen fibrillogenesis.

Several other proteins are present in the extracellular matrix, such as proteases (e.g. plasminogen) and their inhibitors [plasminogen activator inhibitor 1 (PAI-1), α_2-macroglobulin, etc.]. PAI-1 is present at high concentrations around various cells in the quiescent state and is considered important in the regulation of cell migration by controlling the level of cell-associated plasminogen activator required to initiate the degradation of basement membrane proteins. Other important proteins include the matrix metalloproteinases and their inhibitors (TIMP-1 to -3). Some of these proteins are secreted by the cells themselves while others are synthesized predominantly in the liver and reach the extracellular matrix via the plasma.

Some proteins have their action at a distance from the cell, such as fibrillin, a 350-kDa microfibrillar protein that is involved in the assembly of elastin fibrils. Fibrillin is found in the tertiary vitreous and the zonule (see previous section). Mutations in fibrillin are found in Marfan syndrome, a disease of elastic tissue in which dislocation of the lens is a central feature.

Glycosaminoglycans occur in the extracellular matrix bound to core proteins as proteoglycans

Glycosaminoglycans occur in a variety of forms, essentially based on a repeating disaccharide structure (see Box 4.7). The prototype proteoglycan was described in relation to cartilage, in which a series of proteoglycans are linked to a hyaluronic acid backbone (Fig. 4.10). This, however, is not relevant to ocular proteoglycans; for instance, hyaluronic acid in the vitreous is not associated with other proteoglycans that contain glycosaminoglycans (GAGs) but is linked to collagen type IX, which in this

Box 4.7 Structure of glycosaminoglycans

Glycosaminoglycans are long chains of repeating disaccharides based on a common structure: (**A**) heparan sulphate; (**B**) chondroitin 4,6-sulphate. Chondroitin 6 and 4,6 sulphates have additional sulphate groups at the appropriate C atoms (*); dermatan sulphate has the GlcA (glycosamino-) residue replaced in variable lengths of the chain by l-idoA (iduronic acid). Heparan has many more sulphate groups and a higher content of l-idoA than heparin. Keratan sulphate has galactose instead of glucose, and hyaluronic acid has no sulphate groups.

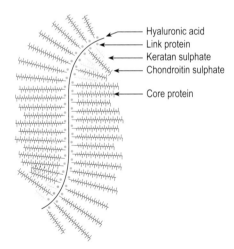

Fig. 4.10 Artist's impression of hyaluronic acid molecule. (After Rosenberg 1975.)

situation is regarded as a proteoglycan. In addition, keratan sulphate proteoglycan occurs in the cornea in the absence of hyaluronic acid, where it appears to regulate collagen fibril diameter (see below). In other tissues, hyaluronan has both structural and cell regulatory activities. For instance, two receptors of the LINK protein family, LYVE-1 and stabilin-1, are important in specific functions of lymphoid cells and endothelial cells respectively. The main cell surface receptor for hyaluronan is CD44 and after internalization, hyaluronan may even have some intracellular functions.

The number of proteoglycans that have been described in relation to other cellular functions has increased greatly (Table 4.4). Many of these have a direct role in specific intercellular interactions while others play a space-filling and/or mechanical supportive role. In the cornea, three proteoglycans, lumican, keratocan and mimecan, are the major keratan sulphate moieties which, together with collagens type VI and XII, are essential for maintaining corneal transparency.

Extracellular matrix molecules are intimately involved in cell adhesion

Cell adhesion is fundamental to many biological processes, such as morphogenesis, development, immune reactions to foreign proteins, etc. Cells adhere both to the matrix and to other cells, and usually do so via specific receptors in the cell membrane known as integrins. Integrins are heterodimeric proteins (they have α and β chains, some of which are common to more than one integrin type), and are described in terms of their chain composition, e.g. $\alpha_3\beta_5$ and $\alpha_1\beta_6$ integrins (Table 4.5; see also Ch. 7 and the role of integrin receptors in leucocyte adhesion). Each cell type adheres preferentially to

Table 4.4 Some tissue proteoglycans

Proteoglycan	GAG	Tissue	Function
Aggrecan	CS, KS	Cartilage	Structural support
Versican	CS	Fibroblasts	Cell migration, support
Decorin	CS/DS	Fibroblasts	Fibrillogenesis
Fibromodulin	KS	? Keratocytes	Fibrillogenesis
α_2 (IX) collagen	CS	Vitreous, cartilage	Collagen binding
Syndecan	CS, HS	Epithelia, fibroblasts	Morphogenesis
Basement membrane	HS	Basement membrane	Support
CD44	CS	Lymphocytes, epithelia, retina	Cell-cell interactions

Table 4.5 Integrin binding to extracellular matrix proteins

- Integrins $\alpha_1\beta_1$, $\alpha_2\beta_1$, $\alpha_6\beta_1$, $\alpha_7\beta_1$, $\alpha_v\beta_4$, $\alpha_6\beta_4$ bind to laminin
- Integrins $\alpha_4\beta_1$, $\alpha_5\beta_1$, $\alpha_v\beta_1$, $\alpha_v\beta_3$, $\alpha_6\beta_4$ bind to fibronectin
- Only integrin $\alpha_3\beta_1$ binds to both laminin and fibronectin

Table 4.6 Proteins associated with cell junctions

Adherens junction	Desmosome
α, β, and γ catenin	Plakoglobin
Plakoglobin	Desmoplakin I and II
Vinculin	Desmoplakin IV
α actinin	Desmoyokinin
Tenuin	Lamin B-like protein
Plectin	Plectin
Radixin	Desmoglein

particular extracellular matrix proteins, depending on the type of integrin receptor it happens to express (see Table 4.5). In addition, cells may express different integrins at different times, depending on their state of activation, as, for instance, with the (myo)fibroblast during wound healing (see below). Differential adhesion by cells is shown clearly in the lens where anterior epithelial cells use the $\alpha_5\beta_1$ integrin to bind fibronectin while the equatorial and posterior fibre cells express the $\alpha_6\beta_1$ integrin.

Binding of the cell to the matrix via integrin receptors not only has a structural role but is also involved in transmembrane signalling, which may be two-way, i.e. the matrix may modify the behaviour of the cell and the cell may transmit information to other cells via the matrix (inside-out signalling) (see p. 189 in relation to profilin and fibronectin).

Epithelial and endothelial cells bind via transmembrane complexes to each other and to the basement membrane

Epithelial and endothelial cells rest on a highly organized basement membrane (see above). Binding of epithelial-type cells occurs predominantly via adherens-type junctions and desmosomes/hemidesmo-

somes, in which several distinct proteins have been identified (Table 4.6). Some of these proteins are members of what is known as the cadherin family of proteins (cell adhesion proteins), a group of transmembrane proteins that regulate intercellular adhesion (see Box 4.5). These proteins are not only important in the mechanical support of intercellular interactions, but also play a role in inter- and intracellular signalling.

Mesenchymal cells bind to the matrix via focal adhesion sites

Mesenchymal cells, such as fibroblasts, keratocytes, chondrocytes, etc., bind to the extracellular matrix via specific focal adhesion sites that contain transmembrane cytoskeletal proteins. Actin stress fibres bind via α actinin and talin to the cytoplasmic side of the integrin receptor and to vinculin, while the extracellular component of the integrin receptor binds to extracellular matrix proteins such as collagen and fibronectin (see Fig. 4.9). Direct reverse signalling takes place through these sites using the signalling protein, focal adhesion kinase, one of the protein tyrosine kinases. Also involved is a further intracellular protein termed VASP (vasodilator-stimulated phosphoprotein) which integrates profilin–actin with talin, vinculin, F-actin and the integrin signalling complex. Certain other mesenchymal cells, such as muscle, have specific proteins in their focal adhesion sites such as dystrophin and paxillin, not only at the site of attachment of the extracellular matrix but also at the neuromuscular junction. A mutation in the dystrophin gene has been identified in patients with muscular dystrophy. An integrin-linked kinase appears to be central to regulation of outside-in and inside-out signalling in adherent cells.

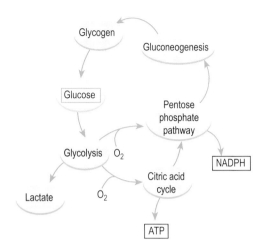

Fig. 4.11 Summary of glucose pathways.

BIOCHEMICAL PATHWAYS THAT AFFECT OCULAR FUNCTION

The eye, particularly the outer retina, is highly metabolically active and requires large amounts of ATP, the universal energy storage molecule, for this purpose. Cells cash in on this energy bank by hydrolysing ATP and coupling this event to cell-specific enzymic reactions that are otherwise energetically unfavourable. ATP is generated by oxidative metabolism, particularly of glucose but also of other molecules such as fats and proteins.

Hydrolysis of ATP is not without risk to the cell: free electrons are produced (H^+), which are normally mopped up by nicotinamide adenine dinucleotide (NAD). Indeed, NADH is the main electron carrier in the oxidation of glucose and other molecules, while NADPH (see below) is used to reduce certain molecules such as free fatty acids to permit them to enter the metabolic pathways.

Oxidative consumption of glucose requires coenzyme A, which is a carrier of acyl groups. Other coenzymes are also required for active metabolism, many of which are derived from vitamins.

GLUCOSE METABOLISM AND TISSUE GLYCATION

Glycolysis is the conversion of glucose to pyruvate in the absence of oxygen, and is accompanied by a net gain of two molecules of ATP. In the presence of oxygen, pyruvate enters the citric acid cycle with the production of 24 molecules of ATP. NAD^+ is regenerated in the mitochondrial electron transport chain. Glucose and other fuel molecules entering the citric acid cycle may thus be consumed to provide energy for synthesis of the building materials for other molecules such as amino acids.

Not all the fuel molecules are utilized immediately but instead are diverted to produce molecules that act as sources of power rather than energy. This is achieved via the pentose phosphate pathway, in which NADPH and ribose are produced, the former for use in reductive processes and the latter in the biosynthesis of nucleotides for RNA and DNA. These different pathways are briefly summarized in Figure 4.11.

The pentose phosphate pathway also permits glucose formation from unrelated precursors (gluconeogenesis) but does not occur in the brain owing to lack of glucose-6-phosphatase; this probably also applies to the retina. However, the pentose phosphate pathway is active in the cornea and lens (see below).

Finally, glucose may be stored in the liver and muscle as glycogen, whence it can be retrieved for energy purposes by glycogenolysis. The Müller cells in the retina also contain stores of glycogen, which may be essential to maintain retinal function (see Ch. 1).

ATP-consuming anabolic pathways and ATP-generating catabolic pathways are under strict regulatory control by a 'master-switch' enzyme system, adenosine monophosphate-activated protein kinase (AMPK), which controls the overall whole body energy metabolism and is involved in loss of neuroprotection in the brain, and possibly the retina, in ischaemic states.

Table 4.7 Distribution of glucose transporters	
Glucose transporter	Tissue
1	Blood–tissue barriers
2	Liver, B cell, kidney
3	Brain, nerves, retina
4	Muscle, heart, fat tissue
5	Small intestine
7	Microsomes in liver

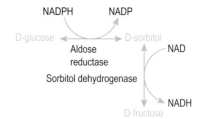

Fig. 4.12 Aldose reductase pathway.

Glucose enters cells by facilitated diffusion

A family of proteins, known as glucose transporters (GLUTs 1–7), permit the facilitated diffusion of glucose into and out of cells down their concentration gradient. Different cells and tissues have different GLUTs, which is relevant to how each tissue handles glucose (Table 4.7). Thus skeletal muscle utilizes GLUT 4, which is dependent for its function in the plasma membrane on insulin; in contrast, brain and retina, which are considered to be insulin-independent tissues, express GLUTs 1 and 3. The liver and adipose tissue also have GLUTs 2 and 7, with several of the other transporters. GLUTs 1, 3 and 4, particularly GLUT 1, can be upregulated in response to hypoxia via the gene hypoxia-inducible factor-1, which also induces other genes such as vascular endothelial cell growth factor, which is important in retinal vessel permeability and new vessel growth.

GLUT 7 is involved in gluconeogenesis and glycogenolysis in the liver, where it is located in the endoplasmic reticulum in association with the glucose-6-phosphatase, the essential enzyme for these reactions.

Excessive levels of glucose may impair cellular metabolism

Glucose metabolism is tightly regulated by insulin released from the pancreatic β cells. In diabetes mellitus, in which there is impaired secretion or utilization of insulin, hyperglycaemia leads to excessive uptake of glucose into cells, despite negative feedback on the expression of GLUTs on the cell surface. This has the effect of overloading the metabolic pathways with activation of alternative routes for glucose handling such as the aldose reductase pathway (Fig. 4.12).

In certain tissues, such as the lens, the effect of increased sorbitol may be to cause damage by osmotic dysregulation because sorbitol cannot be transported out of the cell easily. In this case, even high glucose can have direct osmotic damaging effects on the cell owing to raised intracellular $[Ca^{2+}]_i$ perhaps as a result of cell shrinkage with consequent activation of the stretch receptors. Alternatively, the excessive utilization of NADPH in this pathway might have deleterious effects on the levels of myoinositol, which is required for intracellular signalling, or on the increased generation of reactive oxygen species directly via activation of the phosphoinositol pathway.

It has therefore been suggested that activation of the aldose reductase pathway is not the direct cause of cellular damage but is merely a coincidental perturbation in the cell; instead, excessive production of free radicals may be important during oxidation of the high concentrations of glucose. Whatever the mechanism, aldose reductase is likely to be involved in the lens at least, because inhibitors of this enzyme prevent the development of cataract.

Chronic hyperglycaemia has also been shown to alter cellular metabolism via modulating insulin post-receptor intracellular signalling, involving the cascade insulin receptor substrate 1 (IRS-1)/phosphatidylinositol 3-kinase (PI3K)/Akt, as the result of production of high levels of hexosamine in the cell. This may be one mechanism of induction of insulin resistance in diabetes mellitus.

A more general mechanism for the effects of high ambient glucose concentration on cell behaviour has been the induction of the cytokine TGF-β with its widespread effects on cell function.

Excessive levels of glucose lead to glycation of proteins

Non-enzymatic glycation of proteins also occurs in the presence of high concentrations of glucose. This occurs in two phases: an early reversible phase during which the protein forms a Schiff base and 'Amadori products', followed by a later irreversible phase in which advanced glycation end (AGE) products appear (see Fig. 4.14). This latter process is not fully understood but leads to fluorescent products, which can be detected in tissue extracts. Glycation is linked also to free radical production (see below), during the generation of electrophilic compounds.

Glycation of proteins such as collagen and haemoglobin is well recognized and occurs as part of ageing and pathologically in diabetes mellitus; in addition, important extracellular matrix proteins, such as PAI-1 (see above) may be glycated, leading to defective control of cell behaviour including cell migration and activation. Glycation of cell membrane proteins such as Ca^{2+} channels in pericytes may impair their function, thus rendering them less responsive to endothelin-1-induced contractility. The two processes of non-enzymatic glycation and auto-oxidation of proteins are also directly interrelated and may be important in glucose-derived oxidative stress. This last effect is a direct inducer of apoptosis and mediates neuronal and endothelial cell death in diabetic neuropathy and vasculopathy.

Interestingly, the free radical scavenger vitamin B6 may inhibit AGE production via the inhibition of oxidative degradation of Amadori intermediates and the trapping of reactive oxygen products (see below).

Glucose and lipid metabolism

Glucose and lipid metabolism are also intimately linked via the metabolite acetyl coenzyme A. In the presence of excess glucose, production of fatty acids and cholesterol through acetyl coenzyme A is increased with consequent increases in phospholipids (see below) and circulating levels of very low-density lipoproteins. While this has well-known implications for the development of atherosclerosis, more recently this form of metabolic dysfunction has been suggested to underlie pathologies such as age-related macular degeneration, not simply through the production of abnormal lipid deposits in areas where their removal is difficult, such as the subretinal space, but also by a concomitant increase in lipid-based free radicals (see below).

OXIDATION/REDUCTION AND FREE RADICAL PRODUCTION

Oxidative metabolism and the generation of ATP storage energy molecules are conducted via the cytochrome enzyme system. However, during the

process of oxygen consumption, a small amount of oxygen (< 5%) is metabolized by alternative pathways. Univalent reduction of oxygen produces highly reactive free radicals, namely the superoxide anion and the hydroxyl radical, and the toxic molecule, hydrogen peroxide (Fig. 4.13).

The superoxide anion is generated in mitochondria in the ubiquinone cytochrome b system and in other membranes by auto-oxidation via the cytochrome P_{450}-linked reductases (also part of the drug-metabolizing system), which are rich in the vitamin flavoprotein. Superoxide is then converted by superoxide dismutase to hydrogen peroxide (H_2O_2), which diffuses into the cytosol. Superoxide is also generated in the cytosol itself via recycling of redox enzymes such as xanthine oxidase; conversion to H_2O_2 in the cytosol is rapid. Xanthine, in particular, accumulates in certain tissues during ischaemia, and subsequent reperfusion leads to massive release of free radicals producing extensive tissue damage. This can be prevented by free radical scavengers.

Free radicals can be generated by other mechanisms. Reduction of Fe^{3+} to Fe^{2+} by reducing agents such as ascorbate catalyses the conversion of H_2O_2 to $OH^{\bullet}$, and auto-oxidation of other compounds such as thiols and catecholamines produces free radicals. The Fe^{2+} ion has particular relevance to the problem of retained intraocular metallic foreign bodies. Tissue damage during inflammation is in a large part attributable to the production of free radicals by phagocytic cells during the respiratory burst (see Ch. 7). These interactions are illustrated in Box 4.8.

Free radicals are detoxified by a variety of enzymatic and non-enzymatic mechanisms (Table 4.8). In addition, a critical redox regulatory system involving glutathione and the enzyme glutathione S-transferase is central to cellular homeostasis (Fig. 4.15).

Superoxide dismutases require divalent ions such as Mn^{2+}, Cu^{2+} and/or Zn^{2+} for normal activity; some of

Table 4.8 Detoxification of free radicals	
Mechanism	Agent
Superoxide anion degrading enzymes	Superoxide dismutases
Antioxidants	Ascorbate
Free radical scavengers	Vitamins A and E
H_2O_2 degrading enzymes	Catalase, peroxidase

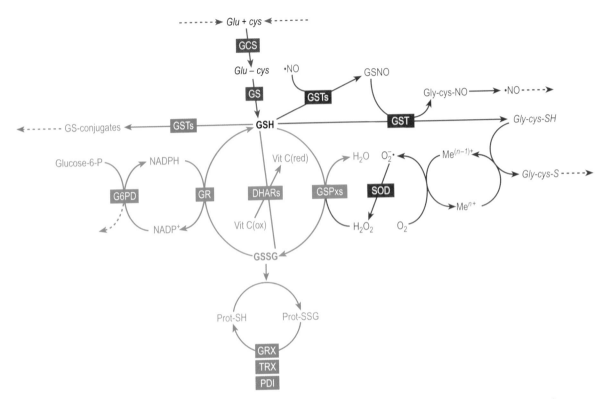

Fig. 4.13 Outline of the interrelations connecting the various roles played by GSH in cellular homeostasis: antitoxic (blue), antioxidant (green), prooxidant (red), modulator (yellow). γ-GCS, γ-glutamyl-cysteine synthetase; DHARs, dehydroascorbate reductases; G6PD, glucose-6-phosphate dehydrogenase; GPxs, glutathione peroxidases; GR, glutathione reductase; GRX, glutaredoxin; GS, glutathione synthetase; GSNO, S-nitrosoglutathione; GSTs, glutathione-S-transferases; Me, metal; PDI, protein disulfide isomerase; SOD, superoxide dismutase; TRX, thioredoxin. (From Pompella et al. 2003, with permission from Elsevier.)

these have been demonstrated in ocular tissues. Further reduction of H_2O_2 is either by enzymatic or non-enzymatic means, and may involve several mechanisms directed towards removal of reactive oxygen species (see Box 4.8).

The mechanism of cell damage varies with each molecular species. Chelated metal ions are important in non-enzymatic degradation of H_2O_2, producing the highly reactive OH• radical, which is particularly damaging to cell membranes. H_2O_2 causes damage by inhibiting glycolysis and glucose uptake.

This information has led to investigation of the value of anti-oxidant free radical scavengers (see below) such as vitamin E as prophylaxis for age-related macular degeneration, but the complex

nature of these biological systems has been demonstrated by the reported increased risk of heart failure in patients taking vitamin E supplementation. Other drugs which may have ocular benefit and possible neuroprotective roles include melatonin, which appears to have some action related to inhibition of free radical damage particularly to mitochondria where the drug reduces mitochondria-based apoptosis.

LIPID PEROXIDATION

Lipids are the structural basis on which cell membranes are built and are generally composed of a hydrophobic tail of two fatty acid chains bound to a hydrophilic (polar) head (see Box 4.9). Fatty acids thus have at least three roles:

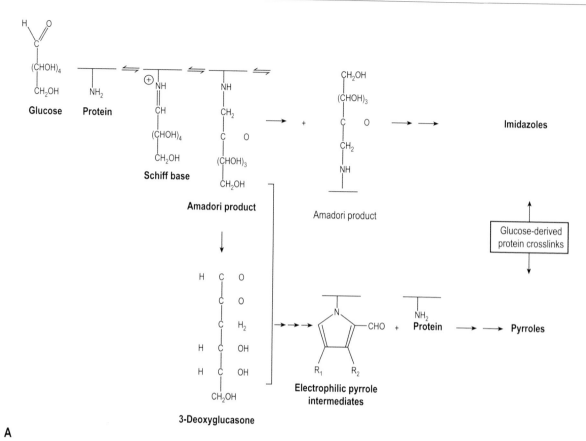

A

B

Fig. 4.14 Process of non-enzymatic glycation. (**A**) Biochemical pathway via Schiff base and Amadori products leading to glucose-derived crosslinks and ultimately advanced glycation end products (AGE). (**B**) Diagrammatic representation of molecular interactions involved in AGE-mediated collagen crosslinks. (Courtesy of A Ceramin and the publishers of Scientific American.)

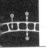

Box 4.8   Generation of free radicals from hydrogen peroxide

The oxidation of hydrogen peroxide (H_2O_2) leads to glutathione consumption via the pentose phosphate pathway and requires a supply of glucose to maintain homeostasis.

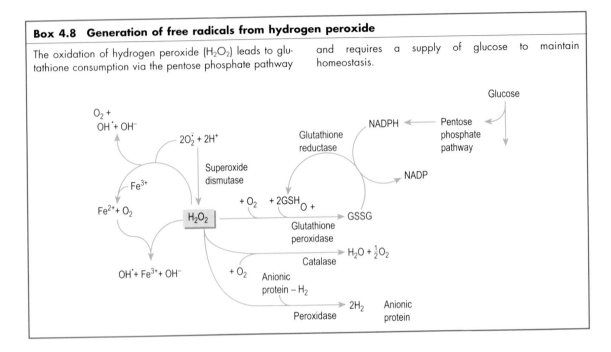

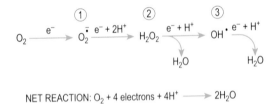

NET REACTION: $O_2 + 4$ electrons $+ 4H^+ \longrightarrow 2H_2O$

Fig. 4.15 Free radical production: (1) superoxide anion; (2) hydrogen peroxide; (3) hydroxyl radical.

- as integral components of phospholipids and glycolipids
- as functional molecules, e.g. hormones and second messengers
- as energy stores in the form of triacylglycerols.

In addition to phospholipids and glycolipids, cholesterol is the third major lipid component of eukaryotic cell membranes; cholesterol is predominantly hydrophobic but has a hydrophilic group on carbon 3 (Fig. 4.16). In an aqueous medium, lipids arrange themselves in such a way that the polar (hydrophilic) groups face the aqueous phase, whereas the hydrophobic groups face each other (a micelle). However, owing to the bulky nature of the two chains of fatty acids, membrane lipids do not readily form micelles but group together as a lipid bilayer (Fig. 4.16). Phospholipid bilayers can reach macroscopic dimensions and are barriers to the diffusion of aqueous solutes but remain quite fluid themselves. Thus they form an ideal material to act as biological membranes. The fluidity of lipid membranes is related to the length of the fatty acid chains, the number and nature of double bonds in the chain and, in eukaryotes, the content of cholesterol. Proteins suspended in lipid bilayers, such as rhodopsin, have very rapid lateral mobility within the membrane unless they are anchored across the membrane to cytoskeletal and/or matrix proteins; in contrast the polarity of the protein in the membrane is fixed.

The formation of lipid bilayers is a spontaneous event, due to the physical hydrophobic interactions between the hydrocarbon tails, assisted by polar interactions between the aqueous phase and the hydrophilic head, and between adjacent polar groups. Furthermore, lipid bilayers form closed compartments in which defects are self-sealing, even after disruption.

Fatty acids undergo physiological degradation during energy consumption by oxidation. Similarly, lipids in cell membranes can be oxidized. Indeed, peroxidation of lipids is one of the main sources of cell damage, and polyunsaturated fatty acids are par-

Box 4.9 General structure of phospholipids

The general composition of lipids is a hydrophobic tail consisting of fatty acids bound to a hydrophilic head, which characterizes the molecule (**A**). Glycolipids differ from phospholipids in having a sugar moiety rather than a phosphorylcholine linked to the fatty acid chain. Sphingomyelin is intermediate between these (**B**).

R_1 and R_2: Fatty acids (usually saturated and unsaturated, respectively)

$\boxed{A_1}$ $\boxed{A_2}$ $\boxed{C}$ $\boxed{D}$: Sites of phospholipase activity

A

Sphingosine

Sphingomyelin

B

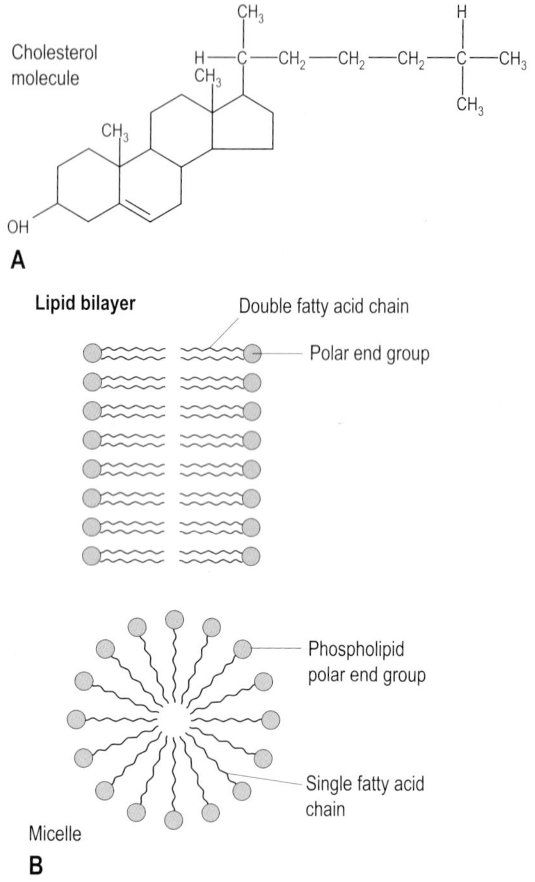

Fig. 4.16 Structure of the cholesterol molecule (**A**) and the lipid bilayer (**B**).

Box 4.10 Oxidation of lipid membranes

Phospholipids, especially those containing arachidonic acid (20:4) and docosohexanoic acid (22:6), a fatty acid abundant in photoreceptor cells, are oxidized to lipid free radicals, which are then conjugated to form dienes. These are then converted to lipid peroxides.

$$RH \rightarrow R\bullet + O_2 \rightarrow ROO\bullet$$

Peroxidation of lipids in cell membranes leads to the release of large quantities of arachidonate, which acts as a substrate for eicosanoid production.

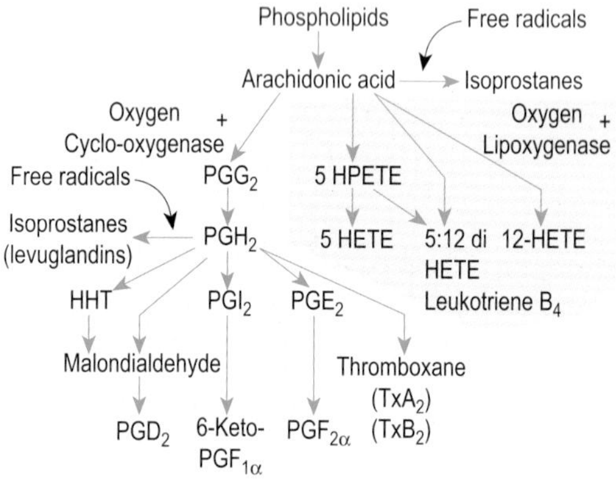

ticularly susceptible to this form of non-enzymatic damage (see Box 4.10).

The lipid peroxides oxidize neighbouring fatty acids and set up chain reactions in the membrane. Phospholipase A_2, by releasing free fatty acids from the membrane, is thought to detoxify this reaction. However, the arachidonate released is then converted to prostaglandins and other eicosanoids (see Box 4.10 and Ch. 6, p. 343). Arachidonates may also be modified by interaction with free radicals in a non-enzymatic reaction. This produces a series of 'prostanoids', prostaglandin-like chemicals termed isoprostanes. In fact, isoprostanes are produced in much larger quantities than prostaglandins and are detectable *in vivo* as a measure of lipid peroxidation, and thus indirectly tissue damage. Isoprostanes occur at low levels in normal healthy individuals, thus reflecting a level of oxidative injury not completely suppressed by natural antioxidants. Isoprostanes have biological and potentially pathological effects on cell function, thus directly contributing to disease.

Release of carbonyl compounds from both carbohydrates and lipids can lead to protein modification by glycation (AGEs, see above) and by lipoxidation (ALEs, advanced lipo-oxygenation end products). These are seen especially in uraemic patients on dialysis. Vitamin B6 (pyridoxamine) may also inhibit ALE production as well as AGE production (see above).

Lipid peroxidation can be limited by vitamin E, a lipid-soluble free radical scavenger that is present within the bilayer (especially photoreceptors) and reacts directly with the lipid free radical to produce the phenoxy radical, or with ascorbic acid in the aqueous phase (see above).

THE OCULAR SURFACE

The ocular surface is composed of the conjunctival and corneal non-keratinized epithelium and is bathed by the tear film. Evaporation of the tear film is clinically measurable as the tear film breakup time, and tear film integrity is restored by blinking. Blink rate and breakup time are therefore linked. Tears provide lubrication for lid closure, assist in 'smoothing out' the irregularities in the ocular surface (which otherwise may have transient effects on light transmission), and also have an antibacterial function.

THE TEAR FILM

The tear film is a protective covering for the cornea composed of three layers: a surface oily layer, an aqueous layer and a deep mucous layer. Previous estimates of tear film thickness suggested that the aqueous layer comprised more than 95% of the tear film, but this has been reduced to 60%, with a larger component being provided by the mucous layer based on evidence from *in vivo* studies using the confocal corneal microscope. In addition, clinical evaluation of the tear film involves an assessment of the 'tear meniscus height' (TMH). The TMH reflects the volume of tears that collects at the contact line between the eyelid margin and the bulbar conjunctiva and has several other names, including the inferior marginal strip and the tear prism or rivus.

The cornea presents a hydrophobic non-wettable surface, which is made wettable by possessing a layer of mucus on its surface. This is overlaid by the aqueous component of the tear film and lastly by a layer of lipid, which prevents evaporation of the tears (Fig. 4.17). Soluble mucus in the aqueous layer and meibomian lipid combine to ensure stability of the tear film by lowering the surface tension and permitting 'spreading' of the tear film on blinking. The breakup time is therefore thought to represent the time it takes for aqueous to evaporate and meibomian lipid to come in contact with the hydrophobic epithelial cell layer.

This view has been modified by the finding that the 30–40% thick mucous layer is not wiped away on blinking. Instead, it is thinned by blinking and may take 30 minutes to reconstitute itself. The mucous layer is composed in part by the glycocalyx of the epithelial cells and by an additional layer of tear mucins produced by the conjunctival goblet cells. Reduced tear film breakup time in dry eye disorders of various types therefore reflects a disturbance in tear mucin/aqueous protein interaction and may be associated with a reduction in goblet cell density.

Tear film lipids have unique characteristics

The lipid layer of the tear film is derived from meibomian gland secretions and is very thin (0.1 µm). It is composed of a mixture of polar and neutral lipids with a melting point (35°C) that ensures it is always fluid on the ocular surface. The polar lipids are in contact with the aqueous phase of the tear film and provide structural stability to the tear film, while the non-polar lipids are the air interface and provide barrier function and thixotropic properties. The lipids include unsaturated and branched-chain fatty acids and alcohols, 8–32 carbon chains in length. They also promote movement of water into the aqueous phase during formation of the tear film, where they bond to tear lipocalins. The functions of the meibomian lipid layer are:

- to prevent evaporation of tears
- to prevent spillover of tears at the lid margin
- to prevent migration of skin lipid onto the ocular surface
- to provide a clear optical medium.

Lacrimal gland secretion provides the aqueous component of tears

The lacrimal gland and its accessory glands (see Ch. 1, pp. 91 and 92) are classic exocrine acinar glands secreting a dilute aqueous solution containing proteins and small molecular weight components and electrolytes (Table 4.9). The principal proteins in tears include immunoglobulin A (IgA), lactoferrin, G-protein, tear-specific prealbumin (lipocalin) and lysozyme. Tear-specific prealbumin is a member of the lipocalin superfamily and together with a further lipocalin, apolipoprotein D, is secreted by the lacrimal gland. The function of tear lipocalin is to interact with meibomian gland lipid and induce surface lipid spreading. It may also have a role in removing harmful lipophilic molecules. Traces of other proteins are often present, particularly serum proteins, depending on how the tears are sampled.

Tear secretion by the lacrimal gland is under neural control: basal tear secretion occurs at a rate

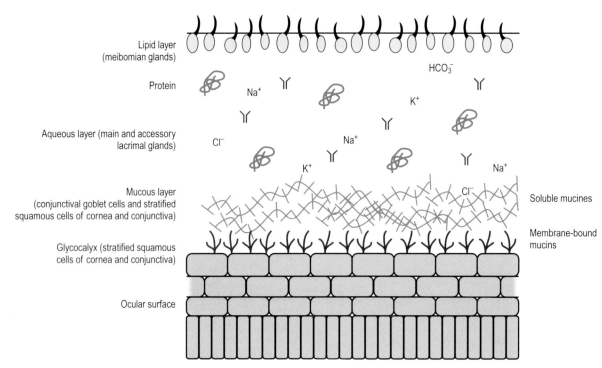

Fig. 4.17 Schematic drawing of the three layers of the tear film. The tear film covers the cells of the ocular surface (cornea and conjunctiva). The upper lipid layer is secreted by the meibomian glands; the middle aqueous layer is secreted by the main and accessory lacrimal glands and the conjunctival epithelium; the inner mucous layer is secreted by the conjunctival goblet cells and stratified squamous cells of the conjunctiva and cornea, and the glycocalyx by the stratified squamous cells of the cornea and conjunctiva. (From Dartt 2004, with permission from Elsevier.)

Table 4.9 Composition of the tear film			
Physical properties	Solutes (μmol/1)	Proteins	Enzymes/inhibitors
98% H_2O_2	Na 120–160	Lysozyme	Glycolytic
6–9 μl volume	Cl 118–135	Lactoferrin	Amylase
pH 7.5	HCO_3 20–25	Tear-specific prealbumin (lipocalin)	Plasminogen activator
310–334 mOsm	K 20–42 Mg 0.7–0.9 Ca 0.5–1.1 Glucose 0.5–0.7 Retinol Urea	G protein (IgA, IgG) (Ceruloplasmin) (Albumin) (Orosomucoid)	(α_2-macroglobulin) (α_1-antitrypsin)

of 1.2 μl/min, but massive tear production can be induced by a variety of mechanical and psychophysical stimuli. Recent studies in mice also show that tears contain the first discovered soluble male pheromone. Neural control is mediated by the autonomic nervous system (see Box 4.11).

The aqueous component contains several proteins with an antibacterial activity (e.g. lactoferrin and lysozyme), and the high levels of IgA may have an immunological role (see Ch. 7). Lactoferrin synergizes with lysozyme in its antibacterial action by binding to lipoteichoic acid on the bacterial surface

Box 4.11 Cellular regulation of tear secretion

Secretion of tears by the lacrimal gland is under parasympathetic control by classic neurotransmitter stimulation involving second messenger systems.

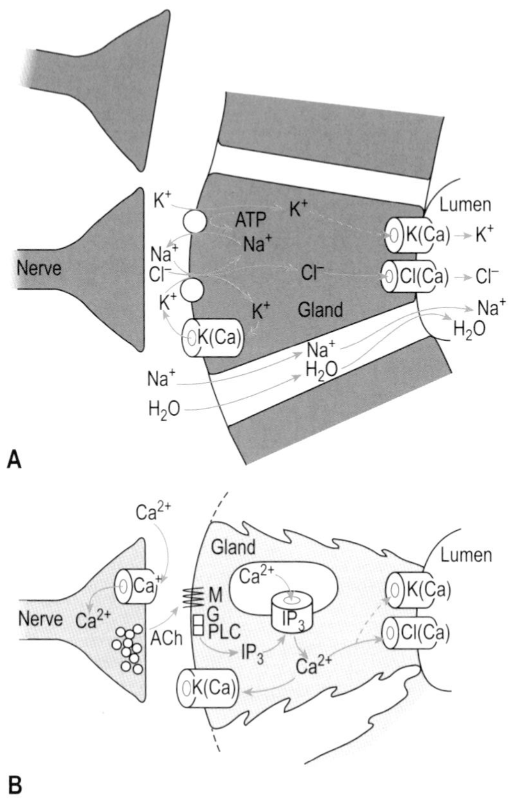

Basal secretion of tears occurs via a Na^+/K^+ ATPase pump, a $Na^+/K^+/2Cl^-$ cotransporter and $K^+(Ca^{2+})$ channels in the basal membrane and $Cl^-(Ca^{2+})$ channels in the apical membrane. Stimulated secretion of tears occurs via release of the neurotransmitter acetylcholine, which interacts with a G-protein-coupled muscarinic (M3) receptor to mobilize intracellular Ca^{2+} stores, causing Cl^- and K^+ channels to open. There may also be a degree of signal network overlap through the epidermal growth factor (EGF) receptor mitogen-activated protein kinase pathway at both the lacrimal gland level and via corneal surface-derived EGF.

Courtesy of B Hille.

and allowing access of lysozyme to the peptidoglycan. The aqueous component also has antiadhesive and lubricant properties, thus ensuring that protein and debris generally do not adhere to the corneal surface (e.g. during prolonged periods of lid closure while sleeping).

The mucous layer stabilizes the aqueous layer by providing a hydrophilic contact surface

The mucous layer is composed of the glycocalyx of the epithelial cell surface and an additional layer of tear-specific mucoproteins (Fig. 4.18). Further tear mucins are secreted by the conjunctival goblet cells.

Mucus imparts viscosity to the tear film and is an inclusive term for the entire secretion from the goblet cells (i.e. glycoproteins, proteins and lipoproteins). Mucins are the glycoprotein components of mucus and vary greatly in molecular size (up to 50×10^6 kDa). The molecular structure of mucin has been likened to a 'bottle-brush,' where the 'hairs' of the brush are represented by multiple *O*-glycosyl-

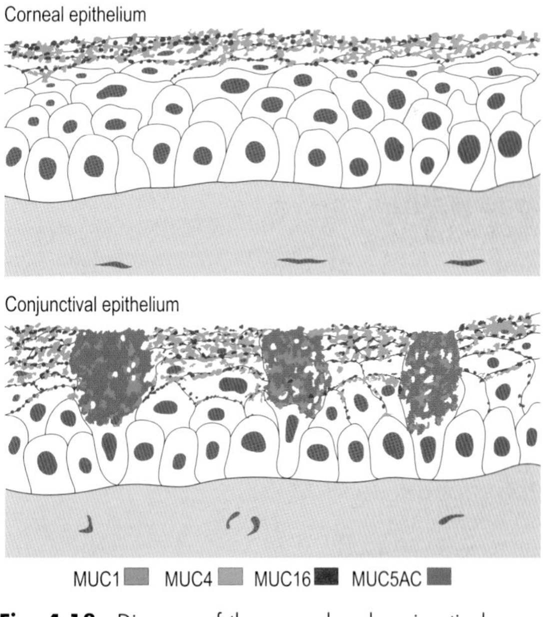

Fig. 4.18 Diagram of the corneal and conjunctival epithelium showing distribution of the membrane-associated mucins MUC1, MUC4 and MUC16 within apical cell membranes, and the secreted mucin MUC5AC within mucin packets in goblet cells. (From Gipson 2004, with permission from Elsevier.)

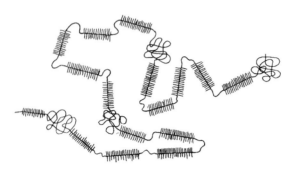

Fig. 4.19 Bottle-brush mucin. (Courtesy of J Tiffany.)

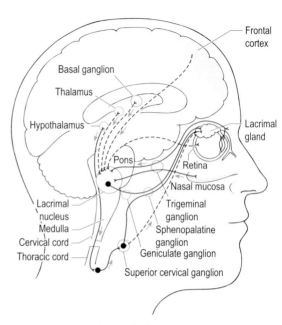

Fig. 4.20 Neural control of tear secretion.

ated short oligosaccharide chains on an elongated protein 'handle' containing many threonine and serine residues (Fig. 4.19). This structure has the capacity to form many interactions with other hydrophobic (lipid) as well as hydrophilic (protein) and charged molecules, thus forming mucus.

There are many mucins produced by cells of mucosal surfaces and there is some tissue specificity concerning the type of mucin on each surface. Mucins in tears are produced by goblet cells (MUC5AC), lacrimal acinar cells (MUC7) and by corneal and conjunctival epithelium. Thus, MUC5AC is the principal tear mucin and is secreted along with 'trefoil' peptides, TFF1 and TFF3, by the goblet cells. MUC1 and MUC4 and the sialomucin complex are also found but are more associated with the glycocalyx. Membrane-bound mucins (MUC1 and MUC4) may be released into the aqueous phase of tears through activity of ADAM-TS-1 (a disintegrin-like metalloproteinase with thrombospondin type 1 motif) metallo-proteases. The importance of mucin in tears has been emphasized by the realization that tears are not predominantly aqueous but are probably a type of mucin-gel, formed especially by MUC5AC.

Tear secretion is under psychoneuroendocrine control

The regulation of tear secretion is shown in Figure 4.20. Most of the control is through the autonomic system and thus tear secretion is affected by instillation of drugs that modulate this system (e.g. pilocarpine, atropine). Apart from direct effects on the acinar cells (see above, intracellular second messengers), the parasympathetic system can markedly increase tear flow via its effects on the myoepi-

thelial cells surrounding the acinar cells (see Ch. 1, p. 94).

Hormonal control of tear secretion is well recognized but not clearly defined. Reduction in tear flow occurs in women after the menopause, while testosterone stimulates secretion of certain tear components, such as IgA.

THE CONJUNCTIVA

The conjunctiva is richly endowed with a variety of specialized cells that allow it to act as a base for and the source of many of the constituents of the tear film. These include immune cells (T and B cells, mast cells, dendritic cells; see Ch. 7) and specialized mucus-secreting goblet cells.

The epithelium is more than a simple covering layer for the conjunctiva

The conjunctival epithelium can be regarded as intermediate in type between the keratinized squamous epithelium of skin and the typical mucosal epithelia of respiratory and gastrointestinal tracts. However, it resembles the latter more closely and may require the multifunctional protein, clusterin, to inhibit keratin production. Clusterin is found in all body fluids including tears, and on the surface of cells lining body cavities. It is involved in transport of lipoproteins, inhibiting complement-mediated lysis, and in modulation of cell–cell interactions.

Although the conjunctiva is non-keratinized, keratins are expressed by the conjunctival epithelium in a typical paired combination (K3/K12). However, there is much more K3/K12 in corneal than in conjunctival epithelium. Several other cytokeratins present in non-keratinized stratified (K4 and K13) or simple (K8 and K19) epithelia are also found.

The epithelium contains numerous intraepithelial lymphocytes and dendritic cells, which resemble similar cells in the other upper respiratory tract epithelium, and is organized as part of the mucosa-associated lymphoid tissue (see Chs 2 and 6). The main function of the epithelium is to act as a barrier to external organisms. However, it also has a major role as the source of tear mucins (see Box 4.11) derived from the intraepithelial goblet cells, which, like the lacrimal gland, are under neuroendocrine control. Mucins act as part of the innate immune defence mechanism and MUC1-deficient mice have a severe inflammatory response to bacterial infections (see Fig. 4.18). In addition, the turnover and health of the epithelial and goblet cells are markedly dependent on vitamin A and the retinoids, and become abnormal in vitamin deficiencies, leading to a severe form of dry eye syndrome. Certain accumulations of goblet cells occur, e.g. on the tarsal (lid) conjunctiva where they occur in crypts (Henle's crypts) and on the bulbar conjunctiva a few millimetres nasal of the limbus (Manz's glands).

In addition to goblet cells there are other types of conjunctival epithelium, distinguished by ultrastructural appearances: secretory epithelia appear in mature and immature forms depending on their content of secretory granules and the presence of a Golgi complex; in contrast, other cells with a high content of RER and/or mitochondria are presumably involved in transport and epithelial regeneration.

The conjunctival stroma is highly vascular and contains aqueous veins

The stroma of the conjunctiva has a superficial 'lymphoid' layer and a deep layer containing a rich plexus of vessels that acts as a watershed between the intraocular circulation and the external circulation of the eye and lids. Through these vessels waste materials from the anterior chamber of the eye are transported to the preauricular draining lymph nodes and venous drainage systems in the neck.

THE LIDS

The lids function to protect the cornea and adnexal structures and have a highly specialized structure that ensures they are properly apposed to the surface of the globe (see Ch. 1, p. 85). Indeed, defects in lid apposition, as occur in diseases such as trachoma where there is scarring and deformation of the lids, lead to significant corneal exposure, ulceration and blindness (see Ch. 9).

Closure of the lids leads to compression of the lipid layer of the tears such that it increases in thickness to about 1.0 mm at the lid margin. When the eyes open, the lipids are dispersed to form a lipid bilayer, with the hydrophilic groups on the phospholipid molecules interacting with the aqueous compartment.

Control of lid movement is via the VII nerve for motor function and the V nerve for afferent input via mechanisms such as the blink reflex (see Ch. 1, pp. 86–87).

The lid also contains specialized mucus-secreting glands [they secrete a different type of mucus, rMUC4, important in eyelid opening during development, from that secreted by the goblet cells (rMUC5AC, see above) in the conjunctiva] and oil-secreting glands that contribute to the makeup of the tear film. Lashes and their hair follicles are also important specialized structures in the lid, where they function to protect the eye from foreign particles.

Incomplete eyelid closure may be physiological during sleep. Control of eyelid closure is under both reflex supranuclear and learned/conditioned (cerebellar) control.

CORNEA AND SCLERA

The outer coat of the eye (cornea/sclera) is a tough non-compressible layer of connective tissue that can withstand considerable deformation and pressure.

THE CORNEA

The cornea is designed not only for light transmission but is also the main light-refracting element in the eye. Its cellular and extracellular matrix components are, however, of the same basic chemical composition as other cells and tissues in the body that normally scatter light extensively, thus rendering them opaque. Light scattering in opaque tissues is the result of the large disparity in refractive index (RI) between matrix components such as collagen (RI = 1.55 in the dry state) and glycosaminoglycans (RI = 1.35). The cornea's ability to transmit light is a function of how the cells and matrix components are organized within the tissue to reduce this RI disparity.

Corneal transparency is a function of its relative acellularity and matrix structure

The epithelium

The six-cell-thick stratified layer that is the corneal epithelium (see Ch. 1, p. 17) presents the first refracting interface to transmitted light. Most of the light-absorbing properties of the cornea take place in this layer, mainly for short-wavelength light. However, the majority of light on the visible spectrum is transmitted through the epithelium.

The cells are typical keratin-expressing epithelial cells containing integrin receptors for basement membrane components such as fibronectin, laminin and collagen. Corneal epithelial cells express a particular combination of paired 55/64-kDa keratins (keratin 3/keratin 12). The 54-kDa protein may have a role in inflammatory eye disease, while the 64-kDa protein appears to be useful as a marker for differentiating cells of the central cornea from limbal stem cells (see below). Keratin 12 may be important in corneal epithelial junctions because K-12 knockout mice are prone to recurrent erosion (epithelial cell loss).

The cells are organized to present few interfaces, the most prominent being at the interface between the basal cells and the basement membrane. Hemidesmosomes affect the adhesion between these cells and the basement membrane. The hemidesmosome is bound to the corneal stroma through a band of anchoring fibrils, which pass through the lamina densa in a woven network (see Fig. 4.9). These fibres are composed of type VII collagen. In addition, trans-plasma membrane collagen type XVI supports firm adhesion in these basal cells.

The epithelium presents an effective barrier to fluid transport, which is achieved by extensive close contacts and tight junctional complexes (Fig. 4.21). The site of the barrier is in the suprabasal epithelium and is mediated by high expression of the tight-junction protein, claudin. Spot desmosomes are numerous and differences in the content of desmosomal proteins have been observed depending on the site. For instance, desmoglein and desmocollin are absent from basal limbal epithelial cells, which may have functional significance in their role as putative stem cells. Recently, it has been suggested that limbal stem cells arise from pouches or stem cell niches in the peripheral corneal epithelium.

Matrix factors affecting transparency: collagen
Several different types of collagen are present in the cornea (Fig. 4.21). In addition to the normal basement membrane, type IV and VII collagens in contact with the epithelial and endothelial cell layers, the two specialized corneal regions, Bowman's layer and Desçemet's membrane, contain collagens not normally found in other matrices. Bowman's layer is a condensation of type I/VI with a high proportion of type III in a matrix containing chondroitin and dermatan sulphate, while Desçemet's membrane contains high levels of novel collagens (types V, VIII, IX and XII) organized in a lattice arrangement. This provides elasticity and deformability to the cornea while maintaining high levels of light transmission. Desçemet's membrane also imparts strength and resilience to the corneal stroma and is the main resistance to normal intraocular pressure.

The regular arrangement of stromal type I collagen (which accounts for 50–55% of stromal collagen; see Ch. 1) fibrils is considered to be important in determining corneal transparency. Transparency was initially attributed by Maurice (1957) to 'destructive interference' in which light is scattered by neighbouring fibrils in predictable and opposing directions, which tend to cancel each other out except along the primary visual axis. However, this concept cannot apply to light transmission in Bowman's layer where the fibrils are irregularly displayed, suggesting that the arrangement of the fibrils is less important than their size. An alternative view therefore is that significant light scatter does not occur within the cornea because the fibril diameter does not exceed 30 nm and the interfibrillar distance is around 55 nm. It is only when the distance between the regions of different refractive index becomes greater than 200 nm that light scatter occurs, as for instance when corneal swelling occurs. In one sense

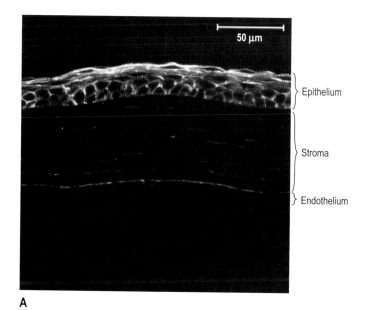

50 μm

Epithelium

Stroma

Endothelium

A

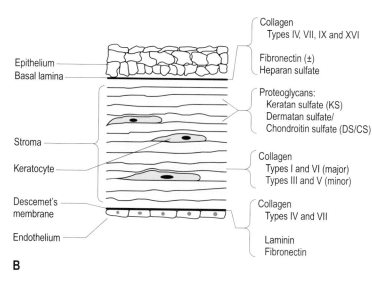

Epithelium
Basal lamina

Collagen
  Types IV, VII, IX and XVI

Fibronectin (±)
Heparan sulfate

Proteoglycans:
  Keratan sulfate (KS)
  Dermatan sulfate/
  Chondroitin sulfate (DS/CS)

Stroma

Keratocyte

Collagen
  Types I and VI (major)
  Types III and V (minor)

Descemet's
membrane

Endothelium

Collagen
  Types IV and VII

Laminin
Fibronectin

B

Fig. 4.21 (**A**) Histological section of the cornea showing the different layers. (**B**) Location of matrix proteins in the different layers of the cornea. (From Sosnová-Netuková *et al.* 2006, with permission from the BMJ Publishing Group.)

this is essentially a paraphrase of Maurice's theory because in both situations the critical factor is inter-fibrillar distance.

Type V (approximately 10%) and some type III (1–2%) collagen also exist in the corneal stroma, while the remainder is made up of type VI collagen. Types I, III and V collagen are fibrillar collagens, but type VI has large non-helical globular polypeptides at both the carboxyl- and N termini of the helical protein backbone (see Table 4.3). It has been suggested that type V collagen is codistributed with type I and is implicated in regulating fibril formation and

thus fibril thickness (Fig. 4.22). However, fibril thickness is also dependent on the nature of the stromal glycosaminoglycans (see below).

The corneal collagen fibrils are arranged in parallel lamellae running at oblique angles to each other (see Ch. 1). Apart from their small size, their uniformity of thickness is likely to be a major factor in light transmission. Studies using X-ray diffraction techniques have shown that the parallel arrangement of the central corneal fibrils extends to the periphery where the fibrils adopt a concentric configuration to form a 'weave' at the limbus (Fig. 4.23) with some

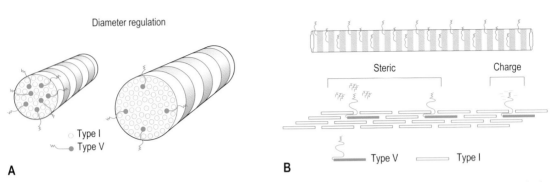

Fig. 4.22 Model for type V regulation of collagen fibril diameter. Collagen fibrils within the cornea contain a high percentage of type V collagen and have small diameters (**A**), while fibrils in other tissues possessing low levels of type V collagen have a large diameter (**A**). The experimental reduction of type V collagen generates fibrils that have the characteristics of those found in tissues with low type V levels. A mechanism by which type V collagen may limit fibril growth is shown in (**B**). Type V N-terminal domains project onto the fibril surface, and when sufficient numbers have accumulated, they block further accretion of collagen monomers and thereby limit growth in diameter. The N-terminal domain is large and possesses a number of acidic residues, and so may affect this block using steric and/or electrostatic hindrance. (Courtesy David E. Birk.)

transversely running fibrils fusing with the circumferential collagen fibrils. This imparts considerable strength to the peripheral cornea and permits it to maintain its curvature and thus its optical properties. Previous studies have shown that the corneal fibrils, running in two preferred orientations in the central cornea, bend as they approach the peripheral cornea to run circumferentially and form the peripheral collagen ring.

Glycosaminoglycans

The corneal stroma is unusual in that it contains no hyaluronic acid, except at the limbus where there is a gradual increase in concentration towards the sclera. The major corneal glycosaminoglycan is keratan sulphate; in the central cornea non-sulphated chondroitin is also present, while towards the periphery chondroitin sulphate is the second major GAG. Chondroitin-4-sulphate and dermatan sulphate are almost identical (see Box 4.7) and many believe that the second major GAG is not chondroitin but dermatan sulphate.

Corneal GAGs exist in the native state as proteoglycans; three major forms exist in the cornea: lumican, keratocan and mimecan. Recent studies in proteoglycan-deficient mice have shown that only lumican is essential for maintenance of corneal transparency, while keratocan maintains overall corneal thickness and less so mimecan. Both corneal dermatan sulphate and keratan sulphate proteoglycans are considered to belong to the class of small non-aggregating proteoglycans.

The critical region in proteoglycans is their linkage sites; for keratan sulphate the link is an N-glycosidic bond between N-acetyl glucosamine and asparagine in the core protein. The terminal sites of the branched oligosaccharide structures contain fucose or mannose, while chondroitin sulphate contains xylose residues.

The interaction between proteoglycans and collagen fibrils has been elegantly demonstrated using cupromeronic blue and $MgCl_2$ at a tightly controlled (3.0 m) concentration (the 'critical electrolyte concentration'). Both dermatan sulphate proteoglycan and keratan sulphate proteoglycan bind to the collagen arrays at specific binding sites (one proteoglycan to one binding site), suggesting that these sites are essential to the spacing of the fibrils and to the thickness of the interfibrillar space. Keratan sulphate proteoglycans appear to bind to the step regions of the fibrils while dermatan sulphate proteoglycans bind to the gap (see Box 4.12). Different binding 'maps' occur in different species, such as the mouse. Therefore, several variations on the theme of proteoglycan–collagen interaction appear to be compatible with transparency. However, small non-aggregating proteoglycans (also known as 'decorins') also appear to be essential. Decorin normally binds dermatan sulphate and promotes angiogenesis, a function that must be suppressed in the normal cornea because it is avascular. Recent studies in human tissue developed this model to reveal a regular hexagonal arrangement of six proteoglycans per collagen fibril interacting with the 'next but one' fibril (Fig. 4.24).

Superior

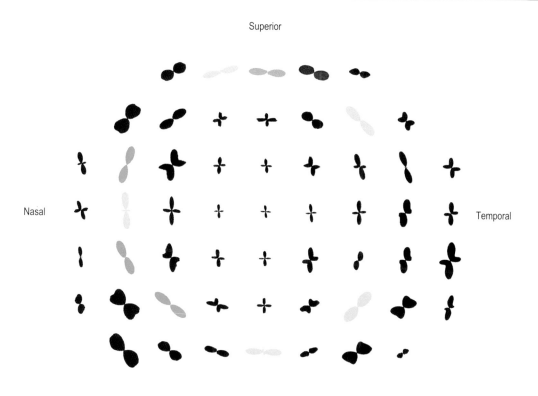

Nasal

Temporal

Inferior

Fig. 4.23 X-ray diffraction of corneal stroma. A detailed map of the preferred orientations of the collagen fibrils across a human corneo-scleral disk using data from synchrotron X-ray diffraction. The measurements were made in a 2 × 2-mm grid across the tissue. The distributions of the preferentially aligned collagen fibrils at each point in the tissue were calculated from these X-ray measurements. It can be seen that the collagen orientation at the centre of the cornea occurs preferentially in the inferior–superior and medial–lateral directions whereas the collagen at the limbus (about 6 mm from the centre) is preferentially tangential to the cornea. The overall dimensions of each orientation pattern represent the quantity of collagen preferentially aligned in a given direction at that point. The mid-grey patterns have been scaled down by a factor of 1.5 and the light grey patterns have been scaled down by a factor of 2 in comparison to the patterns shown in black. (Courtesy Professor Keith Meek and Dr Richard Newton.)

Swelling pressure versus hydration

The cornea is about 80% hydrated. This is higher than other tissues such as the sclera, which is about 70% hydrated. Despite this the corneal stroma 'imbibes' water if it is placed in a solution of saline (this is well demonstrated by the injured, lacerated cornea which swells and becomes opaque); the water-attracting properties are the result of its high content of GAGs. The cornea has been described as 'a slice of water stabilized in three dimensions by a meshwork of fibrils and soluble polymers'. The cornea thus has a swelling pressure and a metabolic pump (the endothelium) designed to maintain it. The swelling pressure generates a level of interfibrillar tension and this may be the biophysical mechanism whereby the fibrils are maintained in their normal arrangement. In addition, the swelling pressure itself may reciprocally activate chloride channels and other transporters that maintain a balance of excess ions in the aqueoues humour.

Cellular factors affecting transparency: keratocytes

Corneal fibroblasts (keratocytes) are important in maintaining transparency because they are the source of stromal collagens and proteoglycans. Although most of the changes that occur in the assembly of the matrix are post-translational, the enzymes that promote these changes are present in the keratocytes in which these genes have been specifically induced (specific enzyme defects are associated with corneal opacification as in the

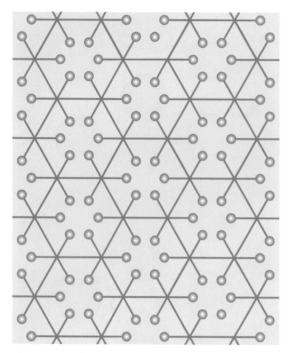

Fig. 4.24 Schematic visualization of the basic components of a new model for the corneal collagen lattice. At equidistant sites along their circumference, six core proteins of proteoglycans are attached to the hexagonally arranged collagen fibrils. GAGs of the proteoglycans as stained by CB are connecting their next nearest neighbour collagen fibrils and form a ring-like structure around each collagen fibril. (From Mueller *et al.* 2004, with permission from Elsevier.)

Box 4.12 Organization of tissue proteoglycans

The organization of proteoglycans in the collagen matrix is probably as shown below: KS-PG (keratan sulphate proteoglycan) double complexes maintain the lateral interfibrillar distance, while CS-PGs (chondroitin sulphate proteoglycan) regulate the overall longitudinal arrangement of the fibrils by spanning three fibrils (**A**). Proteoglycans bind directly to the collagen fibrils, probably through the 'minor' collagens such as V or VI that codistribute with the type I fibrils and have non-collagenous polypeptide domains to interact with the proteoglycans (**A** and **B**). (Courtesy of J Scott and IRL Press.)

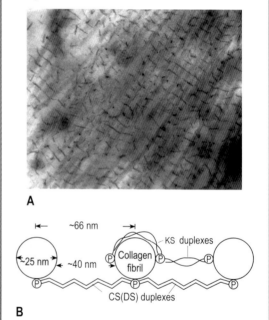

A

B

mucopolysaccharidoses; see Ch. 6). Keratocyte dysfunction may also underlie the corneal haze seen after corneal refractive surgery.

Collagen turnover in early postnatal life is about 24–50 hours, but there is little information on adult collagen metabolism. For both collagen and GAGs, studies on cultured keratocytes have not been very informative because these cells produce a range of GAGs not found *in vivo*. In contrast, organ cultures of cornea produce a panel of GAGs more akin to that found *in vivo*. The preferential production of KS-PG to CS/DS-PG (dermatan sulphate proteoglycan) in corneal cells from different species has been attributed to the relatively hypoxic conditions and to anaerobic glycolysis, which favours the former. In rabbit cornea, the development of transparency correlates with a dramatic increase in the concentration of KS-PG in the early postnatal period.

Keratocytes also express a range of corneal 'crystallins', so called because they are thought to play a role

in light transparency and not because of homology to lens crystallins (see below). Corneal crystallins include *trans*-ketolase and aldehyde dehydrogenase and expression varies from species to species.

The endothelial pump determines the level of hydration of the GAGs and thus transparency
Despite the greater than normal level of hydration of the corneal stroma, its water binding is unsaturated, a condition achieved by an endothelial pump (see Box 4.13), which transports water out of the cornea towards the anterior chamber.

More recent evidence suggests that other mechanisms may be operative in the transport of fluid across the endothelium. These include an Na^+/H^+ exchanger protein which drives an electrogenic

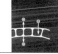

Box 4.13   Corneal endothelial cell pump

The corneal endothelium transports water out of the stroma by an ATP-driven ion pump mechanism.

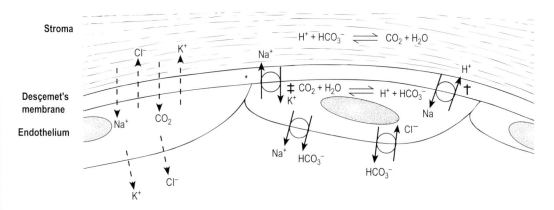

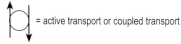

Dashed lines = passive diffusion

= active transport or coupled transport

* Na$^+$/K$^+$ ATPase

† Na$^+$H$^+$exchange

‡ = Carbonic anhydrase in cell promotes HCO$_3^-$ formation

Na$^+$ and HCO$_3^-$ are transported across the endothelium from the stroma to the aqueous, mediated by a Na$^+$/K$^+$-dependent ATPase and a HCO$_3^-$-dependent ATPase, probably involving carbonic anhydrase. The Na$^+$/K$^+$ ATPase is located in the plasma membranes but the HCO$_3^-$-dependent ATPase is in the mitochondria, where its major role in ion transport may be to generate the ATP required for the Na$^+$/K$^+$ ATPase. Carbonic anhydrase may also be involved in the Na$^+$/H$^+$ antiport for maintaining intracellular pH.

coupling between Na$^+$ and HCO$_3^-$ ions. This 'antiport' is essential for maintenance of the intracellular pH by exchanging Na$^+$ (in) with H$^+$ (out) in the cell (see Box 4.13). In addition, the corneal endothelium displays a 'water transporter/channel', aquaporin 1, which is involved in bulk transport of water molecules (see below under Lens) and perhaps also in CO$_2$ transport. Volume changes, especially over short periods, in the endothelial cells may regulate the overall function of each transporter/channel protein.

Transport in the cornea is a two-way process

In addition to the transport of water from the stroma to the aqueous humour, there is a net flux of ions and water towards the epithelium and the tears. For instance, there is a Cl$^-$ pump which appears to be modulated by several receptors including β-adrenergic and serotonergic receptors coupled to the adenylate cyclase and Ca^{2+} second messenger systems, and receptors that involve protein kinase C. Dopamine and α-adrenergic receptors may also be involved in Cl$^-$ transport.

Ion transport into the cornea mediated by Na$^+$/K$^+$ ATPase and Ca^{2+}/Mg^{2+} ATPase in the basolateral plasma membrane of the epithelium is also operational in corneal ion shifts. Na$^+$ movement from the tears into the epithelium is by passive diffusion down a concentration gradient, but from the epithelium into the stroma active transport is required via the Na$^+$K$^+$ ATPase to which Cl$^-$ transport in the opposite direction is coupled. This transport system is sensitive to the eicosanoid metabolite 12(R)HETE (compound C) (see Box 4.10). In addition, this electrolyte flux across the epithelium accounts for the electrical potential difference from (−) outside to (+) inside the cornea of ~ 25–40 μV.

Optical factors affecting image formation

The curvature of the cornea plays a major part in refracting and focusing light to produce an image on the retina. Even with a completely clear cornea, the image can be distorted by abnormalities in curvature, including the various forms of regular and irregular astigmatism, by disease of the cornea such as keratoconus, and the late effects of scarring from wounds such as corneal incisions following cataract surgery, when it can be very difficult to restore preoperative curvature.

While these conditions do not directly affect the transparency of the cornea, they can increase the amount of spherical and chromatic aberration, and diffraction, thus degrading the image.

Metabolism of corneal cells

Oxidative metabolism and glucose utilization

The epithelium takes up most of its glucose from the stroma and converts it to glucose-6-phosphate, after which 85% is metabolized via the glycolytic pathway to pyruvate. The bulk of this is then metabolized to lactic acid, but some is diverted into the citric acid cycle to produce ATP as an energy store. The pentose phosphate pathway accounts for the remainder of glucose utilization by the epithelium, producing an important resource for free radical control, namely NADPH (see Fig. 4.11). This is the main mechanism of generation of reducing agents such as glutathione and ascorbic acid. The corneal epithelium has also developed a unique nuclear ferritin-based mechanism to minimize DNA damage from ultraviolet (UV) light-induced free radical damage. Lactoferrin in tears may also assist in this process.

The metabolism of keratocytes is mostly concerned with generating sufficient energy to produce and maintain stromal components (see above). In the steady state, these cells are not highly metabolically active.

The endothelium has large energy requirements to sustain its pump mechanism and is about five times as active as the epithelium. The major metabolic pathway in the endothelium is anaerobic glycolysis, with the citric acid cycle and the pentose phosphate path also playing a significant role.

Oxygen handling by the cornea

The epithelium obtains its oxygen from the preocular tear film at a rate of 3.5–4.0 µl per cm^2 per hour. The endothelium, however, and the keratocytes in the deep stroma receive their oxygen supply from the circulation via the aqueous humour. Corneal function and health are therefore dependent on local conditions at the surface of the eye and on systemic factors such as cardiopulmonary capacity.

Oxygen is consumed in the citric acid cycle, generating 36–38 molecules of ATP per molecule of glucose. The utilization of the citric acid cycle versus the glycolytic pathway is determined by the energy demands of the tissue, specifically the need for ATP. Thus the endothelium makes greater use of the citric acid cycle than the epithelium. In addition, oxygen consumption by the cornea increases almost twofold when acidosis prevails, as occurs in contact lens wear. This is in part the result of the activation of pH regulatory mechanism, including Na^+/H^+ exchange, which then stimulates Na^+/K^+ ATPase activity.

As discussed above, excess oxygen can be detrimental to the organism if it is converted to the superoxide radical and then to hydrogen peroxide (see Fig. 4.8). In both the epithelium and the endothelium, redox systems involving glutathione and its two enzymes glutathione reductase and glutathione peroxidase depend on the generation of NADPH and thus on a supply of glucose. When the intracellular levels of glutathione are reduced in the cornea by one-third, the clarity of the cornea and its ability to pump fluid decline dramatically.

The aqueous contains high levels of H_2O_2, perhaps by virtue of the reduction of oxygen in the aqueous via ascorbate usage.

Free radical damage to the corneal endothelium induces apoptosis and thus may account for the progressive endothelial cell loss associated with age.

Neurotransmitters and second messengers

Several receptors for neurotransmitters and other agonists are present in the corneal epithelium (see Box 4.14).

In the cornea in particular, cholinergic stimulation of phospholipase C appears to convert phosphatidyl inositol phosphate 2 (PIP$_2$) in preference to phosphatidyl inositol (PI). However, the other enzyme systems, including protein kinase C-mediated breakdown of PI and serotonergically mediated phospholipase C hydrolysis of PIP$_2$, are also significant. Finally there is also evidence for G protein-mediated epithelial second messenger systems in force, reflecting a wealth of signalling systems that occur in this cell layer. Their precise function is not clear but they are probably all essential in the handling of nutrients derived from the tears.

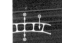

Box 4.14 Agonist receptors in the corneal epithelium

Adrenergic and cholinergic receptors are present in the corneal epithelium and are coupled to a variety of second messenger systems including cAMP, phosphatidyl inositol phosphate 2 (PIP_2), and protein kinase C (PKC) (**A**). They are involved in the transport of fluid out of the cornea in an anterior direction by enhancing the function of the HCO_3^-/Cl^- pump (**B**). Active pumps for outward extrusion of Cl^- (activated by β-adrenergic and other receptors) and inward transport of Na^+ and HCO_3^- are present. Dashed line, passive transport; circles, coupled/active transport. There is also a separate water transporter, aquaporin 5, in the corneal epithelium, which is important for the maintenance of normal corneal stromal thickness.

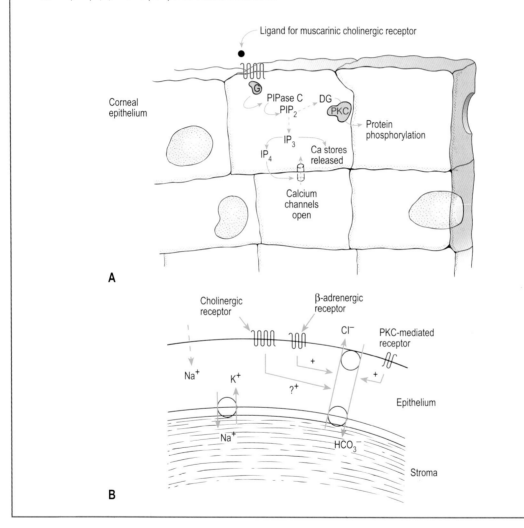

Effects of contact lens wear on corneal physiology

Contact lenses predominantly affect the function of the epithelium. This layer receives its oxygen from the tears and its glucose from the circulation via the aqueous and the limbal vessels (see above). Contact lenses reduce the direct availability of oxygen to the epithelium, thus shifting the balance from aerobic to anaerobic metabolism. Lactate levels in the cornea are doubled with contact lens wear and carbon dioxide production is increased. The induced acidosis has a direct effect on stromal hydration by impairing deturgescence mechanisms (see above).

213

Hard (rigid) contact lenses are usually made from polymethylmethacrylate (PMMA) and have the greatest effect on corneal function; in addition to restricting oxygen availability, hard lenses deplete glycogen stores, even though the level of glucose availability is not reduced. It has been suggested that hard lens-induced inhibition of aerobic enzymes such as hexokinase reduces direct glucose utilization by the cornea. Prolonged wear of hard contact lenses is therefore not possible owing to the damaging effect on corneal transparency induced by the disturbed metabolism. Soft contact lenses are made from polymers of hydroxy ethyl methacrylate (HEMA), poly(HEMA/vinyl pyrrolidones), silicone, or other similar materials, and permit extended wear of the lens owing to their permeability to oxygen and carbon dioxide. However, there is still some degree of lactate accumulation with soft lenses and prolonged use appears to affect the function of the endothelium. Manufacturers of contact lenses continually produce new 'biomimetic'-type lenses with increasing water content (up to 59%) in attempts to support normal corneal physiology (hydrogel lenses).

A popular compromise in contact lens type is the gas-permeable rigid lens, which combines the reduced toxicity of PMMA with high gas-transfer capability. The wide variety of lens types and materials has led to their being characterized on the basis of their 'oxygen flux,' defined as the 'DK' value:

$$\text{Oxygen flux} = DK/L \times \Delta P$$

where D is the diffusion coefficient, K is the solubility, and L is the thickness of the lens material. ΔP is the change in the partial pressure of oxygen across the material. HEMA and PMMA have a low oxygen flux, while hydrogels and silicones have a high flux. Both the thickness of the lens and the DK value determine its suitability for use in terms of its gas permeability. The actual amount of oxygen that reaches the cornea is the most important factor in the design of a contact lens, and most practitioners describe contact lenses in terms of their 'equivalent oxygen performance' (EOP).

Contact lenses may have deleterious effects on the epithelium, causing thinning, reduction in the hemidesmosome density and the number of anchoring fibrils, and reduced adhesion of the epithelium to the basement membrane. This may be a direct effect of low O_2-transmitting lenses on basal epithelial cell proliferation. This is especially true of extended-wear hydrogel lenses. In severe cases, excessive use of contact lenses produces epithelial oedema and keratopathy in the form of punctate epithelial erosions. Rigid contact lenses also produce tear film instability by causing damage to the epithelium and the mucin layer in particular.

Contact lens wear may also induce changes in the corneal stroma (thickening) and the endothelium (polymegathism).

Cell turnover and wound healing in the cornea

The epithelium

The epithelium is constantly being regenerated by mitotic activity in the basal layer of cells. However, after epithelial debridement, the initial response of the epithelium is to migrate as a flattened sheet of single cells across the stroma to close the defect. Hemidesmosomes and intercellular contacts then reform and gradually the single cell layer is restored to its six-layered architecture by mitotic activity in the peripheral basal cells.

Migration of the epithelial cells occurs in a predictable manner as sheets of cells that produce geometric patterns as the advancing sheets meet in the centre (see Box 4.15).

Migration of epithelial cells is achieved by marked cytoskeletal and cell-shape changes involving redistribution of actin–myosin fibrils. Changes in actin distribution in the cell are preceded by changes in actin-binding proteins such as fodrin and E-cadherin, which are under genetic regulation via growth factors.

Migration of the cells is also dependent on matrix-induced intracellular signalling via components such as fibronectin/fibrin, laminin and collagen peptides through cell surface integrins. The role of fibronectin/fibrin in corneal epithelial resurfacing is unclear because these proteins do not appear to be essential for migration *in vitro*. However, it has been suggested that they facilitate healing where the normal basement membrane and, in particular, its laminin component have been lost, but are not essential for wound healing. The clinical application of fibronectin/fibrin to non-healing corneal ulcers has, however, been disappointing.

Adhesion of epithelium to the basement membrane and Bowman's layer is normally achieved via hemidesmosomes, the lamina densa and the anchoring type VII collagen fibrils (see Fig. 4.9). However, while hemidesmosomes form during the early stages of re-epithelialization (18 hours), many days elapse before anchoring fibrils reappear, and many

Box 4.15 Closing epithelial defects in the cornea

Corneal epithelial defects are closed by the migration of single cell sheets of flattened epithelial cells, which advance towards the centre of the defect producing characteristic geometric patterns. The patterns result from contact inhibition of the edges of each advancing sheet.

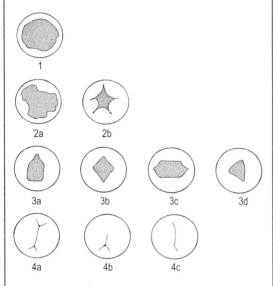

Closure of the defect is dependent on the viability of cells at the peripheral cornea (stem cells). If the original wound involved cells at the limbus, the defect is closed by distant cells converging towards the defect in 'tongues'. Conjunctival epithelium will also try to close this defect but the cells are less effective in producing a stable surface and may also attract blood vessels from the conjunctival stroma.

months pass before full ultrastructural integrity is restored. This may explain in part the phenomenon of recurrent erosion where there has been damage to the superficial stromal layers of the cornea. Proteolytic activity in repairing epithelial defects is also important – both urokinase-type plasminogen activator and matrix metalloproteinases have been implicated.

Most of the mitotic activity in the epithelium takes place at the limbus where 'stem cells' undergo several rounds of division to repopulate the entire corneal surface. However, attempts to promote wound healing using growth-promoting agents such as epidermal growth factor and retinoic acid have not met with great success. Limbal stem cells are believed to reside in 'niches' in the peripheral corneal epithelium, where they differentiate through various stages (Fig. 4.25). At present, there are no specific markers for limbal stem cells.

The stroma

Incisional wounds of the cornea that involve the stroma may be accidental or intentional. The immediate effect is to cause wound gape and imbibition of water from the tears by the GAGs (see above). This causes localized opacification (light scatter) and initiates a series of events in the cornea directed at closing the wound. These include deposition of fibrin within the wound, rapid epithelialization of the wound incision, and activation of the keratocytes to divide and synthesize collagen and GAGs. During the early phase of corneal wound healing, there is loss of specialization in the keratocytes such that they revert to a 'fibroblast'-like function and lay down collagen and GAGs found in any typical wound, e.g. hyaluronic acid, types I and III collagens, and matrix glycoproteins. In addition, the size and arrangement of the fibrils are not regular, further contributing to the corneal opacity. In extensive wounds, this opacification remains permanently; however, in smaller, well-defined wounds there is an attempt by the cornea to restore clarity by producing normal corneal matrix components.

Since the corneal curvature is a function of tension in its circumferential fibres (see Fig. 4.22), restoration of the normal curvature will not be achieved unless the edges of the wound are apposed by surgical reconstruction. This is the basis of refractive corneal surgery where partial-thickness wounds are intentionally left to heal in a gaping configuration; limited incisions in the periphery of the cornea alter its refractive power (Fig. 4.26), the degree of which can be precisely determined by the number and depth of incisions. Various types of laser surgery, such as argon-F1 and ultraviolet laser energy, are used to produce precise customized incisions in the stroma by 'ablating' the tissues. Ablation is thought to be caused by photon–photon interactions derived from thermal reactions or directly by photoablation, whereby molecular disintegration is induced. Further developments in refractive surgery include laser in-situ keratomileusis (LASIK) in which the surface of the cornea is reconfigured by raising a corneal flap, laser ablation of the exposed stromal bed and restoring the corneal flap without sutures. Both these and conventional surgical corneal incisions are fully epithelialized in the normal manner, with epithelial migration into the depths of the

215

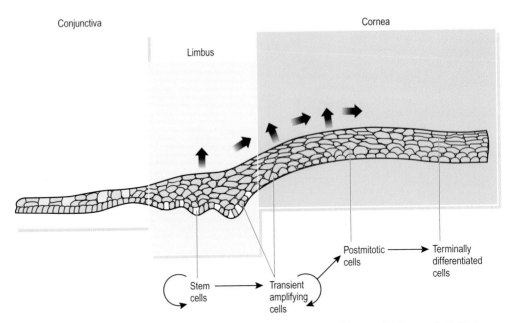

Fig. 4.25 Concept of limbal location of corneal stem cells and transient amplifying cells. Stem cells (white) are exlusively located in the basal limbal epithelium at the bottom of the epithelial papillae forming the palisades of Vogt. Transient amplifying cells occur in the basal epithelia of limbus and peripheral cornea. Postmitotic and terminally differentiated cells make up the suprabasal and superficial layers. (From Schlötzer-Schrehardt and Kruse 2005, with permission from Elsevier.)

wound sometimes producing excessive layers of cells.

Refractive surgery continues to expand both in quantity and in novelty of technique. A new method for assessment of astigmatism uses wavefront technology, which appears to be as effective as standard topographical assessment of the cornea. The fundamental quality of an optical system in for instance the field of astronomy is described in terms of wavefronts of higher and lower order and the eye can be described using such analysis. For instance, images formed by the healthy eye may be blurred for three main reasons: light scatter, diffraction and optical aberrations, e.g. chromatic or spherical. Using wavefront technology, optical aberrations from monochromatic sources such as myopia are selectively addressed and treated with wavefront-based LASIK.

In addition to developments in conventional LASIK therapies, LASIK may also be of considerable value following penetrating keratoplasty where occasional difficult and severe astigmatism may occur.

The endothelium

The corneal endothelium does not normally undergo mitosis in humans even after direct injury as in a perforating corneal wound. With age there is a decline in the number of endothelial cells with an increase in their size and variable morphology (polymegathism). The response to direct wounding is to undergo 'cell slide,' as occurs in the epithelium in the early stages of migration. If sufficient numbers of endothelial cells are lost, the cell layer cannot perform its pumping action and the cornea imbibes water (decompensates) and becomes opaque.

Vascularization

Vascularization of the cornea occurs when vessels from the conjunctiva or the deep episcleral plexus invade the periphery of the cornea during healing of wounds or infected ulcers. When corneal epithelial or stromal defects fail to close promptly, often as a result of infection or during the severe inflammatory response of chemical injury such as acid and alkali corneal burns, the continued release of proteolytic enzymes causes degradation of the stroma and increases the risk of spontaneous perforation. Matrix metalloproteinases such as matrilysin and stromelysin and MMP-9 as well as plasminogen activators (uPA and tPA) are released both by the incoming leucocytes and the resident epithelial and stromal cells (see Ch. 9). Cytokines, such as interleukin 1 (IL-1), IL-6 and IL-8, tumour necrosis factor-α and

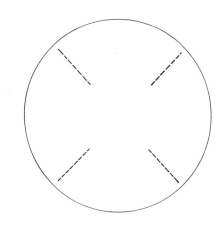

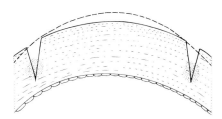

Fig. 4.26 Radial keratotomy. Four relaxing incisions in the circular peripheral band of collagen fibre reduce the curvature of the cornea.

TGF-β, macrophage inflammatory proteins (MIP) 1α and β, and granulocyte–macrophage colony-stimulating factor, liberated from the inflammatory and local cells stimulate further ingress of inflammatory cells and initiate a vascularization response (see Ch. 7). Growth factors such as VEGF, FGF and HGF (hepatocyte growth factor) are also released. Vessels advance across the cornea to the site of injury or infection and contribute to the eventual opaque 'leucoma' of the healed cornea. Inhibitors of angiogenesis are also released during the process, such as endostatin, a degradation product of collagen XVIII, and other products of collagen, fibronectin and even KI5, which is a fragment of plasminogen itself. In addition, thrombospondins (1 and 2) in synergy with a scavenger receptor CD36 are important anti-angiogenic factors present in the normal corneal stroma.

Vitamin A and the cornea

Deficiency of vitamin A leads to impaired corneal and conjunctival epithelial function, with loss of corneal lustre, Bitot's spots, punctate erosions and xerophthalmia, partly as a result of loss of goblet cells in the conjunctiva. Vitamin A or retinol is required for control of epithelial keratin expression and the synthesis of cell surface glycoproteins involved in the glycocalyx. Deficiency of vitamin A leads to a form of 'keratinization' of the corneal epithelium.

Vitamin A is also essential for normal corneal wound healing. A simple abrasion or ulcer that would be dealt with rapidly by a healthy cornea is likely to be complicated by a stromal melting response (kerato-malacia) in vitamin A-deficient humans and animals. Experimentally it has been shown that topical retinoic acid can reverse the effects of vitamin A deficiency. In addition, retinol itself promotes the synthesis of the α-1 proteinase inhibitor, which inhibits a wide range of proteolytic enzymes. Vitamin A has also been shown to have protective antioxidant effects on corneal endothelial cells in culture.

THE SCLERA

The sclera is non-transparent and tough because of its acellularity and matrix components

Matrix factors

The sclera is essentially acellular, containing only a few fibroblasts and non-branching traversing vessels. Recent studies have shown that there are some contractile fibroblasts (myofibroblasts) in the sclera and choroid that may have a role in refractive properties of the eye. It is opaque for the opposite reasons that the cornea is transparent, i.e. that the type I and III collagen fibres are of variable diameter and their distribution is irregular. There are also several other minor collagens in sclera (types V, VI, VIII, XII, XIII). The proteoglycans are predominantly proteo-dermatan and proteochondroitin sulphate of the small non-aggregating type and they are localized to the collagen fibres in a similar manner to corneal proteoglycans. However, there are no proteokeratan sulphates. Other proteoglycans present in sclera include aggrecan, PRELP (proline-arginine-rich and leucine-rich repeat), decorin and biglycan among others. In addition, the amount of proteoglycan in the sclera is considerably less than that in the cornea, with the effect that it is much less hydrated (70%). The sclera, unlike the cornea, also contains elastic fibres around a fibrillin core, accounting for about 2% of toal fibril content in the adult.

The sclera also contains a certain amount of large aggregating proteoglycans, such as versican, neurocan and brevican, combined with hyaluronic acid.

There is a considerable turnover of extracellular matrix constituents in the sclera, and this may determine the shape and size of the eye and thus refraction itself.

Bulk fluid transport and the uveal effusion syndrome

Although most of the bulk transport of fluid out of the eye takes place through the anterior chamber drainage angle and/or the uveoscleral meshwork (see Ch. 1, p. 39), there is appreciable transretinal transport of fluid towards the choroid. Some of this is drained via the normal choroidal vessels but a proportion is drained directly transsclerally. The effect of this transscleral flow is to 'suction on' the retina to its adjoining RPE layer and maintain retinal apposition.

Fluid flowing across the sclera is absorbed by the matrix proteoglycans. Thus, the sclera is maintained in its normal state, by having proteoglycans with a low water-binding capacity. In some conditions, such as the rare uveal effusion syndrome, and in nanophthalmia, the sclera contains high levels of abnormal proteoglycans, especially dermatan-sulphate-containing proteoglycans, which bind and trap large volumes of water. Thus the sclera thickens and may secondarily obstruct the choroidal venous drainage, causing further swelling and water retention.

The disordered collagen/matrix structure in the uveal effusion syndrome has been demonstrated by the cupreolinic blue technique (Fig. 4.27).

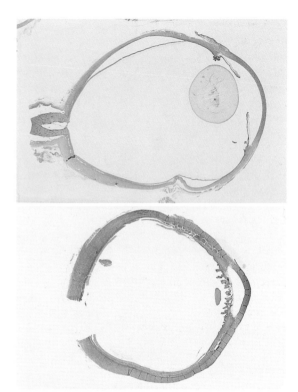

Fig. 4.27 Uveal effusion syndrome. The sclera is grossly thickened in the uveal effusion syndrome (bottom panel) compared to the normal globe (upper panel).

UVEAL TRACT

The uveal tract, comprising the iris, ciliary body and the choroid, is a continuous layer of which the major functions are to regulate the pupil size for optimal visual function and to act as the lymphovascular tissue of the eye. Each component, however, has several other functions.

THE IRIS

Physiology

The iris is derived from neuroectodermal and mesodermal tissue and is designed to function as the lens aperture of the eye. This is achieved by the opposing actions of the sphincter pupillae and the dilator pupillae muscles (see Ch. 1, p. 29). The sphincter is an annular band of true smooth muscle that inserts

close to the pupil margin at the pigment epithelium. The dilator is a highly unique series of myoepithelial cells representing the continuation of the outer layer of ciliary body pigmented epithelial cells. The non-pigmented ciliary body epithelial cells are continuous with the posterior pigmented iris epithelium (see Ch. 1). Between the origin at the ciliary body and the insertion near the sphincter pupillae, the dilator has several side insertions into the stroma of the iris, which allow it to mobilize the iris during dilation.

The functions of the pupil are:

- to regulate the amount of light entering the eye (it increases 16-fold on dilation of the pupil from 2 to 8 mm)
- to increase the depth of focus for near vision
- to minimize optical aberrations.

These functions are mediated by light and near reflexes, whose neural pathways involve autonomic parasympathetic (constriction) and the sympathetic (dilation) mechanisms (see Ch. 6). Unusually large pupil diameters have been linked to the development of myopia through increased optical aberrations.

The neuromuscular junctions of the iris are susceptible to direct pharmacological manipulation by agents that induce miosis (cholinergic agents, sympathetic antagonists) and mydriasis (anticholinergic agents, sympathomimetic agents) (see Ch. 6). In addition, pharmacological agents that induce the release of neurotransmitters from synaptic terminals (e.g. substance P is released after nitrogen mustard exposure) can have a marked effect on pupil responses. There is some evidence that dual innervation exists for iris muscles with excitatory and inhibitory input to each; thus the action of any individual drug may not be entirely predictable, depending on the state of activity at the time of administration of the drug.

Sympathetic activity in the dilator muscles appears to be mediated mainly by α receptors because the effects can be blocked by phenoxybenzene, but some β activity also exists. In some species, such as the cat, the action of sympathetic agents on the sphincter muscle appears to be mediated by β receptors only; in the monkey the action appears to be strongly α-mediated in the sphincter and dilator, thus producing antagonism. Studies on isolated human iris dilator indicate that the excitatory innervation is α-adrenergic while the inhibitor is cholinergically mediated.

Blood flow in the iris

About 5% of the total ocular blood flows through the iris. Iris blood vessels, derived from the major vessel circle, are contained as radial coils within tube-like formations of the stromal tissue, an arrangement that allows them to remain patent when the iris is fully dilated. Iris vessels have tight junctions and lack fenestrations; this renders them relatively impermeable to large molecules, as demonstrated by anterior segment fluorescein angiography. They constitute a second component of the blood–aqueous barrier (see below). Imaging techniques using high-resolution ultrasound allow visualization of iris and ciliary body vessels and indicate that flow velocities as low as 0.6 mm/second can be detected (Fig. 4.28).

THE CILIARY BODY

Functions of the ciliary body

The ciliary body has multiple functions:

- It provides the blood and nerve supply to the anterior segment (see Ch. 1, p. 32).
- It maintains intraocular pressure by secretion of aqueous.

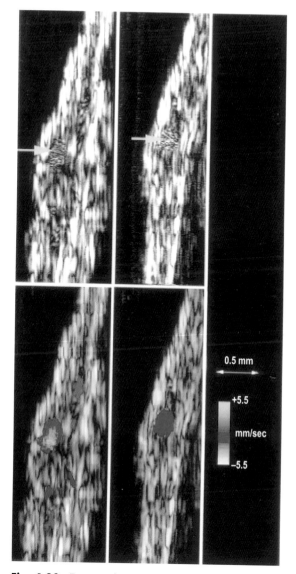

Fig. 4.28 Top panels: swept-mode images of iris and ciliary processes at 37°C (left) and 4°C (right). Arrows indicate position of major arterial circle. Bottom panels: colour flow images derived from swept-mode data shown above. (From Silverman *et al.* 2002, with permission from the World Federation for Ultrasound in Medicine and Biology.)

- It constitutes the major portion of the blood–aqueous barrier.
- Its musculature underlies the process of accommodation.

Blood flow in the ciliary body

The ciliary body receives blood vessels from the long posterior ciliary arteries and the major iris circle (see

Ch. 1). Blood flow through the ciliary body is about 7% of total ocular flow. The vessels are highly fenestrated, leaking most of their plasma components into the stroma. Blood flow in the iris and ciliary body is autoregulated like that of the retina (i.e. it does not alter significantly with changes in perfusion pressure), but it is also under autonomic control and can be modified by a variety of adrenergic and muscarinic inputs. Under normal circumstances, aqueous production is independent of ciliary body blood flow until the latter declines to <75% of normal.

Ciliary muscle and accommodation

In humans, relaxation of the zonule is induced by contraction of the ciliary muscle, which moves forward, thereby allowing the lens to adopt a more spherical shape owing to the elasticity of the lens capsule. There has also been some evidence that contraction of the ciliary muscle steepens the corneal curvature, thus increasing its refractory power, as occurs in lower vertebrates. The parasympathetic neurones mediating this response are carried in the III cranial nerve via the long ciliary nerves (see Ch. 1). It is not clear which of the three sets of ciliary muscle fibres is responsible for the major action in inducing this forward movement but, as for the iris muscles, the effects can be blocked by anticholinergic drugs. Recently, it has been shown that there is a small sympathetic inhibitory component and that this is increased in late-onset myopes. Accommodation produces greater ability to focus on near objects owing to the increased refractive (dioptric) power of the lens. Epidemiological and theoretical quantitative analyses have shown that intense near work for prolonged periods disrupts emmetropization associated with eye growth and induces myopia. In addition, recent studies have shown that young children sleeping in dimly lit, as opposed to completely dark, rooms are at risk of developing myopia because of the persistence of poorly focused images through thin eyelid skin.

Blood–aqueous barrier

Aqueous humour, secreted by non-pigmented ciliary epithelial cells, is derived from plasma but contains different concentrations of electrolytes and other small molecules, and a restricted set of proteins in low concentration (see Table 4.10). Thus a 'barrier' exists between the plasma transudate in the ciliary body stroma and the aqueous in the posterior chamber of the eye. This barrier to the free diffusion of molecules is formed by the tight junctions between non-pigmented ciliary epithelial cells (see Ch. 1). In

Table 4.10 Composition of aqueous humour compared with plasma

Component	Aqueous	Plasma	Units
Glucose	2.7–3.9	5.6–6.4	mmol
Lactate	4.5	0.5–0.8	
Ascorbate	1.1	0.04	
Albumin	5.5–6.5	3400	mg/dl
Transferrin	1.3–1.7		
Fibronectin	0.25	29	
IgG	3.0	1270	
Na	142	130–145	meq/l
K	4	3.5–5.0	
HCO_3	20	24–30	
Mg	1	0.7–1.1	
Ca	1.2	2.0–2.6	
Cl	131	92–125	

contrast, extensive gap junctions between pigmented and non-pigmented cells allow the two layers of the ciliary epithelium to act as a metabolic and transport syncytium. In the iris, where tight junctions between the epithelial cells do not exist, the barrier is formed by tight junctions between the vascular endothelial cells. These endothelial tight junctions contain the same set of proteins as epithelial tight junctions (see Box 4.5), such as occludin and cingulin.

Breakdown of the blood–aqueous barrier occurs in many conditions, including trauma, inflammation, paracentesis and vascular disease. The aqueous humour becomes cloudy (seen as flare in the slit-lamp) because of leakage of plasma proteins into the posterior and anterior chambers – it may even become 'plasmoid' owing to the presence of fibrinogen and other proteins. Inflammatory cells are also likely to be present when the blood–aqueous barrier breaks down. If clotting occurs, as in severe uveitis, the aqueous becomes 'plastic'.

Eicosanoids in the iris/ciliary body

Prostaglandins were first discovered in the eye in 1957 by Ambache, who demonstrated the biological activity in aqueous and named the factor 'irin.' Eicosanoids is the generic term to describe prostaglandins (PGs) and leukotrienes, both of which are metabolites of arachidonic acid (see Ch. 6). Prostaglandins are synthesized in large amounts after trauma or inflammation involving the iris/ciliary body, from arachidonic acid released by esterified sites in membrane phospholipids. Other neuropeptides are involved in this response. For instance, release of substance P from the iris leads to receptor-mediated breakdown of PIP_2 (see Ch. 6) and the formation of large amounts of arachidonic acid in the iris sphincter and synthesis of PGE_2. In the ciliary body, the cyclo-oxygenase pathway is also active in microsomes. PGE_2 is involved in miosis, while $PGF_{2\alpha}$ is involved in the control of intraocular pressure. Interestingly, breakdown of the blood–aqueous barrier in response to PGE_2 agonists, is impaired in PGE-receptor knockout mice. $PGF_{2\alpha}$ is also known to increase vasodilatation and capillary permeabilization in the anterior segment of the eye. Many other peptides are present in the iris/ciliary body and the aqueous including neuropeptide Y, vasoactive intestinal peptide, somatostatin and calcitonin gene-related peptide (CGRP). Nitric oxide is also released during activation of iris/ciliary body tissues. Many of these peptides modulate normal iris/ciliary body functions such as miosis and aqueous humour production. For instance, CGRP relaxes iris dilator smooth muscle via cAMP mechanisms. They also have other functions such as the immunosuppressive role of vasoactive intestinal peptide in ocular immune privilege (see Ch. 7, p. 432).

Drugs that inhibit the cyclo-oxygenase pathway, such as indomethacin and aspirin, may be useful in ocular inflammation. However, steroids act at the level of phospholipase A_2 and may have a more global effect on the response (see Ch. 6). In addition, the lipoxygenase pathway is active in the anterior uvea with synthesis of leukotrienes B_4, C_4 and D_4, and the chemotaxis of polymorphonuclear leucocytes (see Ch. 7). Penetration of drugs into the intraocular environment after topical application occurs more readily through the conjunctiva and the sclera than the cornea, partly as a result of the numerous transport mechanisms available in the conjunctival epthelium but also because of the greater transepithelial permeability of the conjunctiva compared to cornea, which is impermeable even to low-molecular-weight compounds (< 1000 kDa).

Detoxification and antioxidation in the anterior segment

The cytochrome P_{450} system is the major drug detoxification system in the eye
Microsomes contain a group of proteins known as the cytochrome P_{450} proteins, which catalyse the transfer of a single oxygen atom to endogenous and exogenous substances destined for excretion and/or detoxification, such as steroids, phenobarbitone, etc. (see Ch. 6, p. 323). Their main effect is to convert hydrophobic compounds to hydroxylated hydrophilic compounds, which are then more easily metabolized.

The cytochrome P_{450} system is present in the ciliary body (at about 5% of the concentration in liver) where it acts to detoxify many compounds. It does this by either converting the hydroxylated, highly reactive compound to a glucuronide via UDP-glucuronyl transferase or by conjugating it to glutathione via glutathione-S-transferase (see Box 4.16). Most of the enzymes involved in the detoxification process have been identified and/or purified from the ciliary body, in particular the non-pigmented epithelium. There is considerable genetic variation in the induction of the cytochrome P_{450} system in the eye, perhaps explaining the variable toxic effects of drugs in individuals.

The ciliary body is the main source of antioxidant systems in the anterior segment
Although antioxidant systems exist in the lens (see below) and the cornea (see above), the ciliary body is especially rich in antioxidant systems with the highest concentrations of catalase, superoxide dismutase, and glutathione peroxidase types I and II. Type I is selenium-dependent while type II is selenium-independent. Type I is closely linked to glutathione reductase whose main function is the reduction of oxidized glutathione (GSSH) produced by the detoxification of peroxides (see Box 4.16).

Hydrogen peroxide (H_2O_2) is present in normal aqueous, most of it derived from the non-enzymatic interaction between reduced ascorbate and molecular oxygen, and it is reduced to H_2O by glutathione secreted by the ciliary epithelium. Most of these studies have been performed in experimental animals and it is not clear how relevant they are to the human eye. It has been suggested that oxidized ascorbate (via the superoxide anion) is more important in degrading H_2O_2 in humans. Melatonin, a neuropeptide involved in biological circadian rhythms, is also an H_2O_2 scavenger. A role for xanthine oxidase has also been suggested. H_2O_2 can induce norepinephrine release from the iris/ciliary body in the aqueous and has recently been implicated in cataract formation.

Ciliary body tissue also contains a peroxiredoxin, a constituent of a widely distributed family of

Box 4.16 Cytochrome P₄₅₀ and drug detoxification

The cytochrome P_{450} system detoxifies compounds by utilizing the glutathione-S-transferase system and degrading compounds to mercapturic acid.

---

antioxidant enzymes, whose amino acid sequence and tissue distribution are now known. Their role is to degrade H_2O_2 and alkyl peroxides.

THE CHOROID

Functions of the choroid

The function of the choroid is to act as the lymphovascular supply to the posterior segment of the eye.

Blood flow through the choroid

The choroid is almost entirely composed of vessels embedded in a loose connective tissue matrix which has a high content of type III collagen, typical of an expansile or spongy tissue. The blood supply to the choroid has several interesting features:

- 98% of the blood to the eye passes through the uveal tract, of which 85% is through the choroid.
- Blood flow occurs at a rate of 1400 ml/min per 100 g tissue, which is higher than the perfusion of blood through the kidney.
- The choriocapillaris is organized in a lobular architecture, collecting into larger vessels and finally into four vortex veins, one in each quadrant of the globe (see Ch 1).
- Venous blood draining from the choroid is not desaturated, only 5–10% oxygen having been

extracted during passage through the eye. The choroid supplies the outer retina, where the partial pressure of oxygen (Po_2) is highest, rapidly falling towards the retinal inner segments and then rising again, less so, towards the inner retina (Fig. 4.29).

- Blood vessels in the choroid are highly fenestrated and leaky, like ciliary body vessels.
- Choroid and ciliary body blood vessels are sensitive to the Po_2 and Pco_2; in conditions of high Pco_2 the vessels expand greatly in a forward direction, exerting pressure on structures such as the vitreous gel and lens/iris diaphragm.
- Although previously considered to have considerable autoregulation in relation to perfusion pressure, choroidal blood flow, especially around the optic nerve, is sensitive to the effects of nitric oxide and endothelin and other as yet unidentified vasoconstrictors.

Lymphoid function

Intraocular structures lack a recognized lymphatic system. However, the choroid contains a rich network of immune cells including mast cells, macrophages and dendritic cells (see Ch. 1), and this tissue can respond massively to intraocular inflammation (see Ch. 7, p. 433). In addition, choroidal and ciliary body/iris melanocytes are potential antigenic targets for autoimmune disease (see Ch. 7).

AQUEOUS HUMOUR DYNAMICS

A fundamental physiological function of the eye is to maintain an intraocular pressure (IOP) between 10 and 20 mmHg. This is achieved by the circulation of aqueous humour secreted by the ciliary body into the posterior chamber and circulated through the pupil towards the anterior chamber angle where it drains via the outflow apparatus into the episcleral veins (see Ch. 1). Factors affecting IOP include:

- circadian rhythms
- episcleral venous pressure
- rate of flow of aqueous humour
- neural (cranial nerves V and VII) and hormonal influences.

The intraocular pressure as measured clinically actually represents the balance between the inflow and outflow of aqueous and is altered by changes in the gradient of pressure between the posterior chamber and the anterior chamber, and eventually by the episcleral pressure. The uveoscleral outflow is greatly affected by alterations in this gradient of pressure as appears to occur in glaucoma (Fig. 4.30).

AQUEOUS HUMOUR IS SECRETED BY THE CILIARY BODY EPITHELIUM

The rate of aqueous humour formation is about 2–3 μl/min. Aqueous humour is formed by the transport of water and electrolytes from the leaky fenestrated capillaries of the ciliary processes to the epithelial syncytium and thence across the plasma membrane of the non-pigmented epithelium (see Box 4.17).

Composition of aqueous humour

The aqueous humour is composed predominantly of electrolytes and low-molecular-weight compounds with some protein (Table 4.10) and there are significant differences from plasma in several of the

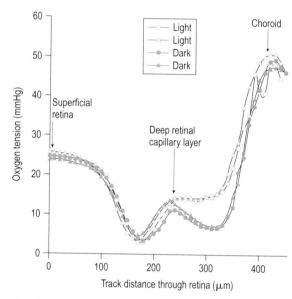

Fig. 4.29 Typical intraretinal oxygen distribution in the normal rat retina under light-adapted and dark-adapted conditions. Oxygen tension is shown as a function of penetration depth of the microelectrode through the retina and choroid. In the outer retina the sudden change in oxygen gradient (at w320 mm penetration depth) is the result of high oxygen consumption of the inner segment of the photoreceptors. The oxygen consumption of this region increases during dark adaptation, resulting in a significant fall in oxygen tension in this region. (From Yu and Cringle 2005, with permission from Elsevier.)

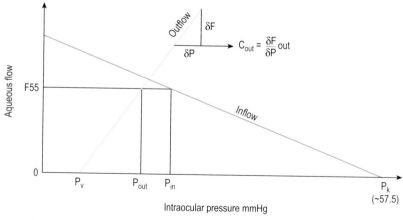

Fig. 4.30 Aqueous inflow declines as intraocular pressure (IOP) rises towards P_k (about 57.5 mmHg). Goldmann estimates pseudofacility as $P_k = 0.58 \times$ Brachial BP. The gradient for inflow is $(F_{55} / P_k - P_{55}) = C_{in} = C_{ps}$ where F_{55} is steady-static flow. C_{ps} is the pseudofacility. (Courtesy D. Woodhouse.)

Box 4.17 Secretion of aqueous humour

Classic theory suggests that passive diffusion of water and ions from the fenestrated vessels of the ciliary body is followed by active transport of Na^+ and Cl^- across the ciliary body syncytium. This is an active secretory process involving Na^+/K^+ ATPase and carbonic anhydrase type II activity. In some respects this has been viewed as ultrafiltration of ions and water and eventually leads to the formation of aqueous humour, which is secreted into the posterior chamber. However, the oncotic pressure of the ciliary stroma is greater than the hydrostatic pressure difference across the ciliary epithelium, so tending towards absorption of water into the ciliary body from the posterior

chamber. Thus active transport of ions in the opposite direction is the main mechanism of aqueous humour formation. This process is also under adrenergic receptor control at the level of the ciliary epithelial cells and possibly also by regulation of blood flow to the ciliary body. More recently, the possibility has been raised that H_2O transport may also be achieved by aquaporin 1 (AqPO1), a water channel protein found in the ciliary non-pigmented epithelium. In addition, some of the K^+ channels are Ca^{2+} sensitive and can be activated by Ca^{2+} entry via Ca^{2+} channels. Release of Cl^- ions into the posterior chamber may also be facilitated by adenosine receptors.

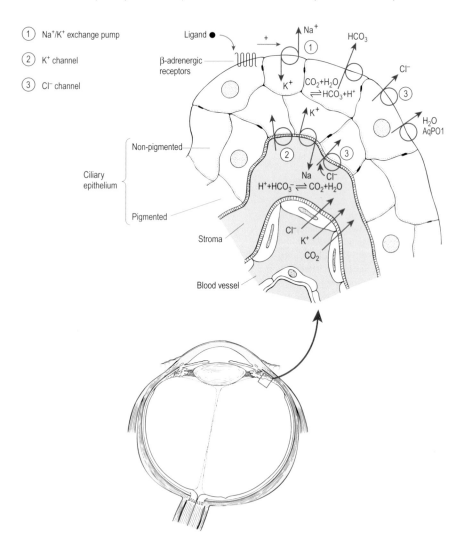

to contribute to bulk flow of water because IOP is reduced in AqPO4/1 knockout mice.

Aquaporin water channels are also present in both the secretory machinery (AqPO4 and AqPO1) and the outflow channel (trabecular meshwork endothelium) and appear

components. Aqueous receives contributions from a variety of sources including the corneal endothelium and the iris/lens, in addition to active secretion from the ciliary body. Several trace compounds are also present in aqueous humour, including steroid sex hormones, enzymes such as carbonic anhydrase, lysozyme, and plasminogen activator, and cytokines such as basic fibroblast growth factor (bFGF) and TGF-β (see Ch. 7, p. 383). Low levels of catecholamines (epinephrine, norepinephrine and dopamine), prostaglandins and cyclic nucleotides are present in normal aqueous, but the source of these compounds is uncertain.

The protein content of aqueous is very low (about 1/500 of plasma), and the major species is albumin. Since immunoglobulins are relatively large molecules, it is unlikely that they gain access to the aqueous via the blood–retinal barrier; local production via iris lymphocytes or plasma cells is a more likely source (see Ch. 7, p. 358). Small amounts of fibronectin are also produced locally.

Aqueous contains detectable amounts of hyaluronic acid, derived as breakdown oligomers from vitreous hyaluronic acid during the normal process of GAG renewal (see below). However, some of the aqueous hyaluronic acid is of higher molecular weight than vitreous, suggesting that it is produced in the anterior segment. Aqueous hyaluronic acid may have a role to play in regulation of IOP because perfusion of the anterior chamber with hyaluronidase leads to a marked drop in pressure. However, it is also possible that intracameral hyaluronidase affects trabecular meshwork cells and extracellular matrix, thus leading to a lowering of the IOP.

NEURAL/AUTONOMIC CONTROL OF AQUEOUS SECRETION

Adrenergic and cholinergic agonists and receptors are present in the iris and ciliary body, and autonomic innervation of this tissue occurs in muscle, vessels and epithelial cells. Adrenergic receptors are present in the ciliary epithelium and regulate IOP via the adenylate cyclase system. β-adrenergic antagonists and α_2-selective adrenergic agonists both suppress aqueous flow. Muscarinic receptors linked to the PIP_2 second messenger system are also present in the ciliary epithelium.

Cholinergic mechanisms are not involved in control of IOP

M_3 muscarinic receptors in the ciliary epithelium linked to phosphatidyl inositol in the cell membrane

Receptor	Agonist	Antagonist	Effect
α_1	Phenylephrine	Prazosin	Stimulatory
α_2	Clonidine	Yohimbine	Adenylate cyclase
β_1	Isoprenaline	Atenolol	Adenylate cyclase
β_2	Epinephrine	Propranolol	Adenylate cyclase

Table 4.11 Types of adrenergic receptor

have been identified, but they do not appear to have a significant role in IOP control. Despite this, cholinergic agents such as pilocarpine are thought to have some action via reduction in aqueous secretion, although the experimental evidence is weak. Most of the action of pilocarpine appears to be mediated via its effect on outflow resistance and uveoscleral flow (see below).

Adrenergic receptors regulate IOP via adenylate cyclase

The majority of α receptors in the ciliary body are α_2 (Table 4.11), while more than 90% of β receptors are β_2. Stimulation of α_2 receptors lowers the IOP via a reduction in aqueous humour production through inhibition of adenylate cyclase. Epinephrine, a preferential α-adrenergic agonist, stimulates prostaglandin synthesis, particularly that of PGE_2 and $PGF_{2\alpha}$, the latter having potent ocular hypotensive activity.

Stimulation of β receptors, particularly β_2 receptors, also leads to an increase in aqueous secretion via activation of adenylate cyclase.

The dual control of aqueous secretion through activation (β) or inhibition of adenylate cyclase (α) is mediated by their respective stimulatory and inhibitory G proteins (see Ch. 6, p. 327). Thus, IOP can be lowered by α_2 agonists (e.g. clonidine) or β_2 antagonists (β-blockers, e.g. timolol). The α_2 receptors are also linked to vasoactive intestinal peptide receptors, which are costimulated and lead to a reduction in cAMP levels, which in itself may also lower IOP. β Antagonists have no effect on aqueous flow when aqueous production is at its lowest, whereas α_2 agonists and carbonic anhydrase inhibitors do.

The mechanism whereby changes in intracellular cAMP levels alter aqueous secretion is not known but appears to involve transport of the HCO_3^- ion across the cells. In addition, a number of other components appear to be involved in aqueous secretion, such as protein kinase C, which is linked to adenylate cyclase activation and thus may act as part of an intracellular signalling network connecting the two main second messenger systems (see Ch. 6, p. 327).

Circadian regulation of aqueous humour formation

It has long been known that there is a diurnal variation in IOP. This is in part the result of a circadian regulation of aqueous humour secretion. Secretion in humans occurs at a rate of 2.6 ml/min during the day and falls to 1.0 ml/min at night. Both β-adrenergic receptor-mediated and neuropeptide-mediated mechanisms, particularly that of vasoactive intestinal peptide, are involved. Activation of G-protein coupled adenylate cyclase leads to cAMP production, which activates protein kinase A thus regulating the cation channels. The process is terminated by hydrolysis of cAMP by phosphodiesterase.

Is guanylate cyclase involved in IOP control?

Large amounts of brain natriuretic peptide (BNP) as well as atrial natriuretic peptide (ANP) are found in the iris/ciliary body and in the aqueous humour of rabbits and humans. The receptor for ANP is linked to membrane-bound guanylate cyclase, and *in vitro* studies have shown that this enzyme can be stimulated by ANP in the ciliary body. In the rabbit this is accompanied by a reduction in IOP but its relevance in humans is not clear because similar levels of peptides are found in both normal subjects and in glaucoma patients.

THE OUTFLOW SYSTEM

The outflow of aqueous from the eye is regulated at several different levels, including the trabecular meshwork, the uveoscleral system and, outside the globe, the episcleral vessels (see Ch. 1).

Regulation of outflow at the trabecular meshwork

Resistance to the outflow of aqueous occurs at the endothelium and within the matrix of the trabecular meshwork itself. The juxtacanalicular cribriform meshwork accounts for a significant proportion of the total resistance to flow. This has been attributed to matrix components, especially the GAGs, present in this region. The trabecular beams, composed of type 1 collagen, with a significant proportion of type III and IV collagen, and other matrix constitutents such as laminin, fibronectin and elastin, are separated by GAG-filled spaces, particularly hyal-

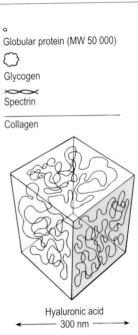

Globular protein (MW 50 000)

Glycogen

Spectrin

Collagen

Hyaluronic acid

300 nm

Fig. 4.31 Model of hyaluronic acid, showing size compared to other 'typical' molecules. (Courtesy of J Alberts.)

uronic acid (Fig. 4.31), that retard the flow of fluid by virtue of hydrophilic properties and large hydrodynamic volume. A wide range of GAGs have been identified in the trabecular meshwork matrix, namely hyaluronic acid, chondroitin sulphate, dermatan sulphate, keratan sulphate and heparan sulphate, with significant variation between species. Some unidentified proteoglycan material has also been detected. Trace amounts of types V and VII collagen have also been detected in the trabecular meshwork.

Trabecular meshwork endothelial cells have special characteristics, namely active phagocytic properties, high levels of cytoskeletal actin, which in cultured cells is particularly sensitive to cytochalasin B, and lower levels of microtubules, which appear to be relatively non-responsive to colchicine. These cells also contain vimentin and desmin, thus showing some similarity to smooth muscle cells. Taken together, these findings suggest that trabecular meshwork endothelial cells are specialized for both endocytic transport of water and solutes, and contractility. Actin mobilization appears to be mediated via adrenergic receptors, probably of the β_2 type, which are highly responsive to epinephrine. Energy metabolism in the trabecular meshwork endothelium is predominantly glycolytic rather than oxidative, although both enzyme systems are present and functional. Transport of water may be achieved not merely by passive transportation of H_2O packets but by activation of a water channel protein, aquaporin 1 (AqPO1), found in corneal endothelial cells.

Metabolism of trabecular meshwork cells

Metabolic labelling studies have shown that most of the matrix components in the trabecular meshwork are synthesized and degraded by the endothelial cells. In addition, these cells have high levels of surface tissue plasminogen activator (tPA), higher even than in vascular endothelial cells, and this is likely to play a role in maintaining patency and reducing the resistance of the outflow passages. Phagocytic activity of trabecular meshwork cells is associated with several other enzymatic activities such as GAG-degrading enzymes and acid phosphatase.

Trabecular meshwork cells have receptors for a variety of agents including epinephrine (β_2 adrenergic receptors, decrease phagocytosis) and glucocorticoids. Both steroids and oxidative damage induce the expression of the trabecular meshwork inducible glucocorticoid response (TIGR) protein. Mutations in the *TIGR* gene have been found in patients with glaucoma. In addition, TGF-β appears to be involved in the glucocorticoid cell response and in the production of trabecular meshwork extracellular material. Steroids inhibit prostaglandin production by trabecular meshwork cells at concentrations as low as 10^{-8} m. Prostaglandin synthesis by trabecular meshwork accounts for a significant proportion of its arachidonic acid metabolism (70% compared with less than 5% in other cells) suggesting that prostaglandins play a major role in trabecular meshwork cell physiology. In addition to substantial amounts of PGE and $PGF_{2\alpha}$, leukotriene B_4 appears to be produced in high amounts.

Trabecular meshwork cells contain the free radical and hydrogen peroxide detoxifying enzyme systems present in other tissues such as the ciliary body (see above). Both a catalase and a glutathione-dependent system are active in handling hydrogen peroxide, which can reach levels as high as 25 μmol/l in the aqueous humour.

Uveoscleral drainage

A variable proportion of aqueous (3–20%) drains directly into the anterior uvea at the ciliary body immediately posterior to the cornea and thence into the suprachoroidal space and towards the posterior pole of the eye (see Ch. 1). The anterior uvea at this point is incompletely lined with endothelial cells. In addition, the localization of MMP-1 (see p. 360) suggests a role for this enzyme in uveoscleral outflow.

Uveoscleral drainage is possible because the pressure in the suprachoroid is 2–4 mmHg lower than in the anterior chamber; this can be reversed after trabeculectomy and can lead to choroidal effusions. This pressure differential is also less with age, leading to greater risk of choroidal effusion in such patients. Prostaglandins may decrease the intraocular pressure by increasing the uveoscleral outflow. Several possible mechanisms have been proposed, including relaxation of the ciliary muscle, cell shape changes, cytoskeletal rearrangements or compaction of the trabecular meshwork matrix.

Episcleral circulation

It was shown many years ago that dye-stained aqueous fluid would not drain out of the eye into the episcleral veins if the IOP was less than 15 mmHg. Thus this represents the combined episcleral venous pressure and the oncotic pressure in the perivenous tissues of the episcleral veins. Aqueous humour draining via the canal of Schlemm into the aqueous veins does so by passing through large transcellular channels and giant vacuoles on the meshwork side of the canal. The canal has direct vascular communications on its outer wall with a network of intrascleral collector channels that drain into the scleral veins (see Ch. 1).

Recently an alternative model for aqueous outflow has been proposed which involves a mechanical pumping mechanism generated in response to small changes in IOP and linked to the ocular pulse. Pumping of aqueous from Schemm's canal into the collecting veins and episcleral veins is assisted by small valves in this model.

Does aqueous contain components that contribute to flow resistance?

Although aqueous has the same viscosity as isotonic saline, its passage through microporous filters *in vitro* is slower than that of saline. This effect can be abolished by proteolytic agents and detergents, but not by hyaluronidase. It has therefore been suggested that some forms of glaucoma may be caused by a build up of a surfactant-like material with age.

THE LENS

The transparency of the lens is a function of the highly ordered state of its cells and extracellular matrix. In essence, the extracellular matrix of the lens is confined to its capsule, while the cells form a syncytium with interlocking cellular processes.

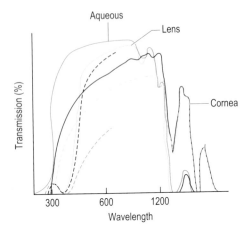

Fig. 4.32 Optical density curves for various ocular components. (With permission of Drs Jaffe and Horwitz and JB Lippincott.)

LENS TRANSPARENCY

The light transmission properties of the ocular media vary to some degree depending on the nature and the age of the tissue. The cornea, aqueous humour and lens all transmit long-wavelength light well above the limit of visible light (about 720 nm). However, short wavelengths below 300 nm are absorbed by the cornea but are transmitted through the aqueous; the lens, however, filters the majority of the short wavelengths below 360 nm and is an absolute barrier to light below 300 nm (Fig. 4.32).

The epithelium

The single-celled epithelium of the lens and its capsule does not scatter or reflect light, essentially because the combined refractive index is the same as that of the aqueous humour (1.336). However, the epithelium is of great importance in the maintenance of fluid and electrolyte balance of the lens syncytium via ion-pump mechanisms (see below). Thus, any agent that disturbs epithelial function and/or viability (such as ionizing radiation to the lens bow region) will have significant effects on lens clarity. This applies to all aspects of lens structure and function.

The organization of the lens fibre cells underpins the transmission properties of the lens

It might be expected that the plasma membranes of the lens fibres would produce interference diffraction patterns that would affect the ability of the lens to transmit light. However, it has been shown that the weak diffraction rings that are produced occur in a repeating pattern with a period of the same dimension as the thickness of an individual lens fibre in the anteroposterior axis. This reduces any scatter by the plasma membranes of the normal epithelium; it has been estimated that the amount of scatter by the epithelium in the human lens is about 5% of the transmitted light.

Lens fibre cells are organized in a densely packed cellular arrangement, with interdigitations like pieces in a three-dimensional jigsaw puzzle (see Ch. 1, p. 36) in which extensive intercellular communication exists via the lens gap-junction-like protein, MIP26 (main intrinsic polypeptide of 26 000 kDa). During development of the lens fibre cells, they become anucleate and specialized for the production of specific lens proteins, the crystallins. These comprise over 90% of the total cellular protein and are embedded within a complex cytoskeletal matrix, some components of which are also lens-specific (e.g. the beaded intermediate filament protein). The high refractive index (RI) of the lens is caused by the crystallins; at the periphery of the lens the RI is slightly less (1.38) than at the nucleus (1.41). The water content of the lens is also greater at the periphery (75–80%) than at the lens nucleus (68%).

The presence of the crystallins is, in itself, insufficient to explain the transparency of the lens. Transparency is predominantly the result of the packing of the crystallins in very high concentration such that they resemble a dense liquid or a glass because of the high level of 'short-range spatial order'; this means that the scatter of light from each individual molecule is related to the scatter from its immediate neighbours and that they tend to cancel each other out. At a macroscopic level, the arrangement of the crescent-like fibre cells in end-to-end concentric shells around a polar axis provides a highly ordered architecture. A series of coaxial refractive surfaces, thus created, promotes transparency of the multicellular structure. However, this general view does not apply to all species and in most there are two types of fibre cell, an S-shaped cell and a concentric cell. Overlapping tails of S-shaped cells form the lens sutures, which paradoxically lie along the visual axis and can affect optical quality and variability in focus.

The crystallins

Crystallins make up 90% of the water-soluble proteins of the lens; there are three types in mammals (see Box 4.18). Some crystallin protein also coex-

Box 4.18 The crystallins

Three types of crystallin have been identified in mammals: α, β and γ, mainly on the basis of molecular weight. The δ crystallins have also been detected in birds. Several other 'taxon-specific' crystallins (ε, τ, ρ, χ, μ, λ, ζ, SIII) are recognized in other species, based on the criterion that they account for at least 10% of the total water-soluble protein. More recent data suggest that in vertebrates there are only two classes of crystallins, α and γβ. Native α crystallin is of two types, αA and αB, each with a molecular weight of about 20 kDa. In the native state, however, the α crystallins form large multimeric aggregates of 300–1200 kDa (average 800 kDa), held together by non-covalent interactions.

β Crystallins range in molecular weight from 23 to 35 kDa and occur in several subtypes: βB_1, βB_2 and βB_3; βA_2, βA_3 and βB_4. Mixed aggregates of between 50 and 200 kDa occur naturally. The γ crystallins are monomeric in the native state; there are six types [γA–E, and γS (formerly known as βS)] differentiated by charge. Not all types are present in human lenses at all ages, some such as γS and γC being present at higher concentrations in fetal than in adult lenses. The relative amounts of α : β : γ crystallin also vary greatly depending on age and other factors; in the 'typical' lens the ratio of α : β : γ is of the order 40 : 35 : 25. Protein sequence analysis has shown homology between the β and γ crystallins; in addition, all three proteins exist as β pleated sheets.

tracts with the urea-soluble protein, indicating that a fraction of the crystallins is strongly bound to the cytoskeletal (urea-soluble) proteins (5% total protein). The water/urea-insoluble protein represents membrane protein (2% total protein) and some crystallin is also found in this fraction when it is solubilized in detergent.

The αA and αB crystallins show about 50% sequence homology. The molecules exist as polydisperse globular proteins in aggregates organized in three concentric layers or as a protein 'micelle'. However, their true quaternary structure is unknown. αA and αB crystallins belong to the family of small heat-shock proteins and display chaperone-like activity. Studies in knockout mice have shown that αA lens-specific crystallin is required for normal lens differentiation and transparency, while αB, which is expressed in neural tissue and upregulated under conditions of stress, is not essential for lens transparency. Homology of lens crystallins to certain enzymes such as aldehyde dehydrogenase class 3 enzymes in corneal epithelial cells suggests that this form of 'gene sharing' is quite widespread.

Recently the crystal structure of the small invertebrate heat-shock protein, Hsp16.9 has been determined, which has allowed a model for lens αA crystalline micelles to be developed (Fig. 4.33). In this model it has been shown that neither αA or αB is necessary to develop the molecular arrangement but that some combination of either will suffice.

Phosphorylation of the αA_2 and the αB_2 chains produces the αA_1 and the αB_1 chains. Spontaneous non-enzymatic cleavage of the molecules also occurs, as does high molecular weight aggregation, especially with age. The α crystallins, acting as molecular chaperones, 'trap' other crystallins and proteins such as intermediate filaments, which may be undergoing denaturation and unfolding. In this way they maintain lens transparency by preventing disruption of the highly ordered structure of the crystallin packing.

The γβ crystallins are thought to have similar structure: four repeating antiparallel β sheets in the form of 'Greek key' motifs (Fig. 4.34). γ Crystallin is a highly stable molecule, attributed to its extensive internal symmetry (Fig. 4.34); it is associated with 'old' cataract and decreases in content with age, except for γS crystallin (see Box 4.18).

Multimeric complexes of β crystallins tend to form between the acidic molecules (βA_2, βA_3, and βA_4) and the basic molecules (βB_1, βB_2, and βB_3), followed by association between similar heterodimers. Homology among the various β crystallins both within and between species is quite variable and sequence analysis is still in progress for most of the human proteins. However, on the basis of γβ sequence homology a predicted structure of β crystallin has been suggested and found to have some basis by X-ray crystallography. In this model, the two γ-like structures are joined by a 'connecting peptide'.

Although the molecular packing of the crystallins and their high refractive index contribute extensively to lens transparency, biophysical studies of molecular interactions between proteins indicate that the crystallins in themselves are not essential but proteins that can adopt the correct state of phase transition and osmotic pressure would do equally well.

Cytoskeletal proteins of the lens

Cytoskeletal proteins are usually to be found in the urea-extractable fraction of lens proteins. In addition to the usual complement of microfilaments, such as

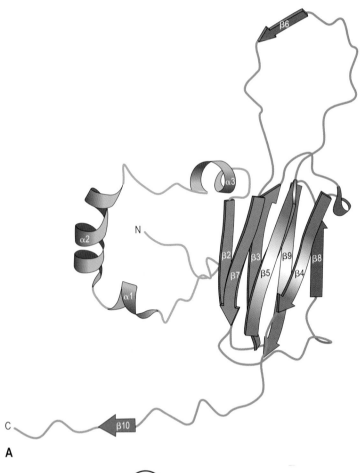

A

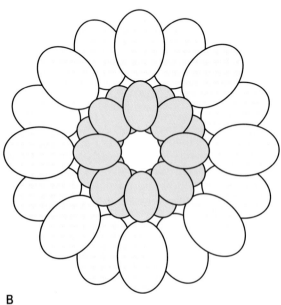

B

Fig. 4.33 (**A**) Secondary structure of the hsp16.9 subunit with an ordered N terminus. The N-terminal domain (green) contains three helical segments, as shown, in half of the subunits. The remaining subunits in hsp16.9 and all subunits in hsp16.5 have unstructured N termini. The α crystallin domain (orange) consists of seven-stranded β-sandwich, an interdomain loop containing one β-strand (β6 at the top) and a C-terminal extension (at the bottom), which is largely unstructured except for the short V10-strand. (Reproduced with permission from Nature Publishing Group.) (**B**) A possible micelle-like structure for α crystallin. The subunits contain two domains and assemble into large aggregates through interactions between their hydrophobic N-terminal domains (lilac), which are located in the centre of the aggregate. The hydrophilic C-terminal (α crystallin) domains (pink) are on the surface of the assembly. (From Augusteyn 2004, with permission from the Optometrists Association Australia.)

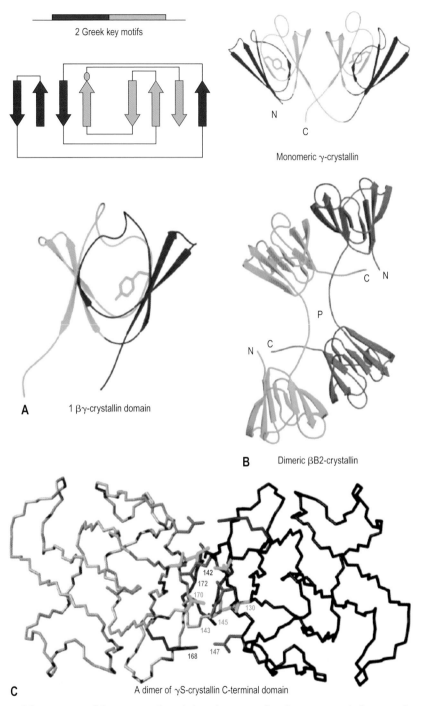

Fig. 4.34 The modular structure of the βγ crystallins. (**A**) Each βγ crystallin domain is made from two linear sequence-related Greek key motifs that intercalate on folding to form two β sheets. The two sheets form a compact and pseudo-symmetric βγ-crystallin domain. (**B**) All lens βγ-crystallins comprise two domains. In the monomeric γ-crystallins the N- and C-terminal domains pair in a symmetrical manner about an approximate dyad using mainly residues from motifs 2 and 4. (**C**) The detail of the N- and C-terminal domain pairing interface is taken from the artifical domain pairing found in the crystal structure of the human γS C-terminal domain. The heart of the interface is formed mainly by two hydrophobic residues from motifs 2 and 4. (From Bloemendal *et al.* 2004; modified from Purkiss *et al.* 2002.)

231

actin, vimentin, and spectrin, and intermediate filaments (see section on cells and tissues above), there are certain lens-specific intermediate filaments such as beaded filaments. Vimentin is the major intermediate filament in the lens cell, and is present in epithelial and cortical fibre cells but not in nuclear fibre cells. A similar distribution has been found for microtubules in lens cells. Cytokeratins are not found in the adult lens. Some differences occur in relative proportions of cytoskeletal elements. Thus talin, α-actinin and the signalling proteins are at high concentration in lens equatorial epithelium while vinculin is prominent in stable fibre cells with strong cell–cell contacts.

The role of the beaded filaments is unclear. There are two classes: 90 kDa and 48 kDa filaments. Their role is likely to be related to crystallin packing and density distribution, perhaps by offering attachment sites for crystallin molecules. More recently, the cytoskeletal protein (CP49) and the novel protein filensin have been identified as 48 kDa and 90 kDa proteins, which together form the beaded filament. CP49 is also known as phakinin. Both proteins coassemble with α crystallin but not with vimentin.

Lenses with targeted deletions of phakinin and filensin are opaque even though lens fibre morphology is normal, indicating that these two proteins, which co-assemble to form beaded filaments, are essential for lens transparency through lens fibre cytoskeletal organization.

Membrane proteins

Membrane proteins are present in detergent-soluble extracts such as sodium dodecyl sulphate (SDS). The lens fibre cell-specific junctional complex protein, MIP26, has been sequenced and its six-turn membrane-spanning arrangement has been suggested (Fig. 4.35).

The MIP26 gene is located on the cen-q14 region of the long arm of chromosome 12. MIP26 is involved in intercellular communication, probably as an ion channel. Indeed, MIP26 is probably responsible in a large part for the lens acting as an ionic and electric syncytium. MIP26 has now been identified as one of the aquaporin genes (AqPO)$_1$. Aquaporins are a recently described family of water transporter proteins that act as osmoreceptors. At least 100 of these genes have been described, 11 of which are present in mammalian systems and five involved in fluid transport through various ocular tissues in and out of the eye (Fig. 4.36). AqPO (MIP26) transports water out of the lens and maintains transparency.

Mutations in this gene cause cataracts in mice. MIP26 is absent from lens epithelial cells and its relationship to gap junction proteins in other cells is unclear. However, AqP1 is present in lens epithelium.

Other membrane proteins include numerous enzymes such as ATPases, and cytoskeletally attached proteins such as calpactin-1 and N-cadherin. Several other high molecular weight proteins also exist in the plasma membrane but their identity and function are unknown.

Extracellular matrix

The only extracellular matrix of any importance in the lens is the capsule. The capsule is constructed as for any epithelial cell basement membrane of type IV collagen and heparan suphate proteoglycan, and acts as a diffusion barrier for the lens. Fibronectin is localized to the anterior capsule while tenascin is present in the posterior capsule. Tenascin is one of a family of matricellular proteins which includes thrombospondin and SPARC (sialo-protein associated with rods and cones, see p. 248), the last being required for lens transparency The $\alpha_5\beta_1$ integrin is present in the anterior lens epithelium while the $\alpha_6\beta_1$ integrin receptor for laminin is present in equatorial and lens fibre cells, both of which are migratory.

Semipermeable membranes and physiology of the lens

As indicated above, the lens behaves like a very large syncytium or single cell, both electrically and chemically. Active pumping mechanisms exist to pump Na^+ ions out of the lens, while chloride and water are transported into the cell (see Box 4.19).

Barriers to transport occur at the capsule and at the plasma membranes of the epithelial and fibre cells. The capsule is permeable to small molecular weight proteins (< 50 000 kDa), including low molecular weight crystallins, but prevents diffusion of large molecules.

At the epithelial barrier, the cells show the typical polarization of other epithelial cells but lack tight junctions at the lateral cell surface. Instead there is an extensive system of gap junctions, which permits rapid intercellular communication, thereby allowing the cells to behave as one.

At the junction between the epithelium and the fibre cell, the main transport mechanism is rapid endocytosis via coated vesicles, while the very extensive system of gap junctions between each lens fibre permits rapid interfibre cell movement of

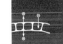

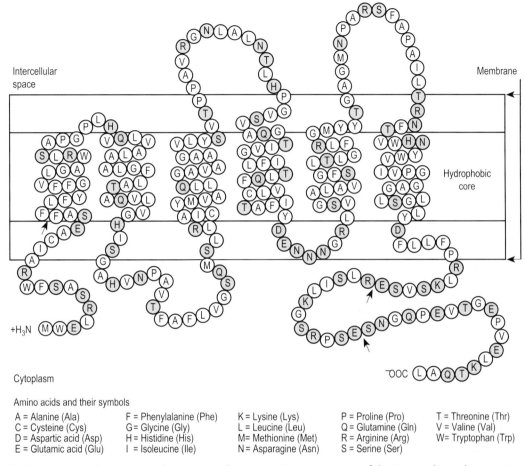

Amino acids and their symbols

A = Alanine (Ala)
C = Cysteine (Cys)
D = Aspartic acid (Asp)

F = Phenylalanine (Phe)
G = Glycine (Gly)
H = Histidine (His)
I = Isoleucine (Ile)

K = Lysine (Lys)
L = Leucine (Leu)
M = Methionine (Met)
N = Asparagine (Asn)

P = Proline (Pro)
Q = Glutamine (Gln)
R = Arginine (Arg)
S = Serine (Ser)

T = Threonine (Thr)
V = Valine (Val)
W = Tryptophan (Trp)

Fig. 4.35 Amino acid sequence and six transmembrane-spanning arrangement of the junctional complex protein MIP26. (Courtesy of J Horwitz.)

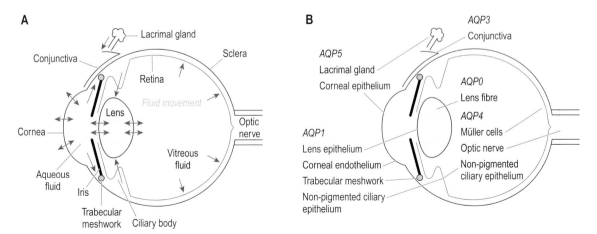

Fig. 4.36 Fluid transport and aquaporin expression in the eye. (**A**) Routes of fluid movement showing secretion by lacrimal gland and ciliary body, absorption by trabecular meshwork and retinal pigment epithelium, and bidirectional movement in cornea and lens. (**B**) Sites of aquaporin (AQP) water channel expression in ocular tissues. (From Verkman 2003, with permission from Elsevier.)

233

Box 4.19 Transport of molecules across the lens surface

The lens behaves like a syncytium in which K^+ is transported into the lens and Na^+ is transported out via Na^+/K^+ ATPase present in the lens epithelium. The lens also contains specific glucose transporters and transporter molecules for ascorbate and water, which ensure adequate metabolism and minimize free radical damage.

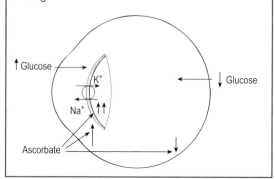

LENS METABOLISM

Carbohydrate

Glucose from the aqueous humour is the main source of energy for lens metabolism. Glucose enters the cell via an insulin-dependent glucose transporter located in the plasma membrane. Both the glycolytic and the pentose phosphate pathways are used, and under conditions of excess glucose the sorbitol pathway is entrained (see Fig. 4.12). About 80% of glucose is consumed by the lens via anaerobic glycolysis. The pentose phosphate pathway uses about 10% of the remaining glucose, providing sugar residues for nucleotide synthesis. Aerobic glycolysis via the citric acid cycle occurs only in the lens epithelium because these are the only lens cells to possess mitochondria. The epithelium also possesses most of the aldose reductase, indicating that any metabolic activity occurring via the sorbitol pathway takes place in this cell. Under normal circumstances less than 5% of glucose is used up in the sorbitol pathway. Indeed, it is unlikely that sorbitol has a significant role in the induction of complications of high ambient glucose (diabetes). Aldose reductase is apparently induced by osmoreceptors and interferes with NADH-binding proteins thus disturbing regulatory free radical scavenger mechanisms (see below).

metabolites. Indeed, 50% of the fibre cell plasma membrane protein consists of MIP26 (AqPO), and the precise nature of the gap junction may be different from that in other cell types, in that MIP26 appears to form channels between the cells.

The Na^+/K^+ ATPase pump in the epithelium actively exchanges Na^+ (pumped out) for K^+ (pumped in). The Na^+ passively diffuses down a concentration gradient in the vitreous, across the posterior lens capsule into the lens body, where it rapidly diffuses to the anterior epithelium and is pumped out into the aqueous. K^+ ions are handled in the reverse direction, eventually diffusing passively across the posterior capsule into the vitreous. While this simple pump–leak model serves to explain ion transport across the lens body, there are several unanswered questions, such as the role of lens fibre Na^+K^+ ATPase which is abundant especially around lens sutures, and the mechanism of Ca^{2+}/Mg^{2+} transport, which also occurs via a specific ATPase. The Ca^{2+}/Mg^{2+} ATPase is most abundant in the lens cortex. In addition, specific transporter proteins for glucose and amino acids exist in the plasma membrane of lens fibre and epithelial cells.

Transport of fluid (H_2O) across the lens has also been shown in an anteroposterior direction at a rate of about 10 µl/h, probably involving AqPO (MIP26) and perhaps acting as a 'rinsing' or washing mechanism to rid the lens of waste products and maintain transparency.

Protein

Synthesis of new protein ceases with lens fibre cell formation, and all changes that occur to lens proteins after this stage are post-translational modifications. Phosphorylation of many proteins occurs, including crystallins, cytoskeletal proteins and MIP26. Several phosphorylation systems exist, including a cAMP-dependent protein kinase A and a phospholipid-dependent protein kinase C. Certain drugs enhance phosphorylation of intermediate filaments, including β-adrenergic compounds.

Numerous enzyme activities have been detected in lens protein extracts but the level of enzyme protein is very low. Some of the taxon-specific crystallins have apparent enzyme activity such as ε crystallin from duck lens (lactic dehydrogenase), ρ crystallin from frog (aldose reductase), and ε crystallin from frog (lung prostaglandin F synthase). These findings are of evolutionary rather than physiological significance but, because several of these enzymes are induced in cells undergoing stress, it has been suggested that stress responses may be the common denominator in these homologies (see above, heat-shock protein and α crystallin). Stress proteins and long-lived lens crystallins may require similar properties to maintain stability and durability in anaerobic conditions. Thus crystallins, especially the α and $\gamma\beta$ series, are among the most conserved proteins known and interestingly are not restricted to the lens (αB has been found in heart, lung, brain and retina). The promotor sequence of the αA gene has been shown to be lens specific and has the capability of driving foreign genes selectively into its sequence. This has been proposed as an explanation for the interchangeability of function for apparently identical proteins from widely divergent sources. Similarly the promotors for χ crystallins are lens specific. During development and growth there is differential expression of the various crystallin genes in a highly regulated manner.

In addition to the evidence for enzymic activity in the crystallin proteins, the lens has several other proteolytic enzymes including endo- and exopeptidase activity and membrane-associated proteases. Interestingly, a parallel has been drawn between apoptosis and lens fibre differentiation because some of the 'death' enzymes such as caspases are activated during this process. The neutral endopeptidases calpain I and II (cysteine Ca^{2+}-dependent enzymes) and their inhibitors, calpactins, have been detected in lens cells. Substrates for these enzymes include cytoskeletal proteins and crystallins, and their role is probably related to protein turnover. Calpain I is present in the epithelium and lens cortex but not in the nucleus. Dysregulation of calpain genes has been suggested as a cause for age-related cataract.

Increased degradation of proteins occurs with age, particularly that of MIP26, which may have significance for coordinated intercellular functions of lens fibres and contribute to cataract. Of interest is the fact that ubiquitin conjugation, a protein degradation system in which the small 8.5-kDa ubiquitin molecule binds to proteins before degradation, is markedly reduced in aged versus young lens nuclei.

Lipid

The plasma membrane of the lens fibre cell has unusually high concentrations of sphingomyelin, cholesterol and saturated fatty acids, imparting rigidity to the cell membrane. This may be important in maintaining intercellular connections.

High levels of phosphatidylinositol are also found in the lens, suggesting significant receptor-mediated second messenger activity in lens cells, e.g. responsiveness to hormones and catecholamines.

Redox systems in the lens microenvironment

The lens is constantly exposed to attack by oxidative agents; indeed there is a high level of hydrogen peroxide in normal aqueous and peroxidase activity is also present in the lens itself. Several enzyme systems are available to minimize or buffer the effects of oxidants, including catalase, superoxide dismutase, glutathione peroxidase and glutathione-S-transferase. The lens contains high levels of glutathione (3.5–5.5 μmol/g wet weight), with the highest concentration in the epithelium, and detoxification via the mercapturic acid pathway is an important pathway in the lens. Glutathione is produced from the interaction between glutamate and cysteine in lens cells. Catalase and low levels of superoxide dismutase have also been identified in lens epithelium, indicating that these systems are also probably important.

Glutathione is also important in protecting thiol groups in proteins, especially cation-transporting membrane proteins in the lens, which additionally accounts for its unusually high concentration in this tissue. More than 95% of glutathione is in the reduced state.

AGEING IN THE LENS AND CATARACT FORMATION

The transmission of light decreases with age, especially for the lower wavelengths (up to a factor of 10), to the point that at low levels of illumination an apparent tritanopia can occur (see Ch. 5). Morphologically, the cells lose cytoskeletal organization and develop vacuolation and electron-dense bodies. An increase in sodium concentration is accompanied by a decline in the membrane potential of the lens, suggesting ion channel dysfunction. Enzymatic activities decline in the lens nucleus but not in the cortex or epithelium. In addition, the appearance of water clefts in the lens as an early sign of cataract suggests decreased function of AqPO (MIP26) and fluid transport.

Ageing of the lens and cataract formation are not synonymous. In age-related nuclear cataract there is extensive oxidation of cystine and methionine residues on lens proteins, while in aged lenses without cataract, oxidation is much less. Glutathione SH (oxidized glutathione) (see Box 4.8 above) is the key.

Post-translational modification of lens proteins continues throughout life. In addition to crosslinking and degradation, which occur in any stable protein system, non-enzymatic glycation is a conspicuous event. In general γ crystallins are synthesized in young lenses, while production of γσ and β crystallins increases with age. In addition, most of the α crystallin is lost from the water-soluble compartment to the water-insoluble compartment, as are some of the β and γ forms.

Non-enzymatic glycation of crystallins occurs at the ε-amino groups of lysine, especially the high molecular weight aggregates of α crystallin. *In vitro*, this reaction produces a yellow fluorescent pigment similar to that seen in the ageing human lens. Interaction between various amino groups and aldehydes released from free radicals, especially lipid, (per)oxidation produces fluorophores and ceroid/lipofuscin. In spite of the colour changes, the amount of protein that is glycated is less than 5% in an aged lens, which is considerably less than for other long-lived proteins such as haemoglobin and collagen. Lens crystallin glycation is more likely to be the result of its interaction with oxidized ascorbic acid than glucose on the basis of intra-lens concentrations, and it is possible that glutathione, by maintaining ascorbic acid in its reduced state, inhibits this process.

MIP26 also undergoes modification with age, losing a 5000-Da peptide to become MIP22 in increasing concentration. Cleavage occurs at both the C- and N-terminal ends of the molecule.

Reduced vision in cataract is caused by increased light scatter by lens proteins

The transmission of light by the lens is reduced when the ordered packing of the lens crystallins is disturbed. This can be induced in many ways, such as increased water accumulation within the lens, formation of high molecular weight lens protein aggregates, and vacuole formation within the lens fibres with age.

Certain metabolic conditions are associated with cataract, the best known being the cataract of diabetes and a similar lens opacity in galactosaemia. In these forms of 'sugar' cataract, accumulation of water in the lens fibres was previously thought to result from the accumulation of non-degradable polyols such as sorbitol and galacticol in the lens fibre cells. However, the role of polyols in water accumulation is less clear and other mechanisms involving MIP26 (see above) are more likely.

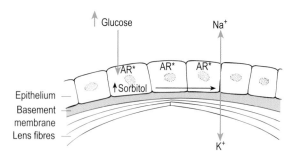

Fig. 4.37 Lens epithelial cell damage and sugar cataract polyol pathway. Polyols in the lens epithelium produce cellular dysfunction and altered ion transport. AR*, aldose reductase induction by high glucose concentration.

High glucose/galactose concentrations in the aqueous lead to increased intracellular accumulation of glucose, which saturates the normal anaerobic glycosis pathways. Accordingly, the polyol pathway is unregulated via aldose reductase, and polyols accumulate in the cells, thereby increasing the osmotic drag of water into the cell (Fig. 4.37). Activation of the osmoreceptor AqPO (MIP26) is then induced.

This causes dysregulation of cellular metabolism, with reduction in the levels of cellular ATP and glutathione, and secondary damage to the cell. In addition, the increased water content of the cell causes phase separation between protein-rich and protein-poor regions of the cells and increased light scatter (cataract).

Osmotic effects may not be the main mechanism of damage in aldose reductase-associated diabetic cataracts because sorbitol can be metabolized to other compounds such as fructose. However, this may still alter the function of the cell by depleting cells of NADP/NADPH and interfering with myoinositol production. Alternatively, the increased levels of fructose, glucose and glucose-6-phosphate could induce non-enzymatic glycation. It has also been suggested that aldose reductase inhibitors have a direct effect on glycated Na^+/K^+ ATPase, leading to restoration of function, and therefore that they are not entirely specific for aldose reductase.

As individual cells loosen their interdigitations with neighbouring cells, water clefts and vacuoles appear within the lens substance. As cells die, there is progressive increase in opacification, which in the lens cortex is seen as 'spoke-like' opacity and in the nucleus is characterized by the accumulation of insoluble protein aggregates and chromophores, causing the nucleus to change colour from yellow to red to black.

Cataract formation is caused by any insult to the lens

Since the lens is designed for the transmission of light, it responds to any insult that disturbs normal development or metabolism by opacification, even if this is only for a temporary period. Thus, certain congenital cataracts appear to affect only the fetal nucleus; radiation cataract may be limited if only a discrete area of the lens bow region is affected; sunflower cataract of trauma may be the result of shearing forces momentarily separating lens fibre cells which then restore their interconnections; and certain forms of cataract such as the 'feather' cataract after vitrectomy are thought to be the result of large volumes of fluid transfused through the vitreous cavity at too low a temperature or an incorrect electrolyte composition. Cold cataract can be induced in young animals and is caused by the reversible precipitation of γ crystallins by phase separation in the fetal nucleus.

Certain forms of cataract have been shown to be the result of mutations (the Philly cataract in mice has deletions in its βB crystallin; a similar mutation has also been seen in guinea-pigs; mutations in MIP26 produce cataracts in mice). Transgenic mice have been developed to study lens physiology using the lens-specific α and γ crystallins.

Age-related cataract formation is multifactorial

A great wealth of studies during the past 20 years has shown many biochemical changes associated with age-related cataract. In essence, these are an increase in the insoluble components of the lens, an increase in chromophores, increased protein crosslinking and aggregation, and oxidation of amino acid groups. There is a concomitant decrease in antioxidant enzyme systems and increased proteolytic activity. The level of glutathione is also reduced. Normal lenses contain a trypsin inhibitory activity, which may regulate age-related proteolytic activity.

The major protein change in cataractous lens is the loss of αA crystallin and the selective loss of γS crystallin. In addition there are numerous degradation peptides detectable in the water-soluble component.

The possibility that UV light might cause or hasten some of the effects of age has been suggested by the observation that 'age' changes appear to be more marked in the region of the visual axis than in the equatorial region of the lens. Current views are that oxidative events are the most likely mechanism of cataract formation. Near-UV light is absorbed by tryptophan, which in sunlight is converted to N-formyl-kynurenine, a fluorescent chromophore similar to 3-hydroxy-kynurenine, a second UV absorbent molecule in the lens. Both these compounds can act as photosensitizers and lead to the production of the free radical, singlet oxygen (see Box 4.20). Free radicals downregulate the function of critical lens enzymes such as Na^+/K^+ ATPase and lead to lens swelling and opacification, at least in the rat model. Other free radicals generated by near-UV light such as hydrogen peroxide have been implicated in the dysfunction of hexokinase, an enzyme central to glucose utilization in the lens.

Oxygen increases the rate of photo-oxidation, and vitamin E, ascorbic acid and glutathione reduce the effects of light damage.

The role of UV light in human cataract is unclear, although some interesting epidemiological evidence has emerged from a study of Chesapeake Bay watermen, which showed the importance of exposure to UV-B in cortical but not in nuclear cataract formation. A similar study found an association between UV-B and posterior subcapsular cataract. Interestingly, aged human lenses appear to absorb more UV-A and even visible light than young lenses.

Certain trace metals and compounds are associated with cataract. Experimental depletion or excess of selenite leads to cataracts by a mechanism that appears to be closely interwoven with Ca^{2+} homeostasis. In contrast, cyanate induces carbamylation of lens proteins and cataract, a process that can be prevented experimentally with aspirin. Interestingly, aspirin usage may also delay the onset of cataracts in humans. Inhibition of cholesterol synthesis also leads to cataract in experimental animals.

In summary, although many factors may contribute to cataract formation, probably the most important is glutathione consumption and unrestricted oxidation of intrinsic lens protein.

Mechanism of age-related cataract formation: a failure of chaperone function

As shown above, there are several processes which can lead to damaged lens proteins. Oxidation, carbamylation, deamidation and other perturbations of βγ crystallins lead to their progressive inability to

Box 4.20   Free radical damage and the lens

Free radical damage in the lens may occur through oxidative metabolism but is considered mostly to be the result of UV damage by activation of endogenous photosensitizers.

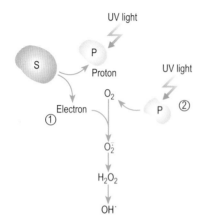

Photosensitizers act by one of two mechanisms: (a) triplet sensitizer absorbs a proton from a substrate, leading to the production of free radicals (SO_2 and H_2O_2); (b) sensitizer reacts with O_2, leading to singlet O_2. Typical photosensitizers include riboflavin, tryptophan and kynurenine (all present in the lens).

sustain normal intermolecular interactions. As they denature and precipitate the α crystallins bind the unfolded proteins, but unlike true chaperones they do not have the ability to refold the βγ crystallins. As a result, the chaperone capacity of the α crystallins is consumed and the complexes precipitate within the fibre cells, forming the insoluble protein fraction that increases with age.

THE VITREOUS

THE VITREOUS BODY IS A TRUE CONNECTIVE TISSUE CONTAINING COLLAGEN, GAGS, AND CELLS

The vitreous is 98% water, 1.0% macromolecules, and the rest solutes and low molecular weight materials.

The matrix

The vitreous transmits light by the same mechanism as the cornea, i.e. its collagen fibrils (10–20 nm) are thinner than half the wavelength of light, and the interfibrillar space is filled with GAGs (hyal-

uronic acid) at intervals that reduce the effects of diffraction in the system. Collagen imparts the gel structure to the vitreous body, is predominantly type II, similar but not identical to cartilage type II collagen (vitreous collagen has more galactosylglucose side chains and a higher content of alanine), and is arranged in a lattice structure in which the fibrils are suspended in a viscous hyaluronic acid solution. This structure is lost with age and in disease by a process known as syneresis in which the hyaluronic acid molecules are degraded to smaller moieties and the collagen fibrils coagmentate to form larger fibrils, becoming visible as 'floaters'. Some type VI and type IX collagens are also present and presumably play structural roles in gel formation. In addition, a hybrid molecule composed of type V/XI α chains has been detected in vitreous in trace amounts and has also been implicated in vitreous fibril formation as for cornea. Recently, a new member of the leucine-rich repeat extracellular matrix protein family, termed opticin, has been identified in vitreous and also in ligament, skin and retina. Its function remains to be elucidated (Reardon *et al.* 2000).

The normal vitreous in the young adult has a distinct architecture (see Ch. 1, p. 39). The cortex has a higher concentration of collagen and hyaluronic acid than the central vitreous, and in addition the cortex contains other GAGs such as chondroitin sulphate, which may be important in vitreo/retinal apposition.

In the central vitreous gel, hyaluronic acid is essentially the sole GAG. Hyaluronic acid occurs as stiff, opencoil disaccharide chains, which in solution become entangled at concentrations above 300 μg/ml and thus add support to the gel matrix. Hyaluronic acid concentrations in human vitreous vary between 100 and 400 μg/ml and the molecule binds to type IX collagen, which acts as a proteoglycan to bind the hyaluronic acid to the collagen fibrils. Type IX collagen is a small non-fibrillar type of collagen that contains several non-collagenous domains; these act as the proteoglycan bridges. In addition, the chondroitin sulphate proteoglycan is present in vitreous at a concentration of approximately 1 : 1 with type IX collagen. Traces of chondroitin sulphate also comprise part of the proteoglycan versican in the vitreous with a molecular weight of 2×10^4 to 4×10^4. Hyaluronic acid is highly polydisperse (variable molecular sizes).

Depolymerization of the hyaluronic acid does not of itself destroy the vitreous gel structure.

Vitreous cells

The vitreous contains a single monolayer of cells (hyalocytes), which line the adult vitreous cortex and are responsible for production of hyaluronic acid in the gel. However, there is no regeneration of collagen in the vitreous and thus there is no reconstitution of the gel after syneresis.

Hyalocytes are of two types: fibrocyte-like and macrophage-like. The role of hyalocytes in health and disease remains obscure.

PHYSICOCHEMICAL PROPERTIES OF THE VITREOUS GEL

The viscoelasticity of the vitreous protects the retina during eye movement and deformations of the globe

The vitreous gel is non-compressible but highly viscoelastic. Thus it responds to deformations of the globe by altering its shape to comply with external forces, but permits rapid restoration of global architecture. In this respect it behaves as a shock absorber, similar to synovial fluid, which also has a very high content of hyaluronic acid. These properties of the vitreous are the result of its matrix structure, particularly its content of high molecular weight hyaluronic acid. This molecule has a very large hydrodynamic volume and at the concentrations present in the human vitreous completely fills the interfibrillar spaces. With age, the vitreous gel detaches from its loose adhesion to the retinal surface except at the vitreous base, where it is firmly adherent and continues to provide support.

Vitreous retards bulk flow of fluid and diffusion of small molecules

The flow of fluid through solutions of GAGs is variably retarded, depending on the nature and molecular weight of the GAG, and is greatest with hyaluronic acid. Flow of aqueous from the posterior chamber towards the retina is therefore slower in young eyes with formed vitreous gel than in older eyes where the vitreous gel has undergone liquefaction. In addition, diffusion of small molecules such as glucose is retarded by the hyaluronic acid in the vitreous. Electrolytes are more affected in their transvitreal transport by electrostatic interactions with hyaluronic acid, which is a polymeric polyelectrolyte (see p. 191).

Transport of fluid and electrolytes in a posterior direction across the retina is an important mechanism in the process of retinal adhesion to the RPE (see next section).

THE RETINA

THE NEURAL RETINA IS HIGHLY ORGANIZED IN LAYERS

The retina has two components, the neural retina and the RPE (see Ch. 1 and Fig. 4.38).

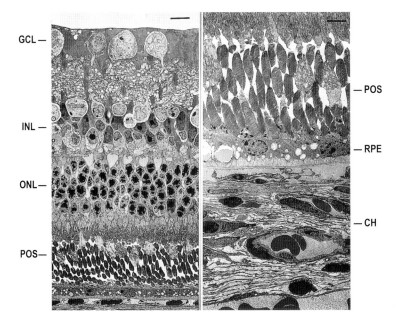

Fig. 4.38 Architecture of the retina: GCL, ganglion cell layer; INL, inner nuclear layer; ONL, outer nuclear layer; POS, photoreceptor outer segments; RPE, retinal pigment epithelium; CH, choroid.

239

Metabolic function in the retina

The retina's metabolism correlates with its blood supply: the outer retina, comprising the photoreceptors and the RPE, has a high metabolic activity and receives most of its blood supply from the choroid while the metabolism of the inner retina is supplied by the retinal circulation and is much less demanding on high energy supplies.

Glucose metabolism in the retina

Despite having the highest rate of aerobic glucose consumption of any tissue, a large proportion of the glucose utilized is converted to lactate. Lactic acid production, oxygen utilization and glucose consumption are also highest in the presence of CO_2/bicarbonate buffering systems, suggesting a role for carbonic anhydrases in the retina. Most of the glucose utilization in the retina is taken by the photoreceptors (> 80%).

The retina can also metabolize other substrates for (ATP) energy stores such as glutamate, glutamic acid, malate and succinate. Retinal glucose is used to produce glutathione via the pentose phosphate pathway, which can be upregulated under conditions of oxidative stress. However, NADPH for glutathione stores is also produced by other non-pentose-dependent systems involving malate and isocitrate. Glucose, glutathione and oxygen are all required for generation of electrical activity, including the ATPase-dependent 'dark currents' (see Ch. 5) in the retina.

The retina is an insulin-independent tissue, i.e. glucose enters retinal cells by transport mechanisms that are regulated directly by the extracellular concentration of glucose rather than indirectly by insulin. Glucose transport occurs by facilitated diffusion via GLUT 1 and GLUT 3 transporter proteins, similar to glucose transport in the brain. GLUT 1 and GLUT 3 are present in cells of the blood–retinal barrier, where much of the transport occurs. Recent studies have shown that retinal cells (photoreceptors) can respond to insulin via a retina-specific insulin receptor, which is similar to brain insulin receptor in that it exists in a 'tonic' state of activity and does not change in conditions of fasting or excess glucose.

Most of the glucose handling described above is dealt with by retinal neurones. However, Müller cells are also likely to be involved in glucose metabolism in the retina, at least as energy stores, because they contain high levels of glycogen, especially in species that lack a retinal blood supply. In addition,

lactate released by Müller cells can be metabolized by photoreceptors. Photoreceptors in turn release glutamate, which is taken up and metabolized by Müller cells.

Protein metabolism in the retina

Many of the neurotransmitters required for normal retinal cell function occur as free amino acids in the retina (see p. 258 and Fig. 4.51). Most of them are generated during glucose metabolism in the citric acid cycle; in addition taurine, which is not a neurotransmitter but appears to be essential for, and is avidly taken up by, photoreceptor cells, is the most abundant amino acid in the retina. Interestingly, taurine may have a protective role for the retina in diabetes. Glutamate is neurotoxic and is therefore converted by the retina to glutamine by glutamine transferase (synthase) localized to the Müller cells (see above). Transport of amino acids is now known to require specific amino acid transporters, for which there are several 'systems' (systems y, b, B, b° and more). Some are linked to Na^+ transport while others are independent of Na^+ intake. Rapid uptake of amino acids is essential not only for the supply of neurotransmitters but also for arginine uptake, which is necessary for the synthesis of nitric oxide, the major regulator of endothelial cell function.

Protein synthesis, as studied by methods such as leucine incorporation, is most active in the photoreceptors during such processes as photoreceptor renewal (see Box 4.21).

In addition to many retina-specific proteins (see below), several proteins common to many tissues are present. For instance, laminin is present in vessel structures, fibronectin in the interphotoreceptor space, and matrix proteoglycans are widely distributed throughout the retina. Tenascin-C is present in the extracellular matrix and is thought to play a role in preventing myelination of retinal neurones. However, tenascin-C knockout mice show no myelination of their retina. Several growth factors are present in the retina, such as insulin-like growth factor 1 (IGF-1) and acidic and basic fibroblast growth factor (bFGF). Basic FGF is not only present in basement membranes of vessels but is also distributed in such regions as the photoreceptor layer, where it may play a trophic role in outer segment renewal.

The retina contains a high content of lipid (20%)

The predominant lipids in the retina are the phospholipids, phosphatidylcholine and phosphotidyl-

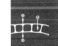

Box 4.21 Photoreceptor renewal

Photoreceptor renewal occurs by synthesis of new protein-rich membrane at the outer limiting membrane, with shedding and phagocytosis of the outer segment tips by the RPE. Disks are formed by the evagination of the plasma membrane ✳ at the junction between the inner and outer segments, while rhodopsin and other proteins synthesized in the ER and Golgi apparatus are transported in vesicles for fusion to the newly formed plasma membrane ✳. Photoreceptor renewal is similar in rods and cones; phagocytosis of the receptor tips occurs in a diurnal manner. The mechanism of phagocytosis is unclear but involves a membrane glycoprotein CD36, which is involved in the uptake of apoptotic neutrophils and oxidized low-density lipoprotein by haematopoietic cells such as macrophages. In addition, rod outer segment (ROS) phagocytosis is associated with induction of cyclo-oxygenase-2 (COX-2), an enzyme involved in prostaglandin synthesis.

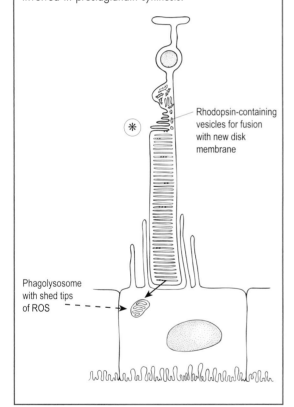

Rhodopsin-containing vesicles for fusion with new disk membrane

Phagolysosome with shed tips of ROS

membranes of photoreceptors are particularly rich in phosphatidylethanolamine while the plasma membrane has higher levels of cholesterol. This is relevant to the activity of rhodopsin because it is inhibited in the presence of the sterol. Thus the older disk membranes at the tip of the photoreceptor (see Box 4.21) have lower levels of cholesterol than the fresh, newly formed disks, allowing easier activation of rhodopsin at the photoreceptor tip.

Lipid metabolism is varied and complex in the retina; thus, in addition to synthetic activities in microsomes, exchange of bases between different lipid species occurs, while frequent acylation–deacylation reactions also occur. Lipids are continually undergoing degradation via phospholipases and modifications including decarboxylation and methylation by the appropriate enzymes.

BLOOD FLOW IN THE RETINA

Blood flow in the retina is autoregulated. To some, this means that the retinal vessel caliber varies with the cardiac output to ensure that blood flow is kept constant; alternatively it has been interpreted as meaning that the blood flow is varied according to the nutritional demands of the tissue. In the adult, the blood flow in the retina is maintained constant over a range of perfusion pressures from 45 to 145 mmHg.

Retinal blood flow comprises about 5% of the total flow to the eye, the majority passing through the choroid.

The blood–retinal barrier regulates the passage of molecules into the retina

The blood–retinal barrier is maintained by tight junctions that exist between the endothelial cells of the retinal vessels and similar tight junctions in the RPE (see pp. 195–201). Thus, the retinal vessels are impermeable to the passage of molecules greater than 20 000–30 000 Da, and small molecules such as glucose amino acids and ascorbate are transported by facilitated diffusion (GLUT 3 in the case of glucose).

Although the retina is considered an insulin-independent tissue, the endothelial cells and pericytes possess high-affinity receptors for insulin, IGF-1 and IGF-2. The role of these receptors in the regulation of glucose transport in the retina is not clear because their effect is delayed for some hours, suggesting that they stimulate protein synthesis and the production of new transporters rather than recruit

ethanolamine (in total around 80%). There is also a high content of polyunsaturated fatty acids in the retina, especially in the outer segments, some containing more than six double bonds (known as 'supraenes'). This renders the retina particularly susceptible to oxidative damage (see p. 195). Disk

existing transporters, as occurs in insulin-dependent tissues such as muscle.

Retinal blood flow may be partly under autonomic control

Retinal vessels possess all four types of high-affinity adrenergic receptors, although in low numbers. In addition there is indirect evidence that, despite well-recognized mechanisms of autoregulation, some degree of autonomic control exists in humans. How this might occur in the absence of nerve fibres is unclear. In addition, the retinal vascular bed may be one of the few systems to lack perivascular mast cells.

Retinal blood flow is responsive to hyperoxia (vasoconstriction) and hypercapnia (vasodilatation), the latter via the prostaglandins PGD_2 and PGE_2. Other mediators of changes in vessel diameter include the eicosanoid, PGI_2, endothelin and nitric oxide. PGI_2 and endothelin have been detected in retinal vessels and presumably are released under appropriate conditions. Nitric oxide is released via endothelial nitric oxide synthase (see Ch. 7, Box 7.6, p. 360) and provides basal levels of vascular dilatation. Retinal illumination induces release of nitric oxide but autoregulation in retinal vessels is not significantly affected by nitric oxide. Contractile activity in the retinal vessels is attributed to the pericytes, whose role therefore may be to regulate blood flow. Their early loss in diabetes may account for the increase in blood flow that occurs in the retina in diabetes, and may contribute to the development of retinopathy.

PHOTORECEPTORS

Photoreceptors are specialized for reception of visual stimuli and have unique characteristics (see Ch. 1, p. 43).

Metabolism and turnover

Photoreceptors are some of the most highly metabolic cells in the body, utilizing glucose both aerobically and anaerobically. Photoreceptor outer segments lie in 'apposition' to the RPE in the interphotoreceptor matrix between the apical microvilli of the RPE cell. Extensive protein and lipid synthesis ensures a continuous turnover of new outer segment membrane at the junction with the inner segment; the tips of the outer segment containing the 'oldest' disks are phagocytosed as small packets of about 200 disks by the RPE cell, a process that occurs in a diurnal manner just after light onset (Fig. 4.39).

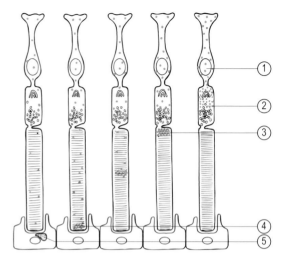

Fig. 4.39 Photoreceptor renewal and points where damage may occur: during (1) transcription; (2) post-translational modification; (3) incorporation into disk membrane; (4) disk shedding; (5) phagocytosis by RPE.

Complete renewal of the rod outer segment takes about 9–10 days. In contrast, although cone outer segments are phagocytosed in a similar manner, the process appears to be more random; cone membranes and their integral proteins are much more stable and long lasting.

Insertion of rhodopsin into the disk plasma membrane follows a well-defined pathway from the inner segment RER to the outer segment plasma membrane infolding (see Box 4.22). Glycosylation of rhodopsin takes place through combined co-translational and post-translational events in a classic lipid-carrier mechanism using dol-p-p-GlcNAc (Fig. 4.40), which can be inhibited by tunicamycin. Acylation of rhodopsin also occurs in the membrane via palmitic acid.

Lipids in photoreceptors are replaced both by membrane turnover and by molecular replacement. The abundant stores of phosphatidylcholine are synthesized from large intracellular pools of free choline and phosphorylation by ATP; the 'activated' choline then reacts with 1,2-diacylglycerol to form phosphatidylcholine. Similar mechanisms operate for the synthesis of phosphatidylserine and phosphatidylethanolamine; all three phospholipids are synthesized in the RER but are transported to the newly forming outer segment membrane by different mechanisms. The role of the high concentrations of docosahexanate phospholipids in photoreceptors has recently been identified as enhancing the

Box 4.22 Rhodopsin synthesis

Insertion of rhodopsin into the outer segment plasma membrane is facilitated by the lack of a signal peptide, which permits integration of opsin into the lipid bilayer by co-translational coupling of glycosylation and asymmetric insertion via specific insertion sequences in the protein.

function of many of the proteins involved in the visual transduction cascade such as GDP-bound transducin (see below).

Several chemical reactions are associated with disk shedding, although the specific stimulus and its site of origin (i.e. the photoreceptor or the RPE cell) are not known. Experimental studies suggest that local factors within each eye regulate the circadian light–dark rhythm of shedding, possibly under the control of melatonin- and/or 5-methoxytryptophol-synthesizing enzymes (Fig. 4.41). Messenger RNA and protein for melatonin receptor (Mel 1a) has been found in retinal neurone and RPE cells. The mammalian retina also appears to possess an autonomous melatonin-responsive circadian oscillator independent of central (suprachiasmatic nucleus) control. In addition, rhodopsin and cone opsin synthesis are in phase with this rhythmic oscillation. However, several other compounds have an effect on disk shedding, such as excitatory amino acids, glutamine and aspartate, while certain divalent ions are also essential (Ca^{2+}, Mn^{2+}). Recent studies in mice lacking the D4 dopamine receptor have shown that this membrane protein may regulate several of the controlling mediators of disk shedding, such as a light-sensitive pool of cAMP.

Phosphoinositide metabolism is considerably greater than phosphatidylcholine or phosphatidylethanolamine metabolism in the photoreceptor but

Table 4.12 Photoreceptor proteins

Integral membrane proteins	Peripheral/cytosolic proteins
Rhodopsin	Arrestin (48-kDa protein, S antigen)
cGMP channel	Transducin
Na^+/Ca^{2+}-K^+ exchanger	Phosphodiesterase
Glucose transporter	Phosducin
Guanylate cyclase	Rhodopsin kinase
Peripherin/rds	Guanylate cyclase
Rom-1	
ABCR/rim protein	
Retinal dehydrogenase	

its precise role in phototransduction is unclear (see p. 257). Cytidine triphosphate is also a product of light transduction and is linked to phosphatidylinositol formation.

Photoreceptor cell-specific proteins

The highly differentiated visual cell contains many unique proteins, including integral membrane proteins, membrane-associated proteins and cytosolic proteins (Table 4.12). The protein composition of the disk membrane is predominantly rhodopsin

243

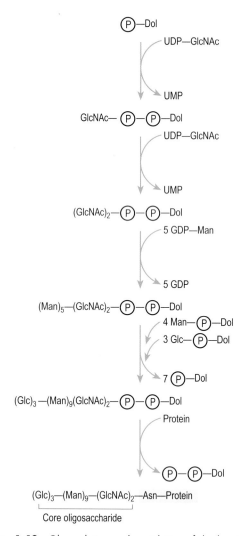

Fig. 4.40 Glycosylation and acetylation of rhodopsin.

(90%), whereas the plasma membrane has a wider range of cell-specific proteins and less rhodopsin (50%).

Rhodopsin is the visual receptor protein; proteins such as peripherin and the spectrin-like protein Rom-1 have structural functions in the maintenance of the photoreceptor shape, similar to those of spectrin/ankyrin-like proteins in red cells. The photoreceptor 'rim' proteins (located in the peripheral rim of the photoreceptor) may have a similar role but are also suggested to have a transporter role. The Na^+/Ca^{2+} exchanger facilitates ionic transport during phototransduction and maintains Ca^{2+} homeostasis. In addition, the spectrin-like protein Rom-1 appears to be linked to a second ion-channel protein of 67 kDa.

In contrast to the integral membrane proteins, many of the peripheral membrane and cytosolic proteins are not exclusive to the photoreceptor and are intimately involved in the light amplification cascade itself (see below). Transducin is a member of the family of G proteins and is composed of three chains (α, β, γ), which dissociate during the light response.

Certain other proteins are located in the photoreceptors as well as in other areas of the retina; these include the IGF-1 receptor, IGF-1 binding protein, and FGF, both of which have been implicated in the induction of proliferative diabetic retinopathy (see Ch. 9). In addition, there is a glucose transporter (GLUT 1) for control of intracellular glucose levels.

Rhodopsin is not the only light-sensitive receptor protein in the retina

Because it was recognized that certain light-sensitive processes such as those entrained in a circadian fashion were likely to reside at a different site from visual photoreception, a search for other photoreceptors was initiated. Early studies indicated that the likely site was intraocular and probably retinal and recently a photopigment, melanopsin, was detected in specialized retinal ganglion cells with large receptive fields (see Ch. 5, p. 284). Further possible photopigments, termed cryptophores, have also been described in plants and related compounds in mammals, but this information is more controversial.

Photoreceptors are easily damaged

The extensive metabolism and rapid turnover of photoreceptor outer segments render them highly susceptible to damage. Damage may occur at any level from synthesis of new membrane to phagocytosis of the outer segment tips (see Fig. 4.39).

Photoreceptors also degenerate when they are separated from the RPE, as in retinal detachment, or when there is a subretinal collection of fluid; photoreceptors are lost in inflammatory and metabolic retinal diseases and are probably highly susceptible to free radical damage. Specific photoreceptor loss occurs in retinitis pigmentosa, a term used for a collection of diseases, for many of which mutations in retinal specific proteins have been described (see Ch. 3, p. 162 and Fig. 4.49).

Damage to the retina also occurs as part of normal physiology via both light- and oxygen-induced

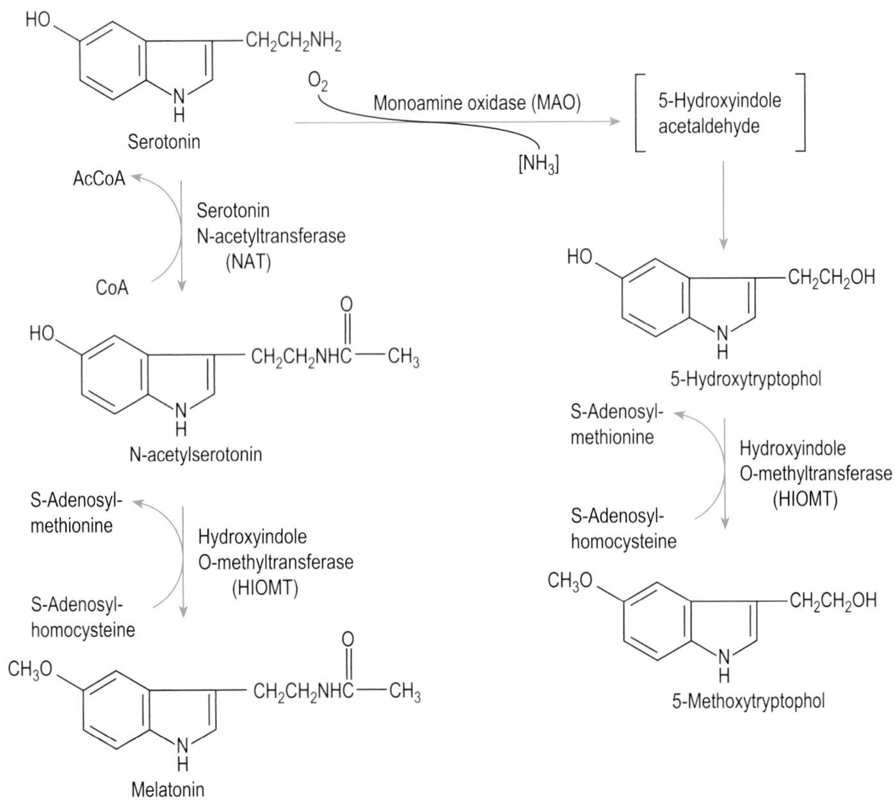

Fig. 4.41 Regulation of disk shedding. Disk shedding may be under the control of melatonin-synthesizing enzymes such as serotonin *N*-acetyltransferase (NAT), which is present in the pineal gland and retina.

mechanisms. Inherited retinal degeneration has also been linked to mutations in the genes for proteins involved in the Wnt signalling pathway. The *Wnt/Drosophila wingless* family of genes express highly conserved secreted glycoproteins which spread across tissues to reach their targets where they interact with the products of two sets of genes (*Frizzled* and genes for low-density lipoprotein-related proteins, LRPs). In *Drosophila*, a species of insect (the fruit fly) that is frequently used to study molecular genetics, Wnt signalling has been shown to be central to normal photoreceptor development as well as to the central nervous system development probably through regulation of the expression of pro-survival factors, such as Dickkopf (*Dkk3*), in cells. In fact this mechanism highlights the fact that photoreceptor damage in retinal degenerations and other conditions is mediated via apoptosis, which may occur by both caspase-dependent and caspase-independent mechanisms. Light-induced retinal damage varies with the intensity, wavelength, duration, cyclical nature and previous antioxidant status.

For instance, it has been shown that cyclical light is less injurious to the retina than constant illumination of equivalent power, an effect associated with higher levels of ascorbic acid, vitamin E and glutathione, and lower levels of 22:6(*n*-3) fatty acids in the tissue. Interestingly, higher levels of cholesterol protect photoreceptor membrane proteins, such as rhodopsin, but reduce their sensitivity to light stimulation. Recent studies on light-damage in rodents have shown that the apoptotic death signal is determined by the rate of rhodopsin regeneration, which itself depends on the level of RPE65, an intrinsic retinal pigment epithelium protein with a critical amino acid residue at position 450. The death signal involves induction of the pro-apoptotic transcription factor AP-1 such that inhibition of regeneration of rhodopsin or suppression of AP-1 can prevent light-induced damage to photoreceptors (Fig. 4.42).

Glutathione peroxidase occurs in two forms related to selenium. The selenium-dependent enzyme does not appear to be functional in the retina. However,

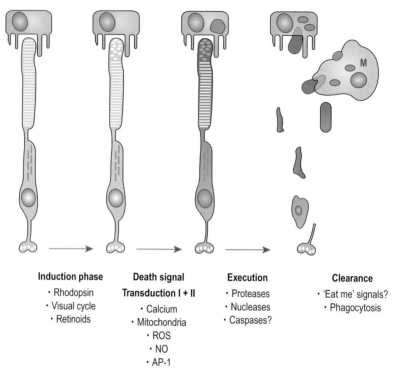

Induction phase	Death signal	Execution	Clearance
· Rhodopsin	Transduction I + II	· Proteases	· 'Eat me' signals?
· Visual cycle	· Calcium	· Nucleases	· Phagocytosis
· Retinoids	· Mitochondria	· Caspases?	
	· ROS		
	· NO		
	· AP-1		

Fig. 4.42 Schematic drawing of major components which contribute to light-induced photoreceptor apoptosis. From Wenzel *et al.* (2005). Induction phase: rhodopsin is essential in this process. Death signal transduction: requires Ca^{2+} and transcription factor AP-1. Execution: mechanism not clear, may require caspases. Clearance: signals inducing phagocytosis by RPE and, in acute light damage, macrophages, are not known. (From Wenzel *et al.* 2005, with permission from Elsevier.)

extensive antioxidant enzyme systems are present in the retina and, under conditions of stress such as light injury, levels of glutathione peroxidase and glutathione-*S*-transferase are markedly raised. Superoxide dismutase (the Cu^{2+}/Zn^{2+} form) is also present in significant amounts in several layers of the retina, but levels of catalase are low.

In addition to the classic mechanisms of free radical damage in the retina, Fe^{2+} ions can interact with hydrogen peroxide to produce high levels of hydroxyl radicals (see Box 4.8, p. 198) and cause retinal injury. Local release of iron may occur in diseases involving retinal haemorrhage and when intraocular foreign bodies are present.

Vitamin E is of major importance in reducing photoreceptor damage, mainly by its role in inhibiting lipid peroxidation at different stages in the free radical damage (see Box 4.23).

The macular region of the retina is particularly susceptible to light damage. Interestingly, this region contains additional yellow pigments lutein and zea-

xanthin and a further pigment meso-zeaxanthin, which may be transported to this region from the blood and whose function is thought to be related to reducing glare from short wavelength blue light. These pigments (carotenoids) also have an antioxidant effect, particularly at low levels of oxygenation. They are referred to as xanthophyll macular pigments and can be measured non-invasively in the retina using Raman spectroscopy. Sustained levels of these pigments are considered protective against macular degeneration.

Finally, melanin in the RPE layer is a very effective free radical scavenger, particularly in the reduced form where it may act as a trap for stray light-induced free radicals emanating from the photoreceptors, but the role of melanin is more likely to be related to protection of the RPE cells themselves because these are terminally differentiated cells. Melanin granules in RPE cells appear to be connected to the lysosomal enzyme system in RPE cells and loss of melanin is associated with age-related macular degeneration.

Box 4.23 Vitamin E as a free radical scavenger

Vitamin E limits free radical damage at several stages in lipid peroxidation.

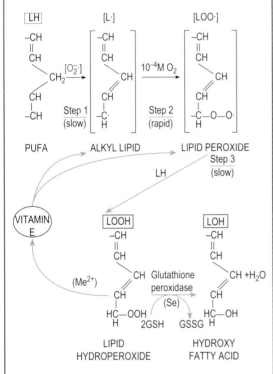

Regeneration of vitamin E under light stress requires ascorbic acid. In experimental vitamin E deficiency there is a marked accumulation of lipofuscin in the RPE, which may be relevant to a similar accumulation of lipofuscin in age-related macular degeneration. PUFA, polyunsaturated fatty acid.

rods. IRBP appears to be essential for photoreceptor survival but is not required for the visual cycle. In addition, there are several cell surface proteins that form part of the glycocalyx of the cell but may also play a part in maintaining retinal apposition. These include fibronectin, intercellular adhesion molecule 1 (ICAM-1) (see Ch. 7) and the CD44 antigen, also known as the hyaluronate receptor. There is also a second hyaluronan binding protein SPARC (sialoprotein associated with rods and cones), which may also be important in providing a scaffold to the matrix.

The interphotoreceptor matrix of the cone is compartmentally separated from that of the rod by an insoluble matrix sheath (Fig. 4.43) containing its own specific proteoglycans, which presumably play a role in the regulation of their different forms of visual excitation. Chondroitin-6-sulphate appears to be the major proteoglycan–GAG in the cone matrix sheath, while a similar but less well-defined sheath around rod outer segments appears to be composed of sialyl conjugates. It has been suggested that these proteoglycan sheaths are important in retinal–RPE adhesion, but the role of specific adhesion molecules such as CD44 and ICAM-1 has yet to be explored.

The interphotoreceptor matrix contains other GAGs including non-sulphated chondroitin and hyaluronic acid (about 14% of total). These are present as proteoglycans and are probably mostly synthesized by the RPE cell.

The interphotoreceptor matrix also contains a number of lysosomal enzyme activities, including matrix metalloproteinases and TIMPs (see p. 359) mostly associated with the RPE cell surface bound to mannose-6-phosphate receptors.

The interphotoreceptor matrix is the biological glue for retinal adhesion

The interphotoreceptor matrix extends from the outer limiting membrane to the surface of the RPE cell. It is an extremely narrow space, almost a potential space, but contains some unique and physiologically important molecules. These include interphotoreceptor retinol binding protein (IRBP; accounts for at least 70% of the interphotoreceptor matrix protein), which transports retinoids between the RPE cell and the photoreceptor, and several species of proteoglycan, which provide a coating for the photoreceptor outer segment. Interestingly, the 6-sulphated (DeltaDi6S) chondroitin species appears to be more prominent around cones than around

THE RETINAL PIGMENT EPITHELIUM

The RPE is a pluripotent cell

The RPE is a multifunctional pluripotent cell, which befits its embryological origins. It expresses many of the proteins considered characteristic of other cell types. Thus it possesses several cytokeratins characteristic of epithelial cells, yet also contains vimentin, which is a mesenchymal cell protein. One group of microfilaments, namely actin, myosin, α actinin and vimentin, is organized as a ring (or belt) around the cell and inserts into typical zonulae occludens; a second type of microfilament bundle, containing actin, myosin, fodrin and vimentin, occurs in the apical processes and may be involved in photoreceptor renewal.

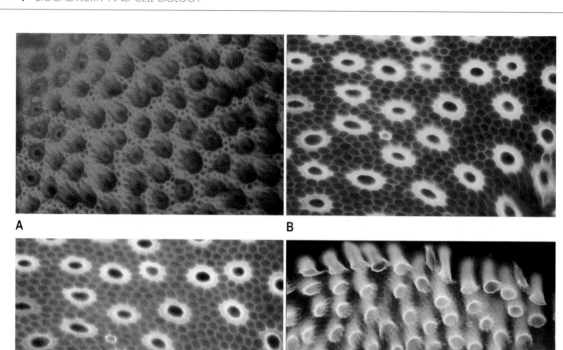

Fig. 4.43 Lectin staining of the interphotoreceptor matrix. (**A**) Wheat germ agglutinin – red labels the rod IPM. (**B**) Peanut agglutinin – green labels cone IPM. (**C**) Double label with WGA and PNA. (**D**) Oblique view to show cone IPM 'sheath'. IPM, interphotoreceptor matrix; PNA, peanut agglutinin; WGA, wheatgerm agglutinin. (Courtesy of JG Hollyfield.)

Under conditions of stress, RPE cells may express proteins more typical of macrophages and other myeloid cells. These include receptors for the Fc portion of immunoglobulin, the CD68 molecule and inducible nitric oxide synthase (see Ch. 7). RPE cells also express the leucocyte marker CD36, which may be involved in ROS phagocytosis. In addition, RPE cells contain high quantities of phosphatidylcholine and phosphatidylinositol with high levels of saturated fatty acids and a high content of arachidonic acid. This may explain to some extent their ready ability to generate prostaglandins with immunosuppressive properties. The high content of cholesterol in RPE membranes indicates a low plasma membrane fluidity compared, for instance, with rod outer segment membranes, whose cholesterol content is low.

Turnover in normal RPE is similar to that in endothelial cells (i.e. very slow or nil), but under certain circumstances RPE cells can proliferate and contribute to pathological processes as in retinal detachment (see Ch. 9). When appropriately stimulated, RPE cells can synthesize and secrete growth factors such as FGF, IGF-1 and interleukin-1, which most likely have a role in the normal physiology of the retina. In addition, RPE cells are an important inducible source of vascular endothelial growth factor. The production of growth factors by the RPE is not fully understood teleologically and it may play a part in regulating other tissues, such as the choroid and sclera, and thus indirectly have a role in the development of myopia. However, in pathological situations this may contribute to conditions such as diabetic retinopathy and subretinal neovascularization. To offset this risk, RPE cells constitutionally secrete a specific anti-angiogenic protein, pigment epithelium-derived factor (PEDF).

The role of the RPE as the second site of the blood–retinal barrier (see Ch. 1, p. 54) is based on the presence of tight junctions (see above); accordingly it is not surprising to find glucose transporter proteins in its plasma membrane, in this case GLUT 1 and GLUT 3. Bidirectional transport of various metabolites occurs but the main bulk flow of fluid is from the retinal side to the choriocapillaris, facilitated in part by aquaporin 1 (see Fig. 4.36); the cell is therefore a polarized epithelium with its apical microvilli in apposition to the photoreceptor cell and its basal infoldings towards the choroid. RPE cells express proteins on their apical surface that would be basolaterally expressed in other epithelia. These include N-CAM (a cell adhesion molecule) and EMMPRIN (extracellular matrix metalloproteinase inducer), which are likely to be involved in photoreceptor adhesion and phagocytosis, respectively. In addition, phagocytosis receptor $\alpha_v\beta_5$ integrin is expressed on the apical surface with the Na^+-K^+ ATPase. Other apical membrane-associated proteins include ezrin, which is associated with long apical microvilli, radixin and moesin. Reversed apical polarization occurs postnatally and is the result of suppressed decoding of specific basolateral signals.

The RPE sits on a prominent basement membrance, Bruch's membrance, composed of five discrete layers, part of which incorporates the basement membranes of the RPE and the choriocapillaris respectively. In addition to proteoglycans and matrix proteins typical of any basement membrane, Bruch's membrane contains hyaluronic acid and chondroitin sulphate plus types I, III, VI and VII collagen, and elastin.

Photoreceptor function is critically dependent on a healthy RPE layer

The RPE has multiple functions (Table 4.13) but its essential role is to maintain the physiology of the photoreceptors. Thus it removes 'spent' photoreceptor tips in the diurnal process of receptor renewal and participates in 11-*cis* retinol recycling. Indeed, it

Table 4.13 Functions of the RPE

Photoreceptor renewal
Retinal attachment
Interphotoreceptor matrix production
Transport of water and metabolites
Retinoid metabolism
Blood–retinal barrier
Immunoregulation
Free radical scavenging

has been known for over 100 years that contact with the RPE was necessary for the bleached retina to regain its 'visual purple'.

As stated above, during the process of photoreceptor disk renewal the outer segment tips are shed in a diurnal manner and removed by the RPE cells in a short burst of phagocytic activity. Cone outer segments are similarly removed by the RPE cells but the process is considerably slower. Phagocytosed outer segment tips are digested in the extensive RPE phagolysosomal system, a process that continues throughout life. Solubilized waste material is then transported across the extensive basal infoldings of the cell into the choriocapillaris. It is not surprising therefore that, with age, there is accumulation of lysosomal bodies and lipofuscin pigment, which may reflect the declining ability of the RPE cell to handle large amounts of relatively indigestible material. This may be linked to reduced melanin production with age (see above). Although this material has been implicated in the development of age-related macular degeneration, there is as yet little firm evidence.

Although some retinoid material will be incorporated in the phagocytosed outer segment tip, this material is not used for regeneration of bleached rhodopsin. Instead this occurs in the cytosol of the RPE cell. The conversion of 11-*cis* retinal to the all-*trans* retinal during phototransduction is accompanied by release of the chromophore into the interphotoreceptor matrix (see below). Regeneration of the 11-*cis* retinal from the all-*trans* retinal takes place only in the RPE, since retinol isomerase is unique to this cell. Therefore, the all-*trans* retinal must somehow enter the RPE cell by a means other than outer segment tip phagocytosis.

How this is achieved is not yet clear, but it is probably more subtle than the proposed mechanism of retinoid shuttling in which IRBP 'transports' the retinoids between the two cells; rather it is dependent upon the 'buffering' effect of IRBP, in which low-affinity binding of retinoid to IRBP permits its release at the appropriate site depending on the local concentration and amount of chromophore bleach. This notion is indirectly supported by evidence from the IRBP-knockout mouse; this mouse has a fully functional neurochemical visual cycle but an accelerated dark adaptation response. In contrast, the exclusive localization of the high-affinity binding protein cellular retinol binding protein (CRBP) to the RPE cell will help to drive the 'flow' of all-*trans* retinol in this direction and assist in the

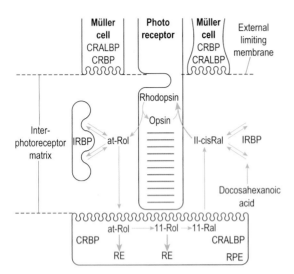

Fig. 4.44 Retinoid shuttling: buffering of all-*trans* retinol (at-Rol) by interphotoreceptor retinol binding protein (IRBP) in the interphotoreceptor matrix. CRBP, cell retinol binding protein; CRALBP, cell retinaldehyde binding protein. (Courtesy of J Saari.)

development of concentration gradients (Fig. 4.44). A recently described regulator of IRBP retinoid transport is docosahexanoic acid, which, in contra-distinction to palmitic acid, induces a rapid and specific release of 11-*cis* retinal from one of the two retinoid binding sites on IRPB. Interestingly, disturbed fatty acid metabolism has been linked to various types of retinitis pigmentosa. The function of Müller cell retinal binding proteins in this system is unclear at present.

The RPE is polarized with tight junctions, but transport is bidirectional

The transport function of the RPE is bidirectional in that, as shown above, retinoid transport, and probably also glucose transport, is achieved through polarized distribution of specific receptors. In contrast, the bulk of transport occurs from the retina to the choriocapillaris, particularly for digested outer segment material. There is also a significant bulk flow of fluid from the retina to the choroid probably via 'solute drag' through mechanisms such as a Na^+/K^+ ATPase pump located in the apical plasma membrane of the RPE and by transport of non-ionic solutes such as amino acids and glucose. Interestingly, RPE cells do not appear to express the water transporters aquaporin 3–5, unlike Müller cells and astrocytes, but do express mRNA for aquaporin 1 (see Fig. 4.36). However, active HCO_3^- transport appears to be the major ion linked to fluid transport

and is mediated by a carbonic anhydrase-regulated system (see section on ciliary body above). There are six isoforms of carbonic anhydrase in the RPE cell. The exchange of ions (and bulk water) establishes an electrical potential across the RPE, positive on the retinal side, of 5–15 mV, and also maintains steady pH regulation (Fig. 4.45) in the face of high lactic acid production by the outer segments of the photoreceptor cell.

The net rate of fluid transport across the RPE is about 4–6 $\mu l/cm^2$ per hour. Transretinal fluid flow has been proposed as a major mechanism for maintaining retinal apposition; indeed, it has been suggested that clinical RPE detachments may result from a breakdown of the transport mechanisms for fluid across the RPE as a result of focal damage.

Thus any process that impairs retinol transport into the RPE from central stores in the liver will affect vision; because vitamin A requirements are supplied through the diet, any condition affecting this, such as protein–calorie malnutrition or one of the malabsorption syndromes, may produce visual symptoms. One of the earliest symptoms of severe malnutrition, endemic in the Third World, is night blindness caused by lack of vitamin A.

The RPE also contains α and β_2 adrenergic receptors, plus enzymes of the cytochrome P_{450} drug-metabolizing system. In addition, melanin, a major constituent of RPE cells (see Box 4.24), is effective in drug detoxification. The melanin content of RPE cells decreases with age.

RETINAL NEUROCHEMISTRY

The main function of the retina is to convert light energy into an interpretable signal for cortical cells in the brain. This process begins with photochemical events in the photoreceptor.

PHOTOCHEMICAL REACTIONS IN THE RETINA

Rhodopsin, vitamin A and photoreceptor turnover

Rhodopsin is the major integral cell membrane protein in rod photoreceptor outer segments and its full 348 amino acid sequence has been determined. There are three glycosylation sites containing various branched combinations of N-acetylglucosamine and mannose residues. Opsin is a seven-turn (α helix) membrane-spanning protein containing a

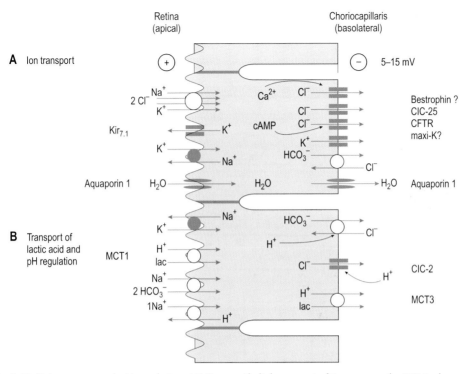

Retina
(apical)

Choriocapillaris
(basolateral)

A Ion transport

Fig. 4.45 Epithelial transport and pH regulation. (**A**) Transepithelial transport of ions across the RPE is shown. Cl⁻ is predominantly transported from the subretinal space to the choriocapillaris. This transport drives the water through aquaporins from the subretinal space to the choriocapillaris. (**B**) Transport of lactic acid and pH regulation is also shown. Lactic acid is removed from the subretinal space by the lac#-H⁺ cotransporter through the basolateral membrane, lactic acid leaves the cell using a different subtype of lac#-H⁺ cotransporter. CIC-2, voltage-dependent Cl⁻ channels of the CIC family; CFTR, cystic fibrosis transmembrane conductance regulator; Kir7.1, inwardly rectifying K⁺ channel 7.1; maxi-K, large-conductance Ca²⁺-dependent K⁺ channel; MCT1, monocarboxylate transporter 1; MCT3, monocarboxylate transporter 3. (From Strauss 2005, with permission from the American Physiological Society.)

serine- and threonine-rich cytosol-exposed C terminus, which is variably phosphorylated, and an intradisk N terminus (Fig. 4.46). This structure follows the general pattern for certain types of membrane receptor such as the adrenergic and muscarinic receptors. Such receptors induce cell signalling on binding of their specific ligand by activating adenyl cyclase to raise intracellular concentrations of the second messenger cAMP (see p. 179 and Ch. 6, p. 327).

Rhodopsin behaves like a genuine receptor, but with differences: in the resting state (i.e. in the dark), Na⁺ channels in the rod outer segment plasma membrane are held 'open' by cGMP, synthesized by guanylate cyclase. This provides the electrochemical basis for the relative depolarization of the photoreceptor cell compared with other cells (-57 versus -78 mV). On stimulation of rhodopsin with light, transdisk membrane signalling occurs via sequen-

tial activation of other membrane-bound proteins, transducin and phosphodiesterase, to lower the cytosolic concentration of cGMP, i.e. it acts like a second messenger in reverse (see below). This has the effect of closing the leaky Na⁺ channels in the plasma membrane and causing a relative hyperpolarization (to -87 mV), thereby generating the electrical response (see below).

Activation of rhodopsin is achieved via isomerization of retinol, a vitamin A compound that lies 'nested' between the first and last transmembrane loops of the rhodopsin molecule, with its long axis in the plane of the membrane (Fig. 4.46). Modelling studies clearly show the relationship between the chromophore pocket and the opsin molecule (Fig. 4.47). In this reaction, the tail of 11-*cis* retinal on conversion to all-*trans* retinal (see p. 255) becomes elongated and more perpendicularly disposed to the

Box 4.24　Melanogenesis

Melanogenesis is dependent on the enzyme tyrosinase, which is present in melanosomes.

Tyrosine

Tyrosinase (in melanosomes)

DOPA

Dopaquinone

+ Cysteine (non-enzymatic)

Alanine–DOPA compounds

5,6-Dihydroxyindole

+ Protein

Polymerized melanin–protein complex

Phaeomelanins (yellow and red pigments)

Eumelanins (black and brown pigments)

taken up by the RPE cell; in the dark it undergoes isomerization within the RPE cell (see Box 4.25) to 11-*cis* retinol, which binds to cellular retinal binding protein (CRALBP) and becomes converted to 11-*cis* retinal-CRALBP, which is transported to the cell membrane and is transferred to interphotoreceptor retinal binding protein (IRBP) on which it is shuttled back to the photoreceptor to reattach to rhodopsin and recommence the cycle (see Box 4.25).

The conversion of 11-*cis* retinal to all-*trans* retinal and then to all-*trans* retinol is the fundamental chemical reaction to take place during the visual impulse, and the chemical reaction has been known for many years. Laser flash photolysis studies have chemically identified the intermediates that occur in the breakdown of vitamin A (Fig. 4.48). Normal vision depends on a plentiful supply of vitamin A, which must be provided exogenously because humans cannot synthesize it. Thus visual deterioration, especially at low illumination (night blindness), is an early sign of malnutrition and malabsorption syndromes, but sensitive electrophysiological tests may be required to reveal its full extent. All *trans* retinol to 11-*cis* retinol isomerization is regulated by palmitoylation under the control of the RPE-specific protein RPE-65, whose role serves to switch off the visual cycle in the dark.

Rhodopsin is synthesized in the ER and Golgi apparatus of the inner segments and transported in protein-rich vesicles to the outer segment, where fusion occurs with the newly formed disk membranes in the periciliary ridge complex.

Phototransduction: the conversion of light energy to an electrochemical response

The conversion of the energy stored in a single photon of light to an electrical response is possible because of the extensive amplification of the molecular cascade involved in closure of the Na^+ channels (see Box 4.26). These channels are kept open by cGMP, which acts as a second messenger in this system.

In the dark, open Na^+ channels allow Na^+ to exit and Ca^{2+} to enter and maintain a relative depolarization. This is linked to a Na^+/Ca^{2+} exchanger, which in the dark maintains a steady intracellular concentration of Ca^{2+}. In the light, the Na^+ channels are closed, leading to a relative hyperpolarization and a decline in the intracellular Ca^{2+} concentration. Closure of the Na^+ channels is achieved by hydrolysis of cGMP by phosphodiesterase, one of the responses that is

isoprene retinal ring structure; this has the effect of generating greater interaction between the retinal and its binding sites to the side-chains of amino acids Lys206 and Lys296, thereby heightening the energy state of the rhodopsin molecule. All-*trans* retinal becomes converted to all-*trans* retinol, which does not fit within the rhodopsin transmembrane loops and thus detaches from rhodopsin and diffuses away into the interphotoreceptor matrix and is

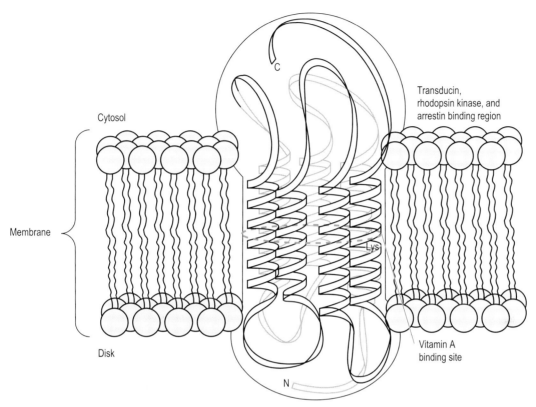

Fig. 4.46 Rhodopsin molecule. The dashed circle in the centre of the transmembrane region indicates the site and plane of 11-*cis* retinal to the lysine residues at position 206 and 209. (Courtesy L Stryer and KW Yau and WH Freeman.)

greatly amplified in the cascade. Signal amplification is achieved by activation of many molecules of transducin by one molecule of metarhodopsin (R*), probably in the region of 300× (Fig 4.49). Similarly, around 600 molecules of cGMP are hydrolysed by a single molecule of PDE and indeed the limitation of its activity is determined by the availability of cGMP. There is a further three-fold amplification of channel opening by one cGMP molecule.

Phototransduction is a biological cascade

The mechanism of cGMP hydrolysis in phototransduction has been extensively investigated; the sequence of events in this response is outlined in Figure 4.49.

Certain enzymes play important roles in this process, including guanylate cyclase and cGMP phosphodiesterase. Guanylate cyclase activation restores cGMP levels with the help of recoverin (see Fig. 4.49), while R* is deactivated to the phosphorylated form R–P and bound by arrestin (S antigen). During these changes there is considerable redistribution of photoreceptor molecules in the shift from light to dark (Fig. 4.50).

Amplification is therefore a function of the time interval at each of the stages of processing.

Does phosphoinositide metabolism have a role in phototransduction?

From the above it would appear that much of the transduction mechanism has been deduced; however, the role and mechanism of Ca^{2+} influx are unclear. Ca^{2+} mobilization is the product of a major second messenger system in many cells, and is activated via receptor-mediated activation of phospholipase C and G proteins. This results in the hydrolysis of phosphatidylinositol 4,5-biphosphate (PIP_2) to form inositol trisphosphate (IP_3) and diacylglycerol (DAG). IP_3 induces mobilization of calcium stores while DAG activates protein kinase C. Two major calcium-binding proteins, calmodulin and GCAP1 and 2 (calcium-dependent modulator of guanylate cyclase) are involved in phototransduction.

253

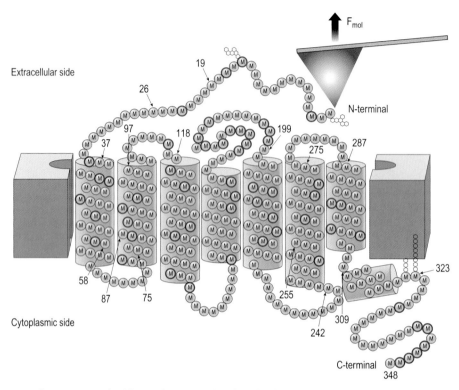

Fig. 4.47 Secondary structure of wild-type Rho mapped with molecular interactions detected by single-molecule force spectroscopy. Arrows and numbers indicate the beginning and end of each structural segment stabilized by molecular interactions. Highly conserved residues (> 80%) are highlighted in gold. Residues framed by dark red circles indicate the positions of mutations associated with retinitis pigmentosa. (From Fotiadis *et al.* 2006, with permission from Elsevier.)

In the invertebrate retina, light induces hydrolysis of PIP_2 with production of IP_3 and DAG, but its role in the transduction cascade is unclear. However, there is evidence that an integral transmembrane phosphatidylinositol transfer protein prevents retinal degeneration in *Drosophila* (the rdg B protein). The evidence in the vertebrate retina is even less convincing. It is possible that this mechanism may have some other function related to membrane conductance and mobilization of ion stores, but un-related to transmission of an electric impulse. However, there is little doubt that phosphoinositide metabolism and turnover is a major pathway in the photoreceptor cell.

Renewal of photoreceptors is associated with accumulation of lipofuscin pigment in the RPE cells

Estimates suggest that RPE cells phagocytose about 2000–4000 disks per day. To cope with this phagocytic load, the RPE cell has an extensive lysosomal enzyme system that can digest about 50% of its load within 1–2 hours (important in terms of cyclic rod

outer segment tip shedding). Uptake of shed rod outer segment tips is receptor mediated, through the $\alpha_v\beta_0$ integrin receptor signalling through the receptor tyrosine kinase Mer. Several other candidates have been proposed including the mannose receptor, fibronectin and intercellular adhesion molecule-1, Toll-like receptor 4, $\alpha_v\beta_3$ integrin and the leucocyte surface molecule CD36, which is also expressed on RPE cells. CD36 recognizes oxidized phosphatidyl choline, a product of aged outer segment tips and may be involved in the engulfment process rather than initial binding. Interestingly, the $\alpha_v\beta_5$ receptor is also involved in retinal adhesion to the RPE layer, functioning in a different diurnal cycle for phagocytosis.

RPE lysosomes contain a battery of enzymes capable of degrading complex lipid–glycoprotein aggregates
(Table 4.14)
Phagocytosis of rod outer segment tips takes place in stages. First, there is formation of the primary phagolysosome by fusion of the endosome with the

Box 4.25 Conversion of 11-*cis* retinal to all-*trans* retinal to all-*trans* retinol and uptake by the RPE cell

11-*cis* retinal is converted to all-*trans* retinal within pico-seconds of absorbing a photon of light. However, at this stage, the all-*trans* retinal is still undergoing some molecular rearrangements in its interactions with the opsin molecule; this 'strained' intermediate is known as bathorhodopsin. Further intermediates are formed at later times and can be followed spectrophotometrically by their peak absorbance as the molecule readjusts itself within the opsin nest to its new conformation. Metarhodopsin II, otherwise known as activated rhodopsin (R*), is eventually converted to opsin and all-*trans* retinal (see text). Metarhodopsin II is a highly efficient initiator of the phototransduction response because it stores 27 kcal/mol of the energy of the incident photon of light. All-*trans* retinal is converted to all-*trans* retinol and taken up by the RPE cell for conversion back to 11-*cis* retinal as detailed in the diagram below.

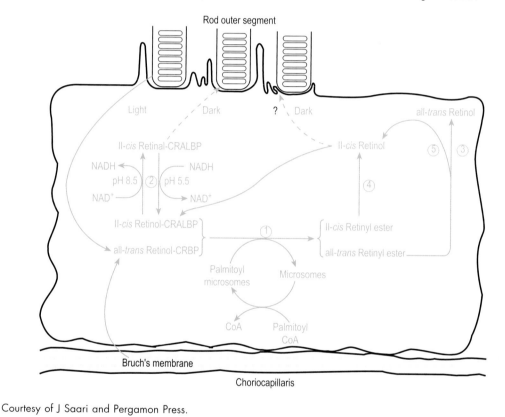

Courtesy of J Saari and Pergamon Press.

Table 4.14 Lysosomal enzymes of the RPE
Acid phosphatase
N-acetyl-β-glucosaminidase
β-galactosidase
Glycosidase, e.g. α mannosidase
Phospholipases A, B and C
Acid lipase
Cathepsin D

lysosome. This may then fuse with lipofuscin granules or with melanosomes to form melanolipofuscin bodies. With age, and experimentally in vitamin E deficiency, there is a greater shift towards fusion with lipofuscin granules. Eventually these bodies are degraded and their products are transported out of the cell. However, the accumulation of insoluble material between the basement membrane and the RPE cell has been attributed to a breakdown in the capacity of the cell to deal with this load. In addition, accumulation of lipofuscin is associated with reduced phagocytic capacity of RPE cells.

255

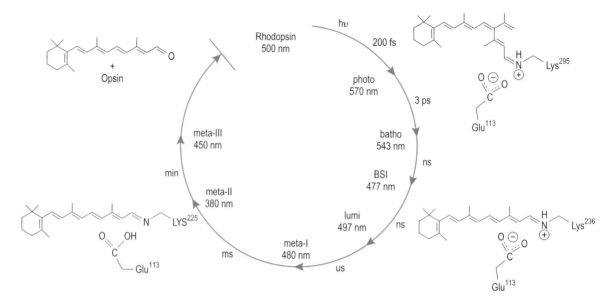

Fig. 4.48 The Rho photocycle. Photoisomerization of the RET chromophore to its 11-*trans* form is the only light-dependent event in vertebrate vision. The RET chromophore is a derivative of vitamin A₁ with a total of 20 carbon atoms. Photoisomerization in Rho occurs on an ultrafast time-scale with photorhodopsin as the photoproduct formed on a femtosecond time-scale. The photolysed pigment then proceeds through a number of well-characterized spectral intermediates. As the protein gradually relaxes around 11-*trans*-RET, protein–chromophore interactions change and distinct λ_{max} values are observed. The Schiff base imine remains protonated, presumably as the result of stabilization by its counter-ion, Glu-113, through meta-rhodopsin I (meta-I). Meta-I is in a dynamic equilibrium under physiological conditions with meta-rhodopsin-II (meta-II), which is characterized by an unproteinated Schiff base imine and a dramatically blue-shifted λ_{max} value (380 nm). Meta-II is the photoproduct that is able to catalyse guanine nucleotide exchange by G_t. Meta-II eventually decays to free 11-*trans*-RET and opsin apoprotein. Important photochemical properties of Rho in the rod cell disk membrane include a very high quantum efficiency (<0.67 for Rho versus <0.20 for RET in solution) and an extremely low rate of thermal isomerization. Some fish, reptiles or aquatic mammals use a derivative of vitamin A₂ (11-*cis*-3,4-didehydroretinylidene), which contains an additional carbon-carbon double bond in the ring. In contrast to vertebrate vision, invertebrate vision is generally photochromic; a photoactivate invertebrate pigment can be inactivated by absorption of a second photon that includes isomerization to the ground state *cis* conformation. (Courtesy of the American Physiological Society.)

Box 4.26 Phototransduction cascade and channel opening

Activation of a single molecule of rhodopsin generates an amplification cascade that leads to the opening of many channels, and the induction of a change in the resting potential of the photoreceptor.

hυ

Rh → Rh* —τ_1→ Rh*-P

G-GDP → G*-GDP —τ_2→ G-GDP

PDE$_i$ → PDE* —τ_3→ PDE$_i$

ΔcG = 0 ... ΔcG < 0 —τ_4→ ΔcG = 0
(CHANNEL open) (CHANNEL closed) (CHANNEL open)

SYNAPTIC EVENTS BETWEEN PHOTORECEPTORS AND CELLS OF THE INNER NUCLEAR LAYER

In the resting state, the dark currents produced by the open cation channels in the outer segment (see Box 5.6, p. 278) are accompanied by high levels of neurotransmitter release at the synaptic junction with the bipolar cells. In the light, there is a decrease in transmitter release, which alters the transmission of electric potentials in the bipolar cells. However, the situation is more complex than this.

Two types of bipolar cell

Synaptic transmission at neuromuscular junctions is mediated by acetylcholine, released from the nerve ending when the action potential wave arrives. Binding of acetylcholine to its receptor on the muscle

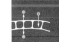

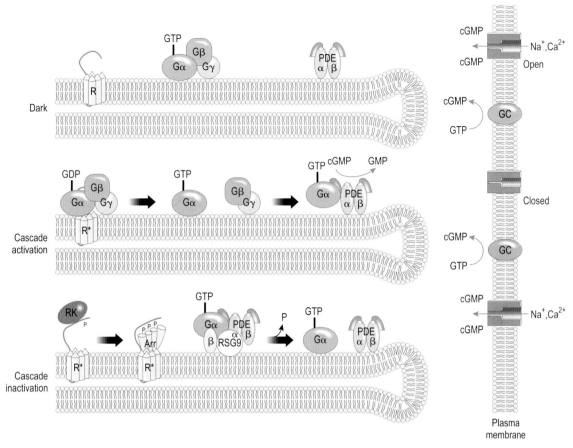

Fig. 4.49 Schematic of phototransduction cascade activation and inactivation. The upper disk illustrates inactive rhodopsin (R), transducin (Gα, Gβ and Gγ subunits), and PDE (α, β and γ subunits), in the dark. The reactions in the middle disk illustrate light-induced transducin and PDE activation. The reactions in the lower disk represent R* inactivation via phosphorylation by rhodopsin kinase (RK) followed by arrestin (Arr) binding and transducin/PDE inactivation by RGS9–Gαβ-PDEαβ complex. (From Burns *et al.* 2005, with permission from Elsevier.)

initiates a second message, which causes a depolarization in the cell owing to opening of the voltage-gated Na^+ channels.

At the synaptic junction between the photoreceptor cell and the bipolar cell, a different type of reaction occurs. First, the photoreceptor does not transmit an action potential wave, but presents a graded hyperpolarization response, which depends on the intensity of the light stimulus. In the dark, while the photoreceptor is in a relatively depolarized state, the neurotransmitter glutamate is released from the presynaptic photoreceptor terminal and binds to a retina-specific metabotropic receptor (see next section for definitions) on one type of bipolar cell (the ON-bipolar), which produces hyperpolarization and keeps the bipolar Na^+ channel closed. When light

activates the photoreceptor, glutamate release ceases and the intracellular concentration of cGMP rises, thus opening the Na^+ channels and causing depolarization of the cell membrane, allowing the ON-bipolar cell to transmit a signal (see Table 4.15).

In contrast, glutamate binding to the ionotropic receptor on a second type of bipolar cell (the OFF-bipolar; see Ch. 5) has the reverse effect of inducing hyperpolarization. To summarize, therefore, when light activates the photoreceptor and transmits the message to the bipolar cell, ON-bipolar cells are depolarized by reduction in glutamate release and OFF-bipolar cells are hyperpolarized by an increase in glutamate release. Additionally, glutamate may bind to horizontal cells where it also produces hyperpolarization.

257

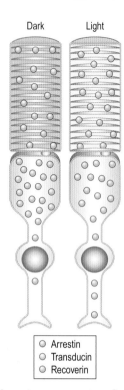

Dark   Light

○ Arrestin
○ Transducin
○ Recoverin

Fig. 4.50 Schematic representation of transducin, arrestin and recoverin subcellular distribution in the dark-adapted and light-adapted rod. (From Burns *et al.* 2005, with permission from Elsevier.)

Glutamate is unlike acetylcholine in that there is no enzyme that rapidly degrades the neurotransmitter and shuts down the response; instead, the glutamate merely diffuses away or is taken up by nearby glial cells and inactivated.

The differential binding of glutamate to ON- and OFF-bipolar cells via specific receptors (see below) is a direct chemical correlate of the electrophysiological and psychophysical responses that can be obtained from these cells, and is a good demonstration of nature's use of a binary (ON–OFF) system to process complex sensory phenomena. Apparently, the segregation of response at the bipolar cell level is retained to the level of the visual cortex.

Neurotransmitters and neuromodulators

Neurotransmitters have a rapid excitatory or inhibitory action at the synaptic junction; in contrast, neuromodulators have a much longer action, often mediated through second messenger systems in the cell. There are many different types of neurotransmitter, most of which are amino acids or amino acid derivatives, and the majority are active in transmis-

Table 4.15 Retinal neurotransmitters and neuromodulatory peptides

Agent	Site of action
Neurotransmitters	
Glutamate	Photoreceptor
γ-aminobutyric acid	Horizontal amacrine cells
Glycine	Amacrine cell
Taurine	
Tyrosine derivatives	
Dopamine	Horizontal amacrine cells
Norepinephrine	
Epinephrine	
Tryptophan derivatives	
Serotonin	Photoreceptor
Aspartate	Photoreceptor
β-alanine	
Histidine derivative	
Histamine	
Neuromodulators	
Peptides	
Vasoactive intestinal peptide	Amacrine, ganglion cells
Angiotensin I and II	Amacrine, ganglion cells
Substance P	Amacrine, ganglion cells
Luteinizing hormone releasing hormone and thyrotrophin releasing hormone	Amacrine, ganglion cells
Leu-and metenkephalin	Amacrine cell
β-endorphin	Amacrine, ganglion cells
Somatostatin	Amacrine, ganglion cells
Neurotensin	Amacrine cell
Glucagon	Amacrine cell

sion of electric impulses within the mammalian retina. Typical excitatory transmitters include acetylcholine and glutamate, while γ-aminobutyric acid (GABA) and glycine are inhibitory. There are a number of neuromodulatory peptides that have direct or indirect effects on neural impulses. Dopamine is probably the best known of these (see below). In addition, recent studies indicate that neuronal nitric oxide synthase may modulate retinal signalling via release of nitric oxide.

Glutamate is the major neurotransmitter in the retina

As indicated above, glutamate (Fig. 4.51) is the major mediator of synaptic transmission between the photoreceptor and the bipolar and horizontal cells. The functional organization of the retina is centred around the specificity of glutamate for four discrete types of receptor on different types of cells (ON- and OFF-bipolar cells, and two types of

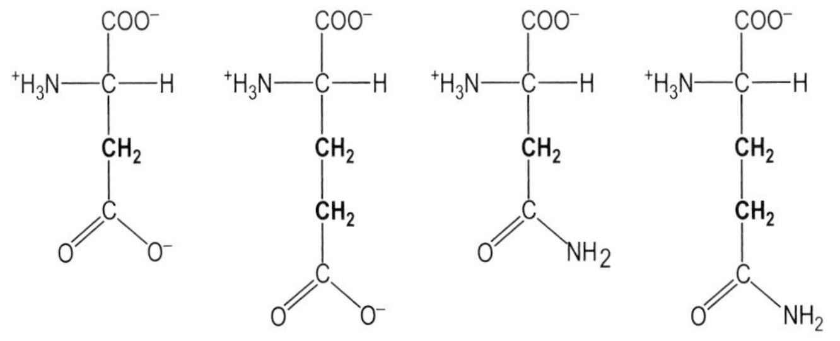

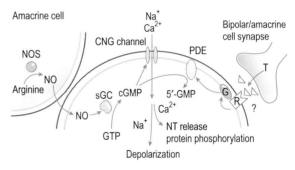

Aspartate (Asp, D) Glutamate (Glu, E) Asparagine (Asn, N) Glutamine (Gln, Q)

Fig. 4.51 Chemical structure of the acidic amino acid glutamate.

horizontal cell). These receptors have been identified using specific blocking agents and are classified according to type:

- *N*-methyl-d-aspartate (NMDA) receptors
- quisqualate receptors
- kainate receptors
- APB (sign-inverting glutamate receptor agonist) receptors.

Each of these receptors has specific characteristics related to whether they are ionotropic (directly affecting ion channels, e.g. NMDA) or metabotropic (primarily affecting aspects of neuronal cell metabolism, such as cGMP levels, and secondarily altering ion-channel permeability, e.g. APB receptors) (see Fig. 5.4). Synaptic transmission in ganglion cells may also utilize glutamate. However, for some time it has been proposed that small cyclic nucleotides may confer gating activity and recent studies have confirmed this (Fig. 4.52). The cAMP and cGMP appear to have opposing gating effects in their interactions with horizontal/amacrine cells and ganglion cells in the regulation of Ca^{2+} influx and in addition appear to be modulated themselves by neuronal nitric oxide synthase derived from neighbouring cells.

Horizontal and amacrine cells

Horizontal and amacrine cells directly modify the rate of electrical firing in bipolar cells by release of excitatory (horizontal cells) and inhibitory (horizontal and amacrine cells) neurotransmitters. Glutamate is the major excitatory transmitter of horizontal cells, while GABA, a derivative of glutamate distributed widely throughout the retina, functions particularly in the horizontal and amacrine cells as an inhibitory mediator. Recently, it has been shown that some horizontal cell negative feedback to cones can be mediated via glutamate-gated Ca^{2+} channels. Glycine is also an inhibitory neurotransmitter in amacrine cells, which have a significant role in

Fig. 4.52 Schematic representation of pathways that might regulate the activity of the cGMP-gated channel in retinal ganglion cells. The cGMP synthesis could be stimulated by nitric oxide adjacent amacrine cells. Activation of cGMP-gated channels will increase Ca^{2+} influx and enhance Ca^{2+}-driven processes. At the same time, G-protein coupled receptors activated by neurotransmitters from bipolar and amacrine cell terminals may regulate the activity of one or more PDEs which control hydrolysis of cGMP and thus the activity of the cGMP-gated channels. From Barnstable *et al.* (2004); modified from Ahmad *et al.* (1994).

determining the size of receptive fields of individual ganglion cells (see Ch. 5).

Acetylcholine is a major excitatory neurotransmitter of amacrine cells and often colocalizes in GABAergic starburst cells, suggesting that these cells can act in a complex excitatory/inhibitory manner in relation to ganglion cell receptive fields. Ganglion cells are thought to utilize glutamate as a major transmitter.

Dopamine exerts a neuromodulatory effect on retinal function

Dopamine occurs in amacrine cells and interplexiform cells in the inner retinal layers and clearly has

259

a role to play in visual function because the reduced and delayed b-wave electroretinogram responses (see Ch. 5) seen in patients with Parkinson's disease are normalized on treatment with l-DOPA. Dopamine receptors (there are two broad classes and several subclasses) are present on all retinal neurones and therefore dopamine probably has many as yet undetermined effects, one of which is to uncouple photoreceptor-driven horizontal cell gap junctions. Horizontal cells are probably the source of activity in the surround region in bipolar cell centre-surround receptive fields, suggesting that regulation of spatial contrast sensitivity may be under dopaminergic control.

Dopamine may have many other effects including regulation of A11-type amacrine cells which couple rod-associated bipolar cells and ganglion cells, and it may even have a paracrine role in altering the level of photoreceptor cytoplasmic cAMP. Dopamine has also been implicated in development in retinal neurones because it has been shown that apomorphine inhibits form-deprivation myopia in experimental animals by a dopamine D_2-receptor mechanism acting within either the retina or the RPE.

Dopamine is inactivated by cellular reuptake, a process mediated by specific Na^+-dependent membrane transporter proteins, which have been cloned. Dopamine may also be antagonized by melatonin, which is synthesized and released by photoreceptors, accounting for the photopic to scotopic transition in rod responsiveness. It is also counteracted by NMDA, which may induce impaired dopamine synthesis.

It can be seen therefore that, while much remains to be determined concerning the mediators of neural function in the retina and visual cortex, a view is already emerging of differential stimulation and inhibition of function induced by a variety of interacting neuromodulators and transmitters, which correlates with observed psychophysical events.

CONCLUSION

The rich variety of biochemical processes that occur within the eye encompasses many aspects of general physicochemical reactions. The general principles that apply to other systems apply also to the eye. Where differences exist, they assist in highlighting the properties and functions of molecules and reactions, while introducing us to the specific mecha-

nisms in the eye. In this way, a greater understanding of the general principles is achieved.

FURTHER READING

Ahmad I, Leinders-Zufall T, Kocsis JD, Shepherd GM, Zufall F, Barnstable CJ. Retinal ganglion cells express a cGMP-gated cation conductance activatable by nitric oxide donors. Neuron 1994; 12:155–165.

Albert DM, Jakobiec FA. Principles and practice of ophthalmology. VI: Basic sciences. London: WB Saunders; 1999.

Augusteyn RC. α-crystallin: a revew of its structure and function. Clin Exp Optom 2004; 87:356–366.

Barnstable CJ, Wei, J-Y, Han M-H. Modulation of synaptic function by cGMP and cGMP-gated cation channels. Neurochem Int 2004; 45:875–884.

Bloemendal H, de Jong W, Jaenicke R, Lubsen NH, Slingsby C, Tardieu A. Ageing and vision: structure, stability and function of lens crystallins. Prog Biophy Mol Biol 2004; 86:407–485.

Burns ME, Arshavsky VY. Beyond counting photons: trials and trends in vertebrate visual transduction. Neuron 2005; 48:387–401.

Dartt DA. Control of mucin production by ocular surface epithelial cells. Exp Eye Res 2004; 78:173–185.

Davson H. Physiology of the eye, 5th edn. New York: Pergamon Press; 1990.

Engelman DM. Membranes are more mosaic than fluid. Nature 2005; 438:578–580.

Fotiadis D, Jastrzebska B, Philippsen A, Muller DJ, Palczewski K, Engel A. Structure of the rhodopsin dimer: a working model for G-protein coupled receptors. Curr Opin Struct Biol 2006; 16:252–259.

Gelman L, Michalik L, Desvergne, B, Wahli W. Kinase signalling cascades that modulate peroxisome proliferator-activated receptors. Curr Opin Cell Biol 2005; 17:216–222.

Gipson IK. Distribution of mucins at the ocular surface. Exp Eye Res 2004; 78:379–388.

Harding JJ. Biochemistry of the Eye. London: Chapman and Hall Medical; 1997.

Ihanamaki T, Pelliniemi LJ, Vuorio E. Collagens and collagen-related matrix proteins in the human and mouse eye. Prog Retin Eye Res 2004; 23:403–434.

Mao Y, Schwarzbauer JE. Fibronectin fibrillogenesis, a cell-mediated matrix assembly process. Matrix Biology 2005; 24:389–399.

Maxfield FR. Plasma membrane microdomains. Curr Opin Cell Biol 2002; 14:483–487.

Menon ST, Han M, Sakmar TP. Rhodopsin: structural basis of molecular physiology. Physiol Rev 2001; 81:1659–1688.

Meyer T, Teruel M. Fluorescence imaging of signalling networks. Trends Cell Biol 2003; 13:101–106.

Mueller LJ, Pels E, Schurmans LR, Vrensen GF. A new three-dimensional model of the organization of proteoglycans and collagen fibrils in the human corneal stroma. Exp Eye Res 2004; 78:493–501.

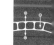

Orth JD, McNiven MA. Dynamin at the actin–membrane interface. Curr Opin Cell Biol 2003; 15:31–39.

Pompella A, Visvikis A, Paolicci A *et al.* The changing faces of glutathione: a cellular protagonist. Biochem Pharmacol 2003;66:1499–1503.

Purkiss AG, Bateman OA, Goodfellow JM, Lubsen NH, Slingsby C. The X-ray crystal structure of human γS-crystallin C-terminal domain. J Biol Chem 2002; 277:4199–4205.

Schlötzer-Schrehardt U, Kruse FE. Identification and characterization of limbal stem cells. Exp Eye Res 2005; 81:247–264.

Silverman RH, Ursea R, Kruse D, Ferrara KW, Rondeau MJ, Coleman DJ. Ultrasound measurement of the effect of temperature on microperfusion in the eye. Ultrasound Med Biol 2002; 28:1413–1419.

Sosnová-Netuková M, Kuchynka P, Forrester JV. The suprabasal layer of corneal epithelial cells represents the major barrier site to the passive movement of small molecules and trafficking leukocytes. Br J Ophthalmol 2006.

Söti C, Pàl C, Papp B, Csermely P. Curr Opin Biol 2005; 17:210–215.

Stein GS, Zaidi SK, Braastad CD, Montecino M, van Wijnen AJ, Choi JY, Stein JL, Lian JB, Javed A. Functional architecture of the nucleus: organizing the regulatory machinery for gene expression, replication and repair. Trends Cell Biol 2003; 13:584–592.

Strauss O. The retinal pigment epithelium in visual function. Physiol Rev 2005, 85:845–881.

Toivola DM, Tao G-Z, Habetzion A, Liao J, Omary MB. Cellular integrity plus: organelle-related and protein-targeting functions of intermediate filaments. Trends Cell Biol 2005; 15:608–617.

Verkman AS. Exp Eye Res 2003; 76:137–143.

Wenzel A, Grimm C, Samardzija M, Reme CE. Molecular mechanisms of light-induced photoreceptor apoptosis and neuroprotection for retinal degeneration. Prog Retin Eye Res 2005; 24:275–306.

Yu D-Y, Cringle SJ. Retinal degeneration and local oxygen metabolism. Exp Eye Res 2005; 80:745–751.

5 PHYSIOLOGY OF VISION AND THE VISUAL SYSTEM

INTRODUCTION

It goes without saying that the ability to detect, recognize and discriminate objects in space is fundamental to survival and is achieved not simply through detection of luminance or contrast sensitivity (visual acuity) but also by discrimination of texture, colour, depth and motion disparities. Most of these functions are located in the higher cortical centres where the retinal 'sensation' (image) is converted into a perception of the outside world. What is seen may not be the same as what is perceived and the latter may be extensively edited through input from other non-visual centres, especially memory and previous visual experience.

As Zeki (1992) has put it: 'To obtain knowledge of what is visible, the brain (does not) merely analyse the images presented to the retina; it must actively construct a visual world.' As will be seen later, the brain builds up a picture of a visual scene by segregation of the image into its component parts; thus there are cortical cells that are directionally selective (motion detectors), others that are orientation selective, and still others that are specific for colour. On face value it might be thought that spatial resolution would be most important to survival but in fact it has been shown that colour is what we see best.

There are further subtleties to the business of seeing. For instance, how do we detect form? Is this simply a computation of input from orientation selective neurones, or does it involve other input? What about that most highly developed function, recognition of faces? What about texture? This chapter addresses

263

some of these aspects of the sensory and psycho-physical responses to visual stimuli, but of necessity in the most superficial of detail.

WHAT DO WE MEAN BY GOOD VISION?

It is important that we have a concept of the limits of our visual capabilities. Vision can be considered in two ways: the optical requirements to achieve an image (i.e. refraction of light by the eye to focus the image on the retina, also known as physiological optics) and the neural processing of visual stimuli by the retina and the brain. The visual process is initiated by the detection of a light signal by photo-receptor cells in the outer retina. These cells convert light energy to an electric stimulus, which is then transmitted to the bipolar cells and onwards to the ganglion cells in the retina (see Ch. 1). The information is further transmitted in the axons of these cells (the optic nerves which, after 50% crossover in the optic chiasma, become the optic tracts) to the visual thalamic organ, the lateral geniculate nucleus (LGN). Synaptic contact with neurones in the LGN that project to the cerebral cortex permits onward transmission of the signals via optic radiation to the visual or striate cortex (V1), where they interact with many other neuronal connections from visual cortical cells in the prestriate cortex (V3–V5), and where parcelling out and processing of the signals takes place to build up the final perceived visual image. Input is also received by the visual cortex from many other areas, particularly those controlling general motor function and eye movement, cerebellar and spatial sense, memory and many other functions.

In biophysical terms a photoreceptor is theoretically capable of detecting a single photon of light (see below), but in practice what are the limits of detection of a visual stimulus? This depends on the nature of the stimulus and the nature of the ambient conditions in which it is presented. Sensing light is a function of all regions of the retina but the foveal region is specialized for high spatial resolution (visual acuity) and colour detection, served by the small 'midget', slow-transmitting ganglion cells (the parvocellular or P system). In contrast, luminance and motion detection are served by the large, fast transmitting ganglion cells (the magnocellular or M system) that dominate the remaining retina and thus incorporate the entire visual field. According to Barlow's single neurone doctrine, it should take only one neurone to detect a visual stimulus. However,

psychophysical studies have shown that both the luminance and colour thresholds for vision are different by orders of magnitude for P neurones between monkeys and humans, suggesting that more than one neurone is involved. In fact, the current view is that continuous pooling of information occurs both in the excitatory and inhibitory neuronal activity that is present at all times and that, after a visual stimulus, the changes in the response rate of many neurones are 'sampled' by the brain until they reach a certain threshold level, at which point they register and the stimulus is 'recognized' (Hurlbert and Derrington, 1993). This perhaps explains how we can sometimes look at an object and yet not 'see' it; furthermore, these psychophysical considerations are highly relevant to methods for testing vision, for instance with regard to setting luminance thresholds for studies of visual fields using small transient targets.

Underpinning good vision therefore, are the concepts of awareness, consciousness and attention to visual stimuli. It has also become known that these may vary for different stimuli; the time taken to detect a moving stimulus is significantly different to that required to detect a colour.

Flicker can be used to determine limits of vision

Detection of a stationary target or spot depends on the size and brightness of the spot relative to the background. The limits of detectability of the target are therefore determined by the spatial resolution and the anatomical relationships between stimulated receptors (see below). Spatial resolution is highest at the fovea and declines sharply towards the peripheral retina; this is clearly demonstrated by the detection threshold at different eccentricities in the visual field.

The threshold for spatial resolution is, however, considerably higher than that for detecting light; this latter parameter can be measured by flicker detection, which is the ability to detect two stimuli separated in time. This function is normally subserved by rod photoreceptors, while spatial resolution is subserved by cones, with some input from rods.

Use of the critical flicker fusion (CFF) frequency test has recently been shown to be a useful predictor of cataract surgery outcome in cases of co-morbidity of lens opacity and macular disease because the CFF (see below) is relatively unaffected by image degradation due to cataract but would be affected by foveal disease.

Motion detection is also a feature of rod vision

It is clear, therefore, that the ability to detect a standard small bright spot in specified regions of the visual field is in fact a much more complex task than would at first appear. Not only does it depend on the absolute brightness of the stimulus, but also on the background on which the stimulus is presented and thus on contrast. It also depends on whether the target is moving or stationary and, if stationary, for how long the target is presented. Its detection depends on the density of photoreceptors and thus the region of retina stimulated. If it is a moving target it will stimulate different cortical neurones depending on which direction it is moving. This functional segregation of visual input is retained at several levels within the cortex before construction of the final visual image.

SENSING COLOUR

Colour is detected by cone photoreceptors, of which there are three types: long (L, red), medium (M, green) and short (S, blue) wavelengths. Early evidence for this was based partly on colour matching experiments, which show that the colour of a test stimulus can be matched by adding together stimuli composed of the three primary colours (see below, colorimetry). This is known as the trichromatic theory of colour vision. Each colour has properties such as hue and chromaticity.

There are many hues but only three primary colours

Hue is an idealized term for the colour produced by light of a single wavelength. In spite of having only three cone photoreceptors, we are able to distinguish many hues of colour, e.g. lilac and violet. It is therefore clear that any single colour is recognized by a mixture of the three primaries and that there must be overlap in the spectral sensitivity for each primary colour (see below). Theoretically it should be possible to produce light of a single wavelength using a narrow slit on a device such as a monochrometer, but photoreceptor sensitivity is also subject to the intensity of the light, and narrow wavebands of this degree of selectivity are not sufficiently intense to produce a stimulus.

The hue-discrimination curve (Fig. 5.1) describes the physiological limits at which a shift in wavelength can be discriminated as a change in colour. Monochromatic light therefore is not a practical reality; most colours are in fact tints, i.e. they are

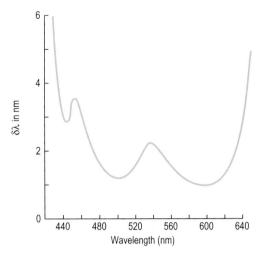

Fig. 5.1 Hue-discrimination curve comparing wavelength discrimination (y-axis) with changing wavelength (x-axis). Discrimination of hues varies for any given wavelength, being best at 455 and 535 nm.

unsaturated hues, the degree of unsaturation being determined by the amount of additional white light they require to match them to a hue.

Chromaticity is semiquantified 'colouredness'

Chromaticity refers to 'colouredness' and depends on hue, saturation and intensity of light (luminosity). Indeed, hue itself is not independent of the luminosity of the stimulus and chromatic shifts occur as the intensity increases till all hues appear yellow–white (the Bezold–Brucke phenomenon) or as the intensity decreases, when all hues appear achromatic (the Purkinje shift; see below). Any colour can thus be matched by a mixture of the three primary colours plus or minus a proportion of white light to account for unsaturation; these are formally described in the chromaticity chart (Fig. 5.2).

Similar colour-mixing techniques are used routinely in computer programs for producing different 'colours' digitally for image creation and other purposes, and have been developed into a computerized colour vision test. Clinically, colour vision can be tested using hue-discrimination techniques (e.g. the Farnsworth–Munsel 100 hue test) and normal values vary with age, peak ability occurring around the age of 19 years. Some effect by rods on cone vision has also been shown by rod function studies.

265

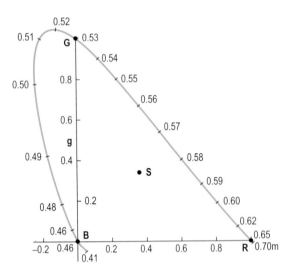

Fig. 5.2 Chromaticity chart. This 'nomogram' allows an estimate of the amount of red (R), green (G) and blue (B) required to produce a value of '1' which is equivalent to standard white (S).

VISION IS ALSO ABOUT SHAPE, FORM AND DEPTH PERCEPTION

The discrimination of shape and form is highly developed in primate vision and much research in the last decade has been devoted to determining the cortical localization of these functions. The appreciation of the complexity and sophistication of this aspect of visual perception has in part developed from the realization that the brain recognizes and can categorize objects according to shape irrespective of the angle or distance from which they are viewed or of the ambient lighting conditions, etc.

Shape processing is achieved by specialized orientation-sensitive cells in the visual cortex, but the extra dimension of form recognition, as in recognition of facial features, requires additional processing, possibly in the inferotemporal cortex. Studies of patients with specific visual defects such as prosopagnosia (inability to recognize familiar faces), however, are powerful indicators of the localization of visual functional sites.

Much is also known about depth perception. For instance it has been shown that there are specific cortical cells responsive only to disparate but simultaneous orientations of an object, presented to non-corresponding regions of the retina. However, no specific 'depth appreciation' cortical region has been identified since these cells have been found in

several defined cortical centres. In addition, multiple other cues also contribute to the appreciation of depth (see below). An understanding of these mechanisms can only come after a description and appreciation of the different types of visual stimuli that separately induce discrete responses in the brain.

LIGHT DETECTION AND DARK ADAPTATION

WHAT ARE THE LIMITS OF DETECTABLE LIGHT?

As in all biological systems, there is no precise answer to the above question. Light energy comes in quanta (small packets) and it has been estimated that between 50 and 150 quanta of light are required to strike the cornea for a discrete signal to be detected. Of these quanta, only about 10% actually reach the photoreceptors. The detection of this stimulus is not simply a function of photoreceptor stimulation but is also dependent on higher neural function, and the concept of a visual 'threshold' is more or less a statistical function dependent on how large the stimulus has to be to reach a level of 'recognition'. This is well recognized by anyone who performs a visual field test using an automated visual field analyser.

Thresholds and the frequency of seeing

A distinction must be made between the theoretical estimate of the number of quanta required to produce an electric stimulus in a patch-clamped photoreceptor cell and the psychophysical conversion of the light stimulus to a perceived sensation. The latter depends on the 'frequency of seeing' a repetitively presented minimal stimulus and is a probability function that varies between and within individual observers.

The former is theoretically a single photon of light. However, there is considerable 'noise' in the system owing, for instance, to random opening and closing of ion channels as a result of thermal isomerization of rhodopsin, or to scatter from background and/or stray light energy from the stimulus itself. These effects can account for up to 1000 quanta/degree, which is well above the absolute threshold for light stimulation. It is thought that some of this is 'smoothed' by coupling between photoreceptors.

What is the minimal stimulus for vision?

Even when theoretical biophysical considerations such as signal-to-noise ratio are taken into account, this deceptively simple question depends on many factors such as background illumination, spatial frequency, summation, wavelength, dark adaptation and optical qualities of the image-gathering system. The specific conditions have to be stated, therefore, before this quantity can be expressed.

In addition, consideration of whether a single rod can detect a single photon of light *in vivo* has to take into account the different routes that a rod can take to stimulate a ganglion cell and convert this into a behavioural response (see pp. 276–285).

DARK ADAPTATION CURVE AND RETINAL SENSITIVITY

The minimum visual stimulus varies depending on whether the stimulus is viewed in the dark or under normal/bright light conditions. In the dark, the eye becomes progressively more sensitive to light stimulation until the light threshold reaches a minimum after about 30 minutes. This is demonstrated in the dark adaptation curve (see Box 5.1), which has two components: an early one resulting from increases in the cone sensitivity and a second produced by increases in rod sensitivity. There is also a light adaptation curve for cones in which the sensitivity to light varies as the luminosity increases or decreases within a wide range of high ambient illumination (see below). Thus the shape of the curve can be varied by altering the conditions.

Light and dark adaptation are the psychophysical correlates of visual pigment bleaching and regeneration, and can be measured by reflection densitometry. This technique is based on the assumption that light reflected from the unbleached retina will contain lower amounts of 500-nm (peak sensitivity for rods) light than that reflected from the bleached retina, since there will be considerable absorption of 500-nm light by the dark-adapted retina. Reflection densitometry studies permit an evaluation of the photosensitivity of the retina, i.e. the rate at which bleaching takes place for a given intensity of illumination. It has been estimated that the normal retina absorbs 50% of the quanta of light striking the retina but, as discussed above, this is not necessarily associated with a perceived visual stimulus because the absorption by a single rod of a photon of light can have at least three outcomes.

Regeneration of rhodopsin after dark adaptation is slow, taking 30 minutes for completion with a half-time in humans of 5 min. This varies significantly between species. Clearly, the sensitivity of the retina

---

Box 5.1 Dark adaptation

The normal dark adaptation curve (a) varies if the conditions are varied: with a very small central white target, rods fail to become stimulated at all and the curve flattens out (b). If the cones are first light adapted by weakly stimulating them to maximum sensitivity or by adapting subjects to red light before placing them in the dark, the cone component can be 'lost' (c); subjects without cone vision also have no cone component (rod monochromats).

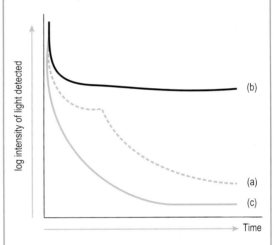

Figure outlining dark/light adaptation responses: (a) mixed rod and cone response of physiological dark adaptation, (b) pure cone response, (c) pure rod response. (Courtesy of H Dawson.)

---

in any individual will depend on the total amount of rhodopsin, and this relationship has been delineated in the Dowling–Rushton equation:

$$\log(z)/A = aB$$

where A is the threshold in complete dark adaptation, B is the fraction of bleached rhodopsin, and a is a constant of proportionality. This sort of mathematical relationship has been used to estimate the rhodopsin content of the retinas of patients with certain forms of retinal disease, such as Oguchi disease, fundus albipunctatus and especially vitamin A deficiency. However, it is important to realize that receptor sensitivity and rhodopsin content are not equivalent and that sensitivity to light is markedly reduced after partial bleaching, long before there is a reduction in rhodopsin content. This is clear in the isolated retina where photosensitivity is permanently reduced even after full recovery in the dark. These changes reflect the level of rhodopsin intermediates

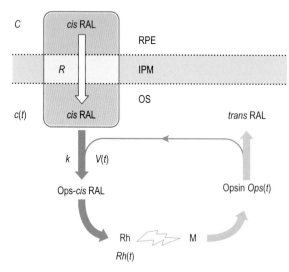

Fig. 5.3 Schematic of the MLP rate-limited model. Removal of photoproduct and regeneration of visual pigment is rate-limited by the delivery of 11-*cis* retinal (*cis* RAL) from the retinal pigmented epitehium (RPE) to opsin in the outer segment (OS). (From Lamb and Pugh 2004, with permission from Elsevier.) IPM, interphotoreceptor matrix; Rh, rhodopsin; M, metarhodopsin.

(metarhodopsin I and II) in the retina, which remain after bleaching (see Fig. 4.48, p. 256).

These effects are important in the determination of photosensitivity of discrete regions of the retina where it has been shown that reduced sensitivity can be detected in regions of the retina not exposed to point sources of light. Although this has been attributed to light scatter, there are probably other mechanisms operative here, particularly related to convergence of neural input (see below).

What does adaptation mean at a molecular level? There is considerable evidence to show that dark adaptation and regeneration of rhodopsin are dependent on the local concentration of 11-*cis* retinal, and the limiting factor for recovery after a large bleach is the rate at which 11-*cis* retinal is delivered to opsin in the bleached photoreceptors (Fig. 5.3). Thus, because a healthy retinal pigment epithelium is central to this process, age-related decline in dark adaptation can be explained on this basis.

In summary, adaptation is exactly what it means: that the retina rapidly adapts to changes in background illumination such that it can respond to increasingly strong or weak stimuli. However, the dynamic range of responses (normally a range from zero to a few hundred impulses per second) over which it functions at any specific level of illumina-

tion remains the same and the intensity of the response when it makes one is also the same. Put simply, the retina adapts rapidly to new lighting conditions when there is plenty of light about but slowly when light levels are low.

Melatonin and circadian rhythms

The light dark cycle, generated in the suprachiasmatic nuclei, drives the production of the pineal gland secretory product, melatonin. Melatonin may also be produced at other sites including the retina and bone marrow. It is synthesized from tryptophan via serotonin in two steps involving the enzymes serotonin-N-acetyl transferase (NAT) and hydroxyindole-O-methyl transferase (HIOMT). Secretion is either suppressed or synchronized by light and can adjust to night length. Melatonin provides information to the organisms to permit organization of various physiological functions and because it can adapt to night length it can promote a seasonal as well as a diurnal rhythmicity (Fig. 5.4; melatonin). Apart from its obvious physiological functions, such as sleep–wake patterns, melatonin influences immune diurnal variations in innate immune defence functions such as antioxidation, glucose regulation, blood coagulation enzyme systems and ocular functions such as control of aqueous secretion.

Melatonin is a methoxyindole synthesized and secreted principally by the pineal gland at night under normal environmental conditions. The endogenous rhythm of secretion is generated by the suprachiasmatic nuclei and entrained to the light/dark cycle. Light is able to either suppress or synchronize melatonin production according to the light schedule. The nyctohemeral rhythm of this hormone can be determined by repeated measurement of plasma or saliva melatonin or urine sulphatoxymelatonin, the main hepatic metabolite.

The primary physiological function of melatonin, whose secretion adjusts to night length, is to convey information concerning the daily cycle of light and darkness to body physiology. This information is used for the organization of functions, which respond to changes in the photoperiod such as the seasonal rhythms. There is still, however, only limited evidence for seasonal rhythmicity of physiological functions in humans related to possible alteration of the melatonin message in temperate areas under field conditions. Also, the daily melatonin secretion, which is a very robust biochemical signal of night, can be used for the organization of circadian rhythms. Although functions of this

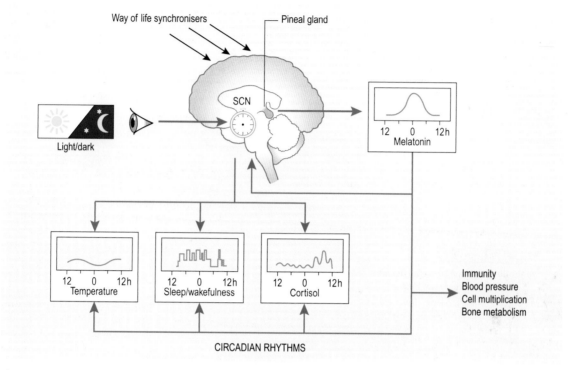

Fig. 5.4 Melatonin acts as an endogenous synchronizer. (From Claustrat *et al.* 2005, with permission from Elsevier.)

hormone in humans are mainly based on correlative observations, there is some evidence that melatonin stabilizes and strengthens the coupling of circadian rhythms, especially of core temperature and sleep–wake rhythms. The circadian organization of other physiological functions could depend on the melatonin signal, for instance immune, antioxidative defences, haemostasis and glucose regulation.

As the regulating system of melatonin secretion is complex, following central and autonomic pathways, there are many pathophysiological situations where the melatonin secretion can be disturbed. The resulting alteration could increase predisposition to disease, add to the severity of symptoms or modify the course and outcome of the disorder.

ARE TWO SMALL STIMULI EQUIVALENT TO ONE LARGE ONE (SUMMATION)?

The threshold for light detection can be measured arbitrarily by setting certain conditions of stimulus size, brightness, pupil size and level of background illumination, and recording how often a subject detects the stimulus. An empirically set level of 'hits'

or positive detection responses (e.g. 55%) can then be set and expressed in trolands (see Box 5.2). Experimentally it has been estimated that at the limit of light detection in the fully dark-adapted eye, the retina is illuminated to a level of 4.4×10^{-5} trolands, which is equivalent to the stimulation of only 1/5000 rods per second. However, if the light is concentrated on one area it will more readily elicit a response and it therefore becomes less practical to think of light energy in terms of area of retinal illumination; instead the minimum flux in light energy required to induce a detectable response is commonly accepted as the threshold and is around 120 quanta per second or, if the stimulus is instantaneous, between 5 and 15 quanta of light.

From this it is clear that stimulation of a single rod is insufficient to produce a visual sensation (even though an electrical response may occur in terms of a change in hyperpolarization of the cell membrane). Approximately 10–15 rods must be stimulated and the summed response must be collected either at the bipolar cell level or within the ganglion cells to induce a visual sensation. These determinations are approximate as fluctuations occur at all levels from the stimulus itself to the responses in each of the different cell types, and the final analysis is based on probabilities of a response taking place.

Spatial summation

As indicated above, the empirical determination of the absolute threshold of light detection depends on the stimulus size; therefore spatial summation must be important in setting this threshold. Each ganglion cell has a receptive field in which a light stimulus falling on a point within that field will produce a response. Receptive fields are the result of convergence of several photoreceptors to synapse with one bipolar cell and of several bipolar cells to synapse with a single ganglion cell (see next section).

Some limited general rules have therefore emerged concerning summation. Ricco's law states that the threshold intensity of a stimulus is inversely proportional to the area of the stimulus, provided the total stimulus area is sufficiently small to fit within the receptive field of a single ganglion cell. In terms of quanta, however, the amount of energy is independent of the area. As the receptive field size increases at greater distances from the fovea, Ricco's law also varies in the area in which it can be applied. In overlapping receptive fields, Ricco's law applies only partially in that larger stimuli require more quanta

to reach the absolute threshold. This has led to further attempts to formulate equations that would provide a general solution for these phenomena, but in practice no simple solution covers all possibilities and summation is best explained by probability theory (see above).

Temporal summation

When the retina is stimulated in rapid succession by a target, the level of response is the same as when the target is presented continuously for the same total period of time. This is known as temporal summation and is formulated by Bloch's law, which states: the intensity of the threshold stimulus is inversely proportional to the duration of the stimulus. Clearly this holds true only for a defined period of time as, if the interval between the stimuli were long, the effect would be rapidly lost. In practice the time interval is of the order of about 100 ms. Beyond this time there is still some degree of summation, known as partial summation, which decays exponentially.

Binocular summation

Summation may occur in visual stimuli received by corresponding retinal regions when using both eyes. In practice mostly because of optical aberrations (see below), the effect is not considered significant. However, it can be demonstrated using wavefront technologies to remove aberrations and indeed it has been shown that such aberrations account for between 5 and 15% of loss in visual discrimination. In a recent study, binocular summation and inhibition, defined as seeing five or more or fewer than five letters on the ETDRS visual acuity chart with both eyes compared with best visual acuity with each eye individually occurred at a prevalence rate of 21% and 2% respectively, which has considerable relevance to driving vision. In addition, the effect of amblyopia may be such that the loss of binocular summation has a distinct effect on overall visual acuity.

VISUAL ACUITY AND CONTRAST SENSITIVITY

VISUAL ACUITY IS NOT SIMPLY A FUNCTION OF CONE ACTIVITY

Visual acuity is a measure of the ability to discriminate two stimuli separated in space. Clinically, this is determined by discriminating letters on a chart, but this task also requires recognition of the form and shape of the letters, processes that involve higher centres of visual perception. Discrimination at a retinal level may therefore be determined by less complex stimuli such as contrast sensitivity gratings. Recent studies have in fact shown that the visual processes that allow discrimination between letters and gratings are fundamentally the same. Interestingly, testing visual acuity in older people using low luminance or low contrast charts, such as the SKILL test (Smith–Kettlewell Institute Low Luminance test), may be a good predictor of eventual development of macular degeneration.

Theoretically, the resolving power of the eye could be derived from an estimate of the angle subtended by a single photoreceptor [about 1.5 µ or 20 minutes (20′) of arc in the case of cones], as this represents the smallest unit distance separating two individually stimulated photoreceptors. However, it is well recognized that the resolving power of the eye can be as great as 0.5′ of arc, for instance when viewing a Landholt C target, or 4″ of arc when viewing a thin line on an illuminated background. This hyperacuity, or Vernier acuity, is achieved by the complexities of retinal neuronal synaptic organization, but the limits of acuity are still determined to some extent by the retinal mosaic or 'grain'.

The highest discriminatory capacity is subserved by cones, although a certain degree of resolution can be achieved by rods. The level of acuity, however, falls off rapidly the greater the distance from the fovea, such that at 5° from the central fovea visual acuity is only one-quarter of foveal acuity. As rod and cone longitudinal dimensions are not sufficiently different to explain the marked difference in acuity, and as the resolving power of the eye is greater than the theoretical limits based on cell size, other mechanisms must underpin acuity. Visual acuity is affected by the luminance of the test object and the degree of adaptation of the observer; dark adaptation increases both rod and cone acuity and therefore is not affected by the sensitivity of cones *per se*. In contrast, light adaptation increases sensitivity of cones but not rods (see above).

Vernier acuity, also known as hyperacuity, is used in everyday life, for instance in measuring distance with a ruler or detecting the time on a mechanical clock. Vernier acuity is not present in infancy but reaches its highest level of function around the age of 14. It is absent in strabismic amblyopia but may be present in patients with anisometropic amblyopia. Vernier acuity, is different from the recently recognized state of supervision, which has been revealed by the use of adaptive optics. Adaptive optics were developed for use in astronomy to minimize optical aberrations and correct higher order dynamic aberrations caused by such aspects as angle of viewing and accommodation, as compared with correction of static aberrations such as astigmatism and defocus (see below). When applied to the eye, for instance in the use of wavefront aberrometers and wavefront guided vision correction in refractive corneal surgery, adaptive optics can theoretically increase acuity to 'supervision' levels.

LIMITS OF AND LIMITATIONS ON ACUITY

The letters on reading charts such as the Snellen's test type and the ETDRS chart (see Box 5.3) have been constructed on the assumption that the average person can resolve two points separated by 1′ of arc. If the limit on acuity is in part determined by the single photoreceptor theory (above) then a one-to-one relationship between the photoreceptor and the nerve cell must exist if there is to be no downstream loss of acuity. For foveal cones such a relationship exists between cone cells, midget bipolar cells and midget ganglion cells (see section on retinal connections, pp. 279–285), but even midget cells have some interconnections with diffuse bipolar and ganglion cells. In spite of these connections, summation of information should not occur for cells subserving the highest levels of acuity and indeed is absent from foveal cone cells but is characteristic of rod cells; furthermore, it has been suggested that the improved visual acuity that occurs under conditions of light adaptation is the result of inhibition of these subsidiary connections.

Visual acuity is also limited by the physical behaviour of light, such as diffraction and chromatic/spheric aberration. A single point of light small enough to stimulate a single cone will produce diffraction rings in its traverse through the pupil sufficient to stimulate more than one cone. Similarly the prismatic separation of white light into its constituent wavelengths will lead to the stimulation of several cones of different types. It is clear therefore that resolution of images must be achieved at a postreceptor level and is in fact a function of the receptive field of each ganglion cell unit. Where there is minimal convergence of information from each receptor, i.e. where the one-to-one relationship between receptor and bipolar cell is maintained, then resolution is at its highest and this occurs at

Box 5.3 Assessment of visual acuity using standard letter charts

Visual acuity in clinical practice is determined as an empirical value based on the assumption that the cone photoreceptor has the ability to discriminate two objects in space subtended by an angle of 1 minute of arc at the nodal point of the eye (**A**). This is measured using a set of charts (optotypes) and standard normal visual acuity equates to the vision of 6/6 or 20/20 (i.e. 1.0 or 100%) when viewing a predetermined standard target (size of optotype letter) at 6 m (UK) or 20 feet (USA). Test conditions describing the ambient illumination, and the illumination of the letters on the chart to provide contrast are also arbitrarily set. The Snellen chart is based on the concept that the smallest spatial target that can be resolved subtends 1 minute of arc at the nodal point of the eye (see above) and although theoretically inaccurate, it serves as a useful parameter (**A**). The Snellen chart has rows of letters of decreasing size and is arbitrarily

set to produce the standard test at 6 m, although other charts with proportionally smaller letters can be used at shorter distances. The LOGMAR (LOGarithm of the Minimal Angle of Resolution (**B**) is more precisely designed with definitive sizing and spacing of the letters and can provide a more quantitative evaluation of visual acuity. It therefore tends to be the standard for use in clinical trials. As indicated in the text, spatial acuity better than 100% can be achieved, for instance when discriminating the 'offset' of a line or edge (**C**). This is termed Vernier acuity. In addition, visual acuity is modified by such factors as glare and contrast, and indeed can be measured as in the contrast sensitivity test using a sine wave grating as shown in (**D**), where diffraction and aberrations have degraded the contrast of a sinusoidal grating pattern. (From Schweigerling 2000, with permission from Elsevier.)

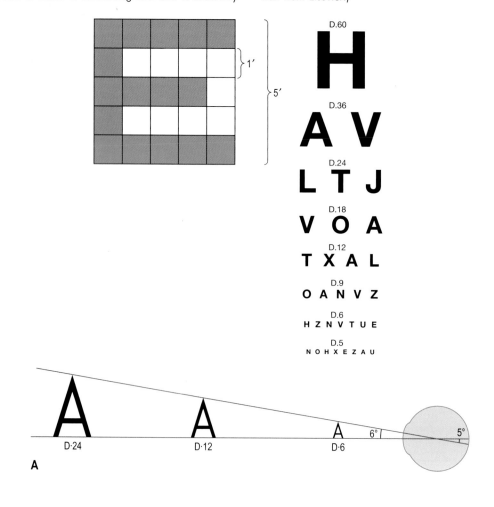

A

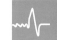

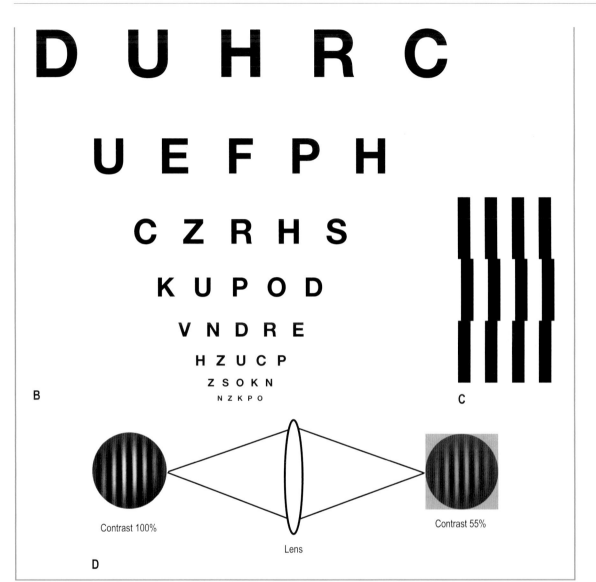

B

C

D

Contrast 100%

Contrast 55%

Lens

Box 5.4 Differential activation of neighbouring cones determines the limits of visual acuity

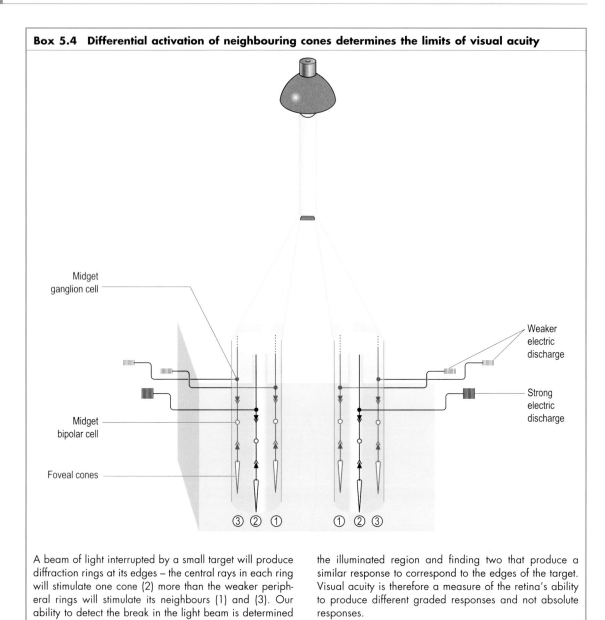

Midget ganglion cell

Midget bipolar cell

Foveal cones

Weaker electric discharge

Strong electric discharge

③ ② ①   ① ② ③

A beam of light interrupted by a small target will produce diffraction rings at its edges – the central rays in each ring will stimulate one cone (2) more than the weaker peripheral rings will stimulate its neighbours (1) and (3). Our ability to detect the break in the light beam is determined by comparing the differential responses in all the cones in the illuminated region and finding two that produce a similar response to correspond to the edges of the target. Visual acuity is therefore a measure of the retina's ability to produce different graded responses and not absolute responses.

the fovea. However, where there is increasing convergence of information, such as with several parafoveal cones synapsing with one bipolar cell, resolution obviously decreases.

The one-to-one relationship, however, does not adequately explain hyperacuity or Vernier acuity. Diffraction and spheric/chromatic aberrations have ruled out the concept of single unstimulated cones occurring between neighbouring stimulated cells; however, it is likely that discrimination is more a matter of degree than absolute responses, i.e. that resolution is achieved by certain receptors being *less stimulated* than their neighbouring receptors on either side. This is likely to occur with diffraction, where alternating light and dark rings emanate from a point source of light, and with chromatic aberration where different wavelengths of light are likely to stimulate their respective neighbouring cones to different degrees (see Box 5.4). This differential stimulation can be registered with the respective bipolar and ganglion cells and, if combined with a minimal degree of receptor convergence, can explain high levels of discrimination. In this way diffraction could explain, at least partly, the ability to resolve a break in a line subtending less than 10° of arc, since partial diffraction lines deriving from the edge of the break would ensure differential stimulation of cone receptors over a very small area. Stimulation of any particular cone is also likely to induce local inhibition (via receptive field mechanisms; see below) in neighbouring cones, thus enhancing resolution further.

These considerations have a number of implications. In particular, the resolving power of the eye is limited by the distance between two images such that a single cone or set of cones is appreciably less stimulated than the rest; the limit of resolution is therefore not an absolute determinant, but depends on conditions such as light and dark adaptation, background illumination, and other factors. Most importantly, it depends on the degree of dendritic connections that occur between the affected cones and the neural cells.

The resolving power of the eye therefore depends on:

- the distance between two objects
- the degree of light and dark adaptation
- the background illumination
- the dendritic connections between the cone and neurones.

CONTRAST SENSITIVITY

Visual acuity is also affected by contrast. The finest limits of resolution have been determined by the ability to discriminate a thin white line against a uniform background illumination (0.5′ of arc). The effects of diffraction are such that detection of this line depends on the liminal brightness increment (l.b.i.). This increment represents the endpoint at which the differential in brightness between the individual dark/bright oval diffraction rings produced at the edge of the line can be detected; if they are not sufficiently different from the background luminosity, then the line will not be detected. The l.b.i. is determined by the contrast between the light and dark lines, and can be measured quantitatively with a sinusoidal grating: a spatial pattern where the average luminance remains the same but the contrast between the light and shaded areas can differ.

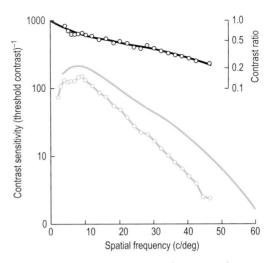

Fig. 5.5 Contrast sensitivity curve showing peak response at midspatial frequencies.

The degree of contrast (C) is described in terms of the maximum (I_{max}) and the minimum I_{min}) as follows:

$$C = (I_{max} - I_{min}) \,/\, (I_{max} + I_{min})$$

Discrimination of the grating is described in cycles per degree (the grating frequency) and visual acuity is equivalent to 1/grating frequency. Using this method it has been shown that there is a peak response in the middle range of frequencies (Fig. 5.5).

Contrast sensitivity is therefore set by the limits of the grating frequency and is affected by both the optics of the system and the direction of the grating lines, being most sensitive in vertical or horizontal directions. As for other methods of determining visual acuity, contrast sensitivity is affected by luminance. In addition, bar width, length and grating motion all affect sensitivity. In the latter there is likely to be significant cortical processing at this level, as there is for 'line modulation sensitivity', a technique whereby grating bars are composed of wavy lines and the subject is asked to determine whether the line is straight or not. This technique can provide highly sensitive measures of acuity.

Contrast sensitivity measurements, while an excellent measure of acuity, are sensitive to phase shifts and grating orientation and for absolute measures of object detection, object contrast is critical. In this context, mesopic low-contrast letter acuity is the most sensitive method for revealing small differences in retinal image 'quality', which influences 'recognition' as opposed to 'detection' of an object.

Wavelength also affects contrast sensitivity such that at high spatial frequencies the gratings appear to be of the same colour whereas at low frequencies (i.e. with coarse gratings), colour differences can be detected. Discrimination is poorest with red–green, however, suggesting that for low frequencies rod–cone interactions are important in achieving best visual acuity. Interestingly, contrast sensitivity appears to induce more electrical signal responses in M cells, generally thought to subserve rod function, than in P cells, which are linked to cone function (see below).

Does the retinotopic arrangement of fibres in the cortex have a bearing on acuity?

The representation of retinal ganglion cells in the LGN and cortex is disproportionately larger for foveal midget cells than for ganglion cells elsewhere in the retina. This produces a 'cortical magnification factor' for foveal cones over other cones. However, the magnification factor is not related solely to the reduced convergence of foveal cones on ganglion cells (see below), but also to a disproportionate LGN and cortical representation of neurones served by foveal cones.

BEST CORRECTED VISUAL ACUITY: EFFECTS OF EXTERNAL FACTORS

Visual acuity is, of course, affected by factors that do not relate directly to the retinal stimulus. These include pupil size, eye movements and binocular viewing.

Pupil size and visual acuity testing in infants

The size of the pupil affects the level of visual acuity in that a reduction in pupil size reduces aberrations but increases the effects of diffraction. Below 3 mm these effects tend to cancel each other out, and visual acuity is independent of pupil size, although wavefront aberrometry reveals that a pupil size of 2.5–3.0 mm produces the best image quality.

The level of visual acuity attained may also have the reverse effect on the size of the pupil. Luminance affects the level of acuity and the size of the pupil is affected by the light level via well-characterized pupil reflexes (see Box 5.5). The size of the pupil also indirectly affects the visual acuity by reducing the amount of light entering the eye when the light

---

Box 5.5 Pupillary light reflexes

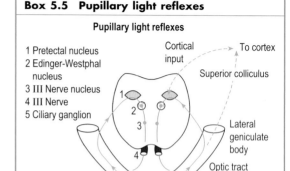

Pupillary light reflexes

1 Pretectal nucleus
2 Edinger-Westphal nucleus
3 III Nerve nucleus
4 III Nerve
5 Ciliary ganglion

- The afferent response commences in photoreceptors, is transmitted to retinal ganglion cells, enters the optic nerve, decussates at the chiasm and traverses the optic tract and terminates in the pretectal nucleus (bypassing the lateral geniculate nucleus).
- Both crossed (via posterior commissure) and uncrossed fibres pass from pretectal nucleus to Edinger–Westphal nucleus (parasympathetic).
- Parasympathetic fibres pass to the III nerve nucleus and leave the brainstem via the III nerve. Fibres synapse in the ciliary ganglion before supplying sphincter pupillae of iris (constriction) via short ciliary nerves.
- Uniocular light stimulus therefore gives rises to bilateral and symmetrical pupillary constriction.

---

stimulus is intense, and conversely increasing light capture under dim lighting conditions. This three-way relationship has been used to develop an objective measure of visual acuity, which may be useful in assessing vision in infants and others who are not able to cooperate in standard visual acuity testing. The test uses a high-resolution infrared pupillometry device to show changes in the amplitude of constriction in response to sine-wave gratings presented on a uniformly illuminated test background. As for contrast sensitivity, there is a peak response in the middle range of frequencies and the threshold for response correlates well with contrast sensitivity estimates of acuity. This pupil response is governed by higher visual pathways, being altered in patients with hemianopia but normal pupil light reflexes;

indeed, the phenomenon is well recognized by clinical neuro-ophthalmologists. Infrared pupillometry has been shown to be valuable in studies of delayed visual maturation and to be significantly more reliable than the Rosenbaum card method in which subjective comparisons of pupil size are made.

Eye movements

The concept that the continuous fine eye movements that occur as part of normal viewing are important in ensuring constant stimulation of the photoreceptors to maintain image perception remains popular. Indeed, it has been shown that images received by peripheral receptors fade rapidly if fixation is deliberately maintained in one position – the Troxler phenomenon. Although this was originally considered to be a mechanism for enhancing the central image by inhibiting peripheral images, use of a 'stabilized retinal image' has shown that elimination of these fine movements does not necessarily lead to a reduction in visual acuity. However, these findings were obtained using high-frequency gratings and it is possible that fine eye movements may be important at lower spatial frequencies in improving contrast.

Binocular viewing and the probability theory of visual perception

Perception is a relative occurrence and depends on many factors to achieve optimal levels (there is a significant element of chance in achieving this optimum). It follows therefore that two eyes are better than one at least in increasing the chances of the highest level of visual processing of the same image.

ELECTROPHYSIOLOGY OF THE VISUAL SYSTEM

As for any sensory system, the transmission of nerve impulses in retinal receptors and neurones is mediated by changes in electric potential across the cell membrane (see Ch. 3) and is accompanied by electric discharge. The action potential is usually an all-or-nothing event and, in muscle tissue, does not occur in the resting state. However, in neural tissue continuous discharge may be taking place and information is relayed by changes in the frequency or rate of electric discharge in the nerve, an increase in frequency usually representing stimulation and a decrease representing inhibition, thus emphasizing the essential binary nature of biological information systems similar to computers. This applies for all nerves in any system: the character of the received

sensation is determined not by the type of nerve but by the site of information relay in the cortex and its subsequent processing in the brain.

In the retina, these general principles hold true for retinal ganglion cells, but in bipolar, horizontal, amacrine and photoreceptor cells the electrical response is more of a tonic or graded response, and the direction of the response can be positive or negative. For instance, it is this graded response that permits spatial discrimination via differential responses to diffraction rings, as described above. However, the graded response in the bipolar cell becomes an on/off response in the ganglion cell. As Ikeda (1993) has put it, retinal information is converted from an analogue signal to a digital signal at the final stage of retinal processing, i.e. at the connection between ganglion and bipolar cells.

THE ELECTRICAL RESPONSE IS INITIATED BY PHOTOTRANSDUCTION

As we have seen (see Ch. 4, p. 256), when a photon of light strikes the photoreceptor outer segment, conversion of rhodopsin to the activated molecule induces a series of molecular events culminating in an electrical response. Cells, and particularly neurones, normally exist in a 'charged' state in that the inside of the cell is 'negative' with respect to the extracellular environment, creating an electrical potential difference across the cell membrane. This condition is maintained by differential distribution of Na^+ and K^+ ions on either side of the cell membrane (see Box 5.6). When a neurone is stimulated, there is an initial period of gradually increasing positivity (the generator potential), which culminates in a spike discharge characterized by a rapid depolarization response of the cell. This is achieved by the rapid influx of Na^+ through ion channels that are 'opened'.

In the photoreceptor the reverse situation occurs. Under resting conditions in the dark, the outer segment is maintained in a depolarized state through open ('leaky') Na^+ channels, which permit the influx of sodium ions from the extracellular space. When light stimulates the outer segment, the sodium channels are abruptly closed, stopping the influx of sodium and thereby leading to a reduced level of depolarization, i.e. a relative hyperpolarization. This is a direct result of rhodopsin isomerization and is mediated by amplification mechanisms involving cyclic guanosine monophosphate (cGMP) (see Ch. 4, p. 257).

The hyperpolarization response is transmitted by a flux in calcium ions along the length of the photoreceptor to the synapse with the bipolar cell (Ca^{2+} wave), which is then induced to release its transmitter (glutamate) (see below). Bipolar cells may then adapt to one of two responses to glutamate depending on the receptor induced: an ON response, which is a hyperpolarized state, and an OFF response, which is a depolarization response (see below). Indeed, the hyperpolarized state conferred on the bipolar cell is also transmitted to the horizontal cells in the same region, as has been shown experimentally using microelectrodes. However, hyperpolarization of the bipolar cell is not as steep as that of the photoreceptor in the excited state.

It will be obvious, therefore, that not only is there a resting potential difference across the photoreceptor cell membrane but there is also a potential difference along the length of the photoreceptor in the dark between the relatively depolarized outer segment tip and the hyperpolarized synaptic region of the cell at its interaction with the bipolar cell. This generates the 'dark currents' in the eye, which are reversed by the photic current on light stimulation when the photoreceptor becomes hyperpolarized (see Box 5.6).

ELECTROPHYSIOLOGY OF SINGLE RETINAL CELLS

Early studies in this field concentrated on the large single neurones that could be obtained from invertebrate eyes and showed that typical action potentials could be obtained, usually preceded by a generator potential (see Box 5.7). Surrounding neurones were usually inhibited when action potentials occurred in a single nerve.

Later studies of electrode-impaled optic nerves in vertebrates showed that the rate of discharge in certain nerve fibres increased (ON response) when a light stimulus was presented to the eye, while it decreased in other fibres (OFF response). Yet others produced an ON/OFF response. As it was known that there were 150×10^6 photoreceptors but only 1×10^6 optic nerve fibres, it followed that many receptors must feed information into a single neurone, i.e. there must be convergence of signals and some of these must be inhibitory while others are stimulatory. On this basis, the concept of receptive fields was developed and confirmed by direct experimental testing on isolated optic nerve fibres using discrete spots of light to stimulate the retina (see Box 5.8). Several phenomena, such as summa-

---

Box 5.6 Dark currents

Dark currents occur in the resting state (dark adapted eye) owing to 'Na⁺-leaking' outer segments.

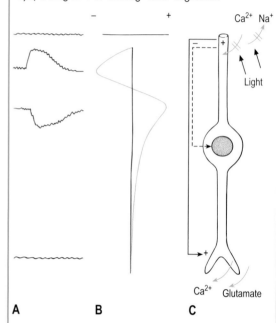

A   B   C

The conversion of light energy to an electric response is dependent on specialized ion channels that tightly control the permeability of the cell membrane to Na^+ and Ca^{2+}. Light stimulation reverses the dark current by closing Na^+ channels in outer segments and releasing Ca^{2+} (and glutamate) at synapses. The cGMP-gated Ca^{2+} channel and the Na^+/Ca^{2+}, K^+ exchanger are located in the plasma membrane of the photoreceptor, not in the disk stack, but are complexed together with peripherin/rds-rom-1, an integral protein of the disk rim.

---

tion, which could previously be inferred only from psychophysical experiments, were directly confirmed. Indeed, summation effects could be compared with the effects of generator potentials in other systems that, in ganglion cells, are called synaptic potentials. The ON/OFF response in the optic nerve fibres has been shown to correlate with the centre/surround organization of the receptive field and is based on interneuronal interactions causing inhibition in surround cells.

Recent studies have provided further information on retinal circuitry and its organization. ON/OFF receptive fields apply to cone–bipolar–ganglion cell circuitry while rod cells synapse directly into cone–cone circuits (see below). ON/OFF receptive field

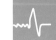

Box 5.7 Generator potentials

Generator potentials

(a) Single neurone responding to single large electric stimulus produces an action potential

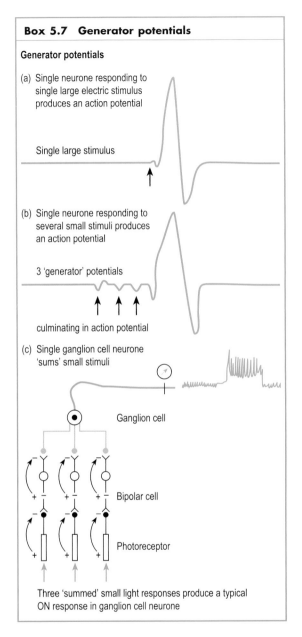

Single large stimulus

(b) Single neurone responding to several small stimuli produces an action potential

3 'generator' potentials

culminating in action potential

(c) Single ganglion cell neurone 'sums' small stimuli

Ganglion cell

Bipolar cell

Photoreceptor

Three 'summed' small light responses produce a typical ON response in ganglion cell neurone

---

gence. P cells have small receptive fields receiving information directly from single or only a few bipolar cells (see below).

How does the photochemical change in the receptor produce the spike discharge in the retinal neurone?

Horizontal cells at the receptor–bipolar cell interface and amacrine cells at the bipolar–ganglion cell interface are integrally involved in the organization of the retinal neuronal response to light. Single-cell recordings have shown that the hyperpolarization response at the receptor level is a graded response (see above, discussion of visual acuity), not an ON/OFF response. Similarly, the hyperpolarizing horizontal cell response is a graded response, but in the horizontal cell there is a longer latency and the potential for summation over a wide range. The bipolar cell response is also graded but with a centre/surround effect where the centre hyperpolarizes and the surround depolarizes. In the amacrine cell transient spikes can be observed, especially if correlated with the ON/OFF response, but only in the ganglion cell is a sustained spike discharge observed with a true depolarization occurring for ON, OFF and ON/OFF responses, depending on which type of ganglion cell is studied. This all-or-none response is graded only in the sense that the frequency or rate of discharge that occurs in the ganglion cell varies with the degree of depolarization.

RETINAL CONNECTIONS, CIRCUITRY AND NEUROTRANSMITTERS

Retinal connections

What is the basis of receptive field organization in the retina? As detailed above, detection and processing of the light stimuli by the retina is founded on the retinal receptor/neuronal network comprising the photoreceptors (rods and cones) and the neurones (bipolar cells and ganglion cells). The information finally transmitted to the lateral geniculate nucleus in the brain by the ganglion cells (ON, OFF and ON/OFF cells) is received directly from the bipolar cells but is modulated by horizontal cells and amacrine cells in the plexiform layers in the retina. This is canonically described in a simple arrangement of direct bipolar cell activity and lateral inhibition by horizontal cells and amacrine cells (see Ch. 1 for details). In reality, retinal microcircuitry is more complex than this, underpinned by the fact that there are several different types of each retinal cell (Fig. 5.6). In addition, the general arrangements

---

organization applies to several different types of signal, including light–dark, blue–yellow and red–green (see below). Amacrine cells and horizontal cells considerably modify the ON/OFF microcircuitry organization and, variably so far, each type of circuit. In addition, the receptive fields of retinal neurones depend on the size of the cell: big ganglion cells (magnocells, M cells) have large receptive fields and small ganglion cells (parvocells, P cells) have small ones. M cells receive from many amacrine and bipolar cells, producing a high degree of conver-

Box 5.8 Organization of visual information into discrete receptive fields

The receptive field of a retinal ganglion cell neurone is the area of retina covered by that cell in which a light stimulus alters the frequency of discharge (**A**). The size of the receptive field varies from 200 to 600 μm in diameter. Receptive fields may have an ON centre (increased rate of discharge) and an OFF surround (decreased rate of discharge), an OFF centre and an ON surround, a double opponent ON/OFF centre/surround organization, or a pseudodouble opponent centre/surround organization (**B**); in addition, each of these arrangements occurs for detection of dark–light, red–green and yellow–blue. It is likely that the receptive fields are arranged in a hexagonal array because this will cover an area most efficiently with minimal overlap (**C**). R, red; G, green.

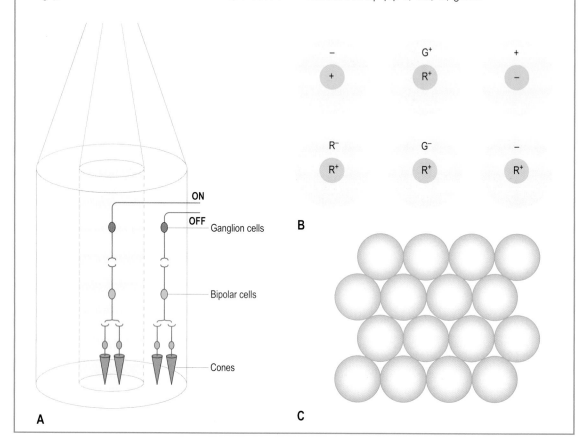

found in most mammalian retinas are complicated by the presence of the fovea in primates, which is characterized by a single type of ganglion cell. An excellent review of this field has been published by Masland (2001).

There are several retinal microcircuits emanating from the photoreceptors acting in parallel, and activating around a dozen cone-driven bipolar cells. Thus cones form several different types of microcircuits with a range of bipolar cells while rod microcircuitry is minimal (Fig. 5.7). In evolutionary terms, cones developed first, even though there are 20 times more rods than cones in the retina. Cone-bipolar cells synapse in the inner plexiform layer in a highly ordered set of stacks, each with a different number of connections and with its unique set of ionotropic, metabotropic (mGlur6), glycinergic and GABAergic receptors and calcium-binding proteins reflecting their inhibitory or excitatory output (translated into ON or OFF responses in the ganglion cell, see Box 5.7 and Figs 5.7 and 5. 8). There are several different types of ON/OFF bipolar cells in part determined by the duration of the response (transient versus sustained); in addition, a single bipolar cell for these types of responses (non-chromatic ON/OFF) takes information from more than one cone (Fig. 5.9).

The organization of colour detection is somewhat different. Wavelength discrimination (see below)

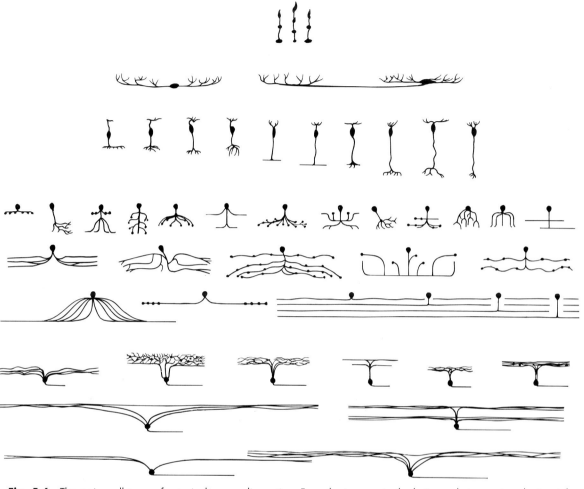

Fig. 5.6 The major cell types of a typical mammalian retina. From the top row to the bottom, photoreceptors, horizontal cells, bipolar cells, amacrine cells and ganglion cells. (From Masland 2001, with permission from Nature Publishing Group.)

requires output from at least two cones to have something to compare against. 'Blue' (short wavelength) cones make synapses with a specialized type of cone-bipolar, while the remainder of the cones (long wavelength red–green cones, comprising around 85%) connect with several different bipolar cells (Figs 5.7 and 5.8). Colour discrimination is therefore made by comparison of light detection by a short wavelength cone (ON/OFF) with that from a long wavelength cone (either red or green, ON/OFF), i.e. essentially a dichromatic system. In most mammalian retinas, there is no red/green discrimination (i.e. true dichromatisim with comparison of only one long wavelength cone with a short wavelength cone) and in 5% of humans this is also true (red–green colour blindness). These concepts are dealt with in more detail later in the chapter (see p. 292).

So where does rod microcircuitry fit into this neuronal organization? Rods detect dim light while cones detect bright light. Detection of dim light by rods is not to be confused with the OFF response of cone bipolar OFF cells (i.e. the response to the absence of light) but is a positive response by rod cells to very low levels of light. Rods connect indirectly with ganglion cells through cone bipolar cells (Fig. 5.7): large numbers of rods synapse with a single rod bipolar cell, which then connects via gap junctions with a cone bipolar cell through a particular type of amacrine cell, the AII cell.

In primates, there is further specialization derived from the system of midget cells: midget ganglion cells connect directly with one cone bipolar cell and through this cell with one cone photoreceptor. Thus

281

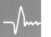

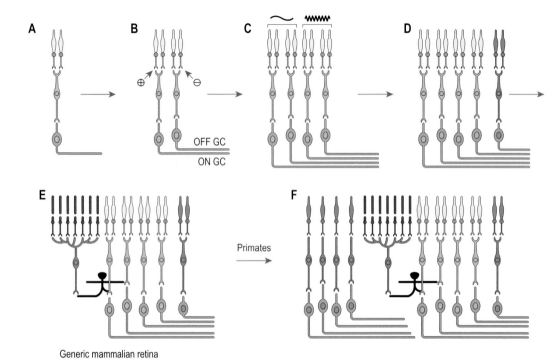

Fig. 5.7 The bipolar cell pathways of mammalian retinas assembled from individual components. This diagram is intended to emphasize the overall organization of the parallel channels. Rods are not as clumped as would be suggested here. For visual clarity, cones are shown contacting only a single bipolar cell each; in fact all cones contact several bipolar cells. (From Masland 2001, with permission from Nature Publishing Group.)

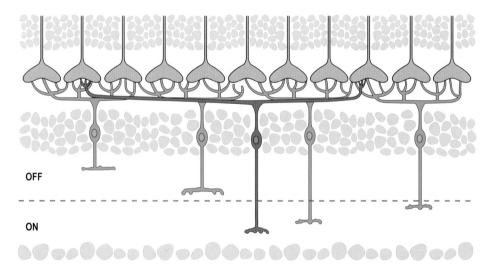

Fig. 5.8 The connections with cones and axonal stratification of different types of bipolar cells. Five different types of bipolar cells are illustrated. Two of them are diffuse (chromatically non-selective) ON bipolar cells terminating in the inner half of the inner plexiform layer. Two are diffuse OFF bipolar cells terminating in the outer half. Each samples indiscriminately from the spectral classes of cones. The blue cone bipolar, however, contacts only blue cones and thus is spectrally tuned to short wavelengths. Within the ON or OFF sublayer, axons of the bipolar cells terminate at different levels, indicating that they contact different sets of postsynaptic partners. (From Masland 2001, with permission from Nature Publishing Group.)

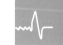

A
B

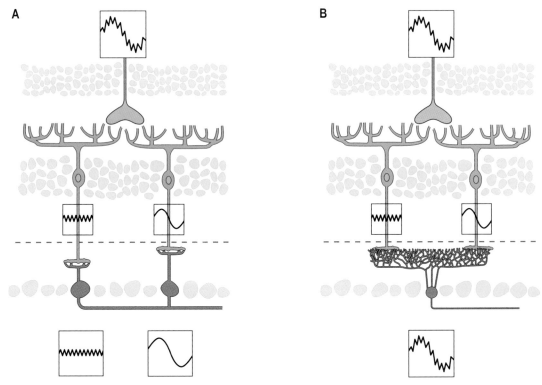

Fig. 5.9 How transient (high-pass) and sustained (low-pass) bipolar cells decompose the output of a cone. The resulting high- and low-frequency channels can contact narrowly stratified ganglion cells (**A**) in which case the two frequency bands are transmitted via separate parallel channels to the brain. A more broadly stratified ganglion cell (such as a beta cell) receives input from both types of bipolar cells. Such a ganglion cell (**B**) has a broadband response. Many such combinations are possible, as are many permutations of input from amacrine cells. (From Masland 2001, with permission from Nature Publishing Group.)

there are a huge number of small bipolar cells and midget ganglion cells at the fovea limited only by the packing of cones in this rod-free area. For instance, midget cells comprise about 70% of the ganglion cells in the monkey fovea. They have a simple centre/surround organization underpinning the excellent spatial resolution of 'supervision'; and it is believed that the midget system also creates the dual circuits required for red–green differentiation added to the existing blue cone system (see Box 5.8 and Figs 5.7 and 5.8).

Horizontal cells (Fig. 5.6) in the outer plexiform layer provide feedback for the rods and cones. For cones, this is classically believed to be in the form of contrast and mostly via generating inhibitory information to ganglion cells surrounding the activated cell (similar to the inhibitory effect of an action potential in a bundle of peripheral neurones on the neighbouring unstimulated neurones, see p. 280). This produces the centre/surround organization of ganglion cells (see Box 5.8). Some also believe that

horizontal cells may mediate their effects based on subtracting the information on the average illumination of the entire retina from that stimulating a restricted set of cones, thus underpinning the mechanism of light adaptation. Rods are separately modified by horizontal cells because of the anatomical location which separates the contact point with the rod far from the rod's contact with the cone-bipolar cell.

In contrast, amacrine cells are much more numerous than horizontal cells (Fig. 5.6) and have a wide range of functions. There are 29 types of amacrine cells, some modifying ganglion cell response over a wide area while others are much more restricted. In addition, they inhibit, enhance, entrain, refine through the large range of neurotransmitters and receptors discussed above (e.g. dopamine, acetylcholine, glutamate, GABA, glycine etc.). They thus affect many functions such as centre/surround organization, orientation selectivity, light–dark effects and colour discrimination. Some amacrine cells

283

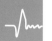

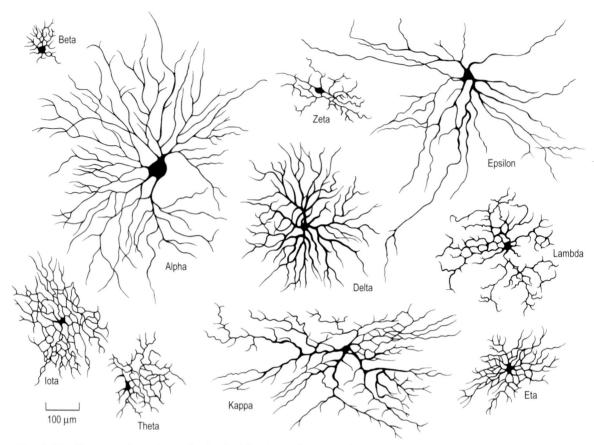

Fig. 5.10 The types of ganglion cells identified thus far in the retina of the cat. Ongoing work in the rabbit and monkey confirms this diversity and many of the cells observed are probably homologues of those seen in the cat. (Courtesy of Dr D Berson.)

may have very small arborizations and function entirely within the receptive fields of a wide-field ganglion cell. Thus some degree of information processing may occur at the ganglion cell level (e.g. in contrast gain control) before it reaches the visual cortex. Recent evidence suggests that retinal information processing can underlie ways in which the human eye can detect changes in moving natural scenes, such as movement of an object relative to its background, which appear to induce correlated firing in a group of retinal neurones. In this way the retina is able to distinguish movements of the object from movements related to fixation movement of the retina as it tracks the object.

Finally there are about 15 different types of ganglion cell (Fig. 5.10). Originally described as X (slow, tonic) and Y (fast, transient) cells in the cat, and P

(parvocellular, midget) and M (magnocellular, parasol) cells in the monkey, several others are now known to be responsible for centre/surround organization and direction/orientation selectivity. In addition, a separate rare population of ganglion cells connects with neurones in the pretectal nucleus and controls pupil light responses (see Box 5.5). There is a further rare set of photosensitive ganglion cells expressing the opsin melanopsin. These cells regulate the production of melatonin by the pineal gland and are thus involved in entrainment of circadian rhythms (see p. 268).

From all of the above it is clear that there is considerable diversity in the retinal microcircuitry in which significant information processing occurs before its transmission to the higher centres in the brain.

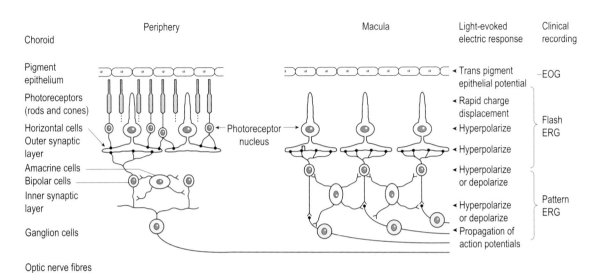

Fig. 5.11 Source of electrophysiological 'traces' from retinal layers. The electro-oculogram lies at the RPE layer while the ERG is retinal. The pattern ERG represents the response after processing in the bipolar cell layer. (Courtesy AM Halliday.)

CLINICAL VISUAL ELECTROPHYSIOLOGY

Clearly it is not possible to determine human electrophysiological responses by direct intracellular recording. However, electrical potentials do exist in the eye and these can be altered by stimulation with bright flashes of light, producing mass responses of the tissue. These responses represent the resultants of many cellular potentials and the source of the discharges can only be inferred. However, extensive studies have located the source of retinal electric responses at different levels in the retina (Fig. 5.11).

Resting potential and the electro-oculogram

Since the eye acts as a dipole, it possesses a measurable resting potential, which is generated at the interface between the retinal pigment epithelium (RPE) and the photoreceptors (the resting retinal potential) and is about 60 mV in height. At a molecular level, the electro-oculogram is representative of the trans-retinal pigment epithelial potential differences generated by separation of ionic gradients across the RPE and maintained by tight junctions. Similar trans-epithelial potential differences occur across all non-leaking epithelial layers. As the eye becomes light adapted there is a steady rise in this potential, which is recordable as a reversible potential on horizontal eye movement and is known as

Box 5.9 The electro-oculogram

The electro-oculogram (EOG) is a record of the electrical dipole occurring between the front and the back of the eye and reversing in current direction when the eye moves from side to side. The height of the potential difference increases in conditions of bright illumination.

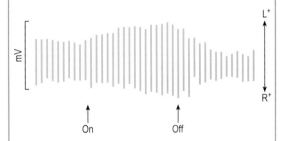

An EOG recording – vertical lines represent the alternating dipole as eyes are moved from left (L) to right (R). The 'light rise' is seen as an increase in the height of the vertical lines as the light is switched 'on'.

the light rise (see Box 5.9). This effect is the result of an extracellular flow of current caused by changes in the potassium concentration in the interphotoreceptor matrix. The electro-oculogram (EOG) is lost in conditions that disrupt the RPE–photoreceptor relationship, such as retinal detachment.

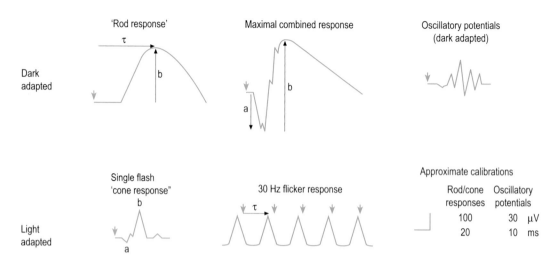

Fig. 5.12 Diagram of the five basic ERG responses defined by the standard. These waveforms are exemplary only and are not intended to indicate minimum, maximum or even average values. Large arrowheads indicate the stimulus flash. Dotted arrows exemplify how to measure time to peak (τ, implicit time), a-wave amplitude and b-wave amplitude.

The electroretinogram

The electroretinogram (ERG) is superimposed on the electro-oculogram and is the cumulative electrical response to a light stimulus from all the retinal elements. It is affected not only by the intensity and duration of the stimulus but also by the stimulus wavelength and pattern, and the level of light–dark adaptation of the retina as for the sensory response itself.

The ERG has several components (Fig. 5.12). Under mesopic conditions, the early receptor potential is barely detectable and becomes apparent only with an extremely high-intensity flash stimulus in a deeply dark-adapted eye. It originates from the photochemical reactions in the rod outer segments on stimulation by light and is dependent on the density of rods and high levels of unbleached rhodopsin. The early receptor potential may therefore be detectable in eyes where the inner retina has been destroyed but the outer retina is substantially intact, e.g. central retinal artery occlusion. However, it is not normally recorded because of the above physiological constraints.

The negative 'a' wave is generated by hyperpolarization in the photoreceptors' inner segments (Granit's PIII component), the a1 component coming from the cones and the a2 from the rods. In contrast, the 'b' wave (Granit's PII component) is believed to come from the bipolar cells either directly or indirectly via signal spread to the Müller cells; b1 is generated by cone-dominated and b2 by rod-dominated bipolar cells. The b wave is lost in certain retinal vascular conditions, such as central retinal vein occlusion.

Oscillatory potentials are thought to be generated by amacrine cells, while the slow rising 'c' wave (Granit's PI) depends on an intact pigment epithelium. However, the electro-oculogram provides a more effective estimate of the integrity of the pigment epithelium. Oscillatory potentials are lost in patients with diabetes.

The ERG as described above is in essence a response to luminous intense stimuli. However, the pattern ERG (PERG), which is the ERG response to a reversing checkerboard of black and white squares of equivalent luminance, is thought to represent the electric response to spatial contrast, probably from ON-centre ganglion cells. Advances in imaging techniques have allowed the confocal scanning laser ophthalmoscope to be used for psychophysical studies in which very narrow beams of light can be directed to discrete receptive field regions in the retina from which an ERG response can be obtained (multifocal ERG).

The visual evoked potential

The visual evoked potential (VEP) records electric activity from the occipital cortex following presentation of a light stimulus to the retina and represents a limited electroencephalogram (EEG). Recordings are taken from a set of six electrodes placed around both left and right occipital cortices, each producing a discrete wave pattern of different amplitudes.

Several types of VEP can be induced, including flash, flash-pattern, pattern-onset, pattern-offset, and pattern-reversal. Considerable individual variability in the wave pattern is seen with the flash VEP, which is composed of two phases: the evoked potential and the after discharge (Fig. 5.13). Variations also occur in the amplitude of response depending on the level of dark adaptation. A pattern-flash VEP is evoked when a black and white checkerboard stimulus is presented. The amplitude of this response is considerably better correlated with the visual acuity. However, a significant electric interference in this response is caused by switching the stimulus on and off (the onset/offset response). The

flash-evoked potential has three components – N1,P1; N2,P2; and N3,P3 – while the pattern-evoked potential is essentially monophasic (see Fig. 5.13). The flash VEP is considered to arise from area V2 of the cortex with retinal origins in the entire papillomacular bundle, while the pattern response is considered to arise in V1 plus ganglia cell receptive fields corresponding to large checks (M cells) and small checks (P cells).

Presentation of a pattern-reversed black and white equiluminant checkerboard can overcome the onset–offset problem if the pattern is reversed at an appropriately short interval, as the effects tend to cancel each other out. Indeed the stimulus can be set to produce pattern-onset, pattern-offset and pattern-reversal VEPs, each of which has a characteristic set of wave patterns depending on the conditions (Fig. 5.14). Considerable ingenuity has been developed in techniques for studying half-field stimulation, macular vision and the effects of age, right versus left eye, etc. However, clinically this test has greatest applicability in assessing the function of the optic nerve by measuring the latency of the response, and in assessing the integrity of foveal vision by evaluation of the pattern and amplitude of the wave forms.

FLICKER

A spoor or beam of light can flicker so fast that the sensation of flicker is lost. The point at which this happens is known as the critical fusion frequency (CFF) and the brightness of the steady-state light is the same as the mean brightness of the flickering

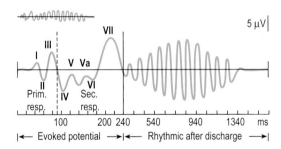

Fig. 5.13 Typical VEP tracing showing several peaks and troughs in the primary and secondary responses with the prominent 'after discharge'.

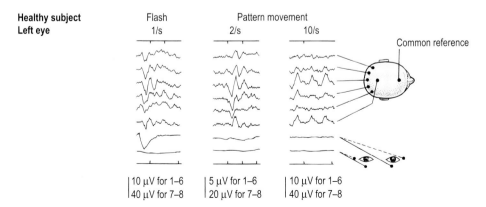

Fig. 5.14 Flash and pattern-averaged VEP responses from each of six electrodes placed over the occipital region of the skull. Pattern reversals were performed at two different rates (middle and right panels). The two lower tracings represent simultaneous ERG recordings. (Courtesy of Dr Ikeda.)

light midway through its cycle. Brighter stimuli have a higher CFF and rods have less ability to achieve fusion than cones (see below).

The fact that fusion occurs at all indicates that there must be some degree of persistence of sensation after the stimulus has ceased, but clearly this is more effective at lower levels of illumination than at higher ones. Fusion is thought to be the result of an after-effect, so that a succeeding stimulus can fall on the retina while it is still responding to the first stimulus. However, it is more probably related to light adaptation in which the response to light is accelerated at higher intensities. In terms of flicker measured by an ERG response, the CFF is seen as a smoothing out of the electric response, which is set at a higher level in millivolts. Presumably it would be possible to induce a second ERG response by presenting a superimposed flash on this new level of illumination.

Subjectively, fusion occurs at 60 cycles/s, but the ERG CFF occurs at 25 cycles/s. Therefore, by setting the flicker cycle at 25 cycles/s one can obtain, through the flicker ERG, a measure of cone function in isolation (see below). Interestingly, direct electrophysiological studies on optic nerve fibres have shown that ganglion cells with a high spike discharge rate also have a high threshold for CFF and vice versa.

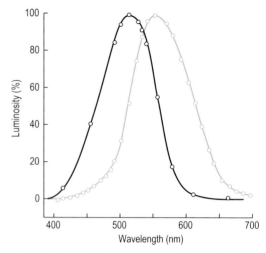

Fig. 5.15 Spectral sensitivity curves showing basis for the Purkinje shift.

COLOUR VISION

COLORIMETRY AND COLOUR DISCRIMINATION

Colorimetry is a measure of function at the photoreceptor level. In contrast, colour discrimination is a cortical function related to perception and the later stages of visual processing. Colorimetry or the measurement of colour is based on techniques of colour matching, which have a long history going back to the days of Newton, Helmholz and particularly Maxwell in the mid-19th century. Indeed, Maxwell, who was recently described in biography as the man who changed the world, is credited with asserting that all vision is colour vision; in a sense, as will be seen later, this is probably a valid perspective. Standards for measuring colour have been established for certain reference conditions of illumination based on the assumption that only a small area of the central fovea is illuminated by the test stimulus; a standard V (λ) or visible wavelength curve was adopted by the Commission Internationale de

l'Eclairage (CIE) in 1964. A colour (C) is specified in terms of the three primary colours by the equation:

$$C = r \cdot (R) + g \cdot (G) + b \cdot (B)$$

and is measured with colour-matching instruments such as the flicker photometer or with spectrophotometers fitted, for instance, with arrays of wavelength-selective photodiode detectors.

DIFFERENT COLOURS HAVE DIFFERENT LUMINOSITY

Spectral sensitivity curves

In the dark-adapted state, light of different wavelengths appears variably bright with a peak luminosity at about 500 nm in the blue–green region, i.e. for lights of equal energy, blue–green appears brightest in the dark (Fig. 5.15). Under photopic conditions, however, peak brightness occurs around 555 nm in the yellow–green. Brightness curves of different wavelengths like this are determined under photopic conditions by flicker photometry. This phenomenon, in which short wavelengths become brighter compared with long wavelengths as luminance is reduced, is known as the Purkinje shift, and begins under mesopic conditions when cone function is still active.

Experimentally, the flicker ERG is useful in studying the Purkinje shift because rod and cone responses can be distinguished by setting the flicker rate above 25 cycles/s, which rod photoreceptors cannot detect (see above). Purkinje shifts are therefore not detectable in guinea-pigs (pure rod) or squirrels (pure cone), but can be detected in cats, which are rod-dominated.

Photochromatic interval

The Purkinje shift underlies the photochromatic interval, which is a measure of the difference in 'brightness' between the absolute threshold at which light of any wavelength is just detected and the brightness at which it appears coloured. Clearly, this interval is vanishingly small at the red end of the visible spectrum and is maximal at about 570 nm.

Cone thresholds

As we have seen above, thresholds are an artificial concept that depend on a critical number of 'hits' on photoreceptors by quanta of light. In practice, under defined conditions light thresholds are measurable and have been well characterized for rods. Cone thresholds can also be measured, for instance by using only the early part of the dark adaptation curve or by using very small bright flash stimuli, which only impinge on the central fovea. By choosing suitable conditions of light adaptation (e.g. by adapting with blue light to desensitize the rods), it is possible to measure cone thresholds with different wavelengths of light. In this way, cone-specific spectral curves can be produced.

COLOUR DETECTION REQUIRES MORE THAN ONE TYPE OF PHOTORECEPTOR

Photoreceptors respond to stimuli by changes in the frequency of electric discharge. Indeed, this is true for all neuronal impulses. Since photoreceptors respond to both luminosity and wavelength, a retina that has a single type of photoreceptor (such as a rod) will not be able to distinguish one stimulus from the other under different circumstances. Wavelength discrimination therefore requires a panel of photoreceptors with peak responsiveness at specific wavelengths independent of their responses to changing luminosity. In theory, the more variety in receptor type with specific spectral sensitivities, the greater the ability to discriminate wavelength, as for any single wavelength stimulus it is the pattern of discharges from the entire panel of receptors that determines this discriminatory ability. Probably through evolutionary constraints, two types of cone photoreceptor provide sufficient discriminatory ability for survival of the species and the additional red–green length wavelength separation is an addi-

tional component restricted to primates (see above under Retinal connections).

Trichromatic theory of colour vision

A specific colour or hue is therefore detected by the summation of responses from a mixture of receptors, and the contribution from each of the three primary photoreceptor types can be deduced from spectral mixing curves (see Box 5.10). Indeed, such colour mixing phenomena are the result of 'confusion', i.e. our inability to differentiate sufficiently narrow wavelengths. This is a reflection of the physiological limits on wavelength discrimination set by our having only three cone photoreceptors. (Certain species of fish have four cone photoreceptors.)

However, hue discrimination is not exclusively a retinal-processing phenomenon. Experiments testing the ability of humans to detect the four unique hues (red, green, yellow and blue) using three chromatic mechanisms in P cells tuned to detect L/M and S-L/M show that hue discrimination requires higher order colour perceptual mechanisms (see below).

Psychophysical evidence for three cone photoreceptors

Experiments using cone thresholds and light adaptation techniques have confirmed that there are three types of cone that respond differently to the same wavelength of light. These are reflected in the spectral sensitivity curves for the three photoreceptors, which form the basis of the chromaticity chart (see pp. 266 and 305). Recent experimental studies have shown that light adaptation is mediated by two mechanisms: (a) changes in intracellular calcium level; and (b) a slower mechanism, possibly involving interaction between dopamine release and melatonin. Studies of colour blind individuals have also provided confirmatory evidence of the trichromatic theory.

Similar results can be obtained using a technique known as the liminal brightness increment, in which the amount of additional light required to produce a detectable difference in the brightness of a target against a changing background luminance is determined. This has been modified by Stiles in a classic study of specific wavelengths of light. The technique can be highly discriminatory by measuring, for instance, the liminal brightness increment in a blue central target against a green background. The studies confirmed that there are indeed single receptors that peak in the red and green regions, but the blue spectral sensitivity curve is more complex and there are probably three components for the

Box 5.10 Spectral mixing curves

Mixing the three primary colours will produce any secondary colour or hue. However, a specific quantity of the primary colour is required to produce each hue and this amount is determined by spectral mixing curves.

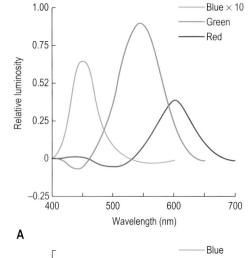

A

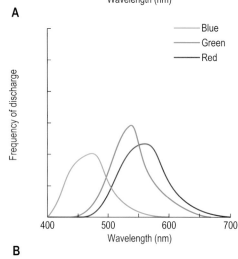

B

(**A**) Graph showing relative amount of each primary colour required to match any specific wavelength.

(**B**) Actual frequency of discharge in retinal neurones for each primary colour at any specific wavelength.

blue mechanism. Whether the influence of rod mechanisms on these tests can be completely eliminated is not clear.

More recently, techniques combining spectral reflectance densitometry and adaptive optics, a technique that removes higher order optical aberrations and allows very high-resolution images of the photore-

ceptors, have been applied to normal individuals and produced remarkable images of the arrangement of S, M and L photoreceptors. Interestingly, despite normal colour vision, the variation in density of L and M cones in particular varies considerably between individuals (Fig. 5.16). It has been suggested that this may represent a compromise between the competing requirements for spatial versus colour vision; and this is reflected in the patchy distribution of the L/M cones at the fovea and their different distribution in the peripheral retina.

Molecular evidence for three receptors

Just as rhodopsin represents the molecular receptor for light energy at the level of the photon, so there are cone pigments that are sensitive to photons of light generated within specific wavebands. The amino acid sequences of these proteins are known (Nathans *et al.*, 1986) and there are surprisingly few differences in the three cone opsins, especially in the transmembrane regions of the proteins that are important for retinal binding (see Ch. 4, p. 253). These differences must, however, account for peak wavelength sensitivity of each of the three opsins, thus revealing the extraordinarily fine spectral tuning that occurs at a molecular level. For instance, a threonine at position 65 correlates with the 'red' opsin, while isoleucine is present at the same position in the 'green' opsin. Although the mechanism of light-induced activation of rhodopsin and cone opsins is in principle similarly based on the conversion of 11-*cis* retinal to all-*trans* retinal (see Ch. 4), the differences in detail are highly physiologically significant. For instance, although the light response by cones is 100 times less sensitive, the cone opsin responses are several-fold faster, in the order of capture of 500 photons of light per second. This is related to the availability of Ca^{2+} ions, regulated by a guanylate cyclase-activating protein. In addition, about 10% of cone opsin may be in the apo-state (i.e. lacking any binding to retinol), but still retains a sufficient level of activity to weakly activate transducin, in what is termed 'dark' noise (see Box 5.6).

Studies using microspectrophotometric techniques and infrared photography (Mollon and Bowmaker, 1992) have shown that the distribution of the photopigments in the short-wave, middle-wave, and long-wave sensitive cones (Fig. 5.17) is not interdependent as might have been expected on the basis of receptive field analyses (see below), but is random or clumped at least for the long and middle wavelength receptors. In the case of short-wave receptors, some degree of organization has been observed from

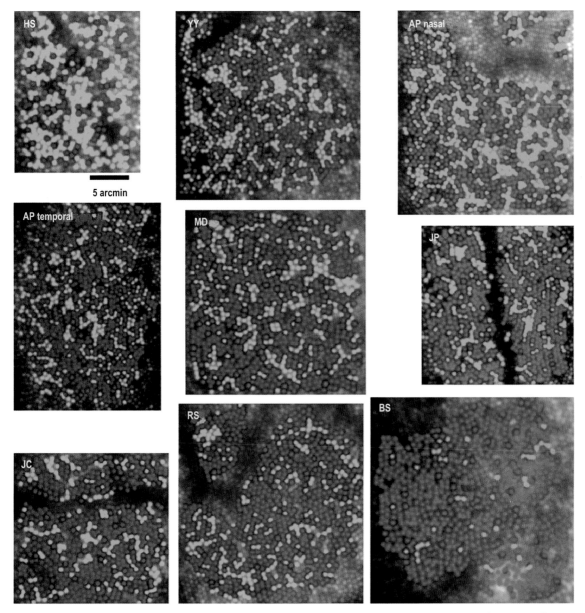

Fig. 5.16 False colour images showing the arrangement of L (red), M (green) and S (blue) cones in the retinas of different human subjects. All images are shown to the same scale. (From Hofer *et al.* 2005, with permission from the Society for Neuroscience.)

immunohistochemistry data, which shows that there are different P ganglion cells for spatial, chromatic and other functions (see section on Retinal connections).

In the foveal region, blue-sensitive cones are by far the most infrequent while, in humans at least, psychophysical studies suggest that long- to middle-waveband cones exist in a ratio of 2 : 1.

CONVERGENCE, YOUNG–HELMHOLZ AND HERING

Responses between photoreceptors and neural cells

Considerable processing of information occurs in the retina between the photoreceptor and the ganglion cell. In the magnocellular pathway, which deals with light and motion detection, M ganglion

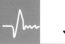

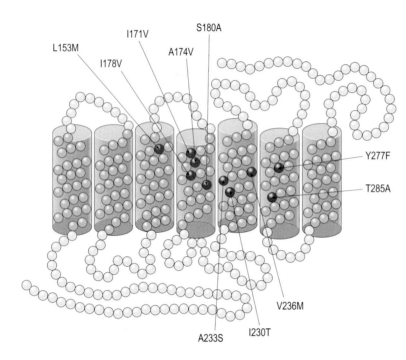

Fig. 5.17 Diagram of the opsin pigment with the seven α-helical barrels that form a ring around the light-trapping chromophore. Each circle on the polypeptide chain represents one of the 364 amino acids that form the L cone opsin pigments. The Y277F and T285A variants distinguish the I_{max} of L and M cone pigments. (From Verrelli and Tishkoff 2004, with permission from the American Society of Human Genetics.)

cells have large receptive fields and many rod photoreceptors feed information indirectly onto a single ganglion cell (see above). In contrast, the parvocellular pathway deals with spatial and colour vision, P cells have small receptive fields, and a single cone cell may have sole input to a single bipolar cell. At a retinal level convergence in the case of colour vision is nonexistent (although there is convergence for colour in the cortex).

In spite of this, sensory perception of colour does not correlate directly with stimulation of a wavelength-specific cone. As we have seen, a red-specific bipolar cell responds simply by producing a change in the firing rate in its nerve terminal, which of itself cannot be distinguished from a similar change in a green-specific bipolar cell, i.e. the bipolar cell cannot distinguish wavelengths although its receptor can. In addition, as there is considerable overlap in the spectral sensitivity of the receptors (see Fig. 5.15 and Box 5.10), some degree of confusion must exist in the initial response, which is smoothed out during processing.

Ganglion cell responses and opponent colour theory

Smoothing out this confusion is achieved by the colour-opponent mechanism based on the receptive field organization of the ganglion cells (see p. 280). In this scheme, there are three colour-opponent arrangements: a reciprocal ON-centre red/OFF-centre green, in which the bipolar cell receives stimulatory or inhibitory input from a single red or green cone; a similar ON-centre blue/OFF-centre yellow; and a third ON-centre white/OFF-centre black in which the bipolar cell receives input from all three cones and in which colour mixing occurs. This has the effect of greatly refining the spectral sensitivity of the ganglion cell responses; it allows the perception of hues and 'unsaturated' colours and accommodates the Young–Helmholtz trichromatic theory of colour vision with Hering's colour-opponent scheme. It also goes some way towards explaining the various colour anomalies found in humans.

Recent studies have shown that blue-ON/yellow-OFF responses arise from a distinctive bistratified ganglion cell type derived from a dual excitatory cone bipolar cell input: an ON-bipolar cell receiving input only from S cones and an OFF-bipolar cell contacting L and M cone inputs. The mechanism of the red–green opponency is still unknown. However, a recently proposed theory that incorporates a contribution of 'white' from rods stimulated under light conditions to the cone input allows a unified concept of how vision is integrated through simultaneous rod and cone input to allow subtle visual perception, such as hue discrimination, motion detection, orientation selectivity and others.

Colour constancy

We use colour to detect and recognize objects. Most of the light we detect is light reflected from objects, and their colour depends mainly on the surface properties of the object and not on the illuminating light. The wavelength of the reflected light clearly varies with the lighting conditions. In spite of this, the colour of an object remains the same, a phenomenon known as colour constancy, which is a function of higher visual processing in the cortex. Colour is therefore a highly complex sensation requiring input from a variety of sources and involving information processing both in the retina and the visual cortex.

COLOUR BLINDNESS

Some of the defined colour vision defects can be explained in simple terms of loss of one or other specific type of receptor. However, in practice the situation is often more complex involving not the loss of one particular receptor but the production of combination genes as the result, for instance, of aberrant crossing over in meiosis (see Ch. 3, p. 144); these produce proteins that are intermediate in their spectral sensitivities thus reducing the range of responsiveness of the protein.

Monochromatism

Rod monochromatism occurs in about 1 in 30 000 of the population; such individuals have true achromatic vision, low visual acuity (0.1–0.3), find high-intensity lights uncomfortable, display nystagmus, and may have some signs of macular dystrophy. These patients do have morphologically normal cones in their outer retina but their functional status is unclear. It has been suggested that they have a single type of blue cone.

Cone monochromatism is very rare (1 in 100 000). These individuals have normal visual acuity but cannot discriminate coloured lights of equal luminosity. Apparently cone monochromats possess all three types of cones, indicating that the defect occurs in cortical processing, probably in area V4.

Dichromatism

Dichromatism occurs when the affected individual matches all colours with mixtures of two primaries. Therefore, the range of secondary colours is restricted. Protanopes are missing the red wavelength, deuteranopes the green, and tritanopes the blue. Mixing of the two colours will produce a sensation of white at certain specificities, which for pro-

tanopes is 495 nm and for deuteranopes is 500 nm. The dichromat cannot distinguish the large range of non-spectral hues from spectral hues as the trichromat can, leading to a much narrower range of colour detection by the isocolour charts.

Anomalous trichromatism

Anomalous trichromats use different proportions of the three primaries to match colour. Protans use more red, deutans more green, and tritans more blue. The colour-anomalous individual differs from the trichromat and the dichromat in that he or she will not accept those matches that the other two agree on. This is the common form of 'colour blindness' occurring in 6% of the male population.

Achromatopsia

Colour blindness may also be the result of defects in cortical processing (area V4). Congenital (rare) or acquired lesions in the lingual or fusiform gyrus are associated with cerebral achromatopsia (also accompanied by prosopagnosia – a failure to recognize familiar faces, i.e. from memory). Similarly, cortical lesions in the superior temporal sulcus (V5) can produce defects in the ability to detect motion (motion blindness or akinetopsia; see p. 303). Isolated defects in form vision have not so far been detected, possibly because they involve more than one cortical area, e.g. V3 and V4, plus connections to other cortical regions involved in psychophysical attributes, and texture analysis.

VISUAL PERCEPTION

Visual perception is the end product of the processing or reinterpretation by the cortex of sensory responses made by the retina to visual stimuli. However, a strict separation of cortical and retinal events does not occur as some degree of processing takes place in the retina and, conversely, certain processes such as instantaneous parallax (see below) occur so quickly that it is difficult to believe they occur exclusively at a cortical level. In addition, perception should not be considered solely as the end product of the processing of sensory information. Instead, it is part of the 'action–perception cycle' (Wexler and Boxtel, 2005), in which perception modifies activity, which then modifies perception in a continuous cyclic pattern, the boundaries of which become indistinct. Motor activity (head and eye positioning etc.) therefore, is central to perception such as stereopsis (see below).

As shown above, there are many different types of visual stimuli, each of which may produce one or more different psychophysical perceptual responses. Sensory perception occurring at an elemental level encompasses visual stimuli such as luminosity, flicker, colour and form, because it involves simple processing of features such as points and lines or wavelengths, but even such an apparently fundamental function as visual acuity determination involves higher levels of processing because it is more than simply a point-to-point projection of the retina on the cortex.

Evidence for higher integrative activity at the cortical level comes from illusions such as the Schrodinger staircase and Rubin vase (see Box 5.11). A clear example of the role of cortical function in visual perception is the phenomenon of colour constancy in which large variations in the chromaticity of an object, induced for instance by changing the wavelength of the illuminating light of the object, do not alter the perceived colour of the object: a yellow banana remains yellow even when illuminated by a green light.

Our understanding of these processes has been greatly advanced by the careful analysis of both the stimuli and the responses, and has allowed specific functions to be attributed to discrete regions of the cortex.

MONOCULAR VERSUS BINOCULAR VISION

Positioning objects in space

Most of the primary visual sensory responses are monocular and are not changed by binocular viewing. Images of objects are projected onto definite positions in space (spatial perception) and each retina has its own delimited visual field. However, the position of an object in space is not an absolute entity but is related to the position of the observer and of other objects. The relative position of objects can be determined only if the retinal sensors are composed of discrete units that have precise 'markers' for localization. This indeed is the basis of the visual field.

In spite of this, objects appear fixed in position even when the observer changes position: simple ray diagrams demonstrate that a new set of retinal receptors must be stimulated every time the relative position of the object to the observer changes, but the observer does not experience the sensation of motion. This 'image stabilization' is achieved by compensatory psychophysical events at the cortical level. Recently, however, it has been shown that a proportion of this neural processing takes place at the retinal level through selective inhibition of ganglion cell firing (see above).

The existence of such mechanisms can be deduced in part from experiments showing that accurate localization of objects does not occur with all forms of eye or head movement. For instance, if the eye of an alert individual is forcibly moved using a surgical instrument such as a squint hook, the image is falsely projected to an incorrect position as if the eye has not moved. Spatial perception on normal eye movement must therefore be integrated with, if not controlled by, higher centres within the brain, such as the frontal cortical eye fields, which influence motor discharge in the ocular muscles. The corol-

---

Box 5.11   Visual illusions

Visual illusions such as the Schrodinger staircase and Rubin vase occur in a cyclical manner in which each of the perceptions regularly alternates. The periodicity of the fluctuations is also alterable with drugs.

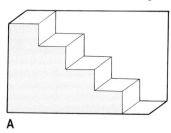

A

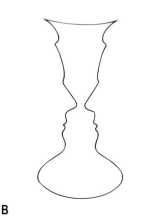

B

(**A**) Schrodinger's structure; (**B**) Rubin's vase.

lary, of course, is that the proprioceptive stretch receptors in the ocular muscles do not have a role in determining eye position as was previously thought, but that their probable role is simply to coordinate muscle tension in opposing muscles at a local 'axon reflex' level. This, however, may not hold true for all situations.

For instance, a problem arises in analysis of images that are perceived during slow visual tracking of a moving object. Despite the fact that no compensation is made for movements of the eyes during tracking, the changing position of the object is accurately observed and followed. This indicates that the higher centres are receiving a continuous flow of information from centres controlling ocular muscle movement, which is assimilated into the total information concerning object positioning: the actual adjustment of speed of eye movement to permit accurate tracking is achieved through visual input, which is ignored by the perceptual process. This means that having initiated a tracking movement, sequential images are interpreted on angular velocity assumptions determined by this initial response, and ignored by the higher integrative centres. These assumptions may, of course, be inaccurate, especially if the velocity of the moving target changes. Thus, any induced errors require repetitive readjustments of the tracking response.

Conclusions derived from experiments such as these are greatly influenced by the design of the experiment. It has been observed that the perception of heading (i.e. the direction taken by the observer under conditions of radial retinal image flow, or optic flow) in a situation where a moving target is also fixated can be achieved accurately only if extraretinal information concerning the position of the eyes is available, i.e. via proprioceptors from extraocular and head and neck muscles. Under special circumstances, such information, termed Structure-from-Motion (SFM) information, can be integrated with purely retinal image information. In addition, the resultant perception can vary significantly depending on whether the object or the observer is moving, even if the relative disparity in motion between them is the same. This sort of information has direct relevance to clinical problems, as in the condition of oscillopsia, where image stabilization is lost and the patient experiences 'retinal slip' (see next section). In such patients it is not clear whether the defect lies in the well-established vestibulo-ocular reflexes or whether loss of a putative cervico-ocular reflex, via neck proprioceptors, is contributory.

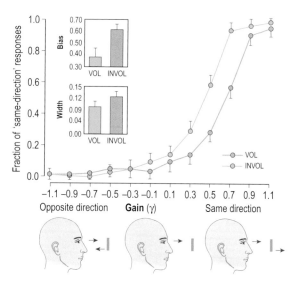

Fig. 5.18 Results of the voluntary (VOL) and involuntary (INVOL) eye movement studies. The curves show responses averaged over subjects, and over all simulated distances (there was no significant effect of distance). Mean bias and width were calculated by fitting the data of individual subjects with the logistic curves and averaging the parameters thus obtained. Bars indicate between-subjects standard errors. (From Wexler 2003, with permission from Blackwell Publishing.)

Thus spatial constancy, i.e. maintaining a 'stationary' percept of moving objects despite their repeated and sudden changes in retinal stimulation, is a fundamental visual perception. Spatial constancy also has a memory component. When an illuminated object is viewed in the dark, the eyes will, after an initial 'searching' response, adopt a position close to fixation (approximately within 2° of the target) when the illumination is switched off (Fig. 5.18). This has been attributed to some element of positional sense from an extraretinal source, such as head–eye position in space and locomotion (egocentric versus allocentric signals). Similarly the constant drift of the eyes towards fixation in the dark has been attributed to a similar mechanism (see next section). 'Place' cells occur in the hypothalamus and thalamus of the brain and correct visual input to active locomotor and possibly navigational (optic flow, see below) input.

Measuring by eye
We frequently use our vision to measure things by eye, e.g. to line up objects in a row or to determine the distance between two points. Simplistically, it might be thought that, for example, the distance

Box 5.12 Aubert's phenomenon

A vertical bright light viewed in a completely dark room will tilt to the left if the head is slowly tilted to the right (**B**). If the head is tilted suddenly or if the line is viewed in the light, the line appears upright in its normal position (**C**).

Thus information on retinal position is fed via the semicircular canals to the object-positioning centre; (**A**) resting position.

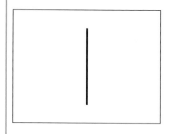
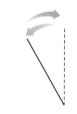
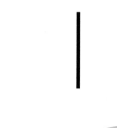
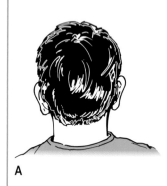
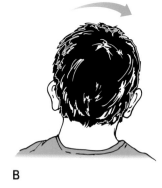
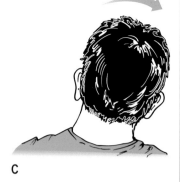

(**A**) Resting position; (**B**) slow head tilt to right, object appears to move to left; (**C**) fast head tilt to right, object stays upright.

between two objects should correlate with a defined distance between stimulated receptors in the retina, or that the length of a line will be determined by stimulation of a fixed number of retinal receptors. However, the psychophysical basis of these abilities is not as simple as it might appear. For instance, two lines of the same length running in different directions may stimulate a different number of receptors as the direction of lines will be distorted by the curvature of the eye and its position on eye movement. In addition, errors will be introduced on head movement since the head rolls further than the eye in the socket (some of this disparity is compensated for by input from the semicircular canals). Attempts have been made to adjust for image distortion due to eye curvature and movement using after-images, which obviously must reflect closely the actual retinal stimulation versus the 'real' direction of the object, but even this is not sufficient to account for the fact that we perceive the object in its true position and not in its distorted position. This is nicely demonstrated by Aubert's phenomenon (see Box 5.12).

A compensatory mechanism based in the higher centres must therefore be in place; it must be highly developed because the accuracy of measuring by eye is extremely high: for detecting the orientation of horizontal lines the error rate is 0.2% and for vertical lines it is 1.0%, as determined with a perceived direction test. The greater accuracy for estimating vertical and horizontal lines over oblique lines is not the result of preferred direction of eye movements or of the numbers of retinal receptors stimulated but is a function of cortical activity.

There is now extensive evidence that the visual cortex contains specific cells that are responsive to the orientation of lines. Indeed, the ability to 'parse

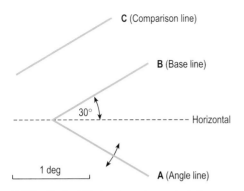

Fig. 5.19 Optical illusion based on orientation detectors in the visual system: as the experimenter moves the 'angle line' the observer attempts to position the comparison line parallel to the 'base line' which is stationary. The bigger the angle, the larger the error made. (Courtesy C. Blakemore.)

visual scenes for the orientation of purely spatial cues,' has been shown to be a fundamental property of even the simple insect brain. Vertical and horizontal orientation detectors occur as simple cortical cells (see below) and are distinct from motion detectors. Orientation detectors are considered essential to the analysis of form.

The patterns of objects also greatly influence our ability to make visual measurements. For instance, two angles can be accurately compared if we can fixate each of them directly and if the sides are parallel. In addition there are numerous examples of optical illusions where objects to be compared appear to be different in length or area/size if one of them has been altered by the addition of other visual cues that are interpreted by the higher visual centres in one particular direction (Fig. 5.19).

Therefore, both patterns and directions are important in visually estimating object dimensions: the retina uses the horizontal and vertical meridians as x and y axes to provide coordinates and thereby to pinpoint objects in space. As these axes are subject to displacement by, for instance, eye movement, it is important that a psychophysical compensatory mechanism exists that will reinterpret the position of the coordinates to project the real position and direction of the object in space.

Are two eyes better than one?

As most 'objects' are three-dimensional, it is clearly important that depth perception is achievable by the visual system. The major advantage obtained by binocular viewing is that it permits depth perception or stereopsis. This occurs in the cortex and depends on the fusion of images from each eye. However, depth perception is a complex event and information from many sources is used to achieve it.

One mechanism for depth perception could be related to the convergence of the eyes. Fixation of an object with both eyes requires a variable degree of convergence depending on the distance of the object, and information derived from this can be utilized to determine object distance. Indeed it has been suggested that variations in convergence can lead to three-dimensional illusions, although these may be caused by other mechanisms.

Is it possible to perceive depth with one eye only? Determination of object position using x and y axes as described above provides two-dimensional information only. Geometrically, it should not be possible to obtain three-dimensional information using one eye. However, certain cues, mostly built upon previous experience, indicate that some sense of depth is possible, e.g. by comparing the relative size of objects (for example, a person and a house), the blue colour of distant mountains (although they should be yellow – they are blue in comparison with the background light blue of the sky), overlapping edges of objects, effects of light and dark shading, effects of texture, and parallax on movement of the observer's head. It has also been suggested that the sensory feedback from the ciliary muscles on accommodation might provide some information centrally regarding depth (similar to the effects of convergence when both eyes are used), but this is unlikely.

When both eyes are used to observe an object in the straight ahead (primary) position, the image is still perceived as one, even though the image of that object must appear positionally but symmetrically different to each eye individually – indeed the image can be treated as if it were projected from a single centrally placed eye (the 'cyclopean' eye). When a second object is presented in the primary position, but closer to the observer than the original object, the second object is seen double when the original object is fixated (Fig. 5.20). Diplopia in this position is described as heteronymous; when the second object is distant from the first, the induced diplopia is described as homonymous. However, this form of diplopia is rarely appreciated because we normally do not attempt to fixate more than one object in the primary position when viewing with both eyes.

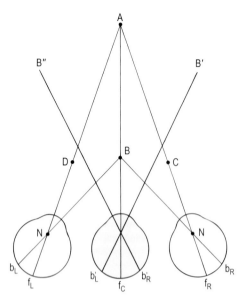

Fig. 5.20 The 'cyclopean eye' (shaded) is the abstract notion representing fusion of the two images from left and right. Image A is fused (fL + fR at fC) but image B cannot be simultaneously viewed without diplopia (heteronymous) (bL + bR at bL' and bR') due to the projected images at B' and B" respectively. Homonymous diplopia would occur if B was distant from A. Using either eye alone for alignment of the object would entail point C aligning with A (right eye) and point D aligning with A for the left eye. N, nodal point. (Courtesy of H Dawson.)

When we aim at a target using a second object to line up fixation, as with the sights of a rifle, we normally do so with one eye only (see Fig. 5.20).

A similar form of diplopia can be induced by a divergent squint, or by placing a base-out prism in front of one eye; both of these conditions have the effect of re-siting the projection of the image to a 'false' position from its normal cyclopean position. False projection in a squinting eye can lead to the development of a 'false' macula, which in fact is a cortical event because the anatomy of the retina remains the same. The development of a false macula reflects the plasticity of the cortex and indicates that projection of the eye through the nodal point is an innate mechanism. A similar 'pseudofovea' may develop in the presence of hemianopia.

The fact that we rarely experience double vision, even when rapidly and simultaneously fixating many objects in a scene, indicates that the images from both eyes are merged or fused; this is not simply a reduplication of information from both eyes but an actual psychophysical event that is used to provide depth information or stereopsis.

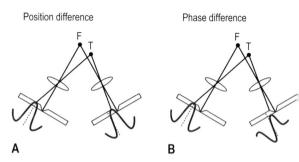

Position difference   Phase difference

A   B

Fig. 5.21 Depth perception based on binocular disparities. The fovea of each eye fixates point F; because object T is closer to the observer than F, the image of T falls at a different retinal location in the two eyes. The dotted line marks the equivalent retinal location in the two eyes. Neurones with receptive fields in both eyes could detect this disparity in two ways. (**A**) Position difference: the right eye receptive field is an exact copy of the left eye receptive field, but in a different retinal location. (**B**) Phase difference: the envelope enclosing the right receptive field profile sits in the same position as for the left receptive field but, within the envelope, the right receptive field has a different structure, responding best to white light on the right-hand side. When tested with a bright bar, both of these mechanisms produce a maximal response to a stimulus with a disparity equal to that of T. (From Cumming 1997, with permission from Elsevier.)

STEREOPSIS AND DEPTH PERCEPTION

The fusion of images to create the perception of depth requires certain conditions: first, the images from each eye must have corresponding points on both retinas. If all points on a sizeable object were exactly corresponding, however, this would merely lead to a reduplication of information and it is likely that only one of these points would register (this would be analogous to allelic dominance in chromosomal gene duplication in which only one gene is expressed transcriptionally while its partner is not; see Ch. 3, p. 153). Single-cell measurements have shown, however, that impulses from both retinas induce electrical activity in cortical neurones.

The second requirement for image fusion is that a certain proportion of points are non-corresponding, and it is the integration of information from corresponding and disparate points that induces the perception of depth. Both position and phase disparity in the corresponding receptive fields are important in the detection of depth cues (Fig. 5.21).

The horopter

Corresponding regions in the retina include both the horizontal and vertical meridia and equidistant points from each of these meridia. Single vision can be achieved only when the images of the object are projected from each eye to the same point in space.

The number of corresponding points can be charted as a 'horopter', in which corresponding points in the retina project to definite single points in space – within the field of binocular single vision. The vertical horopter has a backwards tilt that passes through the fixation point and a point near the feet of the observer and has recently been confirmed to be the result of a shear in binocular retinal correspondence. The true horopter is strictly limited to an area of about 3° from fixation, as determined experimentally. A special form of horopter is one based solely on corresponding points, defined as a circle of projected points in space passing through the fixation point and the nodal point of the eye. This is truly applicable only in the horizontal meridian as the vertical meridians are not exactly parallel. Horizontally placed horopters can form a 'stack of slices', producing a longitudinal horopter named so as to reflect the vertical lines of longitude on the globe of the earth. In practical terms the longitudinal horopter is not a circle but has a well-defined shape, approximately representing the field of binocular single vision (BSV) (see Box 5.13).

The field of BSV is an important parameter, not simply from a physiological standpoint but also for socioeconomic reasons. The normal visual field of each eye is approximately elliptical with a considerable degree of overlap (Fig. 5.22) and the overlapping fields of each eye represent the field of BSV in which full stereopsis is assumed to occur in the context of horopter-related corresponding points on the retina. In the UK, a certain minimum field of BSV is required to qualify for a driver's vehicle licence and is defined as a BSV field of 20° above and below the horizontal meridian and 60° to either side of the vertical meridian (Fig. 5.22). Measurement of visual fields can be performed by many techniques; currently, static automated visual fields are the normal practice, although kinetic and flicker-based fields are also highly informative.

The horizontal horopter is also defined for specific fixation points and therefore certain degrees of convergence; clearly this will change with the distance from the observer. At about 2 m from the observer the horopter is approximately a straight line, while it is concave to the face within this distance and convex beyond.

Box 5.13 Corresponding points of fixation on the retina constitute the 'horopter' field of vision

The horopter circle

A

The binocular single vision horopter field

B

(**A**) The horopter circle

(**B**) The binocular single vision horopter field

Measuring stereopsis

The measurement of stereopsis involves at least two parameters: the degree of convergence required to fuse images from two slightly dissimilar objects, and the limits of dissimilarity between two objects at which the two images can be fused (stereoacuity). The former is relatively easy to measure with an instrument incorporating two base-out prisms, known as a stereoscope. In the stereoscope, two slightly dissimilar but symmetrical images are presented to each eye and the angle of convergence at which the sensation of depth is achieved is recorded. In practice, true stereopsis is not measured by this

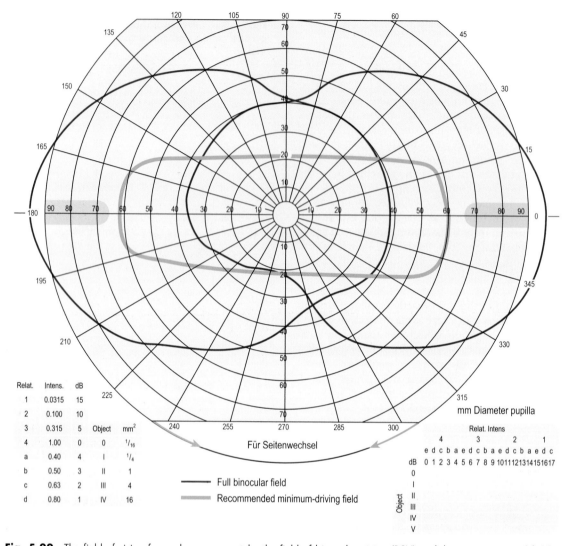

Relat.	Intens.	dB	Object	mm²
1	0.0315	15		
2	0.100	10		
3	0.315	5	Object	mm²
4	1.00	0	0	¹/₁₆
a	0.40	4	I	¹/₄
b	0.50	3	II	1
c	0.63	2	III	4
d	0.80	1	IV	16

Für Seitenwechsel

—— Full binocular field

—— Recommended minimum-driving field

mm Diameter pupilla

Relat. Intens

| | 4 | | | 3 | | | 2 | | | 1 |
| e d c b a | e d c b a | e d c b a | e d c |

dB 0 1 2 3 4 5 6 7 8 9 10 11 12 13 14 15 16 17

Object 0 I II III IV V

Fig. 5.22 The field of vision for each eye separately, the field of binocular vision (BSV) and the minimum visual field required for driving licence purposes in the UK are shown. (Courtesy of H Dawson.)

method because light and shade (i.e. monocular cues) provide considerable amounts of image disparity to the same object viewed by each eye in turn. Other tests that remove the monocular cues but use a camouflaged object include the random-dot stereogram, the random-dot E-test and the Frisby test, in which elements that are non-resolvable monocularly are presented in a random pattern at different disparities and the ability to perceive depth and form in the objects is assessed.

Stereoacuity can be measured as instantaneous parallax, which is the difference in binocular parallax of

both objects (Fig. 5.23). The limits of stereoacuity are in the region of 4′ of arc (range 1.6–24′), which is equivalent to an image disparity less than the diameter of a cone. Instantaneous parallax is lost at a distance of about 450 m but varies with the measurement technique. Conversely, within a certain range of distances, stereoacuity is improved the further away the object is from the observer, although theoretically this should not be so. In this case, the improvement is attributed to greater differences in monocular cues such as relative object size, to which the eye is more sensitive than instantaneous parallax. Stereopsis also improves with duration of the

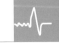

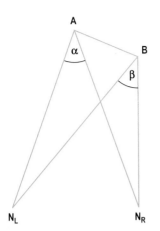

Fig. 5.23 Images A and B cannot be fused; instead they induce 'instantaneous parallax'.

stimulus, which is not the result of small searching or 'image-refreshing' movements of the eye but reflects the minimum time required for neural processing of the stimuli. Indeed, similar but disparate images can be perceived in three dimensions if they are presented to each eye in sequence, but the time interval has to be small (less than 5' of arc).

Image disparity and stereopsis

True stereopsis is dependent on disparities between the two images received by each eye, and therefore a certain number of points must fall on disparate points on the retina. It is also essential that these disparate points are fused like the corresponding points. The position of corresponding versus disparate points can be assessed by determining the actual differences in the stereoscopic projection of a point in space from the separate projections of the point made by each eye (Nouin's technique).

There is a limit to the fusional capacity of projected images, which is a circumscribed area known as Panum's area. It has been shown that it is possible to fuse greater disparities in the horizontal meridian than in the vertical, and therefore Panum's area forms an ellipse. The size of this area varies between individuals while the threshold disparity that can be fused is greatest at the horopter. The extent of Panum's area is reduced by small 'normal' disjunctive eye movements, which can be compensated for by using stabilized retinal images. Double images can be induced outside Panum's area and can be used effectively to estimate depth.

Fusion of disparate images to produce stereopsis tends to invalidate the notion of the cyclopean eye

in which single vision is produced by fusion of corresponding points. However, the cyclopean eye is of value in providing a baseline on which an estimate of the degree of neural processing involved in the fusion of disparate images can be made. Studies of neural circuitry in stereopsis have thus shown that it is possible to perceive depth without monocular cues, for instance by using random-dot stereograms. In these tests, 9×10 picture elements composed of dots, some of which correspond while others are symmetrically disparate, are presented in duplicate to each eye. These studies also reveal that discrete contours or edges are not essential for three-dimensional vision, although the contribution from 'texture analysis' is not clear (see below). Random-dot stereograms are also not quantitative.

The level at which processing for stereopsis occurs has been questioned on many occasions because it is such an instantaneous response and is difficult to separate from a retinal 'sensation'. Stereopsis is also sensitive to certain optical effects such as aniseikonia; horizontally it is affected by as little as a 0.25% change in image size, while vertical magnification disparities are simply transferred to the horizontal meridian of the fellow eye. The Pulfrich phenomenon is an optical illusion based on similar processing events (see Box 5.14). However, true disparity selective cortical neurones have been detected in V1, although the extent to which these neurones are simply 'rivalrous' (see next section) or stereopsis-inducing may depend on the degree of further cortical processing which appears to take place in the middle temporal (MT, V5) area of the visual cortex, an area associated with motion detection (see below). Furthermore, disparity matching appears to be a two-dimensional and not merely a one-dimensional process, involving fusion of images in a vertical as well as horizontal disparity.

RETINAL RIVALRY AND OCULAR DOMINANCE

Retinal rivalry is in essence a term that describes simultaneous perception by each eye individually without fusion of the images. This can be demonstrated as, for instance, when the letters F and L are viewed by each eye separately to produce the letter E. This phenomenon also has a periodicity to it, which is involuntary. It is related to but different from binocular rivalry as illustrated by the Schrodinger staircase or Rubin vase (see Box 5.11). Both are described as 'bistable phenomena' and are processed at retinal and cortical levels respectively.

Box 5.14 The Pulfrich phenomenon

The illusion of depth can be demonstrated by viewing a swinging, luminous pendulum through both eyes, one of which is covered by a red filter and the other by a green filter. It is thought to be the result of disparate images occurring during the movement of the pendulum stimulating corresponding points at fractionally different times

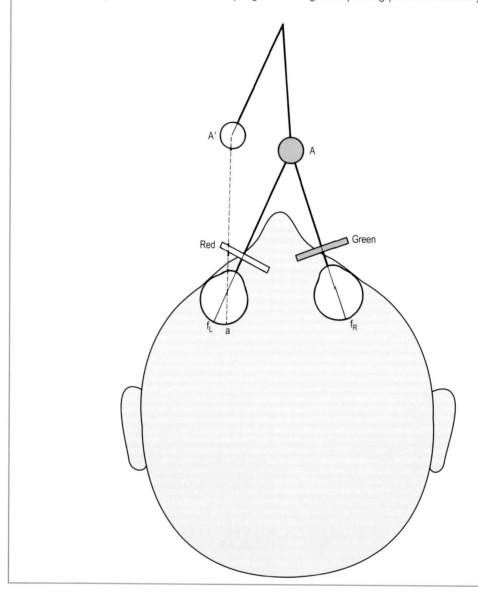

Ocular dominance refers to the preferential use of one eye when performing monocular activities. This can be demonstrated electrophysiologically and is not necessarily related to handedness. However, whether there is evidence for true 'cortical' dominance for preferential use of one eye has not been established. In a perfectly equally sighted individual input from one retina will mirror exactly that from the other retina

Certain involuntary events take place that bear on retinal rivalry and ocular dominance. For instance, if the same image is presented to each eye at different levels of brightness, then the image in one eye may be suppressed (ocular dominance). Or the binocular image may appear less bright than the same image when viewed monocularly (e.g. with a uniocular cataract).

COLOUR PROCESSING

The perception of colour is a complex cortical event that is dependent on input from several sources. The use of mondrians (coloured patterns produced with variably illuminated narrow-waveband light) has shown that the predominance of a given waveband reflected from a surface does not alone determine its colour, but that its colour also depends on the wavelength composition of the light reflected from its surround. Mondrians have been used to demonstrate the phenomenon of colour constancy (see p. 293) but their relative artificiality has been challenged: for instance, demonstration of other phenomena, such as the AMBEGUJAS phenomenon, in which perceived colours can change dramatically depending on the three-dimensional surface of wavelength reflectance (Bergstrom, 2004). Instead, well-defined real colour scenes have been devised that contain cues for the intrinsic surface colours and the recovery of the light source. These studies show that colour constancy is a real phenomenon but is not as absolute as previously thought and depends on input from local and global contrast. This depends on several factors, including spatial configuration and scale, and context. Texture, as in the AMBEGUJAS phenomenon, appears to the most important.

It is clear therefore that the reflectance of light is central to the perception of colour. Although the amount of light reflected from a surface may vary, the brain constructs an image that fits the reflectance, which is a constant physical attribute of the object. Land (1983) suggests therefore that the brain assesses the 'lightness' or 'darkness' of a surface compared with the surround, for each of the three predominant wavelengths in turn, and this permits it to assign a colour to the surface.

Colour is achieved therefore by a comparison of the reflected intensities of lights from one surface with those of surrounding surfaces for lights of different wavebands, followed by a comparison of the comparisons.

SHAPE DETECTION

The detection of form and shape also presents a problem when we consider exactly what we mean by shape. As described above, specialized cells exist that act as edge detectors for vertical and horizontal lines. However, the shapes we perceive are much more complex than can be simply broken down to a series of discrete lines on x- and y-axes. For example, most shapes in the natural world are curvilinear and solid, and require significant processing in the cortex. This has led psychophysicists to develop mathematical algorithms and a 'shape index' to describe these shapes and thus provide insight into how the brain might compute the information (Parker, 1993). These effects can be demonstrated using specially oriented stimuli and show that global orientation detection is not simply the result of input to the primary visual cortex (V1). Second-order orientation detection may therefore also exist as 'collector units' for first-order V1 stimuli. Such collector units may also be affected by brightness texture.

CONTRIBUTION OF TEXTURE ANALYSIS AND MOTION DETECTION TO DEPTH PERCEPTION

Depth perception is, of course, not only about locating objects in space but also about perceiving solid shapes. In fact, some of the early work on depth perception involved studies of aircraft pilots, particularly on take-off and landing. They revealed that motion detection and texture analysis were more relevant for the detection of solid structures, probably the most important aspect of visual perception (Figs 5.24 and 5.25). Many other sources of information combine to produce this effect, including binocular viewing, parallax, illumination and shading, and edge detection. For instance, a random set of dots may assume shape if a group of dots within the set 'moved' in relation to the remaining dots – an image would thus 'pop out' of the page. Similarly, texture and lustre are attributes of an object that relate to discontinuities in colour and/or luminance coming from the edges of the object, and significantly affect perception of its shape.

Most recently it has also been shown that the detection of a shape also depends on previous experience/memory and whether the observer is 'expecting' to see the shape. It is clear therefore that this complex response is built up from multiple inputs and that the search for a shape-detecting centre may prove elusive.

303

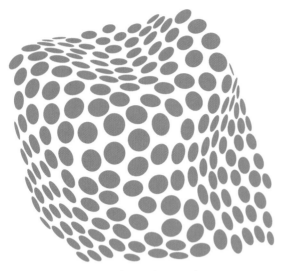

Fig. 5.24 A pattern of optical texture that is perceptually interpreted as a smoothly curved three-dimensional surface. (From Todd *et al.* 2005, with permission from Elsevier.)

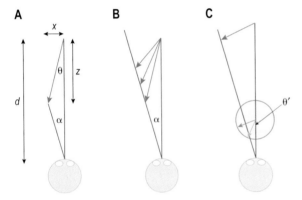

Fig. 5.25 Schematic of stimulus geometry. (**A**) Observer and typical target trajectory (solid arrow) at an angle θ to straight ahead are illustrated. Visual direction of the moving target at the end of its motion is given by angle α. (**B**) Many different trajectories correspond to a single visual direction. (**C**) Location of the pointer (grey circle). If observers used θ to set the pointer, they would respond as shown by the black arrow. The grey arrow shows a typical response if observers used α. From Harris and Drga (2005).

DIVISION OF LABOUR IN THE VISUAL SYSTEM

The sophistication in topographic mapping of brain function is nowhere seen better than in the visual cortex. Zeki (1990) has summarized a conceptual framework for what he describes as the division of labour in the visual cortex. According to this scheme, anatomically discrete areas of cortex subserving different functions are reconstituted to produce a perception of an integrated image. Thus an image should not be regarded as being 'impressed' on the retina like the film in a camera, which is then codified to make it 'understood' by the cortex; rather we should appreciate that the processes of sensing (seeing) and cognition (understanding) are not separate but totally integrated. It is likely that, as additional sensory information is added to the image, a higher level of cognition and thus perception can be achieved.

IMAGING STUDIES

Most of the information about humans has been derived from work on animals. Recently the opportunity to show 'parcelation' in the human visual cortex has come from studies using positron emission tomography (PET), magnetoencephalography and functional magnetic resonance imaging (fMRI) (Fig. 5.26). Normal volunteers, while viewing coloured mondrians or randomly moving dot stimuli, show increases in regional cerebral blood flow (which is an index of activity within an area) in different parts of the prestriatic cortex – V4 for coloured stimuli and V5 for moving targets. In humans, therefore, it can be said that there is a 'colour centre' outside the visual cortex; there is functional specialization as in the monkey. Another intriguing observation is that the effect of coloured stimuli is lateralized in humans and is not necessarily related to handedness or ocular dominance. Similarly, three different 'types' of motion detection have been located to discrete areas of the visual cortex.

THE MAGNOCELLULAR AND PARVOCELLULAR PATHWAYS SUBSERVE DIFFERENT FUNCTIONS

The striate cortex (area V1) contains the entire map of the retina in a highly ordered and predictable distribution. It receives this information via the LGN, where the neuronal organization is also highly ordered (see Ch. 1). At first sight it would seem, therefore, that retinal images should be truly represented in the visual cortex on the basis of a point-to-point topographical representation. In a very limited sense this is true and may even apply to functional differentiations associated with certain

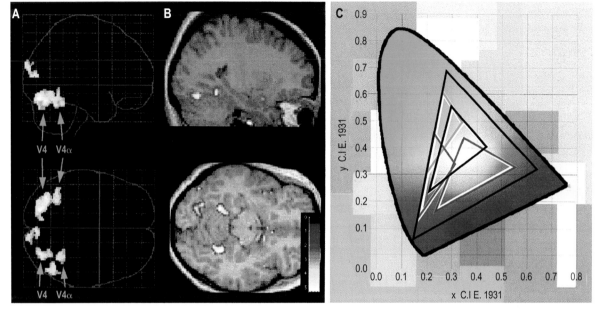

Fig. 5.26 The cortical activity elicited when subjects viewed a dynamically illuminated coloured scene. (**A**) **Left:** Group result of six subjects who viewed a coloured Mondrian, for the comparison of the *varying luminance* and the *varying wavelength composition* mode versus the *static* mode. The perceived colours remained constant at any time. An SPM displayed as a glass-brain reveals that activity was largely constrained to two subdivisions of the V4-complex: V4 and V4α [group of six subjects, random two of whom were scanned twice, thresholded at $P < 0.0001$ ($Z = 3.72$) for height and at 90 voxels for extent of activation, both uncorrected]. There is also activity in the V1/V2 region and lateral to the V4-complex. **Right:** Activity in a single subject for the comparison of *varying wavelength composition* mode versus the *static* mode in a coloured Mondrian. V4 (posterior) is at this threshold only visible in the right hemisphere, V4α in both ($P < 0.001$ uncorrected, slices taken at $x: -26$; $z: -12$ mm). (**B**) This graph contains the Mondrian stimulus used (background) and an overview of the range within which the illuminant changed dynamically (foreground). The latter is displayed in a CIE (Commission Internationale de l'Éclairage) colour flowchart (ellipsoid envelope). The three inner coloured triangles show the range of colour space which four Mondrian patches of the corresponding colours would have occupied during the *varying wavelength condition* had they been viewed on their own (the black triangle depicts the same for the white patch). Even though the wavelength composition of each patch of the Mondrian changed continuously, their perceived colours remained constant in the experiment since they were viewed in context. The range of colour the projection screen is capable of displaying is depicted by the black outer triangle. (From Bartels and Zeki 2000, with permission from Blackwell Publishing.)

neuronal cell types. Thus, the parvocellular (slow) fibres carry information concerning foveal and parafoveal activity such as spatial discrimination and colour, while the magnocellular (fast) fibres act as transmitters of light detection. This explains in part the high sensitivity that we have for light and motion detection, which are served via the peripheral retina, while contrast and colour detection are slower processes.

However, psychophysical phenomena such as colour and spatial constancy indicate that simple representation of images on the visual cortex in a retinotopic fashion is insufficient to explain the resultant perception. Even the briefest consideration of wave-length discrimination, which is an intrinsically colourless event, despite the fact that there are three discrete receptors, would reveal this truth; thus a pillarbox appears red in any condition of illumination even though the actual wavelength of the reflected light from the pillarbox will vary greatly depending on the light source. The perception of colour, and indeed of any visual stimulus, is the result of input from many other cortical sources in addition to the primary visual cortex (see above). A further unexplained problem in studying cortical and indeed lower levels of activity is the constant high level of neuronal 'noise'. It appears that even in the absence of specific stimulation, there is a significant level of endogenous neuronal activity, which

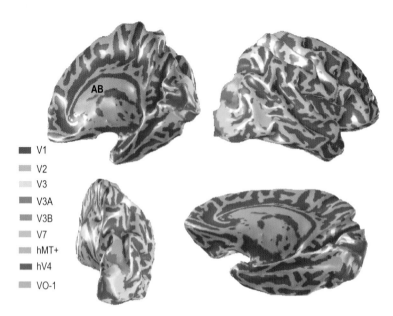

■ V1
■ V2
■ V3
■ V3A
■ V3B
■ V7
■ hMT+
■ hV4
■ VO-1

Fig. 5.27 The locations of nine hemifield maps in the human visual cortex. The maps are shown for one typical subject (AB). (From Wandell *et al.* 2005, with permission from the Royal Society of London.)

is now presumed to modify output (i.e. perception in the case of vision).

THE STRIATE CORTEX AND THE PRESTRIATE CORTEX SHUFFLE INFORMATION BETWEEN THEM IN THE BUILD-UP TO A PERCEIVED IMAGE

The striate cortex (area V1) is connected to the prestriate cortex (areas V3–V8) directly and also via area V2 (Fig. 5.27). Each of these areas has one or more specific functions. For example, all cells in area V5 respond to motion in the visual system, and are directionally selective (i.e. each cell responds to motion in only one direction); none of these cells, however, is specific for colour. This function is subserved by cells in area V4, in which some of the cells act as wavelength discriminators, but some of these cells also respond to orientation of lines and are involved in shape (form) detection. Other studies have, however, shown that contour information can also be derived from motion detection and that this activity takes place in the primary visual cortex. Cells in V3 and V3A are also selective for form but are indifferent to changes in wavelength.

It is clear, therefore, that colour, orientation, motion, stereoacuity, texture, etc., are all processed separately in areas V3–V8. As areas V3–V8 receive their information from V1, V1 (and V2) must also be functionally specialized. Recent studies have suggested that there may be a population of cells that respond to more than one stimulus, such as texture and motion, when these are tested separately. However, this is not the common response.

V2 is likewise organized into areas with thin stripes (for colour detection) and thick stripes (for motion detection) separated by interstripes. Form-selective detectors are present in both the thick and the thin stripes. This form of organization of the visual, and indeed the entire, grey matter into discrete columns of cells responding to specific stimuli has long been known (> 50 years) but its functional significance is not clear.

PARCELLING OUT THE PROCESSING IN V1

The concept of functional/anatomical segregation of visual stimuli into components such as colour, motion and orientation detection, depth perception, and other features is now well established (but see below). The cortical sites of other visual tasks, such as texture analysis and shape recognition, are not so easily located. Still others, such as face recognition, involve regions outside the visual and prestriate cortex, including sites that store memory.

Despite our lack of knowledge, it is still remarkable that such a level of segregation occurs from the retinal ganglion cell input, through the LGN to V1, V2 and V3–V8 in the cortex. Segregation may have developed as a result of the different requirements for generating form, colour and motion (e.g. colour compares input from one part of the visual field to another) but topography for colour may be less important. In contrast, precise topographic localization is important for form analysis and motion detection; in the latter, however, this is assessed only transiently.

Our perception of the external environment may therefore depend on a system of circuits rather like combined and serial parallel processing in computers where there is 'multistage integration', as Zeki (1990) describes it, with feedforward and feedback control. In line with this concept, perception and comprehension of the visual world occur simultaneously and continuous processing of information, both past and present, is ongoing.

IS THE VISUAL CORTEX ORGANIZED FOR HIERARCHICAL NEURAL PROCESSING OR FOR FUNCTIONAL SPECIALIZATION?

The above outline of the organization of visual information at the cortical level may be oversimplistic. In reality, organization of information reception and integration has been considered in two ways, both of which are probably contributory: (a) hierarchical processing of information through the different regions (e.g. sequentially from retinal to LGN to V1, then to V2, and then simultaneously or differentially to V3, 4, 5 etc); and (b) functional specialization in the form of precise topographical localization of aspects of vision to discrete areas of the visual cortex. One of the important recent observations from fMRI work is that the concept of precise retinotopic mapping being restricted to V1 (i.e. representation of the fovea and peripheral retinal regions to precise sites on the striate cortex) may not be accurate. Areas previously considered non-retinotopic such as V4 and for colour and V5 for motion also have retinotopic representation although less exact than in V1. Not only is there region-specific cortical representation for instance of colour, but eccentricity maps (distance from fovea) and polar angular maps (angle from the horizontal meridian) cross each other in their cortical representations allowing a form of mapping of 'visual space' on the cortex (Figs 5.28 and 5.29).

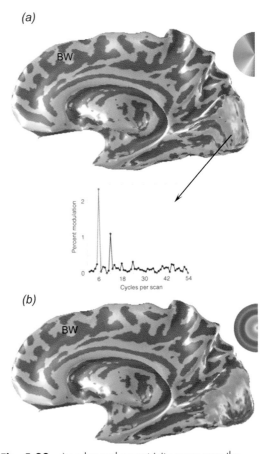

Fig. 5.28 Angular and eccentricity maps near the calcarine cortex. Maps were measured using (**A**) rotating wedges and (**B**) expanding rings comprising contrast-reversing dartboard patterns. The stimuli extended over the central 20° of the visual field and completed six cycles during each experimental scan. The colour overlay indicates the visual field angle (**A**) or eccentricity (**B**) that produces the most powerful response at each cortical location (see the coloured legends on the right). For clarity, only responses near the calcarine cortex are shown. The graph plots the response amplitude as a function of temporal frequency as measured in a 3 mm radius disc located in the calcarine (see arrow). The response is significantly greater at the stimulus repetition frequency (six cycles per scan, shown in red) than other temporal frequencies. The secondary peaks at integer multiples of the stimulus frequency are expected and are also significant. The graph is included in the image to provide the reader with an assessment of the reliability of the responses. The stimulus-driven responses shown here are substantially above the statistical threshold ($P < 0.001$, uncorrected). (From Wandell *et al.* 2005, with permission from the Royal Society of London.)

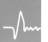

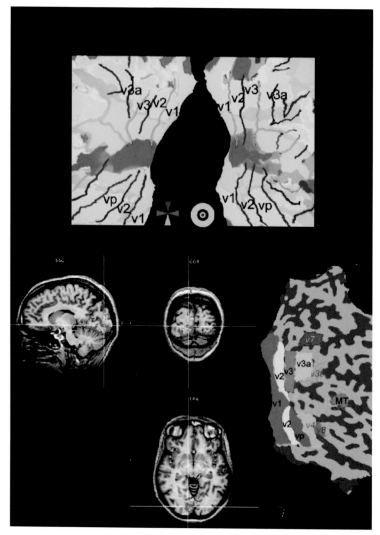

Fig 5.29 Early and mid-level visual areas. *Top*: Superposition of eccentricity and polar angle maps. Yellow, blue, and pink bands indicate eccentricity maps; lines indicate centres of upper, lower, and horizontal representations (see icons). Note that meridian lines cross all eccentricities orthogonally. *Bottom*: Visual areas on a flattened representation and on the brain volume. Visual area names under consensus are denoted in black, and areas currently under debate are marked in blue italics. (From Grill-Spector and Malach 2004, with permission from the publisher of Annual Reviews.)

It has now become clear that perception of colour, motion, form, texture and stereopsis all have varying levels of the following attributes: (a) functional specialization in discrete cortical areas; (b) retinotopic representation within each of those areas; and (c) processing in 'streams' e.g. in a colour stream where neural processing for wavelength discrimination takes place at several levels from the retina, to the LGN to V1 and onwards to the specific cortical region in V4. Similar organization underpins motion detection but less is known about stereopsis or texture appreciation.

However, there is further sophistication in perceptual pathways. Recent fMRI studies have revealed that there are object selective regions localized mainly anterodorsal and anteroventral to the striate cortex (Fig. 5.30, Malach 2004). These regions are not only specialized to detect aspects of vision such as form or colour but also to detect specific objects such as faces, tools, words and even places. Despite this, there is still a strong hierarchical organization for information processing. For instance the receptive fields for the same stimulus are smallest in V1 and increase progressively through V2, to

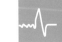

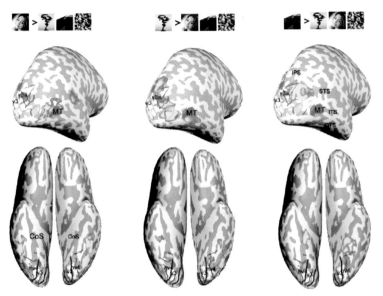

Fig. 5.30 Face-, object-, and place-selective regions in the human brain displayed on an inflated surface representation of the same subject as in Fig. 5.29. Icons indicate the comparison done in the statistical tests. *Left*: areas responding more strongly to faces than objects, places, or textures. *Centre*: areas responding more strongly to objects than faces, places, or textures. *Right*: areas responding more strongly to places (scenes) than faces, objects, or textures. Yellow and orange indicate statistical significance: $P < 10^{-12} < P < 10^{-6}$. Coloured lines indicate borders of retinotopic visual areas. Blue indicates area hMT!, defined as a region in the posterior bank of the inferotemporal sulcus that responds more strongly to moving versus stationary low-contrast gratings (with $P < 10^{-6}$). (From Grill-Spector and Malach 2004, with permission from the publisher of Annual Reviews.)

V3A and V4. To add further complexity to the final percept, there is evidence that top-down processing occurs, for instance activity induced in visual areas V1 and V2 by increased 'expectation' or attention to a region even in the absence of a specific visual object. Even input from emotional stimuli or stereotypical events can modify the visual areas as seen on fMRI.

PHYSIOLOGY OF OCULAR MOVEMENT

Many of the aspects of the visual response described above would not be possible without the coordinated movement of the eyes; indeed eye motion is a fundamental feature of ocular and visual physiology since eyes in the alert state are never at rest. Eye movements are paired even when they move in different directions, as in convergence responses. Neural control of paired eye movements occurs at several levels, as for any neuromuscular event, i.e. at a reflex/subcortical level and via cortical control. The anatomy of the ocular muscles and the innervations of the ocular muscles via the cranial nerves and brainstem nucleus have been reviewed in Chapter 1.

TYPES OF MOVEMENT

Uniocular eye movements

Each eye can be moved in the direction of action of the ocular muscles (see Box 5.15), which are usually described around a centre of rotation of the globe placed about 14 mm behind the cornea. Rotation is either in a vertical (z-axis) or a horizontal (x-axis) plane, otherwise known as Listing's plane. Torsional motion of the eye occurs around a median or vertical plane through the midline of the skull; this movement can also be described in most circumstances in reference to the retinal horizon (the x,y-plane). Rolling movements of the eye occur along an antero-posterior axis, while intermediate movements between any of these axes are possible.

BINOCULAR EYE MOVEMENTS

The extent of movement of one eye is equal and symmetric to the other (Hering's rule); in conjugate movements the eyes move in parallel while in dysjunctive movements (convergence and divergence) they move in opposite directions. In the fusion-free or physiological position of rest (not the primary position of gaze, as this requires fixation on a target) the eyes are slightly divergent.

309

Box 5.15 Evaluation of extraocular muscle function

The direction of action of the extraocular muscles is complex and should be considered in three dimenstions. The diagram indicates the action of the muscles when they are to be tested clinically for their function, as explained below.

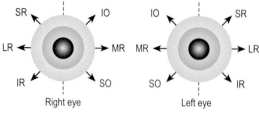

Right eye   Left eye

For instance, in order to test the function of the SO, the simplest way is to test its depressor function when the eye is in a position where the other depressor cannot act, i.e. when the eye is adducted. Adducting the eye in effect 'shortens' the IR (the other depressor of the eye, thereby compromising its role as a depressor – muscles are less efficient if their muscle belly is shortened). The SO is thus the only depressor in the adducted position and vice versa for IR. IR, inferior rectus; SO, superior oblique; IO, inferior oblique; LR, lateral rectus; MR, medial rectus.

Conjugate movements require reciprocal innervation of the muscles, which can therefore be described as conjugate pairs of muscles for each direction of gaze (see Box 5.15). This is limited in that the excursion of each muscle is usually greater than that of the pair. The effect is to produce a field of binocular single vision, a parameter of great practical significance with respect to standards of normal visual function for the purposes of vehicle licence regulations (see Fig. 5.22).

Convergence movements require the combined action of both medial recti; the extent of movement is limited by the near point (5–10 cm from the eyes; not affected by age unlike the near point of accommodation) and the far point of convergence (determined in the position of rest as the projected intersection). The converging power of the eye is measured by the metre angle, which depends on the interpupillary distance and can be assessed using graded prisms. From this, the amplitude of convergence can be calculated, which is the difference between the converging power of the eye for the near and far points of convergence. The fusional drive can add a component to the converging power of the eye – the fusion supplement.

Conjugate movements of the eye may be in the form of short sharp movements (saccades) or continuous tracking movements (smooth pursuit). Even when under apparent steady fixation, there are small conjugate movements (microsaccades). Voluntary gaze or 'search' movements (i.e. directed towards non-defined targets) are under higher cortical control (see below). Experimental studies have shown that visual input is required for saccadic movements and is linked to image latency. Tracking movements, however, require visual input plus object speed to be no greater than 30–40° per second and to match that of the eye movement.

Saccades
- Rapid voluntary relocation of fixation
- Under supranuclear contralateral control
- Latency of 100 ms
- Velocity of 800–1000°/s.

Pursuit
- Slower tracking movements
- Under supranuclear ipsilateral cortical control
- Latency of 150 ms
- Velocity of 30–50°/s.

During saccades, there is selective suppression of motion detection over other stimuli, suggesting that saccades suppress only the magnocellular pathway. It is also important to consider the concept of optic flow, in which an object moving in relation to a static observer generates a pattern of relative motion in the retinal image. The control of eye movements under these conditions may be difficult to analyse, particularly if the observer is tracking a slowly moving object against a faster moving background. The situation becomes even more complex if the observer is also moving.

CONTROL OF EYE MOVEMENT

The eye muscles in the primary position of gaze are in a state of tonic activity. Each muscle, however, is activated when the eye moves in its field of action and is inhibited in the opposite direction. The final pathway for neuronal control of eye movement occurs via the cranial nerves (see Ch. 1 and Ch. 3), which are the motor neurone equivalent of the spinal nerves subserving reflex responses. As for any muscle, however, the ocular muscles are under both reflex and 'higher centre' control, with the frontal cortex regulating voluntary activity and the occipital cortex and superior colliculus serving as 'coordinating centres'. In addition, there are numerous interneurones and connections with other pathways at the cortical level, e.g. via the paramedian pontine reticular formation (PPRF), and at the reflex level, e.g. the vestibulo-ocular reflex and the cervico-ocular reflex. The generation of horizontal and vertical saccades (gaze) and the fine-tuning of eye movements involve the integrated supranuclear network within the midbrain [PPRF and rostral interstitial nucleus of medial longitudinal fasciculus (riMLF)] and brainstem (vestibulo-ocular and cervico-ocular reflexes), which will be discussed in more detail below.

The fixation reflex

The ability to fixate a bright light is a basic reflex that is evident within a few days of birth, but the binocular reflex involving conjugate eye movements and a sustained response takes several months to be fully developed. Foveal fixation is the endpoint of the searching movement of the muscles and may be considered the point of peak activity in the nerve/muscle response. The nerve response can therefore be said to be 'tuned' to foveal fixation. In addition, the very small fine eye movements (microsaccades) that occur with sustained foveal fixation are the result of reflex attempts by the oculomotor centre to achieve the best perceived image, as this falls off rapidly unless a new set of cones is stimulated (see above).

The fixation reflex can be demonstrated easily by testing for optokinetic nystagmus, where either the stationary subject views a moving scene or a moving subject views a stationary scene. The nystagmus has a slow phase when the eyes follow the target and a fast flick when they readjust to the new target position. The optokinetic nystagmus response in humans requires an intact cortex, although there may be a subcortical pathway via the superior colliculus especially for the 'involuntary' searching component of the response. Lesions of the cerebral cortex, for example in the temporal lobe, are associated with defects in the optokinetic nystagmus response. The nystagmus is preserved in parietal lobe lesions, and this test is therefore clinically useful in localizing lesions.

Oculovestibular reflexes are eye movement responses to positional changes in the relationship between the head and the trunk

The vestibular apparatus has structures that convey static head/trunk positional reflex information (i.e. when the subject is not in motion) – the utricle and saccule – and kinetic positional information under conditions of head/trunk acceleration and decelera-

tion – the semicircular canals. In the utricle and saccule, stimulation of the receptor may occur simply on changing position of the head with respect to gravity, but the ampullae in the semicircular canals are stimulated via inertial forces in the endolymph surrounding the hair cells (viscous drag). The semicircular canals are arranged so that they act in synergistic pairs on each side of the head in the x, y and z-axes. Vertical and torsional movements involve all four vertical canals. Recent techniques in three-dimensional analysis of ocular movements allow the possible location of defects to, for instance, a single semicircular canal. The techniques are based on mathematical models containing information on rotation vectors, reference frames, coordinate systems and Listing's law, and use magnetic search coils in preference to video-based systems.

Listing's law states that, when the head is fixed, the primary position of the eye is such that there is a restricted degree of orientation that can be reached by a single rotation about an axis in Listing's plane (see above) (nine positions of gaze; Box 5.15 and Figs 5.31 and 5.32). Listing's law applies during fixation, saccades, smooth pursuit and vergence movements but not during sleep or during vestibulo-ocular reflexes.

The oculovestibular reflex can be demonstrated by the ability of a rotating observer to maintain fixation on a stationary target by reflex movement of the eyes at the same angular rotation (up to 300°/s) as the observer in the opposite direction. In this way there is stabilization of the retinal image. The reflex can also occur in the dark but is less accurate in its predicted excursion.

Rolling eye movements are due to oculovestibular and oculocervical reflexes

Compensatory eye movements during tilting of the head towards the shoulders initially involve the semicircular canals but, if the movement is sustained, static (utricle and saccule) responses participate. However, this compensatory movement of the eyes also involves information about neck position from proprioceptors in the neck (oculocervical reflex). Lateral movement of the head about a vertical axis will induce predominantly oculocervical reflexes, while movement of the head in the median plane with the eyes fixated produces predominantly oculovestibular reflexes (doll's head movement). Doll's head movements are an important clinical sign to test for intact brainstem reflexes in cases of cortical damage and loss of supranuclear control.

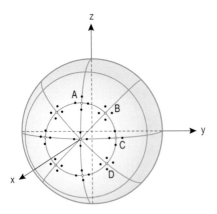

Fig. 5.31 Primary position and Listing's plane. There is a unique orientation of the eye, called 'primary position' or 'primary gaze direction' (direction parallel to the x-axis), such that pure vertical and pure horizontal movements that move the eye or gaze line from primary to secondary positions do not change ocular torsion (eye rotations along the respective meridians through A or through C). Similarly, any movement that rotates the eye/gaze line from primary to tertiary positions on oblique meridian planes does not change torsion (e.g. movements along the meridians through B to D). The axes of single rotations that move the eye from primary to secondary or tertiary positions lie all in one plane, called Listing's plane, (the plane containing the y- and z-axes). Tertiary positions cannot be reached from secondary positions by any combination of horizontal and vertical ocular rotations (a torsional component is also needed; see half-angle rule). (From Angelaki and Hess 2004, with permission from Blackwell Publishing.)

The midbrain is a coordinating centre for reflex eye movement and connects input from multiple sources

Voluntary eye movements (saccades) are initiated in the contralateral motor strip of the frontal cortex (see Fig. 1.62) and pass down to the midbrain via the anterior limb of the internal capsule to synapse in the horizontal gaze centre within the PPRF (Fig. 5.33). Neurones then pass to the ipsilateral VI nerve and interneurones cross to the opposite medial longitudinal fasciculus to subserve the contralateral III nerve. Within the PPRF are burst cells, which have a high but transient rate of discharge (1000 Hz/s) and, when fired, generate the saccade. Normally the burst cells are continuously inhibited by pause cells, until this inhibition is released by discharge from neurones from the frontal eye fields.

Once the saccade has been generated, eye position and fixation are maintained via the tonic neural integrators, also situated within the PPRF. The PPRF also receives inputs from vestibular nuclei, cerebel-

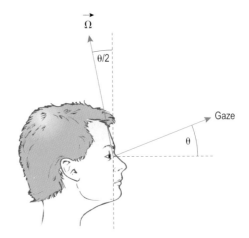

Fig. 5.32 According to Listing's law, the axis of rotation of the eye (Ω) is neither head-fixed nor eye-fixed, but rotates in the same direction as gaze through half the gaze angle (θ/2; the half-angle rule). Thus, at eccentric eye positions, during a horizontal saccade or pursuit eye movement, the axis of rotation of the eye is not purely horizontal (head-vertical dashed line) but also has a torsional component (head-horizontal dashed line). (From Angelaki and Hess 2004, with permission from Blackwell Publishing.)

lum, basal ganglia and cervical proprioceptors, giving rise to fine accurate control of gaze, and their contributions will be discussed below.

The vertical gaze centre is located in the reticular medial longitudinal fasciculus (RMLF), opposite the superior colliculus and above the level of the IIIn nucleus. Unlike its horizontal counterpart, the vertical centre has no identifiable cortical control, neurones from which cross to the III and IVn nuclei to subserve vertical gaze. The medial longitudinal fasciculus, as already mentioned, carries fibres of conjugate horizontal eye movement (involving the VIn and IIIn) and also signals for holding vertical eye position, vertical smooth pursuit and vertical vestibulo-ocular reflexes.

Loss of supranuclear control by lesions affecting the midbrain and brainstem can give rise to a variety of clinical features, the commonest being involvement of the medial longitudinal fasciculus in multiple sclerosis, giving rise to abnormal horizontal saccades (Fig. 5.33).

The superior colliculus is involved in both perception and eye movement control

A small number of fast (M) fibres relay from the retina to the superior colliculus, and thence

CONTROL OF GAZE/OCULAR MOVEMENT

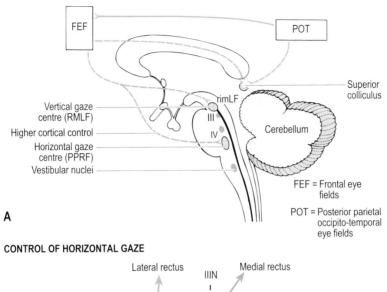

FEF

POT

Superior
colliculus

rimLF

Vertical gaze
centre (RMLF)

III

Higher cortical control

IV

Cerebellum

Horizontal gaze
centre (PPRF)

Vestibular nuclei

FEF = Frontal eye
fields

POT = Posterior parietal
occipito-temporal
eye fields

A

CONTROL OF HORIZONTAL GAZE

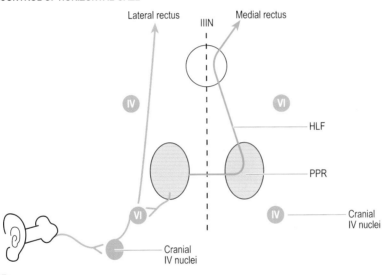

Lateral rectus

IIIN

Medial rectus

IV

VI

HLF

PPR

VI

IV

Cranial
IV nuclei

Cranial
IV nuclei

B

Fig. 5.33 Outline diagrams for integrated control of ocular movements: (**A**) 'higher centre' regulation; (**B**) brainstem, nuclear control.

to the pulvinar and finally the cortex. These fibres bypass the LGN and are described as the extrageniculostriate pathway. The fibres have crossed chiasmal representation, like optic tract fibres, and synapse in the superior colliculus in retinotopic structured layers, as occurs in fibres to the LGN. The organization, however, is less clearly demarcated, being in broad superficial and deep categories of fibres.

The function of these fibres is not entirely clear. There is evidence for neuronal delay to and from the

visual cortex via the posterior pulvinar system and also to the pretectal region where the pupillary fibres relay (Fig. 5.34). The cells also have a receptive field organization and a preference for motion detection (a 'movement field'), particularly the rapid 'reflex' locking-on eye movement that occurs in the initiation of tracking a moving target or in automatic scanning during reading. In certain patients with occipital cortex lesions, 'blindsight' (the patient can detect motion or adjudge orientation without perceptually 'seeing' the object) may be present through preservation of this extrageniculostriate pathway. 313

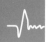

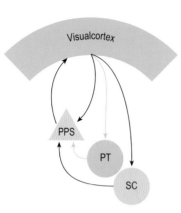

Fig. 5.34 The extrageniculostriate pathway. Neuronal information to the superior colliculus (SC) is relayed to the posterior pulvinar system (PPS) and on to the visual cortex. From there it relays back to the PPS, the SC and the pretectal nucleus (PT), which completes the reverberating loop with the PPS.

Cells in the superficial layers respond to visual input, while those in the deeper layers respond to motion stimuli, although the cells in both layers are in register with each other. The pulvinar also receives many other subcortical inputs and acts as an 'early processing centre' receiving feedback and feedforward information from the cortex and the retina. Lesions in the pulvinar may thus affect such diverse functions as pattern recognition, eye movement and cerebellar integration in visual responses (see below). The current view of the role of the colliculus–pulvinar–cortex relay system, therefore, is that it is a priming system for ocular movement and for reducing errors in the localization response by linking visual and saccadic activity. It should be noted that the colliculus does not send out information that can modify the saccade but receives information in response to the intended saccadic movement.

Cortical centres regulate complex eye movements
Voluntary saccadic gaze movements are initiated by centres in the frontal cortex. Most of the fibres cross the midline in the anterior limb of the internal capsule to end in the gaze centres for motor neurone control of eye movement, but some pass to the ipsilateral superior colliculus where they inhibit automatic gaze responses (see above). In addition, cortical efferents remove tonic inhibitory impulses from collicular output to the ocular muscles, which are present between saccades, as if to 'free them up' for full-excursion eye movements.

Cortical voluntary saccades are 'tuned' as for automatic saccades, controlled by the superior colliculus; in the cortex, tuning is broad and appears to depend on recruitment of a precise number of neurones rather than a selected number of highly tuned neurones responsive to motion and visual activity. Single-cell recording studies have also shown that there are cells that exhibit presaccadic activity, while others respond only to the visual stimuli. A third group appears to show complex responses and may be involved in the integration of the response through a direct connection with the PPRF. The frontal eye fields also have an oculomotor loop to the substantia nigra in the basal ganglia, which contains high levels of dopamine. Loss of cells in the substantia nigra and a consequent decrease in dopamine concentration is a characteristic feature of Parkinson's disease. This can be tested using the 'antisaccadic task' test, in which the urge to fix on objects in the peripheral field is voluntarily suppressed through frontal eye field and superior collicular activity. Patients with this disorder characteristically have difficulties with voluntary gaze movements and the anti-saccadic task.

Tracking, smooth-pursuit eye movements are under cortical control through relay of object position information from the occipital cortex to the posterior parietal cortex (motor cortex of smooth pursuit, posterior parietal occipitotemporal regions) and thence to the PPRF. Here the information is integrated with retinal information on object velocity via the optic tract and with impulses from the head and neck on observer position, before being forwarded to the conjugate gaze centre for horizontal eye movement. In addition, recent studies have revealed that the frontal eye fields have control over pursuits as well as saccades.

The temporal cortex, as a centre for relay of motion detection information (see above), might be expected to be involved in the control of eye movement. Thus lesions in this area affect saccades to moving targets but not to stationary ones, while smooth-pursuit movements are also impaired. Recent studies have shown that the inferior temporal cortex is involved in the initial detection of objects to which we wish to direct our voluntary attention and fixate.

THE CEREBELLUM

Afferent input from the extraocular muscles (the stretch fibres and proprioceptors) is carried in the trigeminal nerve to synapse with cells in the granu-

---

lar cell layer (the Purkinje cell layer; see Ch. 1). There are two, and in some species three, different types of proprioceptor: muscle spindles, Golgi tendon organs and palisade endings, each restricted to the orbital, global and marginal layers of the ocular muscle respectively. However, some direct cerebellar afferent input is also visual via slit-like, narrow, vertical receptive fields.

The bulk of information connecting the cerebellum with the visual system is transferred via two-way traffic with brainstem centres. The oculomotor cerebellar centre, located in lobules VI and VII, produces saccade-type movements for which Purkinje cells are essential. Input is derived via the PPRF, the vestibular nucleus and the mesencephalic reticular formation. The output from the cerebellum predominantly concerns positional sense, and some of it is inhibitory/regulatory. Positional information applies not only to the position of the observer with relation to the object, but also to the velocity of the eye movement with relation to the target and the position of the head. Most of this is derived from the vestibular apparatus and not from visual or proprioceptive input.

This combined input also contributes to tracking movements. Experimental data have shown that cells in lobules VI and VII respond with bursts of activity during smooth pursuit movement when the eye is not actually fixating on a target.

Compensatory eye movements during movements of the head (e.g. during walking or running) are mediated mostly by the vestibulo-ocular reflex and less so by the cervico-ocular reflex through neck proprioceptors. The effect of these reflexes is to stabilize the retinal image by preventing 'retinal slip,' but the control is imperfect. The perceptual system can cope with a certain amount of retinal slip, but if this is too great (more than 5°/s) symptoms of oscillopsia appear. The cerebellum may contribute to control of the vestibulo-ocular reflex via input from the retina to the flocculus. It has been suggested that the cerebellum is the seat of a control mechanism for integration of information on spatial displacement during eye movement.

Ocular movements during natural activity

Most of the information regarding eye movement has come from studies that were designed to evaluate a particular movement, e.g. saccades or smooth pursuit movements. There have been many attempts to investigate eye movements during normal activi-

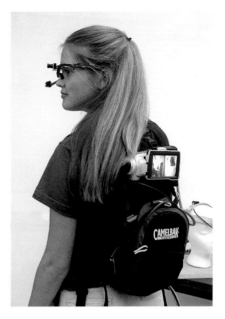

Fig. 5.35 Portable, head mounted eye-tracker developed by Pelz and colleagues, based on commercially available systems that use an infrared videocamera to image pupil and the corneal reflection. A camera mounted on the frame of the glasses records the scene from the observer's viewpoint. Eye position is then superimposed on the video record. (From Hayhoe and Ballard 2005, with permission from Elsevier.)

ties but these have only recently come to fruition because of the development of suitable eye tracking devices (Fig. 5.35). This has revealed the complex pattern of eye movements involved in performing specific tasks (Fig. 5.36) and has shown how extensively higher cortical information guides eye movements. In particular, the strong component of 'prior knowledge' to perform a fixation movement, and the concept of reward when the movement is achieved are now seen to be major drivers of gaze selection.

Neural versus mechanical control of eye movement?

A continuing issue in studies of gaze control is to understand how much regulation of muscle function is mediated via neural control and how much can be attributed to mechanical effects of the muscles. Gaze control involves rotational three-dimensional movements, which obey Listing's law when the head is fixed but do not when the head is moving, plus other movements such as optokinetic nystagmus and those generated via the vestibulo-

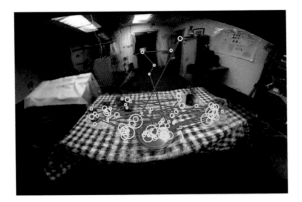

Fig. 5.36 Fixations made by an observer while making a peanut butter and jam sandwich. Images were taken from a camera mounted on the head, and a composite image mosaic was formed by integrating over different head positions using a method described in Rothkopf and Pelz (2004). (The reconstructed panorama shows artefacts due to the incomplete imaging model that does not take the translational motion of the subject into account.) Fixations are shown as yellow circles, with diameter proportional to fixation duration. Red lines indicate the saccades. Note that almost all fixations fall on task-relevant objects. (From Hayhoe and Ballard 2005, with permission from Elsevier.)

ocular reflex, to achieve image stabilization. Not all movements under control of the vestibulo-ocular reflex fail to obey Listing's law, such as the rotational movement that occurs in response to head movement, but the majority do. Movements which do not obey Listing's law, i.e. gaze shifts when the head is not restrained, obey Donder's law: for each position of gaze there is only one three-dimensional orientation (torsional movement).

Recent anatomical studies have suggested that the surrounding muscle sheath with the check ligaments can act like a pulley, allowing fine changes in the pulling direction related to the degree of torsional rotation. The data from these studies are also consistent with Listing's law and have formed the basis of some aspects of management of patients after strabismus surgery using adjustable sutures. However, the major, if not the sole, control of muscle behaviour rests with neural elements at both nuclear and supranuclear levels with considerable regulation coming from higher centres such as the frontal eye fields and the cerebro-cerebellar network (see above). Moreover, some of the neurophysiological control would be consistent with a pulley mechanism while others such as saccades, which also obey Listing's law, are not. What is clear is that both mechanical and neural mechanisms regulate motor

activity, but what remains to be determined is how the three-dimensional perception of space regulates the final motor command.

CONCLUSION

Visual neurophysiology has advanced considerably during the recent past, and our understanding of what constitutes a visual image has greatly increased. Research in this field is extremely active since there are many areas of uncertainty and, possibly more importantly, many potential applications of this knowledge to clinical medicine. The visual system has also served as a model for neural processing and circuitry generally, as it is highly amenable to experimental investigation. This is likely to remain so for many years to come.

The primate visual system is a highly complex arrangement for analysing information concerning the external world derived from a wide array of possible signals, all of which are captured by the retinal sensory receptors. The information is integrated with input from many other sensory systems and stored information from past experience (memory). The final image and its interpretation (perception) are extensively edited by the brain to ensure normality and 'constancy' wherever possible. However, this image is, of course, unique to each individual, despite the fact that we ascribe common definitions to familiar objects. Current research into the psychophysics of vision should ensure that the immediate future, at least, will be richly rewarding.

FURTHER READING

Angelaki D, Hess B. Control of eye orientation: where does the brain's role end and the muscles's begin. Europ J Neurosci 2004; 19:1–10.

Bartels A, Zeki S. The architecture of the colour centre in the human visual brain: new results and a review. Eur J Neurosci 2000; 12:172–193.

Bergstrom SS. The AMBEGUJAS phenomenon and colour constancy. Perception 2004; 33:831–835.

Claustrat B, Brun J, Chazot G. The basic physiology and pathophysiology of melatonin. Sleep Med Rev 2005; 9:11–24.

Cronley-Dillon JR. Vision and visual dysfunction. London: Macmillan; 1991.

Cumming B. Stereopsis: how the brain sees depth. Curr Biol 1997; 7:R645.

Davson H. Physiology of the eye, 5th edn. New York: Pergamon Press; 1990.

Field GD, Sampath AP, Rieke FF. Retinal processing near absolute threshold: from behavior to mechanism. Annu Rev Physiol 2005; 67:491–514.

Frackowiak RSJ, Zeki S. Human brain function, 2nd edn. New York: Academic Press; 2003.

Fu Y, Liao H-W, Do MTH, Yau K-W. Non-image-forming ocular photoreception in vertebrates. Curr Opin Neurobiol 2005; 15:415–422.

Grill-Spector K, Malach, R. The human visual cortex. Annu Rev Neurosci 2004; 27:649–677.

Halliday AM, ed. Evoked potentials in clinical testing, 2nd edn. Edinburgh: Churchill Livingstone; 1993.

Harris JM, Drga VF. Using visual direction in three-dimensional motion perception. Nat Neurosci 2005; 8:229–233.

Hayhoe M, Ballard D. Eye movements in natural behaviour. Trends Cogn Sci 2005; 9:188–194.

Hofer H, Carroll J, Neitz J, Neitz M, Williams DR. Organization of the human trichromatic cone mosaic. J Neurosci 2005; 23:9669–9679.

Hurlbert AC, Derrington AM. How many neurones does it take to see? Curr Biol 1993; 3:510–512.

Ikeda H. Clinical electroretinography. In: Halliday AM, ed. Evoked potentials in clinical testing, 2nd edn. Edinburgh: Churchill Livingstone; 1993:115–139.

Kass JH, Collins CE. The primate visual system. New York: CRC Press; 2003.

Kammermans M, Spekreijse H. The feedback pathway from horizontal cells to cones. Vis Res 1999; 39:2449–2468.

Kaufman PL, Alm A (eds). Adler's physiology of the eye, 10th edn. Chicago: Mosby; 2002.

Lamb TD, Pugh EN Jr. Dark adaptation and the retinoid cycle of vision. Prog Ret Eye Res 2004; 23:307–380.

Land EH. Recent advances in retinex theory and some implications for cortical computations: colour vision and the natural image. Proc Natl Acad Sci USA 1983; 80:5163–5169.

McIlwain JT. An introduction to the biology of vision. New York: Cambridge University Press; 1996.

Mapp AP, Ono H, Barbeito R. What does the dominant eye dominate? A brief and somewhat contentious review. Perception Psychophys 2003; 65:310–317.

Masland RH. The fundamental plan of the retina. Nat Neurosci 2001; 4:877–886.

Mollon JD, Bowmaker JK. The spatial arrangement of cones in the primate fovea. Nature 1992; 360:677–679.

Nathans J, Thomas D, Hogness DS. Molecular genetics of human colour vision: the genes encoding blue, green and red pigments. Science 1986; 232:193–202.

Parker A. Solid shape and the natural world. Curr Biol 1993; 3:401–403.

Schweigerling J. Theoretical limits to visual acuity. Surv Ophthalmol 2000; 45:139–146.

Spekreijse H, Apkarian PA. Visual pathways: electrophysiology and pathology (Documenta Ophthalmologica Proceedings series).

Todd JT, Thaler L, Dijkstra TMH. The effects of field of view on the perception of 3D slant from texture. Vis Res 2005; 45:1501–1517.

Verrelli BC, Tishkoff SA. Signatures of selection and gene conversion associated with human color vision variation. Am J Hum Genet 2004; 75:363–375.

Wandell BA, Brewer AA, Dougherty RF. Visual field map clusters in human cortex. Phil Trans R Soc B 2005; 360:693–707.

Wexler M. Voluntary head movement and allocentric perception of space. Psychol Sci 2003; 14:340–346.

Wexler M, van Boxtel JJA. Depth perception by the active observer. Trends Cogn Sci 2005; 9:431–438.

Zeki S. Colour vision and functional specialisation in the visual cortex. Discussions in neuroscience, vol. VI, no. 2. Amsterdam: Elsevier Science; 1990.

Zeki S. The visual image in mind and brain. Sci Am 1992; 267:42–51.

Zeki S. Inner vision: an exploration of art and the brain. New York: Oxford University Press; 1999.

6 GENERAL AND OCULAR PHARMACOLOGY

INTRODUCTION

This chapter covers the basic principles of clinical pharmacology, with particular reference to drugs used in the management of ophthalmic disorders, methods of ocular drug delivery, and the interactions of drugs and the eye. Although it is generally thought that the medical management of ocular disease is mainly administered through topical therapeutic agents, many systemic drugs and agents are also used. These include diuretics for the control of intraocular pressure, immunosuppressants for control of intraocular inflammatory conditions and antimicrobials for control of infection. Therefore, basic pharmacological principles (pharmacokinetics and pharmacodynamics) are important to ophthalmologists. The basic pharmacology of systemic therapy, including receptor–drug interactions, is reviewed before discussing the more specific topical and systemic therapies in the treatment of ophthalmic disorders.

PHARMACOKINETICS: DRUG TRAFFICKING IN THE BODY

BASIC CONCEPTS

Pharmacokinetics is the mathematical study of the time-course of drug absorption, distribution, metabolism and excretion. One of the simplest parameters to consider when discussing the pharmacokinetics of any drug, is the biological *half-life* of a drug ($t_{1/2}$), which is the time taken for the plasma drug concentration to fall by half after administration. A more accurate method of assessing the efficiency of drug elimination is the estimation of drug clearance from the circulation. For example, after intravenous administration, the $t_{1/2}$ of the drug may be calculated from its plasma concentration–time curve. This

319

simplistic model is based on a single compartment model that states that, following intravenous administration, the distribution of a drug assumes a uniform concentration throughout all compartments (intracellular and extracellular); the elimination by both metabolism and renal excretion is also assumed to be directly proportional to the drug concentration. If this is the case the volume of distribution may be calculated as:

$$V_d = \text{dose}/C_0$$

where C_0 is the estimated (plasma) concentration at the time of injection.

The apparent volume of distribution is defined as the volume of fluid required to contain the total amount of drug in the body at the same concentration as that present in plasma. Drugs in general may be confined to the plasma compartment because they are either too large to cross the capillary wall or are highly protein-bound (e.g. heparin and warfarin respectively). Drugs may also be distributed only to the extracellular compartment because they have low lipid solubility (e.g. gentamicin) or distributed throughout all aqueous compartments if they are lipid soluble. When both the volume of distribution and renal clearance of a drug are known, the $t_{1/2}$ may be estimated. However, when considering a single compartment model, no account is taken of distribution into tissue compartments and metabolism within tissue compartments. When repeated injections of the drug are given, the plasma concentration becomes a function of the rate of both elimination and administration, and the plasma concentration will equilibrate when these two parameters are equal. A steady-state plasma concentration is therefore reached, which in practice may be established after an interval of about three or four plasma half-life lives of the drug given. To reach a steady-state concentration more quickly, loading doses of the drug are often given (for example, antibiotics and warfarin) (Fig. 6.1). In clinical practice the $t_{1/2}$ is important because it will determine the frequency of administration of a drug. If continued intravenous boluses are given, there are frequently large peaks and troughs in drug concentration, which can lead to a greater incidence of toxic side effects.

Bioavailability describes the amount of oral dose that reaches the systemic circulation and becomes available to the site of drug action. However, this blanket term is not sufficiently precise because rapidly absorbed drugs will reach a much higher plasma concentration than those absorbed slowly and, similarly, rapid elimination would also theoretically lead

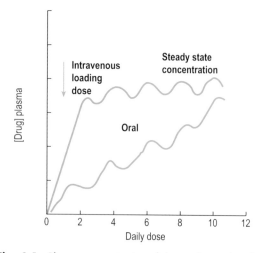

Fig. 6.1 Plasma concentration of drugs after oral and intravenous administration.

to low bioavailability. Bioavailability of a drug is measured as the area under the curve of log plasma concentration against time for both intravenous and oral administration, although the reliability of quantitative drug assessment may be variable for several reasons. For instance, the degree of bioavailability may be altered by incomplete absorption of the drug or destruction of the drug by *first-pass metabolism* before the drug reaches the plasma compartment, irrespective of the rate of absorption from the gastrointestinal tract. Drugs instilled into the eye are absorbed from the nasal and nasopharyngeal mucosae directly into the systemic circulation. As such, they escape first-pass metabolism and have a high bioavailability. Thus, topically administered agents can give rise to quite marked systemic effects (see below).

Drug kinetics can be described as first-order (linear) or zero-order (non-linear, saturation) kinetics (Fig. 6.2). First-order kinetics describes a process where rate is proportional to the amount of drug present and can be defined by linear differential equations. Zero-order kinetics occurs when drug dynamics show *saturation* at high drug concentrations. Saturation may occur, for example, when the capacity of drug-metabolizing liver enzymes is surpassed, leading to unmetabolized drug in the circulation for longer periods. The duration of action of a drug that exhibits saturation kinetics is more dependent on the administering dose than in drugs that exhibit first-order kinetics. Also, there is no direct relationship between drug dose and steady-state plasma

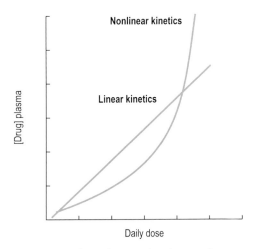

Fig. 6.2 First-order and zero-order pharmacokinetics.

concentration in zero-order kinetics, which may explain sudden unexpected drug toxicity in a number of clinical settings. For this reason, close drug monitoring is required (e.g. phenytoin).

DRUG ABSORPTION

For a drug to reach the site at which it produces its effect, it must first be absorbed from its site of administration. In general, drug penetration of cell membranes increases with lipid solubility. Drugs can cross cell membranes by diffusing directly through lipid, by diffusion through aqueous pores that traverse the lipid, by utilizing carrier molecules, or by pinocytosis by the cell.

The rate of passage (diffusion) through a cell membrane can be predicted by Fick's law

Non-polar substances dissolve freely in lipid and therefore penetrate the cell by diffusion. The lipid solubility, degree of ionization and molecular size of the drug will determine its diffusion coefficient. The rate is determined by Fick's law, which states that the rate at which drugs cross a biological membrane is directly proportional to the concentration gradient across the membrane and the diffusion coefficient, and inversely proportional to the cell membrane thickness (see below).

$$\text{Rate of diffusion} = KA\,(x_1 - x_2)/D$$

where K is the diffusion constant, A is the diffusion area, $x_1 - x_2$ is the concentration difference between

plasma and intracellular compartments, and D is the thickness of the membrane.

Active transport

As for active transport of ions (see Ch. 4), active transport of large polar drugs requires energy-dependent carrier-mediated mechanisms. These transport systems may be disrupted by inhibiting enzyme-dependent carriers or by blocking the carrier mechanism with structurally similar drugs (analogues). Facilitated transport is carrier-mediated transport that does not require energy because it does not proceed against a concentration gradient, for example glucose transport into erythrocytes.

DRUG ABSORPTION IS DEPENDENT ON A DRUG'S LIPID SOLUBILITY

Drug properties

The absorption of a drug depends on its lipid solubility and inversely on its polarity or degree of ionization. An important factor in the degree of penetration of a drug through membranes is that many drugs are weak acids or weak bases. The more the drug is in its un-ionized form, the more likely it is to be lipid-soluble and transferred by passive diffusion through the membrane. For a weak acid or base the pK_a value will determine the degree of ionization, as described by the Henderson–Hasselbalch equation.

For a weak acid the ionizing reaction is:

$$pH = pK_a + \log\{[A^-]/[HA]\}$$

and for a weak base it is:

$$pH = pK_a + \log\{[B]/[BH^+]\}$$

The pK_a is a measure of the relative strength (degree of ionization) of a weak acid or base (the pK_a of a drug is that point at which the compound is 50% ionized). The lipid solubility of the uncharged species also depends on the chemical nature of the drug. For example, although streptomycin and the related aminoglycosides are uncharged, the high percentage of hydrogen-bonding groups within these molecules renders them hydrophilic.

The molecular shape, as well as the charge distribution, of the drug molecule determines which membrane pores it may traverse. Small polar molecules, such as urea, readily traverse small aqueous pores in the membrane, thus accounting for the high permeability of cell membranes to these substances. Most drugs, however, are too large to pass through these pores.

321

The rate of drug absorption varies with the route of administration

The main routes of administration (besides intravenous) are oral, sublingual, rectal, topical (e.g. skin, conjunctival fornix), subcutaneous and intramuscular.

Absorption of orally administered drugs is affected by gastric pH, rate of emptying of gastric contents, presence of food, and surface area of absorptive mucosa (in disorders such as Crohn's disease the absorptive surface area may be reduced). It is important to consider drug interactions during multiple drug therapy and their effect on drug absorption. For example, in migraine gastric emptying is delayed, reducing the absorption of analgesics such as aspirin and paracetamol. This may be overcome with the adjunctive use of parenteral metoclopramide, which increases the rate of gastric emptying. The presence of food is generally unimportant, except in the case of tetracyclines (used to treat certain forms of external eye disease commonly associated with acne rosacea), which form insoluble salts with magnesium and calcium. Some drugs will be inactivated within the gut lumen (e.g. benzylpenicillin and insulin). Most malabsorption syndromes do not affect drug absorption, but in other disorders, such as congestive cardiac failure, drug absorption may be impaired because of the secondary gastrointestinal mucosal oedema. Factors affecting bioavailability are shown in Box 6.1.

DRUG DISTRIBUTION

Once a drug is absorbed, it has the potential to penetrate most compartments of the body so the distribution of the drug depends largely on the route of administration. Intravenous and intramuscular administration of a drug result in high drug availability. Buccal (sublingual) absorption of a drug is used to reduce the extent of first-pass metabolism by the liver (as with topically applied eye drops), which invariably occurs with orally administered drugs that reach the liver via the portal circulation. The distribution of the drug and its ability to penetrate cells is also dependent on its physicochemical properties and thus the extent of binding to tissue proteins or cell membrane receptors (see Box 6.2).

Once the drug has reached the systemic circulation it may become bound to circulating proteins, commonly *albumin* or α_1-*acid glycoproteins* (for basic drugs). Protein-bound drugs are restricted in their distribution into tissues, which reduces the availability of the free drug for pharmacological effect. This, in turn, depends on the affinity of the protein for the drug. High levels of protein binding may occur with acidic drugs that are bound to albumin. If a drug is less than 90% bound to plasma proteins, changes in the plasma protein concentration make little difference to the overall amount of unbound drug in the circulation. In cases of drugs with a high binding affinity for protein, a decrease in the steady-state total concentration of the drug, and as a consequence a comparative increase in the clearance of the increased amount of free drug, would occur if for any reason protein binding was impaired. For instance, impaired plasma protein binding in the case of phenytoin results in peaks of unbound active drug in the plasma.

Basic drugs are bound in varying degrees to α_1-acid glycoprotein, a protein that increases in concentration in certain pathological conditions such as acute inflammation. Under such conditions, the binding of basic drugs (e.g. propranolol) may be increased, thus reducing their effect.

Systemic factors that alter protein binding include hypoalbuminaemia (plasma concentration of albumin less than 25 g/l), renal failure, competition by other highly protein-bound drugs, and changes occurring during the last trimester of pregnancy, such as the diluting effect of the increased plasma volume. In general, competition for binding by other drugs is the major factor affecting distribution because adequate compensatory mechanisms can be initiated to counteract the other causes. The

---

Box 6.1 Factors altering absorption and bioavailability from gut

- Gut motility
- Intestinal pH, mucus, bile salts
- Enterohepatic circulation
- Exercise
- Reduced absorptive area
- Reduced intestinal blood flow
- Intestinal microflora that may metabolize some drugs

Box 6.2 Factors affecting drug distribution

- Physicochemical properties of drug
- Binding to plasma proteins
- Binding to tissue proteins
- Relative blood flow to different tissues

distribution of a drug, as mentioned above, may also be regulated by the binding of a drug to tissue proteins, a process regulated by the abundance of binding sites, affinity constants and the binding of a drug to its receptor. This in turn may give rise to a desired or undesired effect, although receptor numbers are unlikely to be high enough to alter the distribution of the drug appreciably.

In the eye, both the blood–retinal barrier and the blood–aqueous barrier (see Ch. 1) limit the distribution of drugs. Tight junctions between the retinal pigment epithelium (RPE) and endothelium of the retinal vessel endothelium give rise to a relatively impermeable barrier to water solutes and larger molecules. Under normal conditions only lipid-soluble drugs will move between the blood and retina. Similarly, the apical membranes of the non-pigmented ciliary body epithelium and the capillary endothelium of the iris are bound by tight junctions, raising a barrier to all but lipid-soluble drugs (see Ch. 1).

DRUGS ARE METABOLIZED TO FACILITATE CLEARANCE

The metabolism of most drugs occurs almost entirely in the liver, enzymatically altering the drug to increase its water solubility in preparation for excretion, and simultaneously making the compound metabolically and pharmacologically active or inactive. Metabolism can affect the drug in various ways. The first is activation of the parent drug, which may itself be inactive (known as a *prodrug*). The drug may be metabolized to form active metabolites, as for example in the case of diamorphine and diazepam. However, metabolism of a drug can also produce toxic metabolites that may persist in the circulation for longer than the parent molecule and thus restrict the continued use of such drugs (e.g. lignocaine). In general, most drug metabolism modifies the drug so that it can then be excreted, usually in the urine but sometimes in bile.

Drug metabolism takes place in two stages: phase I (oxidation) and phase II (conjugation). Phase I reactions are carried out by a heterogeneous group of microsomal enzymes called cytochrome P_{450}, of which various forms exist (see Box 6.3).

This enzyme system exists in abundance in the liver but is also found in some peripheral organs, including the eye. It is important to note that the activity of these enzymes can be induced by other drugs (e.g. phenytoin and carbamazepine), which accounts for

---

Box 6.3 Drug-metabolizing systems

Phase I metabolism: oxidation
Cytochrome P_{450} (microsomal)

- aromatic hydroxylation
- aliphatic hydroxylation
- *N*-deamination
- *N*-dealkylation
- *S*-oxidation
- desulphuration

Phase II metabolism: conjugation
Conjugation occurs with:

- glucuronic acid
- glycine
- glutamine
- sulphate
- acetate

Box 6.4 Drugs acting as microsomal enzyme manipulators

Enzyme inducers
- barbiturates
- phenytoin
- phenothiazines
- rifampicin
- griseofulvin
- nicotine

Enzyme inhibitors
- isoniazid
- chloramphenicol
- metronidazole
- warfarin
- carbon monoxide

---

many well-recognized drug interactions. Conjugation reactions appear not to be affected by enzyme-inducing drugs to the same extent as oxidative metabolism. There are also other oxidative enzymes that are not part of the cytochrome P_{450} system but which are involved in drug metabolism; these include xanthine oxidase (e.g. purine metabolism), alcohol dehydrogenase and monoamine oxidase (e.g. catecholamine metabolism). Many drugs also affect the function of microsomal enzyme systems (see Box 6.4).

The metabolism of a drug is dependent on several factors. Oxidative metabolism is affected by age. Premature babies metabolize poorly and, similarly in the elderly, oxidative drug metabolism is reduced because of reduced liver size. Smoking may induce certain liver enzymes, necessitating an increased dose of drug for a required effect. Alcohol, on the other hand, inhibits drug metabolism, particularly during and after binge drinking. Both severe liver disease and poor nutrition may markedly impair drug metabolism. An important influence in metabolic reactions is that of genetic control. Different individuals have different capacities to metabolize a drug, but within a population this tends to follow a normal distribution. There are, however, some examples of clear distinctions in the individual's capability to metabolize drugs. This is seen with acetylation of drugs. N-acetylation may be either fast or slow, depending on the amount of enzyme present, which is controlled by a single recessive gene associated with low hepatic acetyltransferase activity (e.g. in isoniazid metabolism). Patients with low acetyltransferase activity are known as *slow acetylators*. Another genetic variation in the rate of drug metabolism is seen with suxamethonium (a depolarizing neuromuscular blocker used in general anaesthesia). About 1 in 3000 individuals fail to inactivate suxamethonium by hydrolysis (pseudocholinesterase), which is the result of a recessive gene giving rise, in homozygotes, to an abnormal cholinesterase with a much lower substrate affinity. Patients who have a hereditary erythrocyte glucose-6-phosphate dehydrogenase enzyme deficiency may develop a haemolytic anaemia when treated with a number of drugs, including chloroquine, vitamin K, acetylsalicylic acid (aspirin) and probenecid.

METABOLIZED DRUGS ARE EXCRETED IN URINE AND BILE

Renal excretion

Drugs differ greatly in their excretion via the kidney. Some drugs are cleared in a single transit through the kidney, while others are poorly cleared. This difference is dependent on the kidney's ability to handle the drug and on physicochemical properties of the drug. Certain drugs may be filtered through the

glomerulus (depending on molecular weight), others are actively secreted by the tubules and still others passively diffuse across the tubular epithelia (reabsorption).

Glomerular filtration

Glomerular excretion of a drug is only possible when drugs are not bound to plasma proteins, and the drug is of a molecular size that can be filtered freely, irrespective of charge (less than 20 000 Da). The clearance of the drug is therefore related to the unbound fraction of the drug and is dependent on the glomerular filtration rate. Glomerular filtration at most removes only about 20% of drug reaching the kidney; the remaining drug passes to the capillaries lining the tubules. Most drugs are presented to the kidney in a carrier form and thus their clearance is slow. Carrier-mediated transport can increase the clearance of the drug even if it is highly bound. Benzylpenicillin is 80% bound and cleared very slowly by glomerular filtration but is almost completely removed by tubular secretion.

Secretion

Drugs may be actively secreted by the tubules into the glomerular filtrate. Different secretory systems, which are relatively non-selective carrier systems, exist for acidic, basic and neutral drug transport into the tubular lumen. Competition for active sites occurs, so that the secretion of drugs can be blocked by other drugs, for example secretion of penicillins is blocked by probenecid, thus decreasing the excretion of the drug.

Reabsorption

If the tubules were freely permeable to drugs, the drug concentration in the filtrate would be similar to that in plasma. Drug reabsorption occurs mainly as a result of the enormous reabsorption of water achieved by the nephron. This builds up a concentration gradient that drives the drug back into the plasma. Thus drugs that are highly lipid soluble are excreted slowly and the reabsorption of drugs, especially those that are weak acids or bases, depends on the drug being in its un-ionized form. Therefore, altering the pH of the urine will increase the elimination of the drug, so that acidic drugs are eliminated more quickly in alkaline urine. This manipulation of urine pH is utilized clinically for the treatment of aspirin overdoses, where forced alkaline diuresis is an effective way of increasing the excretion of the acidic drug. Measurement of glomerular filtration can be achieved with the use of agents that are completely filtered and neither

---

Box 6.5 Factors affecting drug metabolism
• Age
• Smoking
• Alcohol
• Nutritional status
• Pharmacogenetics

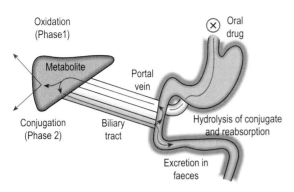

Fig. 6.3 Drug metabolism: enterohepatic circulation.

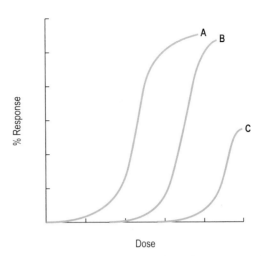

Fig. 6.4 Potency of receptor stimulation by agonists and partial agonists.

secreted nor reabsorbed, for example inulin. Conversely, the clearance of a drug that is completely secreted in one transit through the kidney will correspond to the renal plasma flow, for example *p*-aminohippuric acid.

Biliary excretion

Liver cells also possess transport systems similar to those in the renal tubules, which can transfer drug metabolites from blood to bile. Conjugated drugs (particularly with glucuronate) are concentrated in the bile and delivered to the intestine, where the conjugate may be hydrolysed, releasing the active drug (Fig. 6.3). The drug may then be reabsorbed and its duration of action prolonged (enterohepatic circulation). This is particularly important for digoxin, which is excreted in the bile in an unconjugated form, and for morphine, which is transported as a glucuronide. Some drugs, for example rifampicin, are excreted into the bile and will be excreted unchanged in the faeces.

PHARMACODYNAMICS: DRUG HANDLING BY THE BODY

Pharmacodynamics considers the effects of a drug and the relationship between drug concentration and response. The drug effect is usually initiated by its binding to a cellular membrane receptor, which is specific for the drug, as is the case with autonomic nervous system neurotransmitters, or by non-specific mechanisms, where specific cell membrane receptors do not exist but drug action is dependent solely on its physical properties (i.e. lipid solubility), or by its ability to inhibit specific biochemical enzymes. The effects of enzyme inhibition may be

direct, for example by blocking sodium/potassium ATPase pumps or closing ion channels, or indirect, for example by acting on calcium channels. Some drugs act on intracytoplasmic receptors or cell nucleus receptors. The variety of drug actions is discussed below.

A drug that acts on a receptor may act as an *agonist* or *antagonist*, depending on the response that is elicited. In Fig. 6.4, drugs A and B are both agonists, but drug B is less potent. Drug C, on the other hand, acts as a partial agonist. Antagonists can be either competitive or non-competitive. If the antagonist is displaced by increasing concentrations of the drug (agonist), then competitive inhibition is present. Non-competitive antagonism describes the situation where the antagonist blocks the action of the agonist without competing with the receptor, which may not be overcome by increasing the concentration of the agonist, so shifting the curve to the right and depressing the maximal response (Fig. 6.5).

Drugs often give a graded dose–response curve, where increasing the drug concentration will increase the drug effect. This graded response is seen with drugs that are not permanently bound to the receptor. Thus the *efficacy* of a drug is defined as the maximal response it can give, whereas *potency* describes the amount of drug required to give the desired response. Thus some drugs may be efficacious but not potent, requiring large doses to give an effect. However, if the drug is irreversibly bound to the receptor, its effect will continue well after the

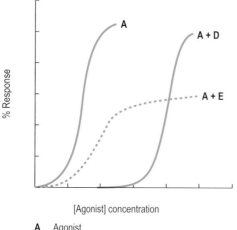

A Agonist
D Competitive antagonist
E Noncompetitive antagonist

Fig. 6.5 The effects of agonist action by competitive and non-competitive antagonists.

elimination of the drug from the bloodstream. Alternatively, the efficacy of a drug may diminish with time, an effect known as *tolerance*, which is thought to be the result of downregulation of specific drug receptors. Some drugs also produce active metabolites that continue to give a pharmacological effect well beyond the half-life of the parent drug. All these effects may complicate the study of pharmacokinetics.

DRUG–RECEPTOR INTERACTIONS

Drugs bind to target molecules on the cell, which then initiate their pharmacological effect. Receptors are proteins that, in general, are situated on the cell surface and are able to bind ligands (e.g. neurotransmitters and hormones) (see Box 6.8). The recognition of a ligand by a receptor is analogous to antibody–antigen binding, that is the lock and key principle (see Ch. 7). The molecular mechanisms involved in this receptor–effector pathway are known as *transduction* mechanisms, where the receptor is linked either directly or indirectly to the effector system altering cell function. Several forms of receptor–effector linkage are recognized, and include:

- Direct regulation of membrane permeability to ions
- Regulation of cell function via an intracellular second messenger

- Regulation of cell function by regulating DNA transcription and protein synthesis.

ION CHANNELS

Receptors can be linked directly with ion channels, which function only when the receptor is occupied by an agonist. This is the fastest type of receptor response, as, for example, when a neurotransmitter acts on a nerve ending. The excitatory neurotransmitters acetylcholine and glutamate cause a direct increase in both sodium and potassium permeability, which results in depolarization of the cell (see Ch. 5). An equilibrium between open and closed ion channels exists and random fluctuations in conductance occur when the ion channels are opened (or closed) after receptor stimulation. The duration of this response can be measured and is referred to as the *mean channel lifetime*.

SECOND MESSENGERS

Receptor binding on extracellular receptors alters intracellular functions by activating a secondary messenger, for example the activation of the enzyme *adenyl cyclase* and calcium ion influx. Activation of these secondary messengers regulates various intracellular activities. In many cases they generate protein kinase activation and phosphorylation of membrane proteins (see Ch. 4). The consequence of any change in protein conformation of the cell membrane may lead to opening of ion channels (e.g. sodium/potassium or calcium channels). Adenyl cyclase may also be activated by G-proteins, which are discussed below.

Cyclic adenosine monophosphate (cAMP)

Cyclic AMP is a nucleotide synthesized within the cell from adenosine triphosphate (ATP) by the enzyme *adenyl cyclase*, and is inactivated enzymatically to 5'AMP by hydroxylation with a group of enzymes called *phosphodiesterases*. The following components are required to generate a secondary messenger. These include a receptor, which faces outwards from the cell, a regulatory protein (G-protein), which faces inward toward the cytoplasm, adenyl cyclase, and a cAMP-dependent protein kinase. Inhibition of the secondary messenger activation can be induced with cholera toxin, which binds specifically to the G-protein in the intestinal mucosa and thus prevents hydrolysis of another membrane nucleotide, guanine triphosphate (GTP) and adenyl cyclase (see Box 6.6).

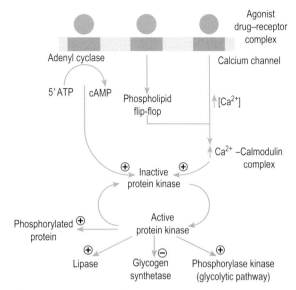

Fig. 6.6 Activation of membrane-associated enzymes by calcium–calmodulin secondary messengers.

Box 6.6 G-proteins regulate second messenger activity

G-proteins are so called because of their affiliation with the guanine nucleotides, GTP and GDP. They consist of three subunits, which catalyse GTP conversion to GDP. In the resting (empty receptor) state the G-protein–GDP complex is associated with the receptor. The presumed conformational change in the cell membrane when the receptor is occupied acts to increase the affinity of the neighbouring G-protein for GTP and to promote the binding of the G-protein–GTP complex to the effector site. This complex can activate ion channels, adenyl cyclase and other secondary messengers, as shown in the figure below.

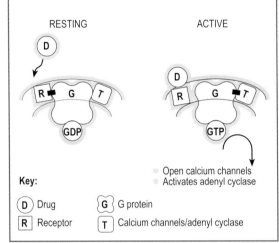

Key:

D	Drug	
R	Receptor	
G	G protein	
T	Calcium channels/adenyl cyclase	

Box 6.7 Hormones and transmitters that act via calcium channels

- Muscarinic agonists
- α_1 agonists
- Histamine
- Serotonin

CALCIUM IS A MAJOR MEDIATOR OF CELLULAR ACTIVITY

Virtually all the calcium in the body is in the skeleton as hydroxyapatite. Intracellular calcium only constitutes 1% of total body calcium. The plasma concentration of calcium is 2.5 mM; 50% is in its ionized form and 50% is bound to proteins or complexed with anions. A rise in the intracellular free calcium concentration can occur as a response to hormones and transmitters, by a net influx of calcium ions into the cell. It may also occur as a result of a release of sequestered calcium without a net influx into the cell. The intracellular calcium concentration is 10^{-7} M, most of which is protein bound, and small changes in free calcium concentration may affect many intracellular processes. Intracellular calcium is normally regulated by an ATP-active transport channel. Accompanying the increase in intracellular calcium level, there is also an increase in the rate of degradation of minor membrane phospholipids (phosphatidyl inositols) by phospholipase C, which in turn alters the membrane permeability and control of membrane phosphorylation, either directly, via its effect on protein kinases, or indirectly, through activation of adenyl cyclase. At the same time a phospholipid flip-flop mechanism occurs within the cell membrane, where methylation of phospholipids converting phosphatidyl ethanolamine to phosphatidyl choline takes place. This further increases calcium permeability, and secondarily regulates adenyl cyclase activation. Intracellular effects of calcium are controlled by an intracellular acidic protein, calmodulin. The calcium–calmodulin complex can thus activate many enzyme systems, including protein kinases, adenyl cyclase, phosphodiesterases and calcium-dependent ATPase (Fig. 6.6). The calcium–calmodulin complex is inactivated via the binding of trifluoperazine (an antipsychotic agent), which can be used to study the mechanism of action of certain therapeutic agents.

REGULATION OF PROTEIN SYNTHESIS

Steroid hormones, because they are lipophilic, can diffuse across the cell membrane and bind to cytoplasmic receptors and nuclear chromatin. Certain regions of the DNA sequence show a high affinity for steroid–receptor complexes, and binding of these complexes generates an increase in RNA polymerase activity and generation of messenger RNA (mRNA) and thus production of proteins (see Ch. 3). One steroid may result in the production of several different species of mRNA within each cell, which may explain the great diversity of steroid actions.

Ligand–receptor affinity determines selectivity

The affinity of a ligand for its receptor is measured by the amount of ligand required to achieve half-maximal binding (EC_{50}). The binding force of the receptor–ligand complex can also be measured by the length of time taken for dissociation of the complex to occur. Low-affinity agonists include those required to potentiate a rapid response (e.g. neurotransmitters), and therefore concentrations of the ligand close to the receptor during stimulation must be high. The *selectivity* of a ligand for receptors is a ratio of the EC_{50} for the receptors being compared. If the ligand (or drug) is more selective for receptor A than for receptor B, it will achieve its clinical effect by stimulation of receptor A at lower

doses, but will still stimulate receptor B if sufficient drug is given. Therefore, clinically, it is important to establish the EC_{50} ratio of a given drug; ratios lower than 50 are considered unsafe for clinical use if stimulation of other receptors is to be avoided.

OCULAR PHARMACOLOGY: DRUG HANDLING BY CELLS AND TISSUES OF THE EYE

This section describes the pharmacokinetics, pharmacodynamics and modes of drug delivery (excluding systemic administration) that are used to treat ocular surface and intraocular conditions.

MECHANISMS OF OCULAR DRUG ABSORPTION

There are several methods of administering ocular medications, including extraocular routes (topical) via either conjunctival/episcleral absorption (non-corneal) or transcorneal absorption, and direct intraocular administration of drugs. The non-corneal route of absorption may be significant for drugs that do not penetrate the cornea well. Corneal absorption still represents the major route of absorption for most ocular medication.

FACTORS INFLUENCING DELIVERY OF DRUGS TO THE EYE

Drugs can be administered in many different topical forms, including solutions, gels and ointments. The efficacy of treatment is usually dependent on intraocular penetration, which in turn is dependent on the permeability of the drug across the cornea, and the anatomical and physiological influences of the local environment, including lacrimation, tear drainage and the composition of the precorneal tear film.

Routes of administration

Conjunctiva
Topical administration into the inferior fornix of the conjunctiva is by far the most common route of ocular drug delivery. Both lacrimation and blinking profoundly influence the residence time of fluid in the fornix. Therefore, the efficacy of such delivery systems depends on the anatomy and physiology of

---

Box 6.8 Receptors

Receptors are unique cell surface proteins capable of binding specific associated substances (ligands). Receptors may be divided into subtypes, depending on the type of agonist or antagonist associated with them. Often receptors can be downregulated or upregulated in different disease states or with chronic drug usage.

A *ligand* is a specific compound (drug or natural substance) that binds to a receptor.

Agonists are substances that, when bound to a receptor, produce a response that may result in stimulation or inhibition of cell function.

Antagonists are substances that prevent receptor activation.

A *partial agonist* is a ligand that possesses both antagonist and agonist properties. As such, its maximal effect is less than that of a pure agonist. However, when occupying a receptor it prevents the actions of other agonists, which are therefore less efficacious.

the lids, the precorneal tear film, and the health of the conjunctiva, cornea and lacrimal system.

The conjunctival sac has a capacity of approximately 15–30 μl (dependent on blinking) and the natural tear film volume is 7–8 μl. The tears turn over at approximately 16% per minute during a normal blink rate of 15–20 blinks per minute. Most solution applicators deliver between 50 and 100 μl per drop so a substantial amount of drug will be lost through overspill on administration. The turnover of tears is also highly dependent on environmental conditions, particularly temperature and humidity. The epithelium of the conjunctiva is continuous with that of the cornea and epidermis of the lids (see Ch. 1) and contains goblet cells, which produce mucus and are integral to the stability of the tear film (see Ch. 4). Drug absorption through the conjunctiva therefore requires transport firstly through the epithelium. In the subconjunctival stroma, which is a highly vascular conjunctiva owing to the rich superficial venous plexus and lid margin vessels, drugs may be absorbed in significant concentrations into the circulation. Also, after administration into the inferior fornix, drugs drain directly through the nasolacrimal duct into the nose, where measurable systemic absorption of drugs via the nasal and nasopharyngeal mucosa occurs. Restricting the entry of a topically applied ophthalmic dose into the nasal cavity by nasolacrimal occlusion for 5 min, or by making appropriate alterations to the vehicle (i.e. from solution to ointment) increases the residence time of the drug in the fornix, and increases ocular absorption (see Table 6.1).

Precorneal tear film and cornea

Tears are considered to act as a buffering system for many substances. The pH of normal tears varies between 6.5 and 7.6, while many drug delivery systems are often formulated at pH of less than 7; the return to physiological pH after drug instillation is, however, more likely to be a function of increased tear turnover than the result of a buffering effect. The precorneal tear film is composed of an outer lipid layer (mixed lipids), a middle aqueous layer (including proteins) and a deeper mucin layer (glycoprotein) (see Ch. 4). The mucin layer contributes to the stability of the tear film, as well as promoting adherence of the tears to the lipophilic corneal and conjunctival epithelium. Any alteration in the components of the tear film will result in instability of the tear film and a reduced conjunctival residence time of the drug. At the same time alteration in the pH of the tear film may affect the ionization of the drug and thus its diffusion capacity. In spite of the extensive losses to the exterior and to systemic absorption, topical (conjunctival) administration of drugs achieves acceptable intraocular levels, mainly because of the very high concentrations that are administered.

The pH of the tear fluid is important in drug formulation because of the physiological homeostatic mechanisms. Drug penetration may be enhanced by changing the degree of drug ionization and enhancing the product stabilization over a range of pH changes. The epithelium of the cornea represents the most important barrier to intraocular transport of drugs via this route. First, the stratified cellular epithelium is bound by desmosomes between the lateral borders of the superficial cells. Second, the corneal epithelium is hydrophobic (as are all cell membranes), and so will allow only lipid-soluble drugs to pass through. In addition, Bowman's membrane, an acellular collagenous sheet (10-μm thick) between the basement membrane of the epithelium and the stroma of the cornea, acts as a further barrier to the penetration of drugs. In contrast, the stroma, which accounts for 90% of the corneal substance and its ground substance (glycosaminoglycans and water), permits ionized water-soluble drugs to pass more efficiently than lipid-soluble drugs. Finally, transport across the single-layer endothelium of the cornea is relatively free because it contains gap junctions that permit good penetration of most drugs into the aqueous humour. Many topical eye medications are weak bases, for example tropicamide, cyclopentolate and atropine, and exist in both ionized and un-ionized forms within the pH range of the tear film (pH 7.4). Altering the solution pH of timolol (pK_a 9.2) from 6.2 to 7.5 increases its corneal penetration and systemic absorption. The partition coefficient (ratio of concentrations in the two compartments) may therefore be increased by raising the pH of the water phase, rendering the drug non-ionized and more lipid soluble. The factors affecting topical drug absorption are summarized in Box 6.9.

Table 6.1 Residence time following topical instillation in rabbit eyes

Drug	Time (min)
Cromoglycate (aqueous)	6.8
Pilocarpine (aqueous)	4.8
Epinephrine (aqueous)	5.9

329

Box 6.9 Factors influencing topical drug absorption

- Environmental conditions – temperature and humidity
- Volume of drug application
- Drug formulation – pH, preservative, vehicle type
- Blink rate
- Stability of tear film
- Absorption through conjunctival vessels and nasal mucosa
- Corneal epithelium and stroma
- Nasolacrimal drainage of tears

DELIVERY METHODS OF OCULAR MEDICATION

RESIDENCE IN THE CONJUNCTIVAL SAC

The bioavailability of ocular medication depends on the precorneal fluid dynamics, drug binding to tear proteins, conjunctival drug absorption, systemic drug absorption, resistance to corneal penetration, drug binding to melanin and intraocular drug metabolism. Both the absorption and the efficacy of the drug can be increased by altering the formulation of the drug and/or by changing the local conditions.

To increase the residence time of the drug in the inferior fornix, and thus its delivery to the corneal epithelium, attempts at reducing the instilled volume of drug and increasing the viscosity of the solution have been made. For instance, polymers that increase solution viscosity include polyvinyl alcohol, hydroxypropylcellulose and other cellulose derivatives. However, increasing the viscosity of the delivery solution only produces a modest gain in ocular drug absorption, particularly for lipid-soluble drugs.

The residence time for many drugs is especially reduced by their pH, tonicity and the direct effect of certain drugs on lacrimation, which all affect the residence time of drugs in the lower fornix. For example, formulation at acidic or alkaline pH is irritant to the eye and increases both lacrimation and the blink rate, and clearance of the drug. Attempts to reduce the tonicity of the drug solution by using dilute buffers (e.g. phosphate buffers) to prevent stinging and lacrimation, and therefore increase

transit time (reduce clearance), have also been employed. Drugs that have a direct pharmacological action on the lacrimal gland, increasing lacrimation and subsequently altering the precorneal fluid dynamics, include muscarinic agonists. Some drugs are also bound to the tear proteins (albumin, globulins and lysozyme), reducing the concentration of the free drug available for absorption.

The corneal epithelium presents a considerably greater barrier to hydrophilic than to lipophilic drugs (10 : 1). Corneal epithelial permeability, however, may be increased during ocular inflammation so that some drugs, for example dexamethasone, are more rapidly absorbed across the corneal epithelium into the eye. Preservatives such as benzalkonium chloride, have also been shown to enhance the ocular absorption of drugs. Benzalkonium chloride and other cationic surfactants increase the ocular absorption of drugs by increasing corneal permeability (by compromising corneal integrity), depending on the molecular size and lipophilicity of the drug. Increased absorption can be obtained with pilocarpine, prednisolone and homatropine. For a drug to penetrate optimally, it must be able to exist in both ionized and un-ionized forms. Drugs will be buffered by the precorneal tear film and any alteration in the pH will change the ratio of ionized to un-ionized forms of the drug, dependent on the pK_a of the drug. In general a drug that exists in a purely ionized form will not penetrate the cornea unless the cornea has been damaged. Once absorbed into the eye, drugs may be bound to melanin within the pigment epithelium of the iris and the ciliary body, which may in turn reduce the bioavailability of the drug and also retard its clearance, leading to increased and prolonged drug levels. Similarly, after penetrating into the eye, drugs may be rendered inactive by intraocular metabolism. Enzymes that participate in ocular drug metabolism include those involved in inactivating neurotransmitters, for example monoamine oxidase, catecholamine O-methyl transferase, esterases, cytochrome P_{450}, and other enzymes including ketone transferase, glucuronidase and aldose reductase within the lens (see Box 6.10). The majority of enzyme activity is microsomal, although some enzymes, for example esterases, are both cytosolic and extracellular. Within the anterior segment, the corneal endothelium, the non-pigmented cells of the iris, and the ciliary body are metabolically most active, so drugs that are good substrates for these enzymes may suffer substantial degradation during absorption.

Box 6.10   Enzymes involved in drug metabolism in the eye

- *Ketone reductase* – this is a cytosolic enzyme dependent on NADPH. It is thought to play a key role in the metabolism of timolol and analogues of propranolol. Found in corneal epithelium, lens, iris and ciliary body.
- *Esterases* – important in the activation of ester prodrugs. Both acetyl- and butyrylcholinesterases are found in rabbits. They are widely distributed throughout the anterior segment.
- *Classic phase I and II oxidizing and conjugating enzymes* – cytochrome P$_{450}$ reductase, demethylase, sulphatase and glucuronidase.

Box 6.11   Drug delivery vehicles

- Solutions
  colloids
  emulsions
  suspensions
- Ointments
- Slow-release preparations
- New ophthalmic delivery systems
- Particulates
- Liposomes

DRUG VEHICLES AFFECT DRUG DELIVERY

Several topical drug delivery systems are used in ophthalmology (see Box 6.11).

Solutions

Solutions are a common mode of delivery because they cause less blurring of vision than ointments. They are easily administered and achieve high intraocular concentrations if applied regularly. They do, however, possess a short contact time and are quickly washed away at a rate proportional to the volume instilled. Polyvinyl alcohol or methylcellulose added to the solution increases the viscosity and/or lowers the surface tension, and will thus prolong contact time. Biologically active drug compounds that are sparingly soluble in water are often formulated as suspensions. Ophthalmic suspensions, particularly steroids, are thought to be useful delivery systems because it is assumed that the drug particles persist in the conjunctival sac and give rise to a sustained-release effect. Suspensions tend to form precipitates and thus need to be resuspended in the mixing bottle before application.

Semisolids (ointments)

Ointments consist of any one or a combination of hydrocarbons, mineral oils, lanolin and polymers such as polyvinyl alcohol, carbopol and methylcellulose. Drugs applied by this method provide an increase in the duration of action because of reduced dilution, reduced drainage and prolonged corneal contact time. Although these preparations melt at the temperature of the ocular tissue and disperse within the tear film, they are still retained longer than other ophthalmic preparations. They do, however, give rise to blurring of the vision and an increased incidence of contact dermatitis, related commonly to the preservative within the preparation.

Slow-release preparations

The problem of short residence times has been addressed by the development of ingenious vehicle supports. For instance, controlled release of ocular medications can be achieved with conjunctival inserts or with hydrophilic soft contact lenses. Slow-release preparations allow the constant release of drug while minimizing the drainage rate of the drug.

Ocular inserts

Controlled-release delivery systems deliver a bioactive agent to the target site at a controlled concentration over a desired time course. Ocular inserts are flexible, elliptical devices, consisting of three layers. The two outer coats of ethylene vinyl acetate enclose an inner coat of drug/alginate mix. The Ocusert with pilocarpine relies on the solubility properties of pilocarpine-free base, which exhibits both hydrophilic and lipophilic properties. Because the drug is miscible in both aqueous and organic solvent media, it will permeate the hydrophobic controlling membranes by diffusion through the pores. Erodible systems such as Lacrisert contain drug within carboxymethylcellulose wafers or polyvinyl alcohol disks or rods. They are manufactured principally for the treatment of dry eyes.

Collagen shields

Collagen is thought to be a suitable carrier of drugs. The three polypeptide α-helical chains are held together by crosslinking between proline and hydroxyproline, which account for 30% of the amino acid content of the molecule. Because of the ability to control the amount of crosslinking in the collagen subunits by exposure to ultraviolet light during manufacture, the time taken to dissolve when placed on the cornea can be altered. Also collagen acts as an ion exchanger and is semipermeable, facilitating controlled release of drugs. Thus, the collagen bandage shields prolong contact between drug and cornea. Drugs can either be incorporated into the collagen matrix, absorbed on to the shield during rehydration, or applied topically over a shield when in the eye. As the shield is erodible, release of the drug occurs gradually into the tear film, maintaining higher concentrations. Several drugs are now delivered using collagen shields (see Box 6.12).

Soft contact lens

In this case the polymer of the contact lens is hydrophilic and thus water-soluble drugs are absorbed into the lens. The lens is hydrated once placed on to the cornea and so releases the drug until an equilibrium is reached between drug concentration in the contact lens and in the conjunctival sac.

A primary concern with all ocular inserts is comfort, while many other criteria determine their usability (see Box 6.13).

ADVANCED OCULAR DELIVERY SYSTEMS

New ophthalmic delivery system (NODS)

NODS is a method of administering a drug as a single unit volume within a water-soluble preservative-free form. The system is easily administered and may offer a significant improvement in bioavailability over drops but full clinical testing has yet to be applied. Essentially the device consists of a water-insoluble drug-loaded flange attached to the end of a water-soluble handle by a soluble membrane film. The flange end is placed into the inferior fornix and the membrane rapidly dissolves, releasing the flange which then hydrates within the inferior fornix and releases the drug.

Particulates

Microspheres and nanoparticles represent promising particulate polymeric drug delivery systems for ophthalmic medications. These systems may avoid the potential disadvantages of other delivery systems, which include discomfort and difficulty of use with inserts, blurring of vision with viscous solutions, and instability of liposomes (see below). They may not represent real particles (capsular wall containing an aqueous or solid core) but are matrix-type structures of lipid base and drug. The particles are formed by polymerization (with ultraviolet light), during or after which the drug may be added. This leads to covalent drug binding to the polymer, so that when the drugs are absorbed into the polymer matrix they form a solid–solution matrix. The binding of the drug depends on its physicochemical properties as well as the nature of the polymer (polybutylcyanoacrylate). Smaller particles are better tolerated by patients than larger ones, and also have increased drug absorption and much slower elimination rates.

Liposomes

Liposomes are vesicles composed of lipid membranes enclosing an aqueous volume. They form spontaneously when a mixture of phospholipids is agitated in an aqueous medium to disperse the two phases, and are composed of phospholipids, including lecithin, phosphatidyl serine and phosphatidyl glycerol. They therefore share the properties of the bilayer of an outer cell membrane. The drugs can be trapped in either the lipid or aqueous phase. They provide the possibility of controlled and selective drug delivery and thus increased ocular bioavailability, although liposomes carry lipophilic drugs more readily than hydrophilic ones. The advantage of liposomes is that they are easily prepared, non-irritant, and do not cause any blurring of vision. Altering their surface charge or binding specific ligands to them increases their adherence to cells and subsequent endocytosis of the liposome–drug complex.

Ocular iontophoresis

Iontophoresis is a method of drug delivery that utilizes an electric current to drive a polar drug across a semipermeable membrane; this may be achieved by either a cathode or an anode depending on whether the molecule is negatively or positively charged. Applications in clinical ophthalmology have yet to be determined but a possibility may be the iontophoretic application of antibiotics in bacterial keratitis, enhancing tissue penetration of the agent. Corneal iontophoresis of gentamicin and aprofloxacin has been successful in treating experimental pseudomonas keratitis. Trans-scleral iontophoresis allows direct drug penetration into the vitreous but has a major disadvantage of discomfort and may produce small areas of retinal necrosis at sites of application.

INTRACAMERAL AND INTRAVITREAL ADMINISTRATION

Despite the considerable ingenuity applied to the development of topical drug preparations, the treatment of many ocular disorders is hampered by poor penetration into the eye. Systemic drug administration also does not guarantee high intraocular drug levels, in part as a result of the integrity of the blood–retinal and blood–aqueous barriers. For instance, the treatment of bacterial endophthalmitis is often inadequate unless vitrectomy and intravitreal antibiotics are used. The recommended dose of intravitreal antibiotics is based on doses that are not toxic to the rabbit or primate retina, but little is known about dose–response in the human vitreous. Experimentally, intravenous administration of the newer cephalosporins produces an incremental increase in the vitreous levels in inflamed eyes (but not in normal eyes). In inflammatory conditions, water-soluble antibiotics (penicillins) have a prolonged half-life as the retinal pump mechanism is damaged in such eyes. However, the commonly used aminoglycosides (see Ch. 8) are more rapidly cleared from inflamed eyes, despite low lipid solubility, because they are eliminated through the aqueous circulation. To achieve continual maximal therapeutic concentrations in the vitreous, repeated injections may be required. This may lead to complications of lens injury, haemorrhage, infection and retinal injury, and methods to reduce the toxicity of this form of treatment have included development of liposome-encapsulated drugs, which may be administered directly into the vitreous, or subcutaneously/subconjunctivally, acting as controlled-release formulations. Similar approaches are being sought both in humans and experimental models with other agents, for example ganciclovir for cytomegalovirus retinitis (see Box 6.14), cyclosporin A for endogenous uveitis (see Box 6.15), and encapsulated anti-fibroblastic drugs (5-fluorouracil) for proliferative vitreoretinopathy.

Box 6.14 Treatment of cytomegalovirus (CMV) retinitis

Ganciclovir was the first agent found to demonstrate therapeutic activity against CMV retinitis (see Ch. 8). At least 80% of patients respond to initial treatment with parenteral ganciclovir. Complications following parenteral administration include thrombocytopaenia and leukopaenia.

Zidovudine (AZT) has no direct antiviral action against CMV but may act by diminishing human immunodeficiency virus (HIV) enhancement of CMV infection and by improving immune function. However, AZT also causes bone marrow suppression, making combined therapy incompatible. Human recombinant granulocyte–macrophage colony-stimulating factor stimulates proliferation, differentiation and chemotaxis of neutrophils and, in combination with anti-CMV and HIV treatment, may prevent neutropaenic episodes.

Cidofovir is a DNA polymerase chain inhibitor that can be used at maintenance dose once a week.

Foscarnet may also be used to treat CMV infection, but up to 30% of patients develop renal toxicity. Despite this it is safer for administration in combination with AZT.

Control of CMV retinitis may occur with intravitreal injections of either ganciclovir or foscarnet. Injections are not directly retinotoxic even though intravitreal levels of these agents are within the toxic range for the drug. Intravitreal injections of liposome-encapsulated drugs reduce the requirement for repeated injection, without any evidence of retinal toxicity. Vitreal slow-release inserts of ganciclovir are now available, but do not protect against systemic infection or infection in the other eye.

DRUGS ADMINISTERED SYSTEMICALLY ALSO PENETRATE THE EYE

The preceding sections focus on the factors that affect the efficacy of topical ophthalmic therapy with minimal systemic side effects. However, drugs for ocular conditions may be administered systemically to achieve sufficient drug concentration in ocular tissue, although in humans the intraocular drug levels that are reached are largely unknown for most substances.

Commonly used drugs in ophthalmology include the carbonic anhydrase inhibitors (acetazolamide

---

Box 6.15 Cyclosporin

Cyclosporins are a group of biologically active metabolites produced by fungi imperfecti. Cyclosporins A and C are the major drugs in this class with immunosuppressive and antifungal activity.

Systemic cyclosporin is used in the treatment of chronic idiopathic intraocular inflammatory conditions (posterior uveitis; see Ch. 7).

Topical cyclosporin may improve the prognosis for corneal allograft rejection.

When applied topically, cyclosporin is bound to corneal and conjunctival epithelial cells, but does not penetrate well into the eye.

Box 6.16 Common preservatives in topical ophthalmic agents

• Benzalkonium chloride
• Chlorbutol
• Phenylmercuric nitrate
• Thiomersal
• Chlorhexidine
• Sorbic acid

---

and dichlorphenamide; see below), which are administered orally or intravenously to reduce intraocular pressure. Various animal studies have also demonstrated the ability of systemic antibiotics to reach intraocular infections in concentrations that are bactericidal to certain pathogens. For example, ciprofloxacin (see Ch. 8) penetrates the aqueous humour following oral administration. Similarly, both non-steroidal anti-inflammatory drugs and steroids penetrate the eye when given orally.

Drugs applied topically may also reach the systemic circulation and affect the contralateral eye. This has been recorded with timolol therapy of chronic open-angled glaucoma with unilateral intraocular pressure rise, which resulted in a significant drop in intraocular pressure in both treated and untreated eyes. In experimental models, a drug effect on the contralateral eye has also been shown with apraclonidine. This phenomenon may occur with a drug possessing a long systemic half-life or unique tissue-binding characteristics within the eye. If supplied in too high a dose or concentration, systemic side effects may occur, as with 10% phenylephrine drops.

TOPICAL MEDICATIONS AND PRESERVATIVES

Ophthalmic solutions and ointments must be sterile, and a wide variety of preservatives are used for this purpose. Most are toxic to the precorneal tear film and epithelium, impeding epithelial healing and disrupting the tear film. The commonly used preservatives are benzalkonium chloride, thiomersal, chlorbutol and organomercuric compounds. Benzalkonium chloride is a surfactant preservative (cationic preservative) which attains its bactericidal activity by attaching to the bacterial cell wall, increasing permeability and eventually rupturing the cell wall. While these preservatives and other cationic surfactants compromise the corneal integrity, they have also been shown to enhance the ocular absorption of drugs. Benzalkonium chloride is most effective at an alkaline pH (approximately pH 8.0) but is inactivated by the presence of soaps and salts, for example magnesium and calcium. As such, some contact lens solutions also combine ethylene diamine tetra-acetic acid (EDTA; a chelating agent) to overcome this problem. Severe toxicity may result from direct cellular damage or from a hypersensitivity reaction to components of the drug, and give rise to papillary conjunctivitis, punctate keratitis and corneal oedema. Chlorbutol also reduces oxygen utilization of the cornea (see Ch. 4) and may result in epithelial desquamation. Mercurial compounds include phenylmercuric acetate and thiomersal. Hypersensitivity to these compounds is the most dramatic and common complication of preservatives in 10% of patients, and mercurial deposits may develop in corneal tissues. All these preservatives are absorbed to various degrees by soft contact lenses.

RECONSTITUTING THE TEAR FILM

With increased knowledge of the anatomy and physiology of the precorneal tear film (Ch. 1 and Ch. 4), tear substitutes have been generated to provide symptomatic relief by artificially reconstituting individual tear film components. Ocular surface disease results from abnormalities in one, but generally more, of the tear film components. *Aqueous* deficiency is observed classically in keratoconjunctivitis sicca, as occurs in, for example, Sjögren syndrome. Instillation of artificial tears is the mainstay of treatment in conjunction with reducing drainage by occluding the lacrimal puncta. *Mucin* deficiency occurs in conditions that affect goblet cell function, for example cicatricial conjunctival disease and hypovitaminosis A, the effect of which is an unstable tear film because the surface tension is reduced and so is insufficient to maintain the aqueous layer. Therefore, areas of non-wetting occur and if left untreated corneal ulceration and scarring can result. Finally, *lipid* abnormalities are associated with chronic inflammation of the meibomian glands (see Ch. 1) and again result in an unstable tear film and inadequate wetting of the cornea.

TEAR SUBSTITUTES

Artificial tears or ocular lubricants are generally formulated as solutions consisting of inorganic ions (0.9% NaCl) and polymers to increase wettability and retention time, i.e. they additionally act to replace one of the actions of the mucin component of the tears. Commonly used polymers include polyvinyl alcohol and semisynthetic celluloses. Methylcellulose, hydoxypropylmethylcellulose and hydroxycellulose are still widely used, although polyvinyl alcohols have additional surfactant properties to further stabilize the tear film for longer periods. Recently, hyaluronic acid has been used, which has much greater retention times than celluloses or polyvinyl alcohols and improves tear film stability. Polyacrylic acid (carbomer) is a gel that is hydrophilic, helping it to form a stable tear film, increasing retention time and thus enabling it to be used less frequently.

Artificial tears are now more commonly available without preservatives. Preservatives affect corneal epithelial stability and thus ability to maintain the precorneal tear film.

MUCOLYTICS

Acetylcysteine, which is a derivative of amino acid L-cysteine, has been used as a mucolytic agent, dissolving the mucous threads that occur in keratoconjunctivitis sicca, but it does not appear to effect corneal wetting so it has to be used in conjunction with other artificial tear preparations.

OCULAR DRUGS AND THE AUTONOMIC NERVOUS SYSTEM

Parasympathetic and sympathetic divisions of the autonomic nervous system supply both ocular and extraocular tissues vital for normal ocular function (see Ch. 1). Agents that influence neurotransmission in the autonomic system are extremely important in the diagnosis and management of many ophthalmic disorders.

THE PARASYMPATHETIC SYSTEM

Acetylcholine is the major neurotransmitter of the parasympathetic system. It is formed enzymatically from choline and acetyl coenzyme A in the nerve endings (Fig. 6.7). Acetylcholine acts on two types of receptors: muscarinic, which are situated at the effector organ (postganglionic), and nicotinic, which are situated at ganglion synapses and also at neuromuscular junctions. In the eye such receptors are found in the motor endplates of extraocular muscles and levator palpebrae superioris, sympathetic and parasympathetic ganglia, iris sphincter, ciliary body and lacrimal glands. The nicotinic–acetylcholine receptor complex consists of two pairs of polypeptide chains and an additional single polypeptide chain (250 000 Da), providing a hydrophilic channel through which ions can traverse the lipid bilayer. This is known as a *ligand-gated ion channel*. As the acetylcholine binds to the receptor in the synaptic cleft the configuration of the polypeptide chains alters, allowing an influx of sodium and potassium ions down the concentration gradient, thus depolarizing the motor endplate. Cobratoxin, bungarotoxin and tubocurarine (active ingredient of curare) block acetylcholine receptors by preventing the opening of these ion channels. Following the release of acetylcholine, it is largely metabolized by hydrolysis, either within the synapses by acetylcholinesterase, or it is absorbed into plasma and then hydrolysed by butyrocholinesterase. Drugs can act as agonists or antagonists at either muscarinic or nicotinic receptors.

Parasympathomimetics mimic the action of acetylcholine

Parasympathomimetics are a group of drugs that act either by directly stimulating the muscarinic receptor, for example pilocarpine and carbachol, or by

> **Box 6.17 Polymer composition of artificial tears**
>
> - Carbomers (polyacrylic acid)
> - Hydroxylethylcellulose
> - Hypromellose (hydroxypropylmethylcellulose)
> - Liquid paraffin
> - Polyvinyl alcohol
> - Polyvinylpyrrolidone
> - Polycarbophil

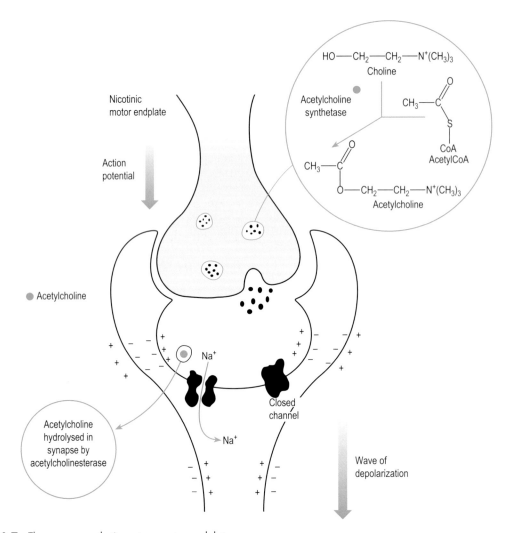

Fig. 6.7 The parasympathetic system: motor endplate.

inhibiting the enzyme acetylcholinesterase, which hydrolyses the acetylcholine in the synapse.

- *Pilocarpine* is used in the treatment of chronic open-angle glaucoma, facilitating aqueous drainage via its miotic action on the iris and contraction of the longitudinal muscle of the ciliary body. This draws on the scleral spur and opens the uveotrabecular meshwork. Parasympathetic stimulation has been shown experimentally to reduce aqueous outflow resistance with concomitant breakdown of the blood–aqueous barrier. Pilocarpine thus not only reduces outflow resistance but also reduces the rate of aqueous secretion. In addition, pilocarpine blocks the uveoscleral drainage route of aqueous (see Ch. 4) so that drainage is confined to the canal of Schlemm. The ocular hypotensive effect of pilocarpine is further achieved by a reduction in blood flow within the ciliary body, which in turn reduces aqueous secretion. Low concentrations of pilocarpine are used in the diagnosis of Adie's tonic pupil, by manifesting the miotic response of the supersensitive iris sphincter caused by loss of postganglionic nerve fibres in this condition.
- *Carbachol* is now infrequently used in the management of glaucoma, except in patients who are refractory to other treatments and hypersensitive to pilocarpine.
- *Edrophonium* (a competitive inhibitor of acetylcholinesterase) is used in the diagnosis of ocular or systemic myasthenia gravis (tensilon test). After

Table 6.2 Antimuscarinic agents

Drug	Maximal mydriasis/ cycloplegia (min)	Duration
Atropine sulphate	40	7–10 days
Homatropine	40	1–2 days
Cyclopentolate	30	12–24 h
Tropicamide	20	3–4 h

Box 6.18 Inhibiting acetylcholine: treatment of focal torsional dystonia

Botulinum toxin
- Effective treatment of essential blepharospasm and other focal torsional dystonias.
- Botulinum toxin is produced as eight different serotypes by the Gram-negative bacteria *Clostridium botulinum*.
- Botulinum toxin A is a 1500-amino-acid protein of molecular weight 142 kDa.
- Botulinum toxin A binds to unmyelinated regions of cholinergic nerve terminals, is internalized and internally prevents the release (by inhibiting exocytosis) of acetylcholine after stimulation of nerve (contraction-dependent blockade).

intravenous administration any improvement in ptosis or diplopia confirms the diagnosis. Longer-acting anticholinesterases (neostigmine) can be used to maintain some neuromuscular function. Immunosuppressive therapies are also used to treat myasthenia because they impair the autoimmune response generated by the acetylcholine receptor antibodies.

- *Longer-acting anticholinesterases* (ecothiopate iodide) are used occasionally in the management of accommodative esotropia, in which they act by abrogating the accommodative response while maintaining convergence and increasing the depth of focus. They are irreversible because they phosphorylate the acetylcholinesterase in the synaptic cleft and regeneration is totally dependent on the generation of new enzyme.
- *Acetylcholine* itself does not penetrate the corneal epithelium well because it is not lipid soluble. However, it may be used (e.g. Miochol) as an intraocular application during surgery to induce miosis.

The side effects of direct muscarinic agonists include conjunctival toxicity, iris cysts, cataracts and systemic absorption, which can give rise to muscarinic stimulation resulting in sweating, salivation, vomiting and bradycardia.

Parasympathetic antagonists affect the pupil and ciliary muscle separately

These drugs block the effect of acetylcholine at muscarinic receptor sites. Their principal effects are those of mydriasis and cycloplegia, but additional effects also include reduction of lacrimal secretions (see Table 6.2).

They are used clinically in the management of iritis (preventing adherence of the iris to the anterior capsule of the lens posterior synechiae), for cycloplegic refraction, to facilitate fundal examination and for the provocation test in narrow-angle glaucoma. The side effects of this group of drugs are seen more often with the longer-acting drugs, for example atropine sulphate. Systemic absorption occurs, particularly with atropine, via conjunctival vessels and via nasal and nasopharyngeal mucosal absorption. Systemic side effects include dry mouth, facial flushing, sweating and tachycardia. Ocular side effects include hypersensitivity reactions and conjunctival hyperaemia, blurring of vision and photophobia, a transient rise in intraocular pressure and, occasionally, precipitation of acute-angled glaucoma.

THE SYMPATHETIC SYSTEM

Acetylcholine, epinephrine and norepinephrine all act as neurotransmitters within the sympathetic autonomic nervous system (Fig. 6.8). Acetylcholine is the neurotransmitter at autonomic ganglia, which includes the sympathetic nervous system. Epinephrine and norepinephrine are generated from hydroxylation of tyrosine to form DOPA, and further modified enzymatically to form dopamine, and finally epinephrine and norepinephrine (Fig. 6.9). Once released from the nerve ending they act on several well-defined subtypes of receptors. The action of the neurotransmitter is terminated by enzyme degradation with monoamine oxidases and catechol-*O*-methyl transferase, and also by active reuptake into the nerve endings (Fig. 6.10).

Adrenergic receptors

Adrenergic receptors are of two types, α and β; two further subtypes exist within each group, classified according to the elicited response and distinguished by selective agonists and antagonists. α_1-receptors mediate excitatory responses: principally smooth muscle contraction. α_2-receptors are located mostly

337

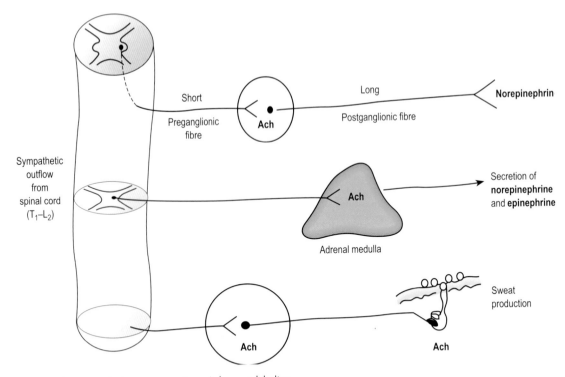

Fig. 6.8 The sympathetic nervous system. Ach, acetylcholine.

on the presynaptic nerve endings and are inhibitory because, when stimulated, they prevent further release of the neurotransmitter from the presynaptic terminal (Fig. 6.10). β_2-receptors can mediate inhibitory responses, relaxing the smooth muscle of blood vessels and bronchi, while β_1-receptors situated in the heart are excitatory and give rise to a positive inotropic and chronotropic response.

The ocular effects of adrenergic agonists include mydriasis, slight ciliary muscle relaxation (probably not relevant in humans), increased formation and increased outflow of aqueous humour (although a stimulation will decrease aqueous humour production), contraction of Müller's muscle and constriction of conjunctival and episcleral vessels (see Table 6.3).

The control of intraocular pressure is facilitated by similar and opposite effects of adrenergic receptors

The control of intraocular pressure (IOP) and aqueous production and outflow has already been discussed (see Ch. 4). It is well documented that certain α-agonists cause lowering of the IOP, for example clonidine, which is principally mediated by

Table 6.3 Profile of adrenergic receptors in the eye

	α	β
Iris dilator	+++	+/–
Iris sphincter	+/–	+
Ciliary process epithelium	+/–	+++
Conjunctival blood vessels	+	+
Müller's muscle	+	–

an α_2-agonist action. On the other hand α_1-agonists (e.g. phenylephrine) cause a rise in IOP with concomitant pupillary dilation. As α_2-agonists produce an immediate fall in IOP, their effect is likely to be central, mediated by stimulation of the medullopontine sympathetic centre. Conversely, α_1-hypertensive effects are thought to be muscular in origin because the effect is antagonized by muscle relaxants.

β-receptors are the predominant receptor on ciliary epithelium, stimulation of which will reduce IOP experimentally. However, β-blockers (e.g. timolol) also reduce IOP. In humans, stimulation of

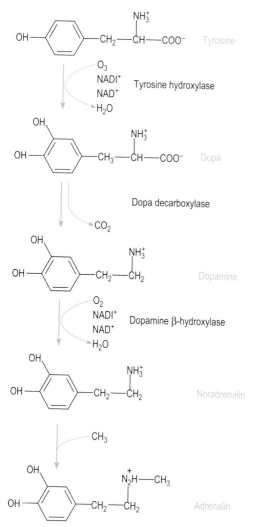

Fig. 6.9 Synthesis of noradrenalin (norepinephrine) and adrenalin (epinephrine).

β-receptors does not cause a reduction in aqueous secretion. Indeed epinephrine (a combined α- and β-agonist) causes an initial rise in IOP that is also associated with an initial rise in aqueous secretion. This effect is mediated by concomitant α_1-receptor stimulation, the hypotensive effect being a purely α_2-agonist action. Experimental evidence suggests that direct application of cAMP also increases aqueous drainage, and adenylate cyclase, which is also activated by β_2-agonists, produces a similar response. Certainly a rise in aqueous cAMP levels correlates well with reduction of IOP, which may be mediated by both α- and β-agonists, but as yet the exact mechanism is unknown.

Adrenergic agonists

- *Epinephrine* stimulates both α- and β-receptors. Adrenergic receptors are found in cell membranes of iris dilator muscle, Müller's muscle, ciliary process epithelium and smooth muscle of ocular blood vessels. Phenylephrine is a synthetic sympathomimetic that acts directly on α-receptors. Mydriasis occurs within 1 hour and lasts 4–6 hours. The mydriasis of phenylephrine can be overcome by the powerful parasympathetic light reflex during fundoscopy. Thus, for maintained pupillary dilation, a combination of phenylephrine and an antimuscarinic, for example cyclopentolate, is used. Systemic absorption is common with phenylephrine and care must be taken when using it in the elderly, in patients with hypertension, or in neonates and children.
- *Hydroxyamphetamine* acts by releasing norepinephrine from the nerve terminals. It is therefore used in the diagnosis of postganglionic Horner syndrome.
- *Cocaine*, whose membrane-stabilizing effect gives rise to its local anaesthetic properties, also prevents the reuptake of norepinephrine into the nerve endings, and is used in the diagnosis of pre- or postganglionic Horner syndrome in cases of anisocoria.
- *Apraclonidine hydrochloride* is a selective α-adrenergic agonist acting mainly on α_2-receptors. It may be applied topically for the prevention and management of raised IOP after anterior segment laser treatment. It lowers IOP by decreasing aqueous humour formation. It does not penetrate the blood–aqueous barrier easily and therefore has minimal systemic side effects, unlike clonidine.
- *Brimonidine* is a selective α_2-receptor antagonist which over longer periods can reduce IOP without significant cardiovascular or pulmonary function effects.
- *β_2-adrenergic agonists* also lower IOP, but their effect is mainly to increase the uveoscleral outflow, and they are often used in combination with β-blocking agents.

Commercially available L-epinephrine (Eppy 1%) can produce local irritation, allergy and adrenochrome deposits in the subconjunctiva. These adrenochrome deposits are most likely to be oxidative products of epinephrine and are most common in the palpebral conjunctiva. Dipivalyl epinephrine (Propine 0.1%) is also used in the treatment of glaucoma. It is a lipophilic prodrug of epinephrine, and can penetrate into the anterior chamber, where it is

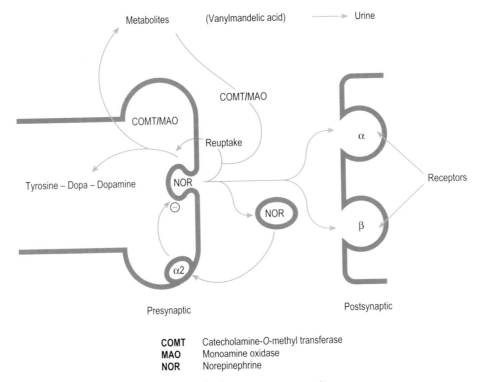

COMT	Catecholamine-O-methyl transferase
MAO	Monoamine oxidase
NOR	Norepinephrine

Fig. 6.10 Adrenergic receptors and metabolism of adrenergic neurotransmitters.

hydrolysed into the active agent. If epinephrine or its prodrug analogues are used to treat aphakic glaucoma, there is a high incidence of cystoid macular oedema. This macular toxicity has been reported to occur in 20–30% of aphakic eyes undergoing epinephrine treatment. The mechanism of cystoid macular oedema is unknown, but the angiographic features are identical to those of other conditions causing macular oedema, such as Irvine–Gass syndrome (vitreous–wound adherence following cataract surgery). Experimental evidence has shown that the high incidence of cystoid macular oedema in aphakic eyes is the result of higher concentrations of epinephrine in the retina of aphakic eyes (Table 6.4).

Adrenergic antagonists

Since the introduction of timolol maleate, topical β-blockers have become the most important therapeutic agents in the medical treatment of glaucoma. The lowering of IOP is a response to a blockade of β-adrenergic receptors in the ciliary epithelium, which produces up to 50% reduction in aqueous production. The site of action probably resides within the ciliary body, but it is not known whether adrenergic

Table 6.4 Sympathomimetic drug receptor profile/action

Sympathomimetic	Receptor/action
Norepinephrine	α and β
Epinephrine	α and β
Phenylephrine	α (non-selective)
Brimonidine	Selective α_2-agonist
Apraclonidine	α_2 partial agonist
Hydroxyamphetamine	Releases norepinephrine from nerve endings: inhibits monoamine oxidases
Cocaine	Inhibits uptake of norepinephrine at nerve endings

antagonists specifically affect ciliary body perfusion or the pumping mechanism of the ciliary epithelium. β-blockers certainly interact with β-adrenergic receptor-coupled adenyl cyclase of the ciliary epithelium. Clinically, there are now many β-blockers available, which vary according to their β-receptor

---

Box 6.19 Adrenergic antagonists

Non-selective β-blockers (β₁ and β₂)
- Carteolol
- Levobunolol
- Timolol

Selective β₁-blockers
- Betaxolol

Box 6.20 Protecting nerve fibres without lowering IOP: Neuroprotection

- *Glutamate-receptor blocking agents* – reduce excessive calcium influx and ATP synthesis inhibiting excitatory cell death. Agents may act at different sites (receptors) inducing amino-acid-induced excitotoxicity.
- *NMDA (N-methyl D-aspartate) receptor inhibition* – NMDA is a postsynaptic ligand-gated ion channel requiring NMDA and glycine for activation. Antagonists can either be competitive or non-competitive, both of which ultimately reduce glutamate secretion and reduce excitotoxicity.
- *Nitric oxide synthase inhibition*
- *Antioxidants*

---

selectivity (see Box 6.19). However, because of the opposing pharmacological actions of epinephrine and β-blockers, these drugs do not have an additive effect in lowering IOP. Timolol maleate is the most commonly used topical β-blocker and is non-selective, acting on both β₁- and β₂-receptors. Timolol binds reversibly with β-receptors and can reduce IOP in normal human eyes by reducing aqueous production by 15–48%. Betaxolol hydrochloride is a lipid-soluble β₁-antagonist that is relatively cardioselective. It reduces IOP by decreasing the production of aqueous at the ciliary body, with no effect on aqueous outflow. Carteolol hydrochloride is a β-blocker that possesses intrinsic sympathomimetic activity, and is thought to be beneficial in glaucoma because it not only lowers IOP but also increases optic nerve head perfusion. Its intrinsic sympathomimetic activity does not appear to confer any protection from systemic side effects of non-selective β-blockade. New β-blockers are frequently under investigation for their effectiveness in reducing IOP and preventing the progression of glaucomatous visual field loss. The ideal β-blocker would block β-receptors in the eye without having any effect on systemic β-receptors.

Systemic side effects of agonist agents include hypotensive episodes, cardiac arrhythmia, headache and anxiety. The systemic effects of β-blockade include bronchospasm, bradycardia, syncopal attacks and central nervous system depression. It is still not confirmed whether systemic absorption of β-blockers raises levels of serum triglycerides and cholesterol, as with systemic β-blockade, which is of particular importance when treating patients with ischaemic heart disease or more widespread vascular disease.

CLINICAL CONTROL OF INTRAOCULAR PRESSURE

Control of IOP is the main aim of therapy in chronic simple glaucoma, a disorder that contributes greatly to the demands on eye healthcare systems. IOP

Box 6.21 Actions of topically applied drugs that lower IOP

β-blockers decrease aqueous production by up to 50% and thus lower IOP, even in normal eyes. Their precise action remains unknown but they are likely to affect either vascular perfusion of the ciliary body or adenyl cyclase of the ciliary epithelium.

Pilocarpine lowers IOP by facilitating aqueous outflow via its direct action on the scleral spur and ciliary body muscle.

Epinephrine stimulates β-receptors located in the trabecular meshwork (increasing both intracellular and aqueous cAMP levels), which increases the facility of outflow. Stimulation of the α-receptors on blood vessels supplying the ciliary body causes vasoconstriction and reduced blood flow, and consequently reduced aqueous production.

Latanoprost is a prostaglandin F₂α analogue and a prostanoid FP receptor (G-protein coupled receptor) agonist which reduces IOP by increasing the outflow of aqueous humour, mainly ureoscleral outflow.

---

control may be achieved surgically or medically and numerous topical therapies based on the pharmacology of the autonomic nervous system are in use, as described above. The common drugs used topically are summarized in Box 6.21.

However, medical treatment of glaucoma may also be achieved by systemic inhibition of carbonic anhydrase, an enzyme central to the formation of aqueous (see Ch. 4).

341

CARBONIC ANHYDRASE IN THE EYE IS A TARGET ENZYME FOR DRUG ACTION

Aqueous humour is secreted actively into the posterior chamber by the non-pigmented epithelium of ciliary processes, which in turn is dependent on the active transport of sodium using the sodium/potassium ATPase pump (see Ch. 4). Aqueous secretion can be decreased by inhibiting bicarbonate formation, an essential component in aqueous production. The production of bicarbonate is catalysed by the ubiquitous enzyme carbonic anhydrase, which exists in at least six isoforms. Carbonic anhydrase catalyses the hydration of carbon dioxide to bicarbonate, which then dissociates to form hydrogen ions and bicarbonate. The subtypes of carbonic anhydrase enzymes located in ocular tissues include carbonic anhydrase isoenzyme II, which is found in the ciliary body, and isoenzyme IV, which is thought to be a membrane-bound fraction of the enzyme found in the apical region of the RPE cells. Inhibition of carbonic anhydrase reduces aqueous production. This may be a direct effect of enzyme inhibition or secondary to the altered intracellular pH and blockade of the sodium/potassium ATPase ion channel. The effect of acetazolamide therapy is perhaps somewhat surprising. Carbonic anhydrase has a high turnover and the drug must not only reach the active site but also remain in high enough concentrations to have a sufficient duration of action. The drug binds avidly to red blood cell carbonic anhydrase and, when saturation is reached, the drug may effectively distribute to other tissue-binding sites, e.g. ciliary processes and proximal tubule of the kidney. Carbonic anhydrase inhibitors are useful in selected cases of glaucoma. However, these drugs are usually sulphonamide derivatives and can have severe systemic side effects, including potassium depletion, dermatitis, renal stones (the incidence is said to be 11 times higher than normal), acidosis and, most commonly, fatigue and paraesthesia of the extremities, which can make up to 50% of patients intolerant to its long-term use. Acetazolamide is the most frequently used agent, and recently a new sustained-release preparation has become available which is said to reduce the incidence of systemic side effects. Dorzolamide is a topical carbonic anhydrase inhibitor used to lower IOP in patients resistant or intolerant to β-blockers. It is irritant to the corneal and conjunctival surface and systemic absorption may rarely give rise to sulphonamide-like side effects.

THE HISTAMINERGIC SYSTEM: HISTAMINE IS RELEASED FROM CONJUNCTIVAL MAST CELLS DURING ALLERGIC REACTIONS

Histamine is synthesized and stored in most tissues. It is derived from the amino acid histidine and excreted in the urine after being enzymatically degraded in the liver by histaminase. Histamine is a modulator of the inflammatory response, particularly in allergic type I hypersensitivity reactions (see Ch. 7). Histamine also plays an integral role in neurotransmission, for example regulating gastric acid secretion. Two common histamine receptors are described, H_1 and H_2, on the basis of the structure of the specific antagonist that binds to them. H_1-receptors are found in abundance in human bronchial muscle and at many other sites. The histamine receptors in these tissues have the same affinity for histamine as for the histamine-competitive antagonist, mepyramine. H_2-receptors are found in the stomach, heart and uterus. The receptors involved have a common affinity for the competitive histamine antagonist, cimetidine. Activation of H_1-receptors results in an increase in intracellular calcium concentration, and activation of H_2-receptors results in stimulation of adenyl cyclase and second messenger production (see Box 6.22).

Mast cells are an abundant source of histamine. Histamine release is mediated by allergen-induced immunoglobulin E (IgE) hypersensitivity responses. Control of this allergic response can be obtained by

---

Box 6.22 Actions of histamine

H_1 actions
- Increases vascular permeability and vasodilatation of arterioles
- Arteriolar dilatation of superficial skin vessels (axon reflex)
- Capillary dilatation and oedema of dermis
- Smooth muscle contraction/bronchospasm
- Increased mucus secretion
- Central nervous system depressant

H_2 actions
- Increased pepsin and acid production
- Increased myocardial stroke volume

H_3 actions
- Receptors associated with neural tissue at presynaptic sites, which, when stimulated, inhibit histamine release, the significance of which is unclear.

preventing mast cell degranulation at the mucous membranes with mast cell stabilizing agents. This is of particular relevance when considering the management of allergic eye disease.

ANTIHISTAMINES

H_1 antihistamines inhibit histamine-induced contraction of smooth bronchial muscles and increased vascular permeability caused by histamine. Some H_1 antagonists have pronounced central nervous system side effects, including drowsiness, but also have the benefit of being antiemetics. The two recently introduced H_1 antihistamines, terfenadine and astemizole, have virtually no sedative or anticholinergic action.

H_2 antagonists are effective in the pharmacological control of gastric acid secretion by decreasing basal and food-stimulated acid secretion (up to 90%). The two drugs commonly used are cimetidine and ranitidine, which are structural analogues of histamine. Cimetidine also inhibits cytochrome P_{450} and decreases the metabolism of drugs (e.g. anticoagulants, phenytoin and aminophylline), thus potentiating their effects. Cimetidine binds to androgen receptors, sometimes leading to gynaecomastia and reduced sexual function.

SODIUM CROMOGLYCATE

Disodium cromoglycate is used in the treatment of allergic hypersensitivity reactions and is administered topically, either into the conjunctival fornix or by inhalation to the bronchial mucosa. It acts by inhibiting the release of histamine and slow-releasing substance of anaphylaxis (SRS-A) from the mast cells within the mucosa, by stabilizing mast cell membranes. It must therefore be administered before mast cell priming with IgE and allergen because it will have no effect once the mast cells have degranulated. Lodoxamide has also been developed recently as a topical application to prevent mast cell degranulation.

Box 6.23 Treating allergic eye disease

Topical antihistamines
- Azelastine
- Levocarbastine

Mast cell stabilizers
- Sodium cromoglycate
- Lodoxamide

EICOSANOIDS AFFECT MULTIPLE OCULAR FUNCTIONS

Eicosanoids are not found preformed in tissues but are generated *de novo* from cellular phospholipids after a wide range of stimuli. They are important mediators of the inflammatory response, and the non-steroidal anti-inflammatory drugs (NSAIDs) owe some of their activity, especially prostaglandin $F_{2\alpha}$, to the inhibition of the synthesis of eicosanoids. The name prostaglandin derives from reports that semen contained a substance that contracted the uterus and was thought to be derived from the prostate gland. However, the first prostaglandins were described in the eye, although not named as such.

The principal eicosanoids are the prostaglandins, thromboxanes and leukotrienes (see Ch. 7). The main source of these substances is from the 20-carbon unsaturated fatty acid, arachidonic acid, which is found esterified in the phospholipids of cell membranes. Figure 6.11 describes the generation of these molecules, where the initial rate-limiting step is the generation of arachidonate by phospholipase A_2 or C. Stimuli that liberate these enzymes include thrombin in platelets, C5a from complement and bradykinin, as well as general cell damage. The free arachidonic acid is then metabolized via two pathways mediated by the enzymes cyclo-oxygenase, generating prostaglandins, and lipoxygenase, generating leukotrienes (see Ch. 7). The anti-inflammatory action of the NSAIDs is mainly the result of the inhibition of cyclo-oxygenase, and thus prostaglandin synthesis (see Box 6.24).

Each prostaglandin appears to act on specific receptors, which have yet to be fully characterized. However, receptor antagonists are gradually being developed for each eicosanoid. A recent example is misoprostol, which reduces gastric acid secretion and gastric erosion by NSAIDs, by the antagonism of prostaglandin E_2 class 1 receptors.

Aspirin, among other compounds, inactivates cyclo-oxygenase and reduces inflammation and pain. Other systemically administered NSAIDs, such as indomethacin and flurbiprofen, are used in an attempt to reduce the inflammatory response in uveitis and scleritis. Indomethacin is used also to reduce cystoid macular oedema, but its effects have yet to be substantiated. Both ibuprofen and diclofenac are now available as topical applications; their principal use is to prevent perioperative miosis during cataract surgery as well as to reduce postoperative inflammation.

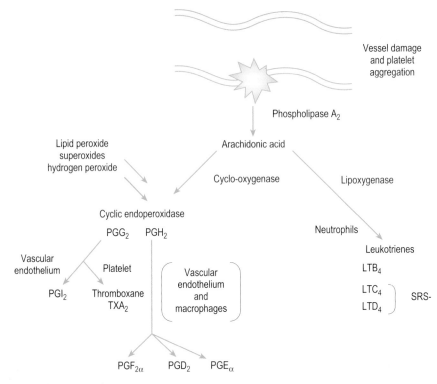

Fig. 6.11 Synthesis of eicosanoids.

Box 6.24   Biological actions of eicosanoids

Prostaglandins
- Prostaglandin I_2 – vasodilatation, decreases platelet adhesion
- Prostaglandin $F_{2\alpha}$ – bronchial smooth muscle contraction
- Prostaglandin E_2 – vasodilatation, bronchodilatation, uterine contraction, pyretic, stimulates release of pituitary hormones, adrenal cortex steroids and insulin from pancreas

Thromboxane
- Thromboxane A_2 – vasoconstriction, platelet aggregation, bronchoconstriction

Leukotrienes
- Leukotriene B_4 – aggregation of neutrophils, chemotactic, stimulation of phospholipase A_2
- Leukotriene C_4
- Leukotriene D_4 – contraction of smooth muscle, bronchoconstriction, vasoconstriction, leukotrienes C_4 and D_4 together form SRS-A.

Box 6.25   Anti-inflammatory topical NSAIDs

- *Diclofenac and flurbiprofen* – inhibit intraoperative miosis and postoperative inflammation
- *Keterolac* – used for prophylaxis and reduction of inflammation following ocular surgery.

More recently prostaglandin analogues have been studied for use in chronic glaucoma, e.g. prostaglandin $F_{2\alpha}$ (see p. 343).

In an attempt to increase the efficacy of NSAIDs and reduce, in particular, gastric mucosal erosions, newer NSAIDs are being generated which are specific for one of the isoenzymes of cyclo-oxygenase, cyclo-oxygenase 2 (COX-2). COX-2 specificity is said to confer a more specific inhibition of inflammatory prostaglandin synthesis, without impairing synthesis of gastroprotecting prostaglandins, e.g. prostaglandin I_2, which is synthesized by COX-1. Conventional NSAIDs are strong inhibitors of COX-1 and less active against COX-2.

SEROTONIN: A POTENT NEUROTRANSMITTER

Neurotransmitters are integral to retinal and cortical function, and drugs that modulate their function may alter visual perception. In addition, some neuromodulatory drugs are used to treat conditions with visual symptoms, such as migraine.

5-Hydroxytryptamine (5-HT; serotonin) is biosynthesized in a manner similar to norepinephrine from the precursor amino acid tryptophan, which is taken up into the nerve endings and converted by tryptophan hydroxylase to 5-hydroxytryptophan, and then decarboxylated to serotonin. Serotonin is degraded by oxidative deamination by the action of a group of enzymes called *monoamine oxidases* to form the aldehydes, 5-hydroxyindoleacetaldehyde and 5-hydroxyindoleacetic acid (5-HIAA), analogous to norepinephrine metabolism. The aldehydes are then excreted in the urine, and may be detected in hypersecretory conditions such as carcinoid syndrome.

SEROTONIN RECEPTOR SUBCLASSES MEDIATE DIFFERENT EFFECTS

Serotonin is a neurotransmitter that is widely distributed throughout the body, particularly in platelets, mucosa of the gastrointestinal tract and neurones of both the central and peripheral nervous system. There are four main types of serotonin receptors, designated 5-HT$_1$, 5-HT$_2$, 5-HT$_3$ and 5-HT$_4$. Although 5-HT is a simple molecule, it has a wide variety of effects in the cardiovascular, gastrointestinal, respiratory and central nervous systems.

5-HT$_1$-receptors can be further divided into subtypes 5-HT$_{1a-d}$. They are differentiated by the kinetics of agonist and antagonist binding to the receptor, and by their regional distribution within the central nervous system. 5-HT$_{1a}$ has been found in the raphe nucleus and the hippocampus, activation of which causes hypotensive attacks and behavioural changes. This has been studied with particular reference to the physiology of anxiety. 5-HT$_{1b}$ is found in rodents and is thought to have an inhibitory effect on the release of 5-HT, similar to the 5-HT$_{1d}$-receptor in humans. 5-HT$_{1c}$ has been localized to the choroidal plexus, but no specific agonist or antagonist has yet been identified. The 5-HT$_2$-receptor is located in the hippocampus, frontal cortex and spinal cord. These receptors are also located on smooth muscle in the bronchus and blood vessels. They have a direct excitatory effect on smooth muscle. 5-HT$_3$-receptors are found in the nerves along the gastrointestinal tract and peripheral nervous system. 5-HT exerts an excitatory effect through these receptors, particularly excitation of nociceptive nerve endings. They are also found in the limbic and cortical areas of the brain, and are thought to play an important role in the development of anxiety and psychotic states. Recently 5-HT$_4$-receptors have been discovered but their clinical significance remains unclear.

5-HT ANTAGONISTS

Selective 5-HT$_2$-receptor antagonists, which are used for the prevention of migraine attacks (e.g. methysergide and pizotifen), probably act by inhibiting the release of serotonin at the aura stage of the attack. During this stage the activation of 5-HT neurones is at its greatest, and thus antagonism of the receptors prevents the sequelae of vascular smooth muscle contraction, local inflammation and nociceptor stimulation. Selective 5-HT$_3$-receptor antagonism (e.g. ondansetron) reduces the 5-HT nociceptive stimulation, and thus the headache of migraine.

GLUCOCORTICOIDS

Steroids are applied topically to suppress the inflammatory reaction of many conditions, commonly anterior uveitis, postoperative inflammation, and corneal graft rejection. They may also be administered subconjunctivally or systemically in more severe intraocular inflammatory conditions. The mechanism of their anti-inflammatory actions is mediated by the drug's effects on both the number and function of lymphocytes, polymorphonuclear leucocytes and macrophages, and an increase in vascular permeability. They also affect inflammatory mediators by inhibiting phospholipase A$_2$, prostaglandin, thromboxane and leukotrienes; they also inhibit histamine release. Steroids have many ocular side effects, including cataract formation, reactivation of viral keratitis or increased incidence of bacterial infection, and steroid-induced rises in IOP. The latter side effect is dependent on the duration and strength (potency) of individual steroid preparations. The rise in IOP is thought to occur via the accumulation of glycosaminoglycans and water in the trabecular meshwork, reducing aqueous outflow. In normal human subjects there appears to be a large genetic influence on steroid responsiveness. Thirty per cent of normal subjects have a hypertensive response when challenged with corticosteroids. This can be characterized further into poor

345

responders, moderate responders (heterozygous responders) and strong responders (homozygous responders). If the individual also has open-angled glaucoma, a greater overall response is seen. It is therefore important that IOP is monitored at regular intervals during the course of prolonged steroid therapy.

The anti-inflammatory potency of any particular steroid is dependent on its ability to penetrate the cornea. Increasing the steroid concentration results in higher intraocular concentrations but this may also be achieved with different formulations of the same parent steroid that increase the contact time of the topically applied drug. Steroids such as prednisolone phosphate are hydrophilic and therefore penetrate the corneal epithelium poorly; in contrast, the acetate forms of both dexamethasone and prednisolone give rise to a much greater intraocular concentration. To date, it is still not established which concentrations of steroids are desirable for low-grade intraocular inflammatory conditions. If this could be established, ocular side effects might be kept to a minimum.

IMMUNOSUPPRESSIVE AGENTS: COMBATING OCULAR INFLAMMATORY DISEASE

Controlling immune responses, particularly T-cell responses (Ch. 7), that mediate allograft rejection, endogenous uveitis, associated or not with other autoimmune conditions, and chronic allergic eye disease may necessitate systemic therapy with immunosuppressants. In addition to steroids there is now a significant armamentarium of agents used in ophthalmology to treat such conditions. Such agents have been generated as a result of our increased understanding of T-cell biology, in particular the interactions of T cells with specific antigens and antigen-presenting cells, activation of T cells and the effects of mediators of inflammation, such as cytokines.

Commonly used agents in addition to the traditional use of steroids for suppressing inflammatory responses (see Box 6.26), include cyclosporin A, purine antagonists and cytotoxic agents such as methotrexate, and occasionally alkylating agents such as cyclophosphamide. Newer generations of similarly acting agents are now used, especially in prevention of solid organ allograft rejection, including tacrolimus (FK 506) and mycophenolate mofetil

---

Box 6.26 Immunosuppressants and their mode of action

- *Corticosteroids* – act on cytosolic receptors and block transcription of cytokine genes (interleukins 1, 2, 3 and 5, tumour necrosis factor-α and interferon-γ)
- *Cyclosporin* – inhibits interleukin-2 production and stimulates transforming growth factor-β production
- *Tacrolimus* – inhibits interleukin-2
- *Azathioprine* – inhibits purine synthesis, blocking RNA and DNA synthesis
- *Methotrexate* – folic acid antagonist, inhibiting dihydrofolate reductase and suppressing DNA synthesis
- *Cellcept* – blocks *de novo* pathway of purine synthesis, which is selective for lymphocytes

---

Box 6.27 Common side effects of immunosuppressants

- *Corticosteroids* – osteoporosis, hypertension, glucose intolerance, altered habitus
- *Cyclosporin and tacrolimus* – nephrotoxicity, hypertension, hyperlipidaemia, glucose intolerance, hirsutism and gingival hyperplasia
- *Azathioprine/Cellcept* – bone marrow suppression, diarrhoea and gastrointestinal upset.

(Cellcept). The mechanism of action of such agents and its effect on T-cell activation are represented in Fig. 6.12.

Although successful, immunosuppressive therapy is limited by its relative non-specificity, the refractiveness of some patients to therapy and the high incidence of side effects (see Box 6.27). To reduce unwanted systemic effects some agents, for example cyclosporin A and tacrolimus, are currently being formulated for topical delivery to treat chronic allergic disease and corneal allograft rejection.

BIOLOGICS

The current expertise in molecular biological and engineering technology has permitted over the past decade the generation of specific molecules that can be engineered to specifically target receptors, membrane proteins or soluble proteins. With reference to eye diseases, this has resulted in newer treatments for ocular inflammatory disorders and retinal choroidal angiogenesis such as 'wet' age-related macular degeneration. For example one of the principal mediators of T-cell responses in autoimmune disorders, such as rheumatoid arthritis, inflamma-

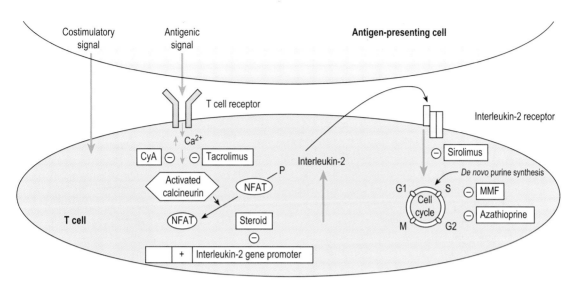

Fig. 6.12 Stages of T-cell activation: multiple targets for immunosuppressive agents. *Signal 1*: stimulation of T-cell receptor (TCR) results in calcineurin activation, a process inhibited by cyclosporin (CyA) and tacrolimus. Calcineurin dephosphorylates nuclear factor of activated T cells (NFAT) enabling it to enter the nucleus and bind to interleukin-2 promoter. Corticosteroids inhibit cytokine gene transcription in lymphocytes and antigen-presenting cells by several mechanisms. *Signal 2*: costimulatory signals are necessary to optimize T-cell interleukin-2 gene transcription, prevent T-cell anergy and inhibit T-cell apoptosis. Experimental agents but not current immunosuppressive agents interrupt these intracellular signals. *Signal 3*: interleukin-2 receptor stimulation induces the cell to enter the cell cycle and proliferate. Signal 3 may be blocked by interleukin-2 receptor antibodies or sirolimus, which inhibits the second messenger signals induced by interleukin-2 receptor ligation. Following progression into the cell cycle, azathioprine and mycophenolate mofetil (MMF) interrupt DNA replication by inhibiting purine synthesis. (From Denton *et al.* 1999, with permission from Elsevier.)

tory bowel disease and posterior uveitis, is tumour necrosis factor-α (TNF-α). Engineering either specific antibodies or immunoadhesins (fusion proteins of their receptors bound to a human immunoglobulin tail) can recognize membrane-bound and soluble TNF-α and neutralize its activity. TNF-α binds two receptors (p55-TNFR1 or p75-TNFR2). The commercially available biologics include *infliximab*, a chimeric antibody (human with mouse-derived variable region recognizing TNF-α) that inhibits TNF-α by neutralizing both membrane-bound and soluble TNF, and *Etenercept*, which is a fusion protein of p75 receptor that successfully binds TNF thereby preventing further binding. Similarly, vascular endothelial growth factor (VEGF) is a principle angiogenic growth factor that mediates angiogenesis and new vessel formation in many conditions including tumours, diabetes and 'wet' age-related macular degeneration. The actions are mediated via the receptors VEGF-R1 and VEGF-R2, although currently none of the commercially available agents are receptor fusion proteins. *Ranibizumab* is a monoclonal recombinant human Fab VEGF; recombinant human FabV2 is a humanized Fab fragment that binds and neutralizes VEGF and *aptamers* (i.e. *pegaptanib sodium*) are nucleic acid ligands that are specific for given proteins and act as decoys, neutralizing their function (Fig. 6.13).

LOCAL ANAESTHETICS: AN INTEGRAL PART OF OPHTHALMIC EXAMINATION AND SURGERY

Local anaesthetics consist biochemically of an aromatic residue linked to an amide or basic side-chain. As such, local anaesthetics are both hydrophobic (aromatic residue) and hydrophilic (amide group), and tend to accumulate at aqueous–non-aqueous interfaces. Because the aromatic residue and side-chain in some local anaesthetics are linked by esters, they are susceptible to metabolic hydrolysis. These compounds are usually inactivated in the liver and plasma by non-specific esterases. As amide links are more stable, this group of anaesthetics has a longer $t_{1/2}$.

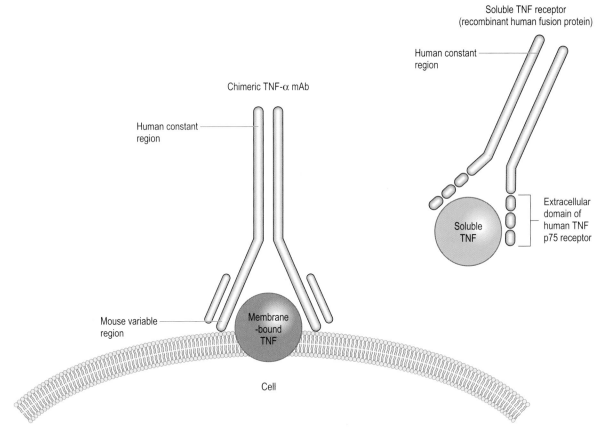

Fig. 6.13 Schematic representation of anti-TNF agents infliximab and the fusion protein etenercept. (From Cochrane and Dick 2007, with permission from Springer Science and Business Media.)

LOCAL ANAESTHETICS AFFECT EXCITABLE MEMBRANES

Local anaesthetics block the initiation and propagation of action potentials by preventing the voltage-dependent increase in sodium conductance via a direct action on sodium channel function and, to a lesser degree, by stabilizing membranes. The action of local anaesthetics is strongly pH dependent. Under alkaline conditions the proportion of the local anaesthetic that is ionized is low but it is also lipid soluble. This allows the anaesthetic to penetrate the myelin of the medullated nerve fibres. However, once inside the myelin sheath, the ionized cationic form of the drug is the active species, giving rise to the local anaesthetic effect. If the local anaesthetic is unable to penetrate the myelin sheath, its action can be mediated only via the node of Ranvier at several sites along the nerve. However, in unmyelinated fibres only a short length of fibre needs to be functionally interrupted to induce anaesthesia. In general, local anaesthetics block small-diameter nerves (myelinated more than unmyelinated) more readily, but practically it is not possible to produce a block of pain sensation without affecting other modalities, and there is no inherent difference between the susceptibility of motor and sensory nerves to local anaesthetics.

Local anaesthetics used in ophthalmology are usually aromatic residues linked to tertiary amide chains (see Box 6.28). These agents are more stable in acidic solutions where they are in their cationic form. However, when applied to the conjunctival sac and orbital tissues (pH 7.4) only 15% will be in the non-cationic form and lipid soluble, allowing the drug to penetrate myelin. Topical application of the anaesthetic blocks parasympathetic and sympathetic fibres first, followed by sensory (pain and temperature), and finally motor (large, myelinated) nerves.

Box 6.28 Local anaesthetic drugs in ophthalmology

Ester-linked
- cocaine
- procaine
- benoxinate

Amide-linked
- lignocaine
- bupivacaine

Box 6.29 Maximal safe doses of regional local anaesthetics

Lignocaine
- 10–15 ml 2% solution (200 mg)
- 20–25 ml 2% solution with epinephrine, 1 : 200 000 (500 mg)

Bupivacaine
- 15–20 ml 0.75% solution (150 mg)

During infiltrative regional anaesthesia for surgery (e.g. retrobulbar or peribulbar anaesthesia for intraocular surgery) a 1 : 200 000 concentration of epinephrine is frequently added to constrict blood vessels and retard vascular absorption and hydrolysis of the agent. Epinephrine is inactivated by heat, so may have reduced potency in precombined formulations. In addition, the pH of the local anaesthetic may be altered when mixing with an epinephrine solution which itself is acidic. This results in a reduced amount of the non-cationic form that is able to penetrate medullated nerve fibres.

LOCAL ANAESTHETICS HAVE BOTH LOCAL AND SYSTEMIC SIDE EFFECTS

Topically applied anaesthetic agents are well recognized as inhibitors of wound healing. They disrupt tight junctions between cells and interfere with corneal epithelial metabolism and, ultimately, the repair of corneal epithelial wounds. Systemic effects include numbness and tingling, dizziness, slurred speech and aggressive behaviour (see Box 6.29). Central nervous system toxicity may ultimately lead to convulsions with respiratory and myocardial depression. In the UK it has been recommended by the Royal College of Ophthalmologists that intravenous access (an infusion line) is available and monitoring of both heart rate and oxygen saturation is performed during infiltrative regional local anaesthesia.

OCULAR TOXICITY FROM SYSTEMIC ADMINISTRATION OF DRUGS

Ocular side effects from the systemic administration of drugs are well recognized (see above in relation to glaucoma treatment and the use of topical steroids). Access to the globe by systemically administered drugs is restricted by the blood–retinal and blood–aqueous barriers, as stated above. In the absence of ocular inflammation, penetration of the drug into the eye is a function of the drug's physicochemical properties. Drugs or their active metabolites may accumulate in the eye, particularly within the melanin of the uveal tract, the cornea (because of its differential solubility characteristics) and the lens.

UVEAL TRACT

Some drugs possess a high affinity for binding to melanin, from which they are only slowly released. A good example of this is chloroquine, which is known to concentrate in the melanin of the RPE and persist in this tissue for prolonged periods. If chloroquine is taken in large enough doses and for a long duration, the drug–melanin complex will result in retinal toxicity, although the exact mechanism remains unknown. The mechanism of drug binding to melanin is complex and involves electrostatic (van der Waal's) forces as well as possible cation exchange, which may displace free radicals from the melanin and in turn give rise to retinal toxicity. However, binding of the drug alone is not sufficient to give rise to retinal toxicity. For instance, β-blockers and benzodiazepines are irreversibly bound to melanin, although the amount of bound drug does not correlate with the damage to the RPE or uveal tract. Indeed, phospholipid metabolism within the RPE is still normal after 6 months of chloroquine treatment. In the case of chloroquine, the retinopathy is seen usually in patients receiving more than 100 g total dose of drug or in patients taking the drug for more than 1 year. In general there is a low incidence of retinal toxicity from hydroxychloroquine, and some centres regard this drug as safe and not requiring monitoring of patients.

Box 6.30 Common oculotoxic drugs

Allopurinol	cataract
Amiodarone	corneal opacity/corneal verticillata
Antidepressants	rise in IOP/acute glaucoma
Chloroquine	corneal opacity/retinal degeneration
Corticosteroids	cataracts/rise in IOP
Ethambutol	optic neuritis
Isoniazid	optic neuritis
Phenothiazines	corneal deposits/retinal degeneration/cataract
Phenytoin	nystagmus
Sulphonamides	Stevens–Johnson syndrome
Tamoxifen	optic atrophy/macular degeneration
Tetracycline	papilloedema
Vitamin A	papilloedema

PHOTOSENSITIZATION

Photosensitizing agents absorb visible and ultraviolet radiation and, as a result, generate free radicals (see Ch. 4). These photosensitizing agents may become bound to macromolecules in the cornea, lens and retina. Amiodarone, phenothiazines and psoralens are well-known examples of photosensitizing agents. The cornea, lens and retina may also act as drug depots. For example, once the therapeutic agent has circulated through the uveal tract into the aqueous it can rapidly penetrate the corneal endothelium and deposit in the stroma or, if lipophilic, accumulate in the corneal epithelium.

Oculotoxic drugs

Examples of oculotoxic drugs include steroids and ethambutol (see Box 6.30). Long-term steroid treatment is well recognized as a cause of both cataracts and glaucoma. Cataract formation correlates well with daily dosage and prednisolone-induced cataracts can be seen in most patients receiving 15 mg prednisolone daily. Topical application of steroids causes glaucoma by decreasing the aqueous humour outflow. The rise in IOP is related to the anti-inflammatory strength of the steroid used and the genetic disposition of the individual (see p. 348).

FURTHER READING

Akingbehin T, Raj PS. Ophthalmic topical beta-blockers: a review of ocular and systemic adverse effects. J Toxicol Cutan Ocul Toxicol 1990; 9:131–147.

Bartlett JD, Janus SD. Clinical Ocular Pharmacology, 3rd edn. New York: Butterworth-Heinemann; 1995.

Bito LZ Prostaglandins. Old concepts and new perspectives. Arch Ophthalmol 1987; 105:1036–1039.

Buckley MMT, Goa KL, Clissold SP. Ocular betaxolol: a review of its pharmacological properties and therapeutic efficacy in glaucoma and ocular hypertension. Drugs 1990; 40:75–90.

Cochrane S, Dick AD. Tumor necrosis factor alpha-targeted therapies in uveitis. In: Pleyer U, Foster CS (eds) Essentials in Ophthalmology. Uveitis and Immunological Disorders. Berlin-Heidelberg: Springer; 2007, pp. 177–192.

Davson H. Physiology of the Eye, 5th edn. New York: Pergamon Press; 1990.

Denton DM, Magee CC, Sayegh MH. Immunosuppressive strategies in transplantation. Lancet 1999; 353:1084.

du Souich P, Verges J, Erill S. Plasma protein binding and pharmacological response. Clin Pharmacokinet 1993; 24:435–440.

Fahy G, Easty D, Collum L, et al. Randomised double-masked trial of lodoxamide and sodium cromoglycate in allergic eye disease: a multicentre study. Eur J Ophthalmol 1992; 2:144–149.

Fechner PU, Teichmann KD. Ocular Therapeutics. New Jersey: Slack; 1998.

Grant WM, Schuman JS. Toxicology of the Eye, 4th edn. Springfield, IL: Charles Thomas; 1993.

Hopkins G, Pearson R. O'Connor Davies's Ophthalmic Drugs, 4th edn. Oxford: Butterworth-Heinemann; 1998.

Lichter PR. Another blockbuster glaucoma drug. Ophthalmology 1993; 100:1281–1282 (editorial).

McGhee CNJ. Pharmacokinetics of ophthalmic corticosteroids. Br J Ophthalmol 1992; 76:681–684.

Mitra AK, ed. Ophthalmic Drug Delivery Systems. New York: Marcel Dekker; 1993.

Pfeiffer N, Hennekes R, Lippa EA, et al. A single dose of the topical carbonic anhydrase inhibitor MK-927 decreases 109 in patients. Br J Ophthalmol 1990; 74:405–408.

Rang HP, Dale MM, Ritter JM. Pharmacology 4th edn. Edinburgh: Churchill Livingstone; 1999.

Urtti A, Salminen L. Drug delivery approaches to minimize systemic concentrations of ocularly administered drugs. Surv Ophthalmol 1993; 37:435–457.

7 IMMUNOLOGY

INTRODUCTION

Immunology is the study of host defence mechanisms. It has developed as a separate discipline during the past 100 years or so, out of the notion that even the simplest organisms have the ability to mount a variety of specific and non-specific responses to invasion or attack by foreign organisms. Immunological concepts are rapidly evolving, with new discoveries occurring at a high frequency. However, as knowledge accrues, the basic mechanisms become clearer and more easily understood.

The eye (and the brain) participate in immune responses, but under certain circumstances the expected response does not occur; this is called 'immune privilege' and is related to the special microenvironment and immunoregulatory mechanisms operating in these tissues. Most of this chapter outlines the basic principles of immune responses, with reference to the eye as appropriate.

OVERVIEW OF THE IMMUNE SYSTEM

Immunity is defined as the ability of the host to protect itself against a foreign organism. To do this it requires an *immune system* comprising the cells and molecules used in the host's defence. For unicellular hosts this may simply mean certain molecules on the cell surface that enable it to recognize foreign organisms. However, for higher-order hosts the immune system is a highly organized network of tissues, cells and molecules.

Hosts defend themselves by mounting an *immune response* involving the recruitment of the cells and molecules of the immune system. Two immune systems are available to the host, the *innate (natural or native) immune system* and the *acquired (adaptive) immune system*. In its first line of defence against

351

attack, the host uses the innate immune system because this is rapidly mobilized and is not dependent on previous exposure to the foreign invader. This form of response is *non-specific* in that the same sort of response occurs to most foreign organisms and even to injury itself. Recent work has shown that qualitatively the innate immune response to different organisms varies to a degree, suggesting some level of specificity. This has led to Janeway's prediction and discovery (Janeway and Medzitor, 2002) of receptors on innate immune cells, such as macrophages, which recognize sets of molecules on foreign organisms, pathogen-associated molecular patterns (PAMPs). Despite an effective innate immune system, it may not be sufficient to protect the host from the initial attack, leading to persistence of foreign material in the host, or from subsequent attacks. In contrast, the acquired immune response is *specific* for that foreign organism and has 'immunological memory' in that each subsequent attack by the same organism induces a faster and stronger specific immune response.

The innate immune system includes:

- Physicochemical barriers such as the skin, eyelids, tears (see Ch. 4).
- Molecules normally present in body fluids such as blood, tears and aqueous humour (e.g. complement, lysozyme, antiproteases). Antibacterial defensins are also on this list of ocular surface proteins.
- Phagocytic and cytotoxic cells such as polymorphonuclear leucocytes, macrophages, eosinophilic granulocytes, natural killer (NK) cells.
- Molecules released by cells responding to attack and acting on other cells (cytokines), such as interleukins and tumour necrosis factor-α (TNF-α) (see below) and complement.

The acquired immune system includes:

- Specific immune systems associated with barrier surfaces (the skin immune system and the mucosa-associated immune system, MALT).
- Cells (lymphocytes) with receptors that specifically recognize foreign organisms and molecules (antigens).
- Molecules that specifically counteract foreign antigens (antibodies); these proteins are known as immunoglobulins and there are five types (see below).
- Non-specific molecules (e.g. cytokines) released by antigen-specific cells (e.g. lymphocytes).

Specific immunity is described as *humoral* when antibodies (derived from B lymphocytes; see below) and complement are involved in removing the antigen or as *cell-mediated* (cellular) when T lymphocytes and macrophages are involved.

Immunity after infection is normally termed *active immunity* in that the host has responded actively to the stimulus. However, immunity may be transferred *passively* by antibodies or cells. Vaccination procedures that involve the administration of antibodies are termed *passive immunization*, while those that involve inducing a response to the antigen or even the attenuated live organism are termed *active immunization* (see Ch. 8).

The development of acquired immunity involves a number of discrete phases, including:

- An afferent phase in which the foreign antigen is transported from the site of entry and presented by specialized antigen-presenting cells (APCs) to the lymphocytes in the lymphoid tissue (see below).
- A phase of T-cell activation in which T cells are transformed from a resting to an active state.
- An effector stage in which T cells induce other cells, such as B cells and macrophages, to remove the antigen. If the antigen remains intracellular as with virus-infected cells, the T cells themselves attack the infected cell (cytotoxic T cells).

This is known as the *primary immune response* and is accompanied by the appearance of antigen-specific T cells and antibody-secreting B cells. On second exposure to the same antigen, antigen-specific memory T and B cells are recruited much sooner and more efficiently, such that antibody levels are considerably higher than on the first exposure. This is known as the *secondary immune response*. In addition, the type (isotype; see below) of antibody in secondary immune responses is different.

Throughout the development of the acquired immune response there are several checkpoints that prevent a runaway overwhelming inflammatory reaction. Most of these regulatory mechanisms are in place to prevent adaptive immune responses to self antigens but they also participate in downregulatory responses to foreign antigens and help to restore homeostasis.

Innate immunity with its early warning, rapid-response system provides a reliable means of protecting the host against most extracellular organisms (pathogens) and is a property of every living being. It might be asked, therefore, why the acquired immune system has evolved? Immune systems are by definition mechanisms that allow the host to remove and destroy foreign organisms while 'self' molecules and cells are not attacked. A difficulty arises, however, when the pathogen resides within the host cell, as in the case of protozoa or, more frequently, viruses. Viruses invade cells by incorporating their genome, or at least parts of it, into the DNA of the cell, which may then lead to the expression of the foreign antigen on the surface of the cell in addition to the self-molecules (also termed antigens because they can induce an immune response). Removal of infected cells thus requires a mechanism in which recognition of foreign antigen occurs in conjunction with self-antigen; this has led to the evolution of the acquired immune system, which is based on the recognition of foreign antigens in the context of self-antigens [the peptide– major histocompatibility complex (MHC); see below].

The innate immune system has thus evolved to deal with extracellular pathogens, while the acquired immune system deals with intracellular pathogens. The acquired immune system has developed a considerable degree of sophistication with a variety of cells (T and B lymphocytes); T-cell subsets [e.g. T helper (Th), T cytotoxic (Tc), T suppressor (Ts) cells]; and even subsets of these (e.g. Th0, Th1 and Th2) (see below), each designed for specific cellular functions. In addition, the T and B cells have evolved in fundamentally different directions – T cells to deal with surface-bound antigen (usually cell-associated) and B cells to deal with soluble (extracellular) antigen. There are also T regulatory (Treg) cells to control the adaptive response. The sophistication and specificity of the acquired immune system involving T cells has thus been harnessed to assist the innate immune system in dealing more efficiently with extracellular organisms via B cells (see Box 7.1).

Certain basic concepts about immune mechanisms can therefore be derived from the above considerations:

- Extracellular foreign antigen is normally cleared by the innate immune system, with some assistance from B-cell activity.
- Intracellular foreign antigen is handled by the acquired immune system in which self and foreign antigens are jointly recognized.
- All cellular defence mechanisms involve interactions of cell surface molecules (receptors) with complementary molecules (ligands).

In addition, acquired immune responses have certain features that are inherent to them:

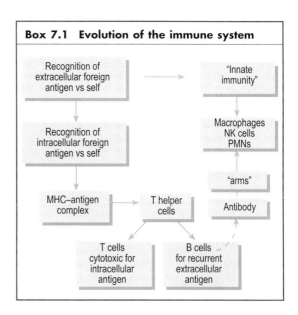

Box 7.1 Evolution of the immune system

- Specificity – based on certain determinants (epitopes) of the antigenic structure
- Differentiation of self from non-self antigens – non-responsiveness to self antigens is known as tolerance and loss of tolerance underpins autoimmune disease
- Diversity – around 10^9 individual epitopes can be distinguished – this is the lymphocyte repertoire
- Memory – the secondary immune response, specific to that antigen and present in both B and T cells
- Specialization – the immune response is customized to different microbes
- Ability to downregulate – the immune response is strictly limited in magnitude and time through specific and non-specific mechanisms.

CELLS AND TISSUES OF THE IMMUNE SYSTEM

The cells and tissues of the immune system can be described in terms of participating in the defence mechanisms of the innate or the acquired immune systems (see Box 7.2). Some cells are central to both.

THE MYELOID SYSTEM AND INNATE IMMUNITY

The cells directly involved in bacterial killing and removal of damaged host tissue at the site of entry

Box 7.2 Cells and tissues of the innate and acquired immune systems

 Mature T or B lymphocyte  6–9 µm; round or slightly indented nucleus; sparse cytoplasm; few granules; few mitochondria

 Plasma cell  5–30 µm; round or oval nucleus; abundant cytoplasm; no granules; abundant endoplasmic reticulum

 NK cell 10–12 µm; round nucleus; abundant cytoplasm; many granules; scattered mitochondria

 NKT cell Phenotypically similar to NK cell

 Monocyte  12–20 µm; round, oval, notched, or horseshoe-shaped nucleus; abundant cytoplasm; abundant granules; well-developed Golgi apparatus; abundant mitochondria

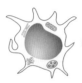 Macrophage  15–80 µm; elongated, indented, or oval nucleus; abundant cyoplasm; many granules and vacuoles; few mitochondria; abundant lysosomes

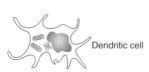 Dendritic cell Irregularly shaped cell and nucleus; many cellular processes; few intracellular organelles; prominent mitochondria

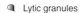 Lytic granules    Mitochondria   Smooth endoplasmic reticulum   Granules

 Phagosomes   Golgi apparatus   Rough endoplasmic reticulum

Box 7.2 *Continued*

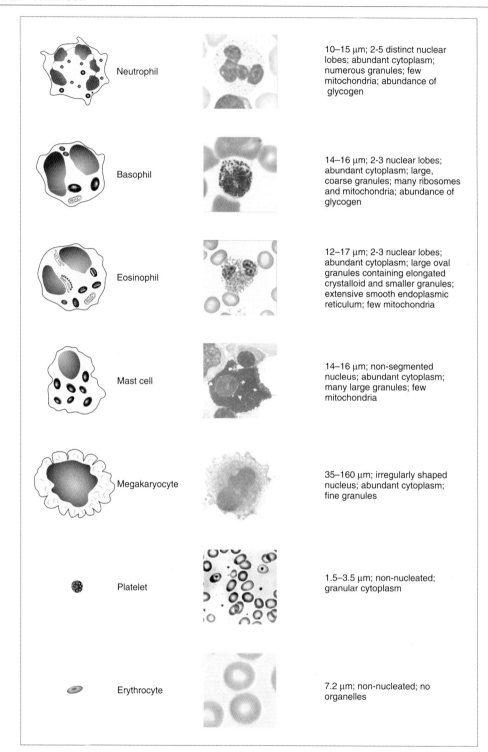

Neutrophil	10–15 µm; 2-5 distinct nuclear lobes; abundant cytoplasm; numerous granules; few mitochondria; abundance of glycogen
Basophil	14–16 µm; 2-3 nuclear lobes; abundant cytoplasm; large, coarse granules; many ribosomes and mitochondria; abundance of glycogen
Eosinophil	12–17 µm; 2-3 nuclear lobes; abundant cytoplasm; large oval granules containing elongated crystalloid and smaller granules; extensive smooth endoplasmic reticulum; few mitochondria
Mast cell	14–16 µm; non-segmented nucleus; abundant cytoplasm; many large granules; few mitochondria
Megakaryocyte	35–160 µm; irregularly shaped nucleus; abundant cytoplasm; fine granules
Platelet	1.5–3.5 µm; non-nucleated; granular cytoplasm
Erythrocyte	7.2 µm; non-nucleated; no organelles

From Mak and Saunders 2006, with permission from Elsevier.

Box 7.3   Generation of macrophages and dendritic cells from myeloid and lymphoid precursors

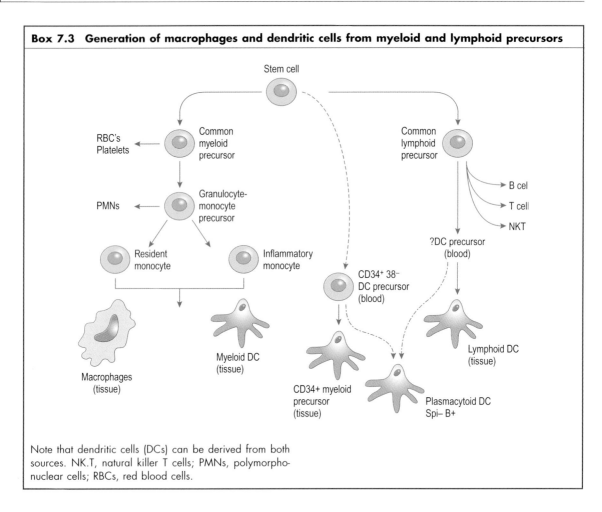

Note that dendritic cells (DCs) can be derived from both sources. NK.T, natural killer T cells; PMNs, polymorphonuclear cells; RBCs, red blood cells.

of the foreign organism are the cells of the myeloid system. Some of these cells are recruited to the site of injury during acute inflammation. Their defining feature is the presence of cytoplasmic organelles (lysosomes) containing a battery of hydrolytic enzymes for both intracellular and extracellular killing.

Neutrophilic granulocytes

Neutrophilic granulocytes (polymorphonuclear leucocytes) are the most common white cell in the circulation and are attracted to sites of inflammation by chemotaxis (see below). These are fully differentiated cells with no capacity for proliferation. They are primary scavengers, causing much of their effect via release of free radicals and proteases from their numerous cytoplasmic granules and lysosomes. These include defensins, lysozyme, lactoferrin and

oxidative enzymes (e.g. NADPH-dependent oxidases, myeloperoxidases and catalase), which are also present in ocular fluids such as tears. The half-life of neutrophils is 1–2 days.

Myeloid mononuclear cells

Monocytes, macrophages and dendritic cells are cells of the mononuclear phagocyte system. Like neutrophils, these cells are derived from marrow stem cells and differentiate into a variety of tissue macrophages (histiocytes) with specific functions (see Box 7.3).

Macrophages have many functions as part of the innate immune system: they phagocytose dead and damaged cells and organisms in inflammatory exudates; they release cytokines of various sorts, which may activate other cells such as lymphocytes and eosinophils; and they are involved in the acquired immune system as APCs, as effector cells in the process of cell lysis, and by removing antibody-coated (opsonized) cells.

Macrophages, like B cells, usually capture antigen for presentation via surface receptors such as immunoglobulin. Macrophages bind the Fc portion of immunoglobulin–antigen complexes (see below) through the Fc receptor while B cells express immunoglobulin on their surface and use the Fab portion to capture antigen. Therefore, to synthesize immunoglobulin the immune system must have already been exposed to antigen. It is clear therefore that macrophages and B cells are only effective as APCs in the context of an ongoing immune response.

In contrast, the most potent APC in the immune system is the dendritic cell, which circulates in the bloodstream to the spleen and to the tissues from where it recirculates in the afferent lymph to the lymph nodes and spleen. The key difference, apart from its greatly increased APC potency, is that the dendritic cell initiates immune responses by taking up antigen *de novo* via endocytosis and presenting the digested products to naïve T cells. This cell therefore acts as an antigen detecting or surveillance system at sites of high antigen exposure such as the skin, conjunctiva, respiratory system and gut.

Other granulocytes

Mast cells/basophils/eosinophils are all part of the granulocyte series of cells. Basophils are the circulating equivalent of mast cells, which occur only in the tissues. However, mast cells and eosinophils have separate lineages. Two types of mast cell are described: the connective tissue mast cells and the mucosal mast cell on the basis of their granule proteases, their susceptibility to degranulation by immunoglobulin E (IgE), and their requirement for different maturation signals (see below).

Eosinophils account for about 0.1% of circulating leucocytes. Their numbers are elevated in chronic allergic disorders, in both the circulation and the tissues. They are also produced in large numbers in response to parasite and helminth infections and contain a panel of particularly potent parasite-specific proteases. Like mast cells they have high-affinity IgE receptors, and are probably effectors of tissue damage in allergic disease including asthma and chronic allergic conjunctival disorders such as atopic keratoconjunctivitis and vernal keratoconjunctivitis (see p. 429).

THE LYMPHOID SYSTEM AND ACQUIRED IMMUNITY

The single most important feature of the acquired immune system is antigen specificity, which is mediated by lymphocytes. In contrast to cells of the myeloid system, which remove debris and organisms by mechanisms that do not have much specificity (thus macrophages will phagocytose broad ranges of organisms dictated by 'pattern recognition receptors'; see p. 352), each clone of lymphoid cell responds to a single antigen. T cells respond to antigen by proliferating and releasing cytokines, while B cells respond by maturing to plasma cells and producing antibodies.

T cells

T cells (for thymus-derived) are lymphoid mononuclear cells that recognize antigen in conjunction with self antigen. T helper (Th) cells respond to antigen in association with MHC class II self-antigen, while T cytotoxic/suppressor (Tc/s) cells respond to antigen combined with MHC class I antigen (see below). T cells release cytokines, which are required for T-cell and B-cell proliferation and differentiation, and also for macrophage activation. T lymphocytes express surface markers (molecules detectable by specific monoclonal antibodies) characteristic of their phenotype. Thus Th cells are described as CD4+ cells and Tc/s cells are known as CD8+ cells (see Box 7.4). Further subsets of T cells occur, such as the rather obscure γδT cells [which possess a T-cell receptor (TCR) with a γ–δ dimer, rather than the αβTCR present on conventional T cells] and T regulatory (Treg) cells, which downregulate the T-cell response.

Cytokines are multifunctional short-acting, short-range mediators of cellular activities, released by T cells and other immune and non-immune cells. Cytokines are distinguished from other mediators as the molecules of 'intercellular communication'.

B cells

B cells are mononuclear lymphoid cells that are specialized for the secretion of antibody. As stated above, there are five types (isotypes) of antibody: IgG, IgA, IgM, IgD and IgE.

During a primary immune response IgM antibody is initially produced by activated B cells. In secondary immune responses, the B cells switch to producing IgG (isotype switching), often with higher binding capacity (affinity) for the antigen, a process termed affinity maturation. During allergic immune responses, a further isotype switch occurs from IgG to IgE. IgA forms part of the mucosal immune system, being present in large amounts in surface secretory fluids including tears. IgA is the most abundant immunoglobulin in the immune system. IgD is present in low amounts in the circulation.

B cells recognize antigen via surface immunoglobulin (sIg). Antigen binds to sIg in the afferent phase of the secondary immune response; in contrast, antigen binds to the secreted form of immunoglobulin (antibody) in the effector phase of the response. Secondary afferent (cognitive) interactions are antigen specific, but effector functions are not (see below).

Natural killer cells

The natural killer (NK) cells are circulating granulocytes but are part of the lymphoid system and are particularly effective against tumour cells and virus-infected cells. Previously called null cells because they lack any of the specific lymphocyte markers, they also contain granules and are thus also known as large granular lymphocytes.

NK cells can be expanded by the T-cell cytokine interleukin-2, whereupon they become LAK cells (lymphokine-acitvated killer cells) for tumours. Similarly they have receptors for antibody allowing them to kill antibody-coated cells. NKT cells are specialized lymphoid cells that only express a single type of TCR.

INITIAL RESPONSE OF THE HOST TO INJURY (THE INNATE IMMUNE RESPONSE)

The host responds to injury or attack by invading microorganisms by mounting an acute inflammatory response. During this response, the pathogens are removed by cells of the innate immune system brought to the site of injury by changes in tissue components such as blood vessels and extracellular matrix. Meanwhile antigen from degraded microorganisms is transported to lymphoid tissues to activate the acquired immune system.

THE ACUTE INFLAMMATORY RESPONSE

The acute inflammatory response goes through three phases

1. Tissue damage and the acute early response
2. The delayed cellular response and phagocytosis

3. Resolution of the inflammation and tissue remodelling.

The acute early phase has several components:

- tissue damage and release of mediators
- vascular changes
- leucocyte activation and adhesion
- leucocyte emigration.

Tissue damage and the release of mediators

The response to tissue injury (physical, chemical or mediated by microorganisms) is immediate. Reactions occur at several levels, both locally and systemically. Immediate local reactions include the release of tissue factors and chemoattractants from damaged tissue and microorganisms. Vessels are also damaged, inducing venous stasis and the leakage of plasma components; platelet and leucocyte activation with intravascular clotting occurs; plasma/serum transudation and exudation lead to tissue fibrin deposition and activation of serum components such as complement (see p. 385).

There are several classes of inflammatory mediators derived from both inflammatory and damaged tissue cells:

- vasoactive amines (e.g. histamine and serotonin)
- cytokines and chemokines (see p. 373)
- lipids (e.g. prostaglandins, thromboxane and leukotrienes)
- free radicals (see Ch. 4, Box 4.8, p. 198)
- neuropeptides (e.g. substance P, vasoactive intestinal peptide)
- endothelium-derived mediators (endothelin, nitric oxide, prostacyclin, platelet-activating factor, etc.)
- plasma-derived mediators (e.g. complement, kinins and clotting cascade peptides)
- leucocyte-derived mediators (e.g. granule proteases, phospholipase A_2)
- bacterial products (e.g. endotoxin, proteases and chemotactic factors including formylated peptides).

During the first 20 min to 48 h, there is a progressive increase in polymorphonuclear cell infiltration. Degranulation of these cells leads to high tissue levels of several proteases, cytokines and cationic proteins. Neutrophils contain some of the most powerful antibacterial agents, including defensins, which have similarity to defensins from other species including plants and insects (see Table 7.1). Defensins are mediators of non-oxidative bacterial killing and are also produced by epithelial cells such as gut

Table 7.1 Neutrophil antibacterial agents

Class	Agent
Free radicals/gases	Hydrogen peroxide Hypochlorite Chloramine OH radical Nitric oxide
Enzyme	Proteinase 3 Collagenase Elastase Azurocidin Cathepsin G β glucuronidase Myeloperoxidase Lysozyme
Peptide	Defensin β-lysin Vasoactive intestinal peptide
Ion binders	Lactoferrin Calprotectin

and conjunctival mucosal cells. Both α and β defensins have been found in ocular surface cells and tears. Among the proteases released by neutrophils during acute inflammation are a set of enzymes that degrade the extracellular matrix. These enzymes are also released by activated or injured tissue parenchymal cells and are involved in tissue remodelling. More than 24 of these zinc-dependent endopeptidases, known as matrix metalloproteinases (MMPs) have been identified in humans, they are related to the transmembrane proteins that contain disintegration and metalloprotease domains (ADAMTs). The MMPs self-activate and cross-activate each other in a cascade-like fashion, thus permitting maximal tissue degradation as required. Their effects are counteracted by naturally occurring inhibitors (see Table 7.2) termed tissue inhibitors of matrix metalloproteinases. There are four types of TIMP: 1, 2, 3 and 4, TIMP-4 only occurring in the mouse. MMPs are also inhibited by recognized anti-proteases such as α_2-macroglobulin, tissue factor pathway inhibitor 2, and a recently described plasma membrane inhibitor, RECK (reversion-inducing cysteine-rich protein with Kazal motifs).

However, much of the cell and tissue damage is mediated by free radicals, particularly hydrogen peroxide (H_2O_2) and superoxide anions (see Ch.4), which are released as part of the respiratory burst (see Box 7.5). In addition, free radicals may combine

Table 7.2 Matrix metalloproteinases (MMP) and their substrates

MMP	Interstitial collagens	Basement membrane	Elastin	Other proteins
Collagenases				
MMP-1	Types III, I, II, VII, X	⎧ Laminin		
		⎨ Entactin		L selectin
MMP-8	Types I, III, II	⎪ Fibronectin		
MMP-13	Types II, I, III	⎩ (±)Proteoglycan		
Stromelysin				
MMP-3		⎧ Fibronectin	±	⎧ EGF-like proteins
		⎨ Laminin		⎨
MMP-10		⎪ Entactin	±	⎩ Plasminogen
		⎩ Proteoglycan		
Stromelysin-like				
MMP-7		⎧ Fibronectin	+	⎧ Plasminogen
		⎨ Laminin		⎨ ↓
MMP-12		⎪ Entactin	++	⎪ Angiostatin;
		⎩ Proteoglycan		⎩ α_1 antitrypsin
Gelatinases				
MMP-2	Types I, VII, X, XI	⎧ IV/V	++	
		⎨ Fibronectin		
MMP-9		⎪ Laminin	++	
		⎪ Entactin		
		⎩ Proteoglycan		
Membrane-type				
MMP-14	Types I, III, II	⎧ Fibronectin		
MMP-15		⎨ Laminin		
MMP-16		⎪ Entactin		
MMP-17		⎩ Proteoglycan		
MMP-24				
Furin-recognition site				
MMP-11				

with reactive nitrogen species (nitric oxide) released from inflammatory cells (see Box 7.6).

Vascular changes

The immediate cause of inflammation is release of plasma into the extravascular space and the instantaneous coagulation of proteins with activation of inflammatory mediators. Plasma release (vascular leakage) is caused by changes to the blood vessels induced by the inflammatory factors (e.g. trauma, chemical microorganisms, etc.). The immediate response of the vascular endothelium is to undergo retraction and this is associated with transient vasoconstriction. The major vascular response, however, is vasodilatation mediated initially by nitric oxide (NO). The initial vasoconstriction is mediated by several locally released compounds, particularly endothelin, which is released by pericytes and smooth muscle cells to act on the endothelium. The later vasodilatation is also mediated by locally released factors, in this case the gas nitric oxide. NO is synthesized by specific enzymes from the amino acid arginine and has widespread physiological and pathological effects, some of which are related to its role as a free radical (see Box 7.6). This is accompanied by an increased blood flow, the opening of capillary channels and the leakage of plasma into the extracellular space. This in turn leads to an increase in the tissue osmotic pressure, thus attracting further fluid build-up in the tissues (oedema). In response to this, there is an increase in lymphatic drainage from the injured site, thus reducing the tissue swelling and at the same time increasing the flow of antigenic material to the draining lymph nodes (see below). These vascular changes vary in degree with the severity of the tissue injury.

Box 7.5 The neutrophil respiratory burst

The neutrophil respiratory burst describes the activation of neutrophils and their utilization of oxygen during the inflammatory cascade. The stimulus for this response is the release of mediators from injured tissue cells. Tissue damage is caused by free radical release and tissue proteases (see also Ch.4).

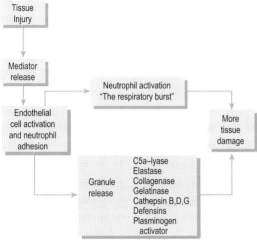

The central component of the respiratory burst is H_2O_2, which is metabolized through several pathways, some of which cause further tissue damage (e.g. superoxide and chloramine) while others reduce it to water. Tissue damage is therefore dependent on the levels of reduced glutathione (GSH) in the milieu. NADP, nicotinamide adenosine dinucleotide phosphate; NADPH, reduced NADP; PKC, protein kinase C.

Hypochlorous acid (HOCl) is a short-lived, highly reactive oxidant that is lipophilic and membrane permeant. It binds proteins and renders them more susceptible to proteases. Chlorinated proteins are more immunogenic and may provide a link between the innate and the acquired immune systems.

Box 7.6 Nitric oxide

Nitric oxide was originally described as endothelium relaxing factor because it was found to be the agent released by the endothelium that was responsible for inducing autocrine vasodilatation in response to insult. Nitric oxide is a gas produced by the activity of the enzyme nitric oxide synthase (NOS) on interaction of the amino acid arginine with oxygen:

$$O_2 + \text{L-arginine} \xrightarrow{\text{NOS}} \text{Citrulline} + NO$$

There are at least three isoforms of nitric oxide synthase, endothelium-derived (eNOS), neuronal (nNOS) and inducible (iNOS). The iNOS is released from inflammatory and other cells, particularly macrophages, and is involved in both immunoregulation and tissue damage through its interaction with superoxide radicals released from activated neutrophils. In its latter role it may also function as an antibacterial agent by damaging bacterial cell membranes. The prostanoids are co-released with NO through induction of cyclo-oxygenase-2.

NO interacts with superoxide anions to produce peroxynitrite, which is believed to be directly involved in membrane damage (see equation below). NO has direct effects on many other proteins such as the important zinc finger regions of many enzymes where it nitrosylates free cysteine SH groups with ejection of the Zn moiety from the configured protein. These damaging effects to parenchymal cells may also be the basis for T-cell apoptosis (cell death), so leading to downregulation of the immune response.

$$O_2^{\bullet} + NO^{\bullet} \rightarrow ONOO^- + H^{\bullet} \rightleftharpoons ONOOH \rightarrow HO^{\bullet} + NO_2^+ \rightarrow NO_3^- + H^+$$

Thus NO produced constitutively in small amounts has a physiological role involving guanyl cyclase and increases in cGMP, while in large amounts it may be cytotoxic, producing depression of mitochondrial respiration, metal enzyme damage with consumption of both Zn and Fe ions and DNA damage.

The vascular endothelium also undergoes significant functional and morphological changes during the inflammatory response. Whereas the normal endothelium presents a non-adhesive surface to circulating cells such as platelets and leucocytes, during inflammation the endothelium becomes much more adhesive, an effect achieved by the expression of specific adhesion molecules on its surface. There are three major classes of adhesion molecules, the selectins, the integrins and the cell adhesion molecules (CAMs), each with different functions (see below and Table 7.3). In addition, the endothelium may undergo a marked morphological transformation, changing from a flat resting cell to a large protrud-

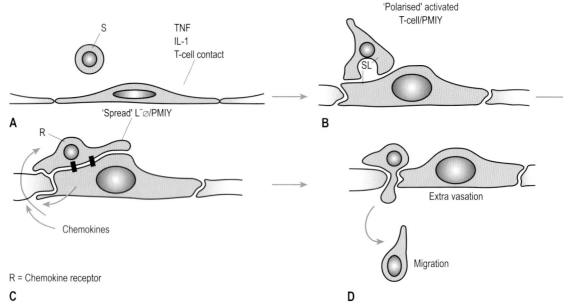

Fig. 7.1 Stages in extravasation of leucocytes from blood vessels during inflammation. (**A**) Rolling, (**B**) rolling and loose adhesion, (**C**) firm adhesion, (**D**) emigration. IL-1, interleukin-1; TNF, tumour necrosis factor; SL, selectin–ligand; R, receptor; L$_\phi$, lymphocyte; PMN, polymorphonuclear leucocyte.

Table 7.3 Adhesion molecules and their ligands		
Type	Cell	Ligand
Selectins		
L selectin	Leucocytes	GlyCAM-1
		MADCAM-1
P selectin	Endothelium	PSGL
E selectin	Endothelium	ESL
Integrins		
LFA-1	Leucocytes	ICAM-1, -2, -3
$\alpha_4\beta_1$	Leucocytes	VCAM-1
$\alpha_4\beta_7$	Leucocytes	VCAM-1
		MADCAM-1
Matrix-binding molecules		
CD44	Leucocytes	Hyaluronate
CD31	Leucocytes	CD31

ing cell with multiple cytoplasmic organelles. In this respect it resembles the high endothelial venule cells in the lymph node, which are specialized for leucocyte adhesion (see below).

Leucocyte activation and adhesion to the endothelium

Neutrophils are attracted to the site of inflammation through a series of discrete events that occur during margination and extravasation of the cell from the

vessel. These involve rolling, loose adhesion, firm adhesion and then migration of the cell through the intercellular junction. Each of these steps is mediated by the reciprocal expression of adhesion molecules and their respective ligands on the surface of leucocytes and the endothelium (see below) (Fig. 7.1). During the later stages of the response (24–72 h) when other inflammatory cells are involved (monocytes and lymphocytes), similar adhesion mechanisms are involved but with a different set of molecules. Thus coordinated expression of adhesion molecules appears to regulate the nature of the inflammatory cell exudate.

Adhesion of leucocytes to the endothelium thus involves a series of molecular events

- Selectin–ligand (S–L) interactions occur during the initial rolling phase of leucocyte endothelial cell interactions. These are initially low-strength interactions and are enhanced by the upregulation of selectins on the endothelium by inflammatory cytokines such as interleukin-1 (IL-1) and TNF-α or by contact with an activated T cell.
- Leucocyte activation by chemokines mediated in part through upregulation of specific chemokine receptors (see later) then occurs and induces polarization and firm adhesion of the cell to the endothelium.

- Integrin–CAM interactions induce spreading of the leucocyte on the endothelium and prevent detachment of the leucocyte.
- Extravasation of leucocytes through the endothelium is mediated by expression of PECAM-1 (CD31) on both the leucocyte and the endothelium, possibly through a 'zipper' mechanism in which disassembly of intercellular tight (occludin) junctions and adherens junctions occurs. A further molecule, CD99, expressed on both leucocytes and endothelium, may be important in transendothelial migration of monocytes.
- Migration of leucocytes through the tissues is the final stage and is induced through binding of chemokines selective for each cell type.

Certain molecules are specific for each type of leucocyte–endothelial cell interaction; for instance, E and P selectins mediate the attachment of polymorphonuclear leucocytes to endothelial cells, while vascular cell adhesion molecule (VCAM) preferentially mediates T lymphocyte–endothelium binding. Both of these interactions have been reported in inflammatory tissue in the eye from cases of sympathetic ophthalmia, a form of autoimmune posterior uveitis (Fig. 7.2).

Leucocyte migration into the tissues and chemotaxis

Many of the mediators released in the earliest stages of tissue injury are attractants for inflammatory cells. Both thrombin and the cleavage product fibrinopeptide B from fibrin lead to leucocyte chemotaxis from the onset of vessel leakage and fibrin formation. Prokaryotic peptides released from bacteria, such as formyl-methionine-leucine-phenylalanine, are powerful neutrophil and monocyte chemotactic agents. Activated complement components (see below) have an important role as chemoattractant agents in the neutrophil/monocyte response. Other important chemoattractants include interleukin-8 (IL-8), a cytokine (chemokine) released from tissue cells including the retinal pigment epithelium (RPE), tumour necrosis factor-α (TNF-α) and platelet release compounds such as platelet-activating factor (PAF), transforming growth factor-β (TGF-β), platelet-derived growth factor, platelet-derived endothelial cell growth factor, and many others. Lipid mediators, such as the leukotrienes, are also important neutrophil chemoattractants, while certain cytokines, such as monocyte chemotactic protein (MCP) and the macrophage inflammatory proteins (MIP-α, MIP-β and the che-

mokines; see below), are selective for mononuclear cell chemotaxis. There is now a large body of information on the cytokines that induce inflammatory cell migration. Collectively these are known as chemokines (inducing movement through chemotaxis) and receptors for different chemokines are present on different cells, thus regulating not only the numbers of cell that migrate into the tissue but also the type of cell (see p. 385, Fig. 7.13).

Cells such as neutrophils and monocytes 'sense' a chemical gradient of these attractants and migrate up the gradient by using specific cell surface receptors clustered preferentially towards the leading, polarized edge of the cell (Fig. 7.3). These receptors (e.g. the C5a receptor) are composed of seven transmembrane segments (in a manner similar to the transmembrane spanning segments of rhodopsin; see Ch. 4, p. 253) that possess a cytoplasmic connection to a G-protein-linked second messenger system. This activates the intracellular machinery (actin–myosin motor) required for forward movement.

Phagocytosis and removal of damaged tissue and microorganisms

Recovery from inflammation requires the removal of dead microorganisms and necrotic tissue by phagocytic cells (polymorphonuclear leucocytes and macrophages). Even in the absence of microorganisms, altered (damaged) self-proteins are recognized by cells of the innate immune system and phagocytosed. In the eye this is classically seen with lens-induced uveitis, in which denatured lens crystallin proteins are released into the anterior chamber in cases of traumatic and hypermature cataract. In the latter circumstance, engorged macrophages may block the outflow channels and produce a 'phacolytic glaucoma' (see Ch. 9).

Phagocytosis, particularly of bacteria, is facilitated by certain molecules of the innate immune system known as opsonins, which are present in plasma and bind to the surface of microorganisms when they are released into the extracellular space. One of the complement components, C3b (see below), acts as an opsonin. Interestingly, different actin cytoskeletal structures are constructed to phagocytose different types of particle, e.g. IgG-coated versus complement-coated particles. In addition, the role of microbial pathogen receptors such as Toll-like receptors (see next section) on maturation of the phagosome is unclear but appears not to play a significant part.

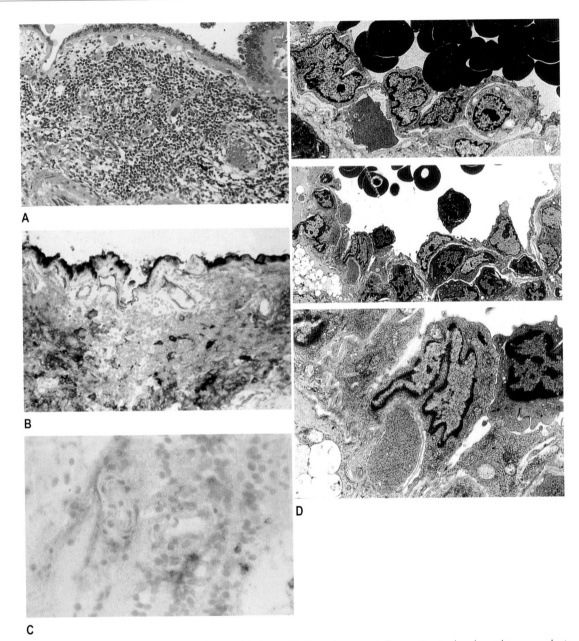

Fig. 7.2 Adhesion molecules in sympathetic ophthalmia. (**A**) Granulomatous inflammation in the choroid in sympathetic ophthalmia, stained with haematoxylin & eosin. (**B**) Expression of intercellular adhesion molecule 1 (ICAM-1) [alkaline phosphatase anti-alkaline phosphatase (APAAP): red/pink stain] on the retinal pigment epithelium and on infiltrating inflammatory cells in the choroid in the same case as (A). (**C**) Expression of endothelial leucocyte adhesion molecule 1 (ELAM-1) (APAAP: pink stain) in the retinal vessels in the same case as (A). (**D**) Endothelial cell activation in experimental autoimmune uveoretinitis, a model for posterior uveitis including sympathetic ophthalmia. Note the marked swelling of the endothelial cells and the attachment and migration of lymphocytes through the endothelial cell barrier. These cells have adopted an appearance similar to high endothelial venules in the lymphoid organs, which are specialized for the adhesion of lymphocytes. L, lymphocyte; M, macrophage/monocyte. (All images courtesy of A Abbas.)

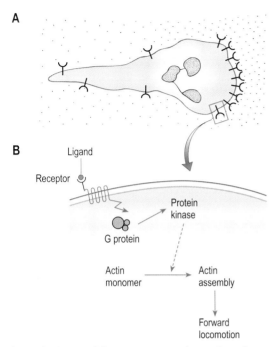

A

B

Ligand

Receptor

Protein kinase

G protein

Actin monomer → Actin assembly

Forward locomotion

Fig. 7.3 Neutrophil migration up a chemical gradient. (**A**) Cells sense the concentration gradient and polarize towards it with a wide leading edge and a trailing tail. Receptors for the chemoattractant cluster in the membrane of the leading edge, increasing the signal at this end of the cell. (**B**) Diagram of the seven-coil transmembrane receptor (the same basic structure as rhodopsin) that mediates the intracellular signal via G-protein links. This activates a protein, tyrosine kinase, to initiate actin assembly and induce forward movement of the cell.

Molecules of the acquired immune system also promote phagocytosis, particularly antibodies which bind avidly to the foreign antigen by specific interaction of their antigen-binding site (the Fab portion of the molecule) but are non-specifically removed by binding of their Fc portion to the phagocyte cell surface (see section on antibodies below, p. 371). Cells that express high levels of surface receptors for C3b and Fc are termed 'professional phagocytes', and include neutrophils and macrophages. Studies in genetically targeted knockout mice suggest that the Fc pathway for phagocytic activation is the major one.

Activation of innate immune cells by microorganisms

Invading microorganisms release factors that attract leucocytes to the site of inflammation and also induce those same leucocytes to engage in attempted removal of the offending agent. How is this innate immune response achieved? Previously this was considered to be a non-specific mechanism, i.e. when the body was under siege from different types of microorganisms the same set of innate immune responses would be set in motion. However, it has long been recognized that responses to different organisms vary greatly, some being virulent or lethal while others are harmless. Janeway proposed that prokaryotic pathogens expressed broad sets of molecules different from any molecules in eukaryotes; he termed these pathogen-associated molecular patterns (PAMPs) and they were recognized by specific pathogen recognition molecules (PRMs). If PRMs were expressed on the cell surface, they were termed pattern recognition receptors (PRRs). Activation of these molecules led to qualitatively different types of response by the cells of the innate immune system, particularly macrophages and dendritic cells. In addition, these responses were critical to the maturation of APCs in the downstream induction of the adaptive immune response.

Janeway's prediction proved to be correct. An explosion of information has revealed that there are several classes of membrane and soluble PRMs, including the Toll-like receptors (TLR), the scavenger receptors and the collectins (see Table 7.4). The components recognized include pathogen cell wall material, bacterial DNA and proteins, viral DNA and RNA, and lipoproteins from microbes.

Lipopolysaccharide is a classic microbial product that complexes with a serum protein lipopolysaccharide-binding protein and binds to the microbial co-receptor CD14. This then complexes with TLR4 and initiates the signalling cascade [most involving myeloid differentiation factor 88 (Myd88) and onto a nuclear factor-κB (NF-κB) core] to activate the macrophage or dendritic cell (Fig. 7.4). There are several TLRs, first described because of their similarity to *Toll* gene of the *Drosophila* fruit fly, which regulates both dorsal-ventral patterning and antifungal/anti-Gram-positive bacterial immunity. Some are membrane receptors while others recognize nucleic acids in the endosome (Fig. 7.4).

TLRs are not so much involved in the phagocytosis and clearance of microorganisms (see section above) as in the maturation of dendritic cells for induction of the adaptive immune response through T-cell activation; for this, different TLRs activate different types of dendritic cell (Fig. 7.5). In contrast, macrophages also express other PRRs, including scavenging receptors, which are primarily involved in phagocytosis. Two main classes of scavenging recep-

Table 7.4 Selected pattern recognition molecules of the innate system

Molecule	Location	Ligand	Function
CD14	Monocytes, macrophages PMNs	LPS, numerous microbial cell wall components	LPS sensitivity; clearance of microbes; proinflammatory cytokine induction
Toll-like receptor family	Splenic and peripheral blood leucocytes	TLR2, bacterial peptidoglycan techoic acid TLR3, viral dsDNA TLR4, bacterial LPS TLR5, bacterial flagellin TLR7/8, viral ssDNA TLR9, bacterial DNA with unmethylated CpG	Induction of IL-1, inflammatory cytokines and costimulatory molecules
Scavenger receptors (A, B and C)	Tissue macrophages, hepatic endothelial cells, high endothelial venules	Bacterial and yeast cell walls	Clearance of LPS and microbes; adhesion
NK activatory receptors	NK cells	Self or non-self protein antigens induced on stressed, transformed or virus-infected host cells	Killing of infected, stressed or transformed host cells; production of inflammatory cytokines
γδTCRs	γδ T cells	Native proteins or unprocessed peptides derived from microbial, viral or damaged host cells	Production of cytokines activating NK cells and macrophages; induction of antimicrobial compounds; production of chemokines
NKT semi-invariant TCR	NKT cells	Glycolipids presented on CD1d	Cytokine secretion and perhaps cytolysis
Collectins (MBI, lung surfactant proteins A and D)	Plasma proteins produced by hepatocytes	Microbial cell wall polysaccharides	Binding of C1q receptor; activation of complement; promotion of phagocytosis; modulation of CD14-induced cytokine production
Acute-phase protein (C-reactive protein)	Plasma proteins produced hepatocytes	Microbial polysaccharides	Activation of complement; enhancement of phagocytosis
Natural antibodies	Secreted by CD5+ cells	Bacterial, viral and fungal components, host nucleic acids and other self-components	Enhancement of phagocytosis; clearance of pathogens; protection of fetus and neonate

LPS, lipopolysaccharide; PMN, polymorphonuclear cells, dsRNA, double-stranded RNA, ssDNA, single-stranded DNA; CpG, cytosine-phosphate-guanine dinucleotide.
From Mak and Saunders (2006).

tors occur in humans, SR-A which binds molecules on aging damaged (e.g. oxidized) cells, such as oxidized low-density lipoprotein, as well as some microorganisms, and SR-B which occurs on other cells as well as macrophages and binds many different types of microorganisms through polyanionic interactions. TLRs are for the most part cell surface receptors, although some, such as TLR3 and TLR9, bind intracellular molecules such as viral genomic messenger RNA and nucleotide degradation products such as CpG molecules. In addition, a further set of molecules deals with intracellular pathogen products, the NOD 1 and NOD 2 proteins (nucleotide-binding oligomerization domain family), which like the TLRs have a leucine-rich repeat domain. These proteins are also known as CARD (caspase recruitment domain) proteins and bind unique peptidoglycan bacterial molecules. They are also involved in

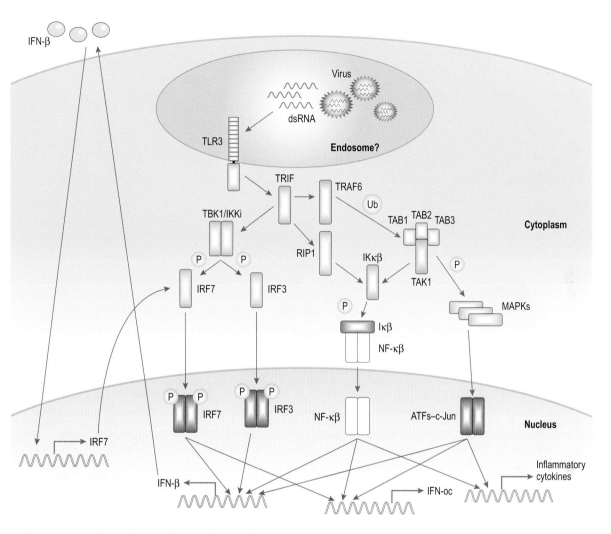

Fig. 7.4 TLR3-dependent signalling pathway. After recognizing extracellular double-stranded RNA, TLR3 transmits signals through TRIF, which interacts with TBK1, RIP1 and TRAF6. TBK1, together with IKKi, phosphorylates (P) IRF3, allowing it to translocate into the nucleus and activate type 1 interferon promoters particularly the IFN-β promoter, Secreted IFN-β stimulates expression of IRF7, which induces IFN-α, probably through a TBK1–IKKi-dependent mechanism. Both TRAF6 and RIP1 are involved in the activation of NF-κB. NF-κB is a central regulator of cell activation (see text). Abbreviations: dsRNA, double-stranded RNA; IFN-β, interferon-β; IKKi, IκB kinase; IRF3, interferon regulatory factor 3; NF-κB, nuclear factor-κB; RIP1, receptor interacting protein 1; TBK1, TANK (Traf family member associated NFκB activator) binding kinase protein 1; TLR, Toll-like receptor; TRAF6, tumour necrosis factor receptor-associated factor; TRIF, Toll/interleukin-1 receptor-domain-containing adapter inducing IFN-β. (From Kawai and Akira 2006, with permission from the Nature Publishing Group.)

autoimmunity, especially the inflammatory bowel disease Crohn's disease, which is linked to certain types of ocular inflammation.

NK, NKT and γδT cells also express PRRs and mediate innate immunity

NK cells recognize self and non-self ligands on virus-infected cells, tumour cells and host cells that have increased levels of stress proteins. MHC class I and MHC class I-like molecules (see below) are involved in these interactions. Using receptors such as Ly49H, natural cytotoxicity receptors and a further receptor termed NKG2D, NK cells recognize a range of viruses such as cytomegalovirus, myxoviruses and influenza viruses. NKG2D is a receptor for tumour proteins and the MHC class I molecules that they recognize in combination are known as MICA and MICB.

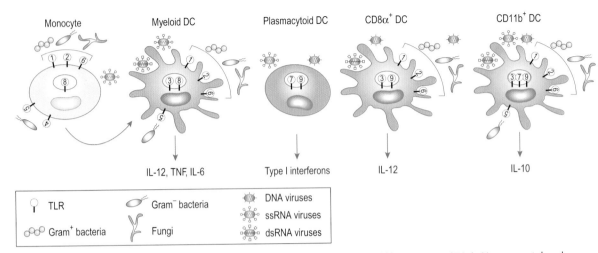

Fig. 7.5 Dendritic cell (DC) populations express non-overlapping sets of Toll-like receptors (TLRs). Human peripheral blood myeloid DCs and monocytes express distinct sets of TLRs on their cell surfaces and in the lysosomal compartment. Myeloid DCs express a variety of surface TLRs and can recognize bacterial, fungal and viral pathogens and secrete the inflammatory cytokines interleukin-12 (IL-12), tumour necrosis factor (TNF) and IL-6. Although they have a similar set of TLRs, monocytes do not express TLRs but upregulate TLRs as they mature into DCs. Both human and mouse plasmacytoid DCs express TLR7 and TLR9, respond to viruses and secrete type 1 interferons. The secondary lymphoid organs blood-derived DC precursors give rise to DCs. TLR number (e.g. TLR3) on each cell type as indicated.

NKT cells in contrast express the T-cell receptor (see p. 368) but unlike normal T cells they only express one form of the receptor and use this to bind glycolipids on a range of organisms such as *Leishmania donovani*, Gram-negative glycosyl ceramides and similar molecules on organisms such as *Plasmodium* and *Trypanosoma*. Two important ocular microorganisms, *Pseudomonas* and *Staphylococcus*, may also be detected by NKT cells. NKT cells used a non-classsical MHC class I molecule, CD1d, to mediate these interactions. The cytolytic function of NK and NKT cells occurs via the release of granule contents such as perforin, granzyme and other proteoglycans (see later under cytotoxic T cells).

γδT cells colonize the skin and gut epithelium and recognize small alkylamines and pyrophosphomonoesters on microbes and tumour cells. The latter are a major component of mycobacteria. In addition, they recognize heat-shock proteins and have been implicated in inflammatory diseases such as Behçet's disease and the ocular inflammation associated with it.

Effector cells in the inflammation response

Much of the tissue damage in the early stages of the response is caused by release of tissue-degrading enzymes from professional phagocytes (see above) and as such they are considered to be important as non-specific effector cells in the inflammatory response. Activation of complement during the early phase of the response also provides the materials for non-antibody-dependent complement-mediated lysis of tissue cells, via the membrane attack complex (MAC) of complement (see p. 388) and other cells such as NK cells. Macrophages also play a major role as effector cells in the acquired response in addition to antigen-specific cytotoxic T cells and NK cells.

Lymphocytes also play a significant part in the initial acute inflammatory response. Even in 'sterile wounds', in which defence against microorganisms does not play a major part, lymphocytes participate in the overall response. Lymphocytes enter into the site of inflammation at the same time as the monocytes, and act as bystanders ready for activation by APCs primed with antigen. This may be from degraded organisms or denatured tissue proteins ('altered self'). Usually, no recognizable immune response occurs.

RESOLUTION OF INFLAMMATION

Resolution of inflammation occurs when the foreign antigens have been completely destroyed and removed, and tissue architecture restored. Macrophages are critically important in the resolution phase of an inflammatory reaction. In addition, resolution involves new vessel formation (angiogenesis) in the early part of wound healing, restoration of epithelial surfaces by cell migration and proliferation (see Ch. 4, cornea), and remodelling of the extracellular matrix by initial deposition of sulphated glycosaminoglycans, followed by influx of fibroblasts and hyaluronate/collagen deposition. Each of these stages is precisely orchestrated to occur in the above sequence, usually regulated by cytokines and matrix components. For instance, angiogenesis is initiated in quiescent endothelial cells by the expression of protease activity on the cell surface, and release of growth factors from surrounding inflammatory cells such as fibroblast growth factor, platelet-derived growth factor, platelet-derived endothelial cell growth factor and vascular endothelial growth factor (VEGF). VEGF is a major player in the overall wound-healing response; it initiates vascular leakage at the onset of inflammation and promotes angiogenesis in the later stages. It also activates a specific endothelial cell receptor (VEGF3) for induction of lymphangiogenesis, essential for transport of antigen to the draining lymph node.

VEGF induction is itself under the control of hypoxia-inducible factor (HIF1a and b), a transcription factor generated by cells in hypoxic tissue, as in a wound, but is also produced by macrophages in the absence of hypoxia. Thus wound healing, acute inflammation, innate immunity and adaptive immunity are all part of a coordinated response by the organism to remove the offending microorganism and restore homeostasis.

In addition, certain chemokines, such as IL-8, involved in recruitment of leucocytes have angiogenic properties. Increases in matrix hyaluronate in the later stages of the response permit fibroblast invasion but inhibit neutrophil and monocyte migration, thereby assisting in resolution of the response.

CHRONIC INFLAMMATION

When the foreign antigen is not completely removed, the inflammatory response enters a chronic state characterized by mononuclear inflammatory cells such as monocytes and lymphocytes, often arranged in granulomas (see Ch. 9). Failure to remove the foreign antigen may occur because of an inadequate initial response or because the antigen is particularly difficult to destroy. Intracellular bacteria that evoke phagocytic destruction are a prominent stimulus for induction of chronic inflammation.

In chronic inflammatory disorders, the acquired immune response also participates, but it too appears to be insufficient to remove the foreign antigen. This may be because the antigen has 'fooled' the immune system by parasitizing the inflammatory cells, as in parasitic and chlamydial disease (see Ch. 8). In autoimmune disease (see p. 422), the 'altered self' antigen is continually present and induces persistent inflammation. In certain circumstances a low-grade lymphocytic activation occurs. Such lymphocytes may release cytokines, which induce fibroblast activity such as TGF-β and connective-tissue-activating peptides (CTAP-1 to CTAP-6). The connective-tissue-activating peptides are low molecular weight compounds released from leucocyte and platelet granules during inflammation and which themselves undergo partial degradation to produce other proinflammatory peptides such as neutrophil-activating peptides (1 and 2), thereby sustaining the inflammatory response. If this response is excessive, subepithelial fibrosis may occur and produce conditions such as benign mucous membrane pemphigoid, an extremely debilitating and blinding anterior segment disease. Recently, connective-tissue-activating peptides have been implicated in the fibrosis of Graves' ophthalmopathy through activation of the insulin-like growth factor receptor on orbital fibroblasts.

In chronic inflammation the distinction between innate and acquired immune responses becomes blurred and such disorders manifest as a mixture of low-grade inflammatory activity with partial attempts at healing (fibrosis).

THE SYSTEMIC RESPONSE TO ACUTE INFLAMMATION: THE ACUTE-PHASE RESPONSE

Although the acute inflammatory response is initiated at the site of tissue injury, systemic effects are produced in proportion to the level of tissue damage and virulence of the organisms (see Ch. 8). These effects are mediated primarily by cytokines acting in this situation at a distance, and are known as the acute-phase response. These cytokines include the 'alarm' cytokines, IL-1 and TNF-α, released mainly from macrophages activated by mast cell and platelet degranulation and/or directly by bacterial products such as endotoxin, peptidoglycan and degraded nucleotides through their PRRs (see above). These cytokines induce adhesion molecule expression on endothelia when they are released into the circulation and initiate further rounds of inflammatory cell accumulation and cytokine release. In addition, changes in vascular tone are caused by release of low molecular weight metabolic products including the prostaglandins PGI_2, PGE_2, PGD_2 and $PGF_{2\alpha}$ (vasodilatation), thromboxane A_2 (vasoconstriction), and leukotrienes C_4, D_4 and E_4 (smooth muscle contraction).

The effect of systemic cytokine release is to induce a fever response by the direct action of IL-1 and IL-6 on the hypothalamic temperature control system, and, second, to induce hepatocyte gene transcription for several 'acute-phase reactants' such as C-reactive protein, serum amyloid components A and P, α_1-glycoprotein, C3 and collectin (see section on complement below); mannan-binding proteins, and haptoglobin. Fibrinogen, α_2-macroglobulin and α_1-antitrypsin are also synthesized.

While many plasma proteins rise in concentration, others such as albumin and transferrin fall. Clinically, the acute-phase response manifests as an elevated erythrocytic sedimentation rate caused by more rapid settling of IL-6-mediated, fibrinogen-mediated rouleaux formation of red blood cells.

Many of the acute-phase proteins enhance existing innate defence mechanisms such as C-reactive protein, which acts as an opsonin and binds complement. Others act to inhibit the effect of inflammatory cytokines such as serum amyloid protein and IL-1.

DEVELOPMENT OF ACQUIRED IMMUNITY AND IMMUNOLOGICAL MEMORY

Normally, initiation of the acquired immune response does not take place at the site of injury or penetration by foreign organisms. Instead antigen is taken up by APCs at the site of inflammation and transported to the regional lymph nodes and/or spleen where it is presented to T and B cells. T and B cells specifically recognize the antigen and respond by proliferating. Effector T cells migrate back to the site of injury where they release mediators (cytokines) that attract cytolytic effector cells (cytotoxic T cells and activated macrophages). B cells differentiate to become antibody-producing plasma cells, some of which migrate to the bone marrow but most of which remain in the draining lymph node follicles and germinal centres, producing high levels of specific antibody, which is released into the circulation (see below).

ANTIGEN RECOGNITION IS MADE POSSIBLE BY ANTIGEN-PRESENTING CELLS

Foreign antigen is *presented* to T cells by three types of cell: macrophages, B cells and dendritic cells. However, antigen is *recognized* by specific T cells only after it has been processed and made presentable in an appropriate form to the T cell. Some antigens are recognized by T cells without processing, but they are very unusual.

There are differences in the type of antigen that each of the three cells can present. Macrophages and B cells usually recognize antigen through the immunoglobulin molecule, macrophages using their Fc receptor to bind the Fc portion of the immunoglobulin molecule (see next section on antibodies) in immune complexes while B cells take up free native antigen via their sIg molecule. Thus, macrophages and B cells can initiate an immune response only if the host has already been exposed to that antigen and has the capacity to mount a memory-type response. In contrast, dendritic cells can process and present antigen to resting, naïve T cells, i.e. cells that have not previously 'seen' the antigen. Accordingly, dendritic cells are important in the initiation of immune responses while macrophages and B cells are implicated in the perpetuation of the response while antigen persists in the tissue.

From the earliest stages of an inflammatory response, dendritic cells at the site of injury (usually derived from bone-marrow-derived circulating monocytes extravasated in the vascular leakage) start to migrate in large numbers from the subepithelial layers into afferent lymphatics to the regional lymph nodes. During this phase, they prepare the antigen by combining it with MHC class I and II molecules so that it can be presented as a complex to T cells. T cells will respond only if they possess the specific receptor (the TCR) for that antigen and if the antigen is sufficiently immunogenic. In the normal course of events it is likely that the great majority of processed antigens never get as far as initiating a perceptible T-cell response.

T CELLS RESPOND TO ANTIGEN BY CLONAL EXPANSION

If the antigen is presented to the specific T cell that recognizes it, in a suitable form and in the presence of the correct costimulatory signals, the T cell responds by clonally proliferating, i.e. it rapidly divides, producing many daughter cells, which are all exactly the same in their recognition of that antigen alone. The stimulated T cells (Th cells) migrate to the B-cell follicles in the lymph nodes (see below) and release a range of cytokines that 'help' B cells to expand, also in an antigen-specific manner. Other T cells migrate to the site of injury where they assist in mounting the antigen-specific effector response that will eliminate the foreign antigen.

T AND B CELLS PARTICIPATE IN THE EFFECTOR RESPONSE

Effector responses are those that actually mediate the immune response. Activated Th cells release cytokines that activate other cells in addition to B cells. These include:

- Cytotoxic T cells that recognize intracellular foreign antigen when it is presented on the surface of tissue cells complexed with MHC class I antigen (see below)
- Macrophages that, when activated, remove foreign antigen and perpetuate the immune response by engaging in local antigen presentation at the site of inflammation (if this goes awry, conditions such as lepromatous leprosy and sarcoidosis can develop)
- B cells that are stimulated to full differentiation as plasma cells with considerable local antibody production (see below); soluble antibody is then available to form immune complexes and participate in further local antigen presentation and antibody-mediated cytotoxic reactions via NK cells (see below).

DENDRITIC CELL APOPTOSIS

While activation of Th cells through MHC class II–peptide complexes on dendritic cells offers an explanation for how immune responses to exogenous antigens occur, initiation of immune responses to intracellular antigen is less well explained unless the organism directly infects the dendritic cell. However, intracellular organisms such as viruses infect many cell types and such cells are killed by sensitized Tc cells recognizing viral peptide on MHC class I surface antigen. An explanation for how these T cells die has now been proposed: apoptotic and dying infected cells containing virus are selectively phagocytosed by dendritic cells at the site of injury and in the draining lymph node if they have migrated

to this site and both self and viral antigens are processed for presentation on dendritic cells through MHC class I antigen. Thus Tc can be directly activated on appropriately conditioned dendritic cells without obligatory help from Th cells.

EFFECTOR MECHANISMS

As outlined in the introductory section, the innate immune system has a variety of non-specific effector cells that remove damaged tissue and dead microorganisms. The acquired immune system also has a variety of effector mechanisms, which it uses to rid the host of specific foreign antigen. These include antibodies and cells, but the acquired immune system also utilizes non-specific mechanisms that are activated by antigen-specific cells and molecules, including complement and cytokines.

ANTIBODIES

Antibodies are distributed in the endoplasmic reticulum, the Golgi apparatus and the surface of B cells, monocytes, mast cells and NK cells, and in secretory fluids. Each antibody binds uniquely to a single antigen, which usually represents a short sequence of an immunogenic molecule and is normally defined as an antigenic epitope.

All five antibody isotypes have similar basic structure

Antibodies are composed of light and heavy chains (Fig. 7.6).

Two identical heavy (H) chains linked by disulphide bridges to two identical light (L) chains, either a κ chain or a λ chain, form the basic structure of antibodies. Each chain is composed of a series of repeating homologous units, about 110 amino acids in length, comprising discrete immunoglobulin domains. Each domain is composed of two layers of β-pleated sheets with three or four strands of antiparallel polypeptides (Fig. 7.7). Many other molecules adopt a similar folded structure and are classed together in the immunoglobulin superfamily. Differences exist in the precise geometry of the molecules as shown by crystallography (Fig. 7.8), which has significance for antigen binding.

There are five immunoglobulin isotypes (see Box 7.7).

A

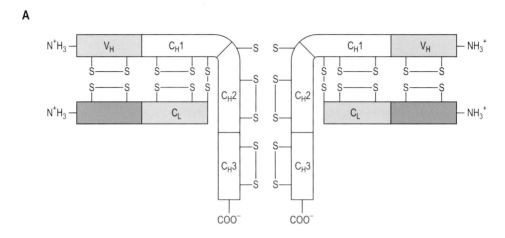

B

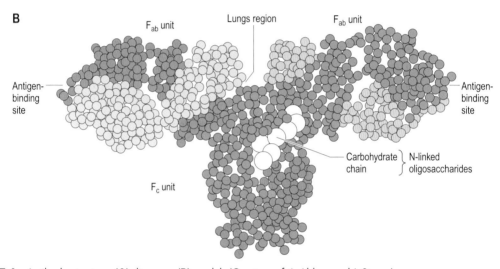

Fig. 7.6 Antibody structure: (**A**) diagram; (**B**) model. (Courtesy of A Abbas and L Stryer.)

Special features of H and L chains

Although not directly involved in antigen binding, the framework region determines the folding of the molecules and thus the amount of complementarity-determining region (CDR) that is presented on the surface of the variable sections of the molecule for interaction with antigen. There are three components or segments to the CDR (CDR-1, -2 and -3) and the third (CDR-3) in both heavy and light chains is the most variable (Fig. 7.6).

The C regions on the heavy chains are globular structures attached to the binding region by a flexible rod-like hinge portion of the molecule (see Fig. 7.6). The hinge region has both rigidity (conferred by proline residues at the top of the C_H rod) and flexibility as the result of a large number of glycine residues. The last C_H domain of immunoglobulin has a transmembrane and cytoplasmic portion, involved in intracellular signalling.

The secretory forms of IgM, IgA and IgD have C-terminal extensions (tail pieces) which allow multimer formation by attachment to the J chain. Finally N-linked oligosaccharides are bound via asparagine residues. These contribute greatly to the differences in the overall conformation. Complement binds to the CH_2 or CH_3 regions of the immunoglobulin molecules.

Limited proteolysis of antibody produces fragments: papain attacks the hinge region producing single Fab fragments which bind one antigen molecule; pepsin attacks the second C_H segment producing $(Fab)_2$ fragments which can bind two antigen molecules (see Fig. 7.6).

Box 7.7 Isotypes of immunoglobulin

Five isotypes of immunoglobulin exist, denoted by their heavy chain (α, γ, δ, ε, μ); there are two light chains (κ, λ), which occur in a ratio of 60:40 in humans. The Fc and C3 binding regions are responsible for the effector functions of antibodies (see below). Three complementarity determining regions (CDRs) are nested within framework regions, in the V and hyper-V regions of the H and L chains, and receive contributions from both chains. Somatic mutations in the CDRs are responsible for the enormous antibody diversity and affinity maturation that occurs on repeated exposure to antigen.

IgG1

IgE

J chain

IgA (dimer)

J chain

IgM

opes or neoepitopes in protein molecules, which are uncovered after changes to the three-dimensional conformation by partial hydrolysis.

Epitopes on protein antigens can be overlapping or non-overlapping. Overlapping epitopes lead to competition for binding; in such circumstances antibodies to an overlapping region might sterically inhibit presentation of a peptide to T cells. This, however, would occur only with MHC class II–peptide complexes where the binding site for the TCR embedded in the MHC groove overlaps with a binding site for antibody. This mechanism has been suggested for the inhibition of experimental uveitis with an antigen-specific monoclonal antibody. Antibodies may also compete by allosteric mechanisms in which binding of the antibody alters the conformation of the molecule so that it does not bind a second antibody.

Antibody production is initiated by binding of antigen to the B cell receptor, namely surface IgG. This induces proliferation and hypermutation of the B-cell variable region CDRs and occurs in the germinal centres of the secondary lymphoid tissue (see below). This is followed by selection and differentiation of the B cells until a single antigen-specific B-cell clone is produced. Differentiation of this clone into a plasma cell takes place either within the lymph node or after the clone has trafficked to the site of inflammation or to the bone marrow.

As indicated above, antigen specificity is determined by complementarity between the epitope on the antigen and the CDR. However, this is not exclusive and other neighbouring regions on the antigen (paratopes) and on the IgG molecule outside the hypervariable region may influence the final antigen specificity and avidity. In addition, antibodies as proteins may have other properties relating to their non-ligand (antigen) binding sites, for instance the recombination of the V_H and V_L chains may fortuitously produce a site that binds ADP or acts in a catalytic fashion. Such antibodies may therefore have additional functions that may be more closely ascribed to innate rather than adaptive immunity. Such antibodies are termed superantibodies.

Monoclonal and polyclonal antibodies

Any single antigen, especially large proteins, may have multiple antibody-binding regions (epitopes). Antibody responses may therefore be polyclonal, oligoclonal or monoclonal depending on the immunodominance of the antigenic determinants. Selection of cells from an immunized mouse under special conditions and fusion of those cells with an immortalized cell line is a powerful technique for producing large quantities of antibody to a specific antigenic epitope (see Box 7.8).

Monoclonal antibodies have revolutionized diagnostic techniques in medicine today and are now having a similar effect on the therapy of diseases such as cancer and autoimmunity.

CYTOKINES ARE THE EFFECTOR ELEMENTS RELEASED BY CELLS DURING INNATE AND ADAPTIVE IMMUNE RESPONSES

Almost all of the biological effects of T cells are mediated by cytokines. More importantly, T cells may alter the characteristics of an immune response by releasing different cocktails of cytokines. Cytokines in the broadest sense, however, are produced

Box 7.8 Monoclonal antibodies

Monoclonal antibodies are produced by the fusion of antibody-secreting B cells from an immunized animal (usually a mouse or rat) with an immortalized myeloma cell line which is defective in an enzyme, hypoxanthine-guanine phosphoribosyltransferase (HGPRT), and therefore cannot utilize hypoxanthine (HAT). When the cells are cultured in aminopterin (to block endogenous purine synthesis) and HAT, only the B cells/myeloma fusion cells survive. Thus an immortalized antibody-secreting cell is produced. Those cells secreting high levels of monoclonal-specific antibody are screened and selectively grown out.

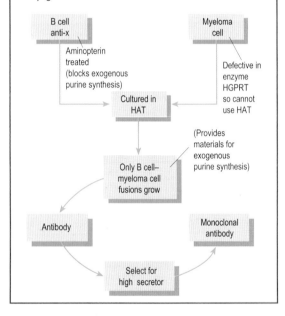

by a wide variety of leucocytes and tissue cells, particularly monocytes/macrophages and fibroblasts. The response of tissues to invasion by viruses and bacteria is to produce cytokines; for example, virus-infected cells activate NK cells, which can be induced to release cytokine by innate recognition of viral double-stranded RNA; bacterial lipid (endotoxin) is recognized by CD14 and TLR4 on monocytes and by complement, all leading to cytokine release.

What makes a cytokine a cytokine?
Cytokines have the following properties:

- They are secreted by cells in response to a specific stimulus.
- They are short-lived and short-range molecules, acting on cells within their neighbourhood.

375

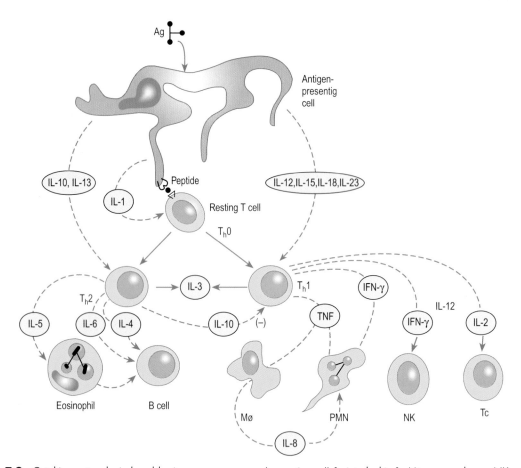

Fig. 7.9 Cytokine networks induced by immune responses. Ag, antigen; IL-1, interleukin-1; Mφ, macrophage; NK, natural killer cell; PMN, polymorphonuclear leucocyte; Tc, T cytotoxic cell; Th, T helper cell; TNF, tumour necrosis factor; • peptide. (Courtesy of A Abbas.)

- They may have effects at a distance if they are liberated into the circulation in sufficient concentration.
- They are effective at very low concentration.
- They may secondarily induce cytokine release by the target cell.
- They may act upon many different cell types (pleiotropism) and may have multiple different effects on the same target cell.
- They may be redundant, may induce cytokine synthesis themselves and may alter the effects of other cytokines.

Cytokines have three general effects.

- They regulate the innate immune response.
- They regulate the adaptive immune response.
- They regulate the growth and differentiation of haematopoietic cells.

Cytokines now include several groups of molecules such as the interleukins, growth factors, colony-stimulating factors, transforming growth factors, interferons, tumour necrosis factors, chemokines and monokines. Considerable functional overlap exists between these groups. Interleukins have now been described, each with a range of actions. IL-1 is produced by almost all nucleated cells, including ocular cells such as the RPE, and is central to the initiation of most inflammatory and immune responses. IL-1 has extensive homology to fibroblast growth factor and may also be implicated in angiogenesis. IL-2 is the major T-cell growth factor and initiates release of cytokines from the cells upon which it acts (Fig. 7.9).

Cytokines function in a vast interconnected network of agonist/antagonistic feedforward and feedback inhibitory and stimulatory loops that ensures fine control over the immune response, mostly to avoid the excessive collateral damage that would occur in an over-robust response to a pathogen.

Cytokines involved in specific immune reactions

The interleukins, interferons and tumour necrosis factors are central to the immune response, and the character of the immune response is determined by the set of cytokines released. Activation of a Th0 cell (a lymphoblast that has recently been presented with antigen) by IL-1 released from the APC drives the T cell to differentiate into a Th1 or Th2 cell. Th1 cells secrete interferon-γ (IFN-γ), in response to IL-23 secreted by macrophages or dendritic cells during the initial innate response to antigen. Th1 cells are involved in delayed-type hypersensitivity responses and tissue damage associated with granuloma formation. This is achieved by activation of macrophages and NK cells, which release reactive oxygen and nitrogen intermediates (free radicals). In addition, release of IL-2 by Th1 cells activates cytotoxic T cells. In contrast, Th2 cells release IL-4, IL-5, IL-6, IL-10 and IL-13, activate B cells and induce antibody production. IL-5 also stimulates eosinophils, which are the effector cells in allergy-associated tissue damage, while IgE avidly binds to mast cells and causes release of the mediators of immediate hypersensitivity. IL-15 and IL-18 are also Th1-type pro-inflammatory cytokines (see Fig. 7.9).

The simple outline given is considerably modified during the event. For instance, IL-1, IL-2 and IL-4 can also activate macrophages directly, while IFN-γ is involved in the production of $IgG_{2\alpha}$ (the only immunoglobulin controlled by this cytokine). It is also not clear how the immune system directs the response down a Th1 or Th2 pathway, but this may involve prior conditioning of the APC. In addition, Tho (naïve) cells may be induced to another type of Th effector cell, the Th17 cell, or to a regulatory cell type, the Treg cell, depending on the conditions (see p. 357).

Cytokines involved in lymphomyeloid cell maturation

Several cytokines are involved in the growth and maturation of lymphomyeloid cell populations from stem cell precursors. These include the colony stimulation factors, granulocyte colony-stimulating factor (G-CSF), macrophage colony-stimulating factor (M-CSF) and granulocyte–macrophage colony-stimulating factor (GM-CSF). In addition, several other cytokines with pleiotropic effects, including TNF-α and IL-1, have important roles in the maturation of these cells.

Cytokine receptors and cytokine receptor antagonists

T-cell activation is antigen specific but the cytokines released are not. However, cells targeted by cytokines require the appropriate receptor for that cytokine to respond. In addition, the targeted cells require a cell-signalling mechanism to mediate the response.

Cytokines utilize a common cell-signalling mechanism involving a cytosolic protein NF-κB, which regulates genes encoding cytokines, their receptors and several other genes involved in the acute inflammatory response. NF-κB is released from its inhibitor (IκB) when the cell is stimulated by cytokine and enters the nucleus bound to the transcription factors p65/p50. These initiate the changes in cell function (Fig. 7.10).

Five families of cytokine receptors are described based on structural motifs in the proteins: the immunoglobulin superfamily (IL-1 and c-kit); a two cystein/WSXWS receptor (type 1 receptor–binds IL-2, IL-3, IL-4, IL-5, IL-6, IL-7, IL-9, IL-11, IL-13, IL-15, GM-CSF, G-CSF); a type II receptor (binds IFNs); a TNF receptor [part of a larger family of receptors involved in apoptosis including Fas–Fas ligand (FasL) mechanisms, TRADD (TNF receptor-associated death domain), TRAF (TNF receptor-associated factor) and CD40, see p. 406]; and seven transmembrane helix family (chemokine) receptors. Some cytokines have more than one receptor and some of the structural motifs are shared between the receptors, for instance, the common γ chain of the IL-2 and IL-15 receptors (Fig. 7.11). Binding of cytokine to the receptor initiates signal transduction pathways such as the Janus family kinases (Jaks) and the signal transducer and activator of transcription (Stats) proteins which act upstream of NF-κB. Several proteins are included in the Jak–Stat families and these intracellular proteins are now targets for drug discovery programmes in attempts to control immune responses (Box 7.9).

Cytokines, when released, do not have a free rein in mediating their activities. Cytokine receptor antagonists (ra) are now being discovered, and the prototype in this field is IL-1ra. This protein is a naturally occurring competitive binding protein for the IL-1 receptor but fails to induce any of the signal transduction events of IL-1. This is important because the uncontrolled activity of IL-1 in large amounts produces severe side effects similar to the acute-phase response. IL-1ra recognizes the separate receptors for IL-1 on T and B cells. IL-1 can also bind to a 'decoy' receptor, IL-1RII, which fails to transmit the signal.

Receptors may be of low or high affinity in their ability to bind ligands and this encroaches somewhat on receptor specificity, allowing certain cytokines to compete for the same receptor. In addition, for certain multichain receptors, such as the IL-2r, one of the chains may be shared by several cytokines (the common γ chain) and so assembly of the appropriate receptor on the membrane may depend on the precise cytokine milieu presented to the cell. The local concentration of any particular cytokine will therefore have an influence on the final cell response. This cytokine redundancy is seen for instance with

GM-CSF, IL-3 and IL-5. GM-CSF and IL-3 have widespread effects, whereas IL-5 is more restricted. By competing for the same receptor on different cell types, the amount and receptor-affinity of any one cytokine can determine the nature of the cellular response.

Tumour necrosis factor

Certain cytokines have a prominent role in tissue damage, one of which is TNF. TNF exists in both soluble and membrane-bound forms and can induce a variety of responses in cells, including activation of polymorphonuclear leucocytes, induction of MHC antigens and adhesion molecule expression, and

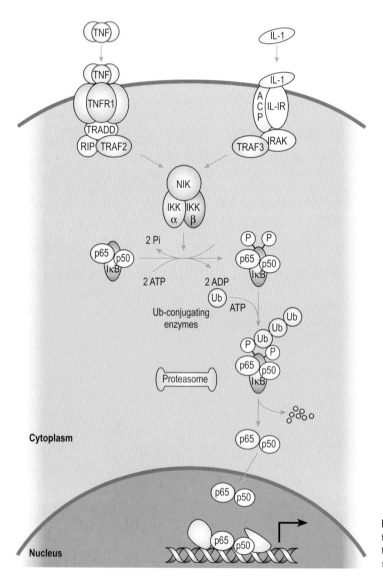

Fig. 7.10 The pro-inflammatory signal transduction pathway. p50 and p65 are the two DNA-binding subunits of the NF-κB dimer. (Adapted from Baeuerle 1998.)

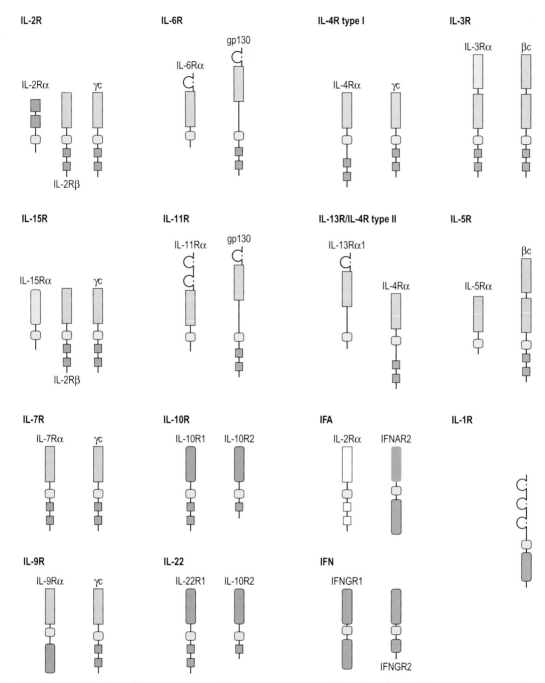

Fig. 7.11 Examples of cytokine receptor complexes. Receptors grouped together share at least one component chain. The interferon receptor (IFNR) chains are not shared. The interleukin-1 receptor (IL-1R) is composed of a single unshared chain. Domains are identified as follows: Box 1/Box 2 motif (small red boxes); Ig-like domain (incomplete loop); transmembrane domain (yellow box); WSXWS domain (red rectangle); death domain (blue rectangle). (From Mak and Saunders 2006, with permission from Elsevier.)

Box 7.9 The JAK / STAT pathway is a major signalling pathway for some cytokines

The linked kinase and kinase-like domains give the JAK molecules their two-faced (Janus)-like activated kinase name while STAT refers to 'signal transduced and activator of transcription'. Four JAKs (JAK1–JAK3 and TYKZ) and six STATs (STAT1–STAT6) are known. Trimer formation of the cytokine proteins brings the loosely associated JAKs and STATs together to crossactivate each other: for instance STAT4 is involved in IL-12 production while STAT6 is involved in IL-6 production.

Interferon-γ is a major cytokine for pro-inflammatory responses and activation of the IFN-γ receptors leads to activation of JAK1, JAK2 and on to STAT1 (see below). STAT1 moves to the nucleus and in collaboration with other transcription factors it activates gene expression. However, JAK–STAT pathways are not induced in isolation: for instance the MAP kinase pathway is activated via Pyk2 and a range of adaptor proteins (e.g. Vav, Cbl, Crk) and other molecules such as Fyn are required for this effect (see Figure).

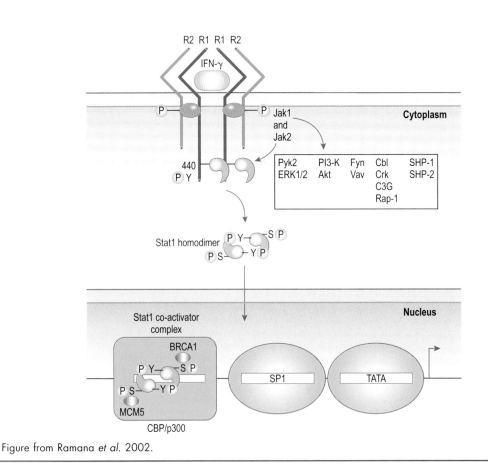

Figure from Ramana et al. 2002.

prostaglandin synthesis. Two forms of TNF exist, TNF-α and TNF-β, the latter also known as lymphotoxin; both forms bind to the same cell receptor.

TNF-α is pro-inflammatory, pro-coagulant, cytotoxic and antiviral, and modulates haematopoiesis. Its inflammatory effects act on both the acute-phase response and locally on cells at sites of inflammation. As such it is a mediator of endotoxic shock. TNF signals through two receptors (p55 and p75), which are members of a larger TNF receptor family involved in several aspects of the immune response (Box 7.10). Many are associated with cell death (apoptosis). Each receptor forms a (p55 or p75) homotrimer before ligand binding. TNF is produced as a pro-protein with a long signalling sequence. When cleaved off, the molecule trimerizes and binds to the trimeric receptor. TNF receptors can be cleaved from the cell surface and persist in the extracellular space and bloodstream, where they can act as competitive inhibitors of TNF itself.

TNF is a pro-inflammatory cytokine that experimentally can cause intraocular inflammation, similar in some respects to endotoxin-induced uveitis.

There are two TNF receptors, TNFRI (p55) and TNFRII (p75). The p55 receptor is the dominant one and is expressed on many cell types.

TRANCE

TRANCE (TNF-related activation-induced cytokine, also known as osteoprotegerin ligand, or OPGL, and receptor activator for NF-κB ligand, or RANKL) activates osteoclasts in bone for bone turnover and innate immune cells, macrophages and dendritic cells for the immune response. Deficiency of TRANCE leads to the severe bone disease osteopetrosis. It is produced by osteoblasts and bone marrow stromal cells, and also by T cells. The receptor, RANK is found on osteoclasts and endothelial cells, and mature dendritic cells and T cells.

Interleukin-1

Interleukins constitute a subclass of cytokine: their name is derived from their ability to effect communication between leucocytes. It has since been shown that many of these mediators are derived from a range of cells and have effects on many cell types

---

Box 7.10 TNF receptor superfamily

The tumour necrosis factor receptor (TNFR) superfamily (also known as the nerve growth factor receptor family) is a very important class of signal transduction molecules in the immune system. Included in this family are the TNF receptors 1 and 2 (TNFR1 and 2), the low-affinity nerve growth factor receptor (NGFR), CD40, CD30, Fas, and others indicated in the table below. Members of the TNF receptor family are generally transmembrane proteins, but many of them can also be secreted as soluble molecules, derived either by proteolytic cleavage from the membrane or by differential mRNA processing. The TNFR family is characterized by the presence of cysteine-rich motifs of 40 amino acids in the extracellular domain that are involved in ligand binding. The ligands for these receptors are type II transmembrane proteins with a 'jelly-roll' β-sandwich structure, many of which can also be secreted.

Some TNF receptor family members are associated with additional signal transduction molecules called TNFR-associated factors

(TRAFs). These proteins contain zinc-binding domains that are thought to mediate the binding of the protein to DNA, leading to transcriptional activation. Signal transduction is initiated by stimulation of oligomerized receptor complexes upon ligand binding. The ligands, such as TNF, are often found in multimeric form, and this multivalency enhances the induction of signalling. Other members of the TNFR family (most notably, the apoptosis-inducing molecule Fas) contain death domains (DDs) in their cytoplasmic tails. For example, the DD sequence allows the interaction of the membrane-bound Fas molecule with the signal-transducing protein FADD (Fas-associated death domain), which in turn delivers signals causing the cell to initiate apoptosis. More recently it has been discovered that several proteins containing the DD sequence are not involved in apoptosis at all but actually promote cell survival. In fact, depending on downstream events, engagement of TNFR1 (which contains a DD sequence) can lead either to cell death or to cell survival.

The functional consequences of ligand engagement by members of the TNF receptor superfamily are very diverse. Fas binding induces apoptosis, which is important in the maintenance of immune self-tolerance. CD27, CD30, 4-1BB, and CD40 signalling enhance the survival, proliferation, and activation of B or T lymphocytes, often playing critical roles as costimulators or signal modulators. Signalling by other TNFR family members results in the activation of NF-κB in macrophages and the induction of an inflammatory response. The TNF receptor superfamily is thus central to many aspects of both innate and acquired immunity and plays fundamental roles in both cell death and survival. A greater understanding of this receptor family, as well as its corresponding family of ligands, holds great potential for the creation of novel drugs and therapeutics that could be used to control many aspects of autoimmunity and other immunopathologies.

Continued

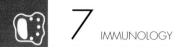

| Box 7.10 | TNF receptor superfamily—*cont'd* | | |

TNFR Superfamily members

Name (alternative name)	Ligand	Downstream signal-transducing molecules	Involved in
TNFR1 (TNFRp55, CD120a)	TNF, LTα	TRADD, FADD, TRAF1, 2	Inflammation, acute-phase response, cell survival and apoptosis, bacterial toxic shock
TNFR2 (TNFRp75, CD120b)	TNF, LTα	TRAF1,2,3	Inflammation, thymocyte proliferation
Fas (CD95, APO-1)	FasL	FADD	Apoptosis
NGFR (p75^NGFR)	NGF, BDNF, NT-3, NT-4/5	TRAF6	Neuronal growth stimulation; NF-κB activation; apoptosis; sensory neuron development and function
CD40	CD40L (CD154, gp39)	TRAF1,2,3,5,6	B cell proliferation, development, and costimulation; isotype switching; apoptosis, cytotoxic T-cell responses
CD30	CD30L (CD153)	TRAF1,2,3,5	Cell death?
DR3	TWEAK (VEGI)	TRADD, FADD	Apoptosis
DR4 (TRAILR-1, CD261)	TRAIL (CD253)	FADD	Apoptosis
DR5 (TRAILR-2, CD262)	TRAIL (CD253)	FADD	Apoptosis
OPGL-R (RANK, ODAR)	OPGL* (RANKL, TRANCE)	TRAF1, 2, 3, 5, 6	Osteoclast differentiation and/or activation; dendritic cell survival and function
4-1BB (CD137)	4-1BBL (CD137L)	TRAF1,2	T-cell costimulation
CD27	CD70 (CD27L)	TRAF2,5	T-cell development and activation
OX40 (CD134)	OX40L(CD252)	TRAF2, 3	B-cell differentiation and secondary Ig responses; adhesion of activated T cells to endothelium

*OPGL is also bound by the antagonist OPG.
LTα lymphotoxin-α; TRADD, TNF receptor-associated death domain; FasL, Fas ligand; FADD, Fas-associated death domain; NGFR, nerve growth factor receptor; NGF, nerve growth factor; BDNF, brain-derived neurotropic factor; NT, neurotropin; DR, death receptor; TWEAK, TNF-related weak inducer of apoptosis; VEGI, vascular endothelial growth inhibitor; TRAIL, TNF-related apoptosis-inducing ligand; OPGL-R, osteoprotegerin ligand receptor; RANK, receptor activator of NF-κB; ODAR, osteoclast differentiation and activation receptor; TRANCE, TNF-related activation-induced cytokine; OPG, osteoprotegerin.

including leucocytes. IL-1 is centrally involved in the inflammatory process as an activator of macrophages and endothelial cells but not of other forms of leucocyte. In particular it induces adhesion molecule expression on endothelial cells and also promotes prostaglandin synthesis by these cells. IL-1 also activates bone cells and accelerates bone turnover, and it induces marrow stromal cells to produce G-CSF and IL-3. Two forms of IL-1 exist, IL-1α and IL-1β, each with its own receptor but receptor usage is not highly restricted. Thus, IL-1α and IL-1β have broadly similar effects on cells. IL-1 is extremely potent and is counteracted by the IL-1 receptor antagonist, which plays a major role in regulating IL-1 activity (see above).

IL-1 activates cells within the eye, particularly the RPE and the retinal vascular endothelium. It has been implicated in the pathogenesis of various forms of uveitis and has been shown to be uveitogenic experimentally and to have significantly greater damaging effects than TNF-α.

IL-1α and IL-1β are produced as pro-proteins without a secretory signal sequence and must be digested by caspase-1 (IL-1β) or other proteases (IL-1α) before they are activated. IL-1 (and IL-18) signal through

Myd88 (like Toll receptors; see above) (TIR: Toll/IL-1R cytoplasmic domain of IL-1R) (Fig. 7.12).

Interleukin-2

IL-2 is the major cytokine involved in T-cell-mediated responses, both Th1 and Th2 (see below), and also induces NK cell activity, in both of which it may act in an autocrine manner. Activated T cells thus express the IL-2 receptor, which has been detected on circulating T cells and lymphocytes from intraocular samples from patients with endogenous uveitis. The receptor is shed from activated cells into the circulation and is present at raised levels in patients with active disease, including uveitis. IL-2 may also act as a 'death' factor, inducing apoptosis in the presence of other death-promoting signals such as Fas. In this respect, IL-2 may be more important as a regulator of the immune response because it promotes T-cell activation-induced cell death and is also crucial for the production of Treg cells, which are important in tolerance (see below).

The interferons

IFN-α and IFN-β are members of the type I interferons, of which there are many, while IFN-γ is the only type II interferon, a classification based on structural differences. IFN-α was the first cytokine to be identified, sequenced, cloned and introduced to clinical therapeutics. It is used in the treatment of multiple sclerosis, hepatitis C and certain forms of retinal vasculitis. It is produced by many cells in response to virus infection but the main source constitutively is a rare population of dendritic cells, the plasmacytoid dendritic cells. Large quantities of this cytokine are produced by plasmacytoid dendritic cells in response to virus infection, leading to maturation of myeloid dendritic cells with strong induction of antiviral cytolytic activity and B-cell isotype switching. IFN-β is produced mainly by fibroblasts.

Recently, two interleukins (IL-28 and IL-29) have been described which have IFN-αβ-like activity and can induce antiviral activity in the absence of IFN.

IFN-γ is released from virally infected cells and has potent antiviral activity. It is also a major pro-inflammatory cytokine and induces MHC and other antigens on cell surfaces, thus promoting acquired immunity via antigen presentation. It has been shown to induce MHC class II on cells in the retina (which does not normally have MHC class II⁺ cells); these may be tissue-specific APCs. It also induces the innate immune response by activating macrophages to produce cytokines like TNF, IL-1β, IL-12

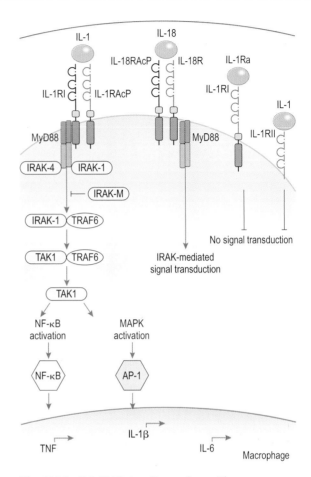

Fig. 7.12 IL-1/IRAK signalling pathway. The engagement of IL-R1 by IL-1 recruits IRAcP into the complex, followed by recruitment and dimerization of myeloid differentiation factor 88 (Myd88). The Myd88 then recruits IRAK-1 and IRAK-4 to the complex, where IRAK-4 induces the phosphorylation of IRAK-1 in an interaction that is negatively regulated by IRAK-M. In a series of events, activated IRAK-1 interacts with TRAF6, which subsequently activates TAK1. The TAK1 induces the activation of both the NF-κB and MAPK signalling pathways, leading to the activation of transcription factors including NF-κB and AP-1 and the transcription of TNF, IL-1β and IL-6 genes. The IL-1-related cytokine IL-18 signals through a similar pathway mediated by IL-18R, IL-18RAcP and Myd88 that leads to IRAK-1 activation. (From Mak and Saunders 2006, with permission from Elsevier.)

and IL-18, and also to engage in cytotoxicity through release of reactive oxygen species and nitric oxide. Like TNF-α and IL-1, IFN-γ, has potent uveitogenic activity. In addition, high levels of IFN-γ have been detected in aqueous samples from patients with acquired immune deficiency syndrome (AIDS) retinitis.

Production of interferons is under the control of interferon-regulating factors (IRFs), which bind to interferon-stimulated regulatory elements (ISRE) on the promoters of the IFN genes.

Transforming growth factor-β

TGF-β is an important immunosuppressive cytokine (see below). There are at least six types of TGF-β, and many cell types elaborate this mediator, including cells within the eye such as ciliary body epithelium and RPE. TGF-β has been suggested to account for part of the immunosuppressive activity normally found within the eye (see pp. 433–434). TGF-β2 appears to be the main isotype found within the eye and is normally secreted in a latent form; however, it is readily converted to the active form by enzymes such as plasmin, which would normally be present in an inflammatory exudate.

TGF-βs have widespread effects on cell adhesion, differentiation, proliferation, migration, maturation, activation and regulation both within and on cells outside the immune system. *In vitro* studies are greatly affected by small changes in the TGF concentrations, and thus many effects require *in vivo* investigation. TGF-βs are essential however, because deletion of the TGF-β gene in mice is lethal for the embryos. Overall, TGF-β1 and TGF-β2 are anti-inflammatory and immunoregulatory, but TGF-β1 is profibrotic. TGF-βs are produced by leucocytes and by parenchymal cells in the central nervous system, kidney and eye. TGF-β receptors comprise three chains, of which I an d II bind to form a high-affinity receptor while III binds either of the other two chains in a regulatory, non-signalling role.

Interleukin-6

IL-6 has pro-inflammatory activity but recent evidence suggests that its major role may be to limit tissue damage. It has multiple and wide-ranging effects, and participates in the acute-phase reaction as well as haematopoiesis. IL-6 is produced by many cell types, both immune and non-immune, including ocular cells such as RPE cells. IL-6 may be instrumental in promoting a Th2-type response with preferential activation of B cells. However, experimentally IL-6 appears to have a marked uveitogenic effect, similar in severity to that of endotoxin. In addition, IL-6 has been detected in the aqueous of patients with endogenous and postsurgical uveitis. Most recently, IL-6 has been shown to combine with TGFβ to promote induction of a newly discovered type of Th effector cell, Th17, which mediates active inflammation including uveitis (see pp. 433–434).

Interleukin-8

IL-8 is regarded as a chemokine for neutrophils but also has chemotactic properties for monocytes and lymphocytes (see above). IL-8 is released by immune and non-immune cells but is somewhat more restricted than IL-6. RPE cells, corneal endothelium and stromal cells will release IL-8 after appropriate stimulation. IL-8 is less uveitogenic than IL-1, which appears to be the main cytokine in this respect. IL-8 binds to the chemokine receptors CXCR1 and CXCR2.

Interleukin-10

IL-10 is an 18-kDa cytokine produced by many cells. It is predominantly an 'immunosuppressive' cytokine and is involved for instance in immunological privilege of the eye and other organs. The effects of IL-10 can override those of many pro-inflammatory cytokines. It does this by inhibiting synthesis or secretion of TNF-α, IL-1, chemokines and IL-12 by macrophages. It also reduces MHC class II expression on APCs, thus downregulating specific and innate immune responses. Certain viruses such as Epstein–Barr virus release an alternative form of IL-10, raising the possibility of virus-induced immune suppression. The heterodimer IL-10 receptor is expressed mainly on haematopoietic cells.

Interleukins 12, 23 and 27

IL-12 rose to prominence as the major mediator of Th1 responses during the time that IL-2 was recognized as having a regulatory as well as a T-cell-activating role. IL-12 is produced by APCs, particularly mature dendritic cells and activated macrophages, and is strongly pro-inflammatory both for Th1 cells and NK cells. IL-12 synergizes with IL-18 to induce IFN-γ production by activated T cells and NK cells. IL-12 is a heterodimer with p35 and p40 chains. It shares the p40 chain with IL-23, in which the p40 chain combines with a separate p19 chain to form the IL-23 heterodimer. There is some evidence that IL-23 is the pro-inflammatory cytokine and that the p35 chain of IL-12 may have some regulatory activity. IL-27 has a p35-like and a p40-like chain and its main function is to induce the IL-12Rβ chain on Th1 cells and is required only for the initiation of the Th1 response not for its maintenance. IL-12, IL-18, IL-23 and IL-27 induce the primary and memory adaptive T-cell response in a coordinated series of reciprocal interactions between the dendritic cells and T cells.

Interleukins 15 and 21

NK cells are absolutely dependent on IL-15. Both IL-15 and IL-12 synergize to activate NK cells. IL-15

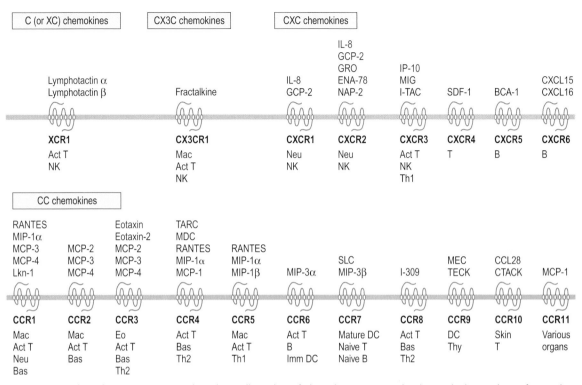

C (or XC) chemokines	CX3C chemokines	CXC chemokines

				IL-8				
				GCP-2				
				GRO	IP-10			
			IL-8	ENA-78	MIG			CXCL15
Lymphotactin α		Fractalkine	GCP-2	NAP-2	I-TAC	SDF-1	BCA-1	CXCL16
Lymphotactin β								

XCR1	CX3CR1	CXCR1	CXCR2	CXCR3	CXCR4	CXCR5	CXCR6
Act T	Mac	Neu	Neu	Act T	T	B	B
NK	Act T	NK	NK	NK			
	NK			Th1			

CC chemokines

RANTES		Eotaxin	TARC							
MIP-1α		Eotaxin-2	MDC							
MCP-3	MCP-2	MCP-2	RANTES	RANTES				MEC	CCL28	
MCP-4	MCP-3	MCP-3	MIP-1α	MIP-1α		SLC		TECK	CTACK	
Lkn-1	MCP-4	MCP-4	MCP-1	MIP-1β	MIP-3α	MIP-3β	I-309			MCP-1

CCR1	CCR2	CCR3	CCR4	CCR5	CCR6	CCR7	CCR8	CCR9	CCR10	CCR11
Mac	Mac	Eo	Act T	Mac	Act T	Mature DC	Act T	DC	Skin	Various
Act T	Act T	Act T	Bas	Act T	B	Naive T	Bas	Thy	T	organs
Neu	Bas	Bas	Th2	Th1	Imm DC	Naive B	Th2			
Bas		Th2								

Fig. 7.13 Chemokine receptors. A relatively small number of chemokine receptors bind to multiple members of a much larger collection of chemokines (blue shading). Cells expressing the chemokine receptor in question are indicated below the name of the receptor (grey shading). Adapted from Hancock *et al.* (2002). (From Mak and Saunders 2006, with permission from Elsevier.)

also activates γδ T cells. IL-15 has similar functions to IL-2 on T cells. However, there are striking differences from IL-2; for instance, IL-15 is not produced by T cells but by bone marrow stromal cells. The IL-15 receptor has a unique α chain but uses the IL-2R β and γδ chains. IL-21 also activates NK cells and induces T-cell activation but unlike IL-2 and IL-15 it inhibits B-cell proliferation.

Interleukin-18

IL-18 has similar functions to IL-1 and IL-12 and induces production of IFN-γ and TNF-α in macrophages. Interestingly IL-18-deficient mice show marked susceptibility to bacterial infections but have no impairment of response to challenge with ocular antigens.

Interleukins 19, 20, 22 and 24

These have similar functions to IL-10, i.e. they are immunosuppressive cytokines.

Chemokines and chemokine receptors

Cells involved in the inflammatory response are targeted by cytokines that induce their migration to the site of inflammation. Such cytokines are termed chemokines and include interleukins and other cytokines with additional functions. Chemokines are small peptides (usually 8–15 kDa) and are classified in two main subsets based on a particular amino acid sequence involving two cysteine residues: –C–C– chemokines and –C–X–C– chemokines in which the latter contains an intervening non-cysteine residue (see Fig. 7.13). Some chemokines do not belong to either category, having either only one C residue or having additional intervening amino acids, but they are unusual.

Regulation of inflammatory cell traffic to sites of inflammation is determined by the set of chemokines released in the tissues and the expression of specific receptors on different cell types. There is considerable redundancy in the system but it has been suggested that, depending on the cytokine milieu in which T-cell activation occurs, particularly IL-27, chemokines and chemokine receptor expression determines whether a particular immune response will adopt a predominantly Th1 or Th2 response (see Fig. 7.14). This is in part achieved at

A

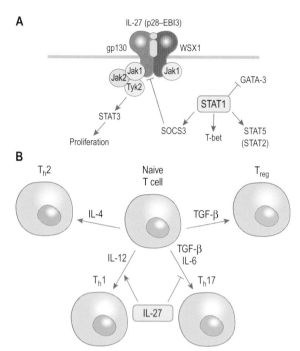

Fig. 7.14 Regulation of CD4⁺ T-cell differentiation by IL-27. (**A**) Components of IL-27 and its receptor. Engagement of the IL-27 receptor recruits JAK kinases. Substrates for the JAK proteins include STAT transcription factors, which enter the nucleus and modulate target gene expression after being phosphorylated. Tyk2, tyrosine kinase 2. (**B**) CD4⁺ T-cell differentiation, emphasizing the involvement of IL-27 and other IL-12 family members (IL-12 and IL-23). TGF-β, transforming growth factor-β; T$_{reg}$, regulatory T cells. (From Colgan and Rothman 2006, with permission from the Nature Publishing Group.)

the level of the endothelial cell before the emigration of the cell into the tissue (see p. 362). Of even greater importance is the evidence that chemokines appear to regulate T-cell, B-cell and dendritic cell interactions in the secondary lymphoid organs, particularly with regard to lymphocyte recirculation and homing (TARC and SLC).

COMPLEMENT

The term 'complement' was coined to describe an activity in sera required for antibody-mediated lysis of bacteria but that was lost after heating to 56°C. Antibody itself was heat-stable and retained the ability to agglutinate the bacteria but could not kill them. This additional activity therefore 'complemented' antibody-mediated cytotoxicity.

What is complement and what does it do?

Complement is a property of serum derived from sequential zymogen activation of a series of plasma proteins (a zymogen is an enzyme that is activated by a second enzyme, which itself has been activated by proteolytic cleavage, i.e. an enzyme cascade as occurs in kinin formation, coagulation and visual transduction).

Two enzyme cascades exist, one initiated by antibody combining with antigen, the classical pathway, and a second initiated directly by bacterial surface components, the alternative pathway (see Box 7.11). Thus, even at this level, a distinction between innate and acquired immunity exists. The classical complement pathway is in fact the major effector mechanism for humoral immunity (see above).

A third mechanism for complement activation has been described. This involves members of a family of molecules called lectins (lectins are non-antibody, non-enzyme carbohydrate-binding proteins, as in the selectin adhesion molecules; see above). Lectins that contain collagen-like domains are known as collectins; these molecules are of considerable importance in innate immune mechanisms against microorganisms. Collectins bind to the same receptor as the C1q component of complement (see below) and are thus able to activate the classical pathway.

A major lectin in this pathway is mannan-binding lectin (MBL), which is linked to serine proteases MASP-1 and MASP-2. These enzymes are responsible for cleaving C4 and C2 respectively.

Complement has the following effects:
- It is involved in the initiation of the acute inflammatory response by release of certain peptides that act as chemotactic factors and induce vasodilatation with increased permeability (anaphylatoxin).
- It mediates antibody-dependent cytolysis by polymerizing on cell surfaces to form pores in the cell membrane.
- It solubilizes and removes immune complexes from the circulation.
- It induces phagocytosis by acting as an opsonin.

Complement proteins in the normal circulation are inactive and are maintained in this state by an elaborate system of inhibitors that not only inhibit activation of the various enzyme systems but also limit the response once activated.

The central axis of the complement pathway is the conversion of C3, activated by C3 convertases, to C5 convertase by the binding of C3b (see Box 7.11). This leads to the sequential addition of a series of complement proteins that result in the membrane attack complex (MAC). Complement proteins are synthesized in the liver and in mononuclear phagocytes.

The classical complement cascade

Activation of C1 is induced by binding to IgM or IgG, but only if the immunoglobulin has bound antigen. Free immunoglobulin does not activate complement. Binding occurs to the C_H3 domain of IgM or the C_H2 domain of IgG, and requires at least two immunoglobulin molecules. Thus a single molecule of IgM, which is a pentamer, is able to 'fix' complement, while several molecules of IgG, usually aggregated together, are required to achieve the same. IgM is therefore known as complement-fixing antibody.

C1 can be activated by antibody-independent mechanisms including contact with retroviruses, mycoplasma, or even polyelectrolytes such as DNA and heparin. These presumably act in a non-specific manner by virtue of their charge. Importantly, the acute-phase proteins, C-reactive protein and serum amyloid protein, can also bind complement non-specifically.

C1 is composed of three molecules, C1q, C1r and C1s. C1q is a collagen-like molecule with a triple-helix conformation, while C1r and C1s are serine proteases. The molecular complex comprises a tetramer of C1s and C1r with six or more C1q molecules (Fig. 7.15).

Box 7.11 Innate immunity: new insights in complement and collectins

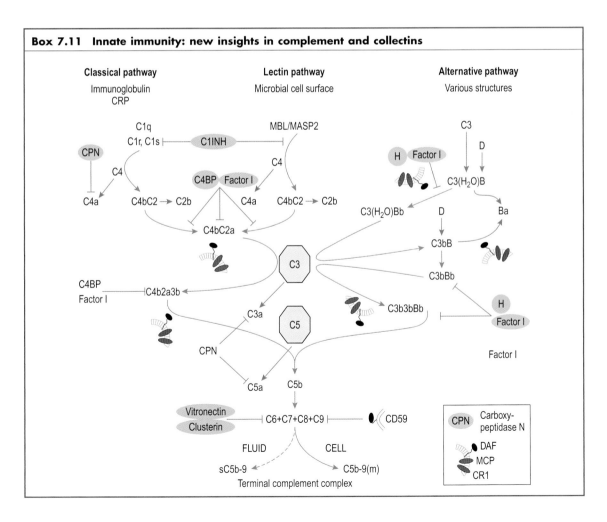

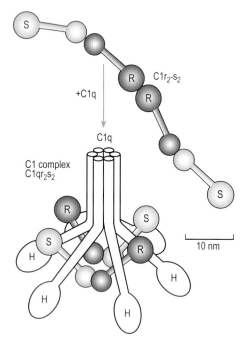

Fig. 7.15 Diagrammatic representation of the generation of the C1 complex comprising a tetramer of C1s and C1r with six molecules of C1q. (Courtesy of A Abbas.)

When two or more globular heads of C1q bind IgM, C1r is cleaved to C1r⁻, which then cleaves C1s to C1s⁻; this activates C4 to C2 to undergo partial proteolysis and bind to form C4b2a⁻. C4b is unstable because it contains an internal thioester bond and is rapidly inactivated by binding a water molecule to form iC4b. If, however, C4b is formed in close contact with a cell membrane it can covalently bind to the surface and remain in an active state. In contrast, C2 is a single-chain molecule that binds to surface-bound C4a in the presence of Mg^{2+} ions. C2b, produced by C1s⁻-induced partial proteolysis of C2, diffuses away while the C2a binds to C4b.

The complex of C4b2a⁻ contains the C3 convertase activity. The C4b component binds to the C3 molecule and brings the C2a moiety into close contact with C3, which it cleaves to C3a and C3b. C3 is a 195-kDa αβ heterodimer with an internal thioester bond similar to C4.

When partially cleaved this molecule is also unstable and is rapidly inactivated to iC3b. However, if in contact with a cell membrane it binds covalently in conjunction with C4b2a to form C4b2a3b⁻, i.e. C5 convertase (see below).

C3a, C4a and C5a are small cationic peptides also known as anaphylatoxins that bind to specific receptors on basophils and mast cells. C3 cleavage products also have a role in antibody production by interacting with follicular dendritic cells in the germinal centre (see later).

The alternative pathway
The alternative pathway is triggered by low levels of C3b, which are spontaneously produced *in vivo* by proteolysis and by $C3(H_2O)$, which is also formed by spontaneous hydrolysis of C3. On normal cells C3b is rapidly deactivated to iC3b by innate regulatory mechanisms (see below), but on foreign surfaces C3b can remain active. C3b binds to factor B on the surface of the cells and is converted by factor D, a serine protease, to C3bBb. This contains the C3 convertase activity and requires a further protein, properdin, to protect it from proteolysis.

Deposition of C3b on foreign surfaces such as bacteria leads to further production of C3b, i.e. a positive feedback amplification loop occurs, which helps to eradicate foreign particles rapidly. C3bBb is combined to form C3bBb3b, which represents the alternative form of C5 convertase (see Box 7.11).

Collectin activation of complement
Collectins include several well-characterized proteins, such as conglutinin and MBL, which directly bind to the C1q receptor on cell surfaces and initiate such phenomena as C4-mediated red cell lysis. MBL directly activates the $C1r_2C1s_2$ tetramer in the absence of C1q. This may be mediated in association with a serine protease (MBP-associated serine protease, or MASP; see above). Collectins also have direct opsonin activity (see below, macular degeneration).

Cytolysis and the membrane attack complex
The membrane attack complex (MAC) is formed by a set of complement proteins inserting themselves into the lipid bilayer and is possible because certain proteins within the complex have a lipophilic core. C5 binds loosely to C5 convertase on the cell membrane, and is split into C5a, which diffuses away, and C5b, which complexes with C6 and then C7. C5b,6,7 is highly lipophilic and burrows into the cell membrane. There it acts as a receptor for C8, an αβγ trimer whose γ chain is lipophilic and also inserts into the bilayer. The C5b,6,7,8 complex is weakly cytolytic but becomes considerably more so when it binds C9, a serum protein that polymerizes to form

the MAC with 12–15 C9 molecules per C5–9 complex. This forms a 'pore' in the cell membrane, similar to the perforin pore of cytotoxic T cells and NK cells (see below). The pore renders the cell permeable to small ions but not to proteins, and is therefore thought to cause cell death by osmosis. It is also possible that the large influx of Ca^{2+} ions poisons the cell.

The effects of the MAC on the cell are dose dependent. Sublethal doses of MAC may 'activate' the cell and induce a protective response against further attack and even cell proliferation. Genes activated in this manner are known as RGCs (response genes to complement) and several have been described.

Regulation of complement activation

Complement activation is an extremely powerful cytolytic mechanism that can be rapidly activated as a first line of defence against invasion by foreign organisms. It is also extremely effective in memory B-cell responses and antibody-dependent cytotoxicity. It can also swiftly remove potentially toxic immune complexes from the circulation. However, it is potentially extremely hazardous if randomly and uncontrollably activated, and there are therefore several inhibitory mechanisms in place to regulate this system (see Box 7.12).

Activation of complement can be induced by many cell types via receptors that exist on their cell surfaces (see Boxes 7.11 and 7.12). Furthermore, some of the biological effects of complement are produced by the cleavage products of complement activation. For instance, C3a and C5a are potent chemoattractants and anaphylatoxins, and mediate early-phase responses in acute inflammation (see p. 358). Anaphylatoxins act directly via C3a and 5a receptors on granulocytes, macrophages and mast cells to induce degranulation and the release of vasoactive mediators (see Box 7.13).

Complement activation is usually incomplete: implications for age-related macular degeneration

As shown in Box 7.11, the multistep complement activation cascade requires the correct conditions for activation of each step and because of instability in many of the molecular intermediates it frequently fails to proceed to formation of the full membrane attack complex (MAC), particularly if activated via the collectins. In addition, the process can be blocked by a range of inhibitors at many stages. What happens to these intermediates? Recently, it has been suggested that while such molecules may not

---

Box 7.12 Regulation of complement activation

Complement proteins comprise around 15% of total serum proteins. Most serum protein is derived from the liver but complement in tissues may derive from epithelial cells and resident macrophages.

Inhibitory activities exist for both fluid-phase activated complement and for surface-bound complement. Regulation also occurs at all stages of activation. Complement component 1 inhibitor (C1INH) is the only known inhibitor of C1r and C1s, and is present in the blood at high concentration. It is classed as a serine protease inhibitor (a serpin), similar to proteins like α_1-antitrypsin and α_1-antiplasmin. C1 circulates in the bloodstream bound to C1INH and is released when it binds an antigen–immunoglobulin complex. Serum also contains C4bp (C4 binding protein) in large amounts.

Factor H inhibits by binding C3b, competing with factor B and Bb. It therefore acts on both the fluid and surface-bound phases. Factor I cleaves C3b, rendering it inactive (iC3b).

Cell-bound inhibitors are a second line of defence should any C bypass the fluid-phase components. Most normal cells possess membrane cofactor protein (MCP, CD46) and type 1 complement receptor (CR1), both of which rapidly degrade active C3b. Cell surface sialic acid also preferentially binds factor H to factor B, conferring anticomplementary activity on materials such as mucin. These mechanisms are important, especially on surfaces such as the tear film. Tears contain measurable levels of complement proteins; these are important in maintaining an organism-free ocular surface. However, C activation on the ocular surface could have significant damaging effects, which are reduced by mucin-bound factor H. Decay-accelerating factor (DAF) is a further cell-bound protein which minimizes the effects of C.

Universal cell surface proteins such as homologous restriction factor (which binds C8), vitronectin or S protein (which binds C5b,6,7), and CD59 (binds C8 and C9) are important in minimizing bystander damage during immune-mediated tissue damage. Glycation of CD59 in diabetes may lead to loss of function and allow endothelial cell damage (see also Box 7.11).

---

cause lysis of the target cell, they may coat the cell and promote apoptosis; this is then followed by the silent (i.e. non-inflammatory) removal of the cell debris by scavenger macrophages. Such a mechanism may be occurring at some level of activity during the normal 'house-keeping' actions of the resident macrophages. Indeed it is likely to take place at sites where there is minimal cell turnover but where removal of cell debris is important, e.g. at

Box 7.13 Complement receptors and immune complexes

Receptors (CRs) for several complement proteins are present on many cell types.

- *CR1* – has a short consensus repeat structure like several of the complement proteins themselves; regulates C activity by binding C3 convertase; acts as the opsonin receptor for phagocytosis of immunoglobulin-coated cells and clearance of immune complexes.
- *CR2* – present on follicular dendritic cells in lymphoid tissue (see below); may act like an 'antigen trap' in this situation for presenting immune complexes to B cells.
- *CR3* – acts as a marker for certain cell types (such as macrophages); it is an integrin receptor and binds iC3b, where it may act as an opsonin, e.g. on iC3b-coated organisms.

the retinal pigment epithelium. Such a fine homeostatic mechanism may be susceptible to dysfunction: indeed, mutations in the complement inhibitory protein, Complement Factor H have been associated with a higher than normal risk of age-related macular degeneration. Factor H provides a check on the complement cascade at two critical points, C3 and C5 induction by their immediate precursors.

CELLULAR MECHANISMS OF TISSUE DAMAGE

Tissue damage in cell-mediated immune reactions may be induced by a variety of cell types including macrophages, cytotoxic T cells and NK cells. In addition, macrophages are involved in the clearance of cell debris in acute inflammatory reactions and in antibody-dependent cytotoxicity.

The delayed-type hypersensitivity reaction is the hallmark of cell-mediated immunity

The delayed-type hypersensitivity reaction is a Th1-mediated reaction to foreign and/or autoantigen and is characterized by the presence of granuloma in the tissues. These accumulations of cells contain a central core of macrophages around a vessel with T cells in the surrounding area. Fibrinoid necrotic material may be present in the centre with giant cells (fused macrophages) and epithelioid cells. Such lesions are typical of reactions to mycobacteria and also occur in less well-defined diseases such as sarcoidosis. Similar microgranulomas are typical of sympathetic ophthalmia (Fig. 7.2) and indeed of

several chronic posterior uveitis syndromes. Such granulomas contain many types of T, B and macrophage-like cells, and also have a high content of dendritic cells. It is possible that these cell collections represent small extralymphatic lymphoid follicles where extensive antigen presentation is in progress. Once the antigen has been removed, the granuloma subsides.

Macrophages are a heterogeneous group of cells

Macrophages cause tissue damage by release of reactive intermediate metabolic products and tissue proteases (see pp. 359–360). However, not all macrophages behave in this manner. In the resting state tissues contain resident macrophages (see Fig. 7.16) that, in certain tissues, may have an immunosuppressive role (such as alveolar macrophages in the lung). In central nervous system tissue, including the retina, specialized resident tissue macrophages occur (microglia) (see Ch. 1). These cells may be induced to express MHC class II antigen during inflammation and become involved in regulating the immune response.

Further differentiation of macrophages may occur during an inflammatory response with the differential expression of adhesion molecules, inducing antigen presentation properties in one type of macrophage and phagocytic activities in another. Differential release of cytokines such as IL-3 and IL-5 by macrophages during parasitic infection may induce a predominantly eosinophilic response. Macrophages are derived from precursors in the bone marrow that circulate as monocytes. Monocytes on activation are induced to enter the tissues and under the influence of cytokines may differentiate into myeloid dendritic cells, whose function is antigen presentation, and phagocytic macrophages, which have a role in tissue damage and clearance of debris.

Do cytotoxic T and NK cells induce cellular damage by making holes in the cell membrane?

Killing by cytotoxic T cells is a multistep process. Initial recognition and binding of a target cell (e.g. an infected or mutated cell) is followed by damage to the cell membrane. This lethal insult induces apoptosis with DNA fragmentation and lysis of the cell. The cytotoxic cell then disengages to attack another target cell.

Membrane damage takes the form of pore formation similar to that induced by the complement

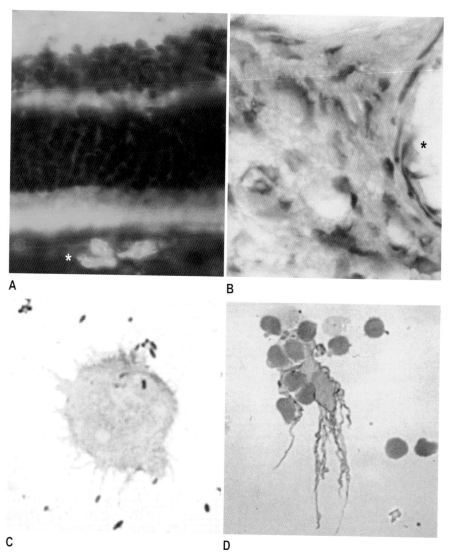

Fig. 7.16 Immunohistochemistry of choroidal dendritic cells in sections from normal rat eyes and in cytospin preparations after culture *in vitro*. (**A**) Immunofluorescence of section of rat eye stained for MHC class II (OX6); note MHC class II-positive cell in the choroid (*). Photoreceptors and bipolar cells also show autofluorescence caused by retinal chromophores. (**B**) Immunoperoxidase-stained sections of choroids showing brown-stained MHC class II (OX6) -positive dendritic cells surrounding a vein (* marks the lumen). (**C**) Slide preparation of cultured human dendritic cell showing moderate positivity for B7 antigen; the rod-like structures also present in the figure are photoreceptor fragments. (**D**) Slide preparation of large veiled MHC class II-positive (immunoperoxidase) rat dendritic cell clustered with T cells in co-culture. (From Forrester *et al.* 2005, with permission from the BMJ Publishing Group.)

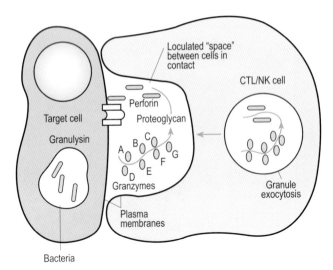

Fig. 7.17 Perforin killing.

membrane attack complex (MAC; see above). In this case, however, it is induced by perforin, a protein released from lysosomes of antigen-activated Tc cells that polymerizes in the cell membrane to form a leaky pore (Fig. 7.17). Perforin is released in association with a granule proteoglycan and serine proteases (granzymes), which are also likely to be involved in the lytic process. However, cell death is not automatically caused by osmotic lysis. Instead prelytic DNA breakup occurs as a result of activation of the apoptosis genes. Therefore there are important differences between MAC-mediated cell lysis and Tc/NK killing.

Alternative mechanisms have also been shown for T-cell cytotoxicity. CD8[+] T cells may recognize non-peptide (e.g. lipid) antigen in the context of CD1. Thus cells containing bacteria are directly recognized by CD8[+] T cells and the bacterial lipid induces the release of a novel enzyme, granulysin, which directly kills the intracellular bacteria.

ORGANIZATION OF THE IMMUNE SYSTEM

The immune system is designed to provide cells that can circulate freely through the tissues and organs of the body in such a way that they are readily available to mount a defence against foreign organisms at short notice. Immune cells are thus highly motile, normally quiescent cells travelling to and from the lymphoid organs; they can be readily activated if required.

Centralized antigen recognition mechanisms provide the most efficient means of rapid response because all the necessary requirements for cell activation can be concentrated at one site. This takes place in the lymphoid organs. Some cells carry afferent information concerning possible breaches in the body's defences to the central lymphoid tissues (particularly dendritic cells and other APCs), while effector cells (T and B cells) remove the invading organism and restore tissue homeostasis. Trafficking of cells to and from the tissues to the lymphoid organs requires specific receptors on the circulating leucocytes and the vascular endothelium in each tissue.

Secondary outposts of local antigen presentation can be set up in sites where normal lymphoid tissues do not exist (such as the brain and eye) or where persistent antigen generates a chronic inflammatory response. Granulomas, the hallmark of chronic inflammation in the tissues, are probably the morphological representation of such antigen presentation 'factories' because they have many similarities to lymphoid follicles and other areas within lymph nodes and spleen. The Dalen–Fuchs nodule in posterior uveitis is a classic granulomatous lesion (see Ch. 9).

FUNCTIONAL ANATOMY OF LYMPHOID ORGANS

During development the main sources of lymphomyeloid cells are the bone marrow and thymus. Ultimately all cells derive from stem cells in the bone marrow. Stem cells are poorly characterized and their existence is based mainly on evidence for cell differentiation, often from *in vitro* cell culture studies. Haematopoietic stem cells have few lineage markers (i.e. they are lin⁻) that give rise to common myeloid progenitors and common lymphoid progenitors. These can be induced to give rise to T and B cells (IL-7) or macrophage/dendritic cells (GM-CSF, M-CSF). B cells mature in the peripheral lymphoid tissues, particularly Peyer's patches, lymphoid tissue in the wall of the small intestine. T-cell precursors colonize the thymus where they undergo selection and lineage differentiation before being distributed to the peripheral lymphoid organs.

Bone marrow stem cells produce all blood cells

Blood cells – including red cells and platelets, granulocytes, monocytes and dendritic cells – are produced in the bone marrow and released directly into the circulation. B cells are also released directly into the circulation and circulate between the lymphoid organs and blood.

The marrow is a loose spongy stromal network whose cells, together with local macrophages, release growth factors (cytokines; see above) that initiate differentiation of each cell type. IL-3, GM-CSF and M-CSF are particularly important. IL-1 and IL-6, released by stromal marrow cells, also participate in T-cell maturation, while IL-7 promotes B-cell development.

The thymus regulates T-cell development and maturation

T-cell precursors enter the thymic cortex (Fig. 7.18). Here they interact with thymic epithelium ('nurse' cells), which encapsulate them in large numbers. At this stage they are still immature cells expressing cell surface markers for Th and Tc cells (CD3⁺, CD4⁺ and CD8⁺: the so-called double-positive cell; see Box 7.4 for explanation of CD numbers). After some time they are released from the nurse cells and migrate through the cortex to the medulla, making contact with macrophages and dendritic cells as they go. Many T cells die during this process (clonal deletion and/or apoptosis) but selected cells differentiate to express one or other T-cell phenotypic marker (CD4 or CD8). Maturation in the medulla also involves contact with the medullary epithelium and thymic dendritic cells, which express high levels of MHC class II antigen. The T cells then enter the blood vessels and migrate to the lymph nodes and spleen.

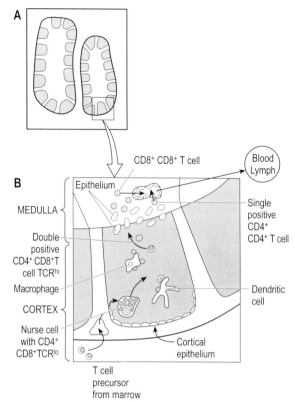

Fig. 7.18 Functional anatomy of the thymus. The bilobed thymus (**A**) is divided into lobules composed of an outer cortex and inner medulla (**B**). T-cell precursors enter the cortex and leave as committed mature T cells via the medulla into the blood or lymph. (Courtesy of A Abbas.)

The medulla of the thymus contains several characteristic whorled bodies (Hassall's corpuscles), which are probably remnants of discarded nurse epithelial cells. In the adult, the thymus involutes but some T-cell maturation continues into adult life, both in the thymic remnant and extrathymically.

Lymph nodes are designed for antigen trapping

Lymphocytes and APCs from the tissues enter the cortex of the lymph node via the afferent lymphatics (Fig. 7.19) where they present antigen to T and B cells (see below). Follicular dendritic cells in germinal centres of the lymph nodes and the spleen present antigen–antibody complexes to B cells in the B-cell areas, while interdigitating dendritic cells present antigenic peptides to T cells in the T-cell area. The eye (and the brain) connect directly with cervical lymph nodes (see Ch. 1 and Ch. 4), but

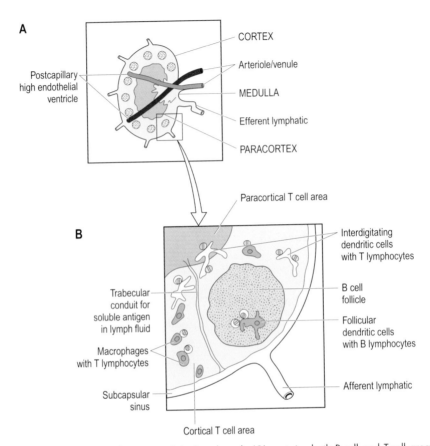

Fig. 7.19 Lymph node architecture. The cortex of the lymph node (**A**) contains both B-cell and T-cell areas, while the paracortex is exclusively a T-cell area. Follicular dendritic cells present antigen to B cells (**B**), while interdigitating dendritic cells present to T cells. B cells traffick through T-cell areas, during which T–B interactions occur (T-cell 'help' for B cells and B-cell antigen presentation to T cells).

lymphocytes and APCs from these tissues also find their way to the spleen through the aqueous veins.

Antigen is carried in soluble form to the lymph node in blind-ended vascular lymphatics from the tissues and in cell-associated form inside APCs (dendritic cells and macrophages). APCs migrating from the tissues to the lymph nodes do not leave the node. However, T and B cells circulate between the lymphatics and the bloodstream. Both resting and activated lymphocytes (lymphoblasts) migrate from the cortex to the medulla and enter the efferent lymphatics on their way to repopulate the tissues.

The spleen receives antigen from all sources (lymphatics and blood)
The spleen is a central lymphoid organ at the interface between the blood and lymphatic circulations.

The bloodstream communicates with the lymphatic system at the thoracic duct where recirculating lymphocytes enter. The spleen receives antigen-primed APCs from all regions including those that may have bypassed their regional lymph node and those derived from tissues that do not have a well-developed lymphatic system, i.e. the eye and brain. For instance, APCs that encounter antigen within the anterior chamber pass through the trabecular meshwork and aqueous veins (see Ch. 2) to enter the conjunctival veins and eventually drain into the lungs and spleen. However, the spleen does not receive lymphocytes from the tissue in lymphatics.

The spleen is organized like a lymph node with the addition of the red pulp (red cell area) and its venous sinuses (Fig. 7.20). T-cell and B-cell areas are separated, with the T-cell areas (white pulp) being par-

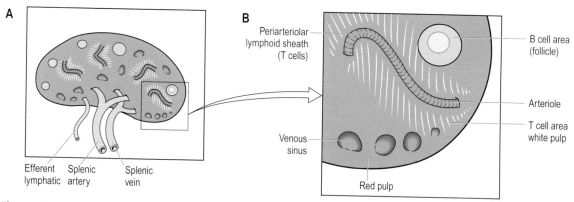

Fig. 7.20 The spleen receives its cells via the bloodstream (**A**); T cells accumulate in the periarteriolar region of the white pulp (**B**), while B cells are arranged in follicles. Activation of a B-cell follicle leads to the appearance of a germinal centre.

ticularly large and aggregated around an arteriole (periarteriolar lymphoid sheath, or PALS) and surrounded by well-defined macrophage/dendritic cell zones (marginal zone).

THE MUCOSAL IMMUNE SYSTEM

Initial contact of the host with exogenous antigen takes place at surfaces such as skin and mucous membranes. The skin provides an effective physical barrier to microorganismal contact unless penetration is achieved, as with insect vectors and trauma. However, the mucous membranes are more easily breached by microorganisms and, not surprisingly, considerable lymphoid tissue is concentrated at these surfaces to deal with new antigens as they arrive. This is termed the mucosa-associated lymphoid tissue (MALT) and is specialized to some degree for each tissue, e.g. bronchus-associated lymphoid tissue (BALT) and conjunctiva-associated lymphoid tissue (CALT). In essence it comprises intraepithelial lymphocytes and APCs (especially dendritic cells) and aggregations of lymphoid follicles in the mucosal layers. These are best exemplified by the Peyer's patches of the gastrointestinal mucosa and the tonsils in he oropharynx. Regional specialization occurs in various compartments of the mucosal immune system with specific homing receptors ('addressins', adhesion molecules) directing movement of cells to different mucosal sites (see below).

As indicated below, MALT is specially adapted for antigen capture and presentation to specific lymphocytes that 'home' to that tissue. In addition, exposure of the host to antigen via the MALT frequently leads to tolerance to that antigen by mechanisms that are as yet poorly understood (see section on tolerance below).

THE IMMUNE SYSTEM AS A POLICE FORCE

The immune system can be regarded as a surveillance system constantly checking for intruders. Cells of the innate immune system, such as neutrophils and monocytes, undertake part of this function but at a relatively non-specific level. The acquired immune system has cells that mediate this function in a much more targeted way. The afferent limb of the immune system uses dendritic cells in this role, while the messengers sent out to do the 'dirty work' are the T and B lymphocytes.

Dendritic cells are the major surveillance cells of the afferent lymphoid system

Dendritic cells are derived from stem cell precursors in the bone marrow and proliferate/differentiate under the influence of cytokines such as GM-CSF, stem cell factor (Flt3 ligand) and TNF-α. They leave the bone marrow and circulate as veiled cells in the bloodstream before entering the tissues, where they remain for a few days to weeks. In the skin, conjunctiva and cornea they can be identified as Langerhans' cells, and they interact closely with tissue cells such as keratinocytes and epithelial cells. In the uveal tract, there is a rich network of dendritic cells in association with tissue macrophages (see Fig. 7.17), 395 which are also ultimately derived from the bone marrow but are longer lived.

Dendritic cells migrate in the afferent lymph to the lymph nodes and spleen in response to appropriate stimulation (e.g. TNF-α); they interact with T cells in the T-cell areas of these tissues (interdigitating dendritic cells). Other specialized dendritic cells, which possess Fc receptors and serve as antigen traps because they have the ability to bind immune complexes, occupy the follicles in lymphoid tissue where they present antigen to B cells (follicular dendritic cells). Dendritic cells do not leave the lymphoid tissue; they are short-lived cells with a half-life of a few days and their numbers are replenished from the bone marrow.

Trafficking of cells to and from the lymphoid system depends on specific cell surface adhesion molecules

In contrast to dendritic cells, T and B cells recirculate through the lymphoid organs many times. They do this by binding to specific regions of the lymphoid vasculature, the high endothelial venules (HEVs) (see Fig. 7.2), which are specialized for lymphocyte capture by the expression of specific adhesion molecules on their surface. About 25% of the lymphocytes passing through a lymph node will leave the bloodstream and any given naïve lymphocyte can traverse each lymph node at least once a day. However, in practice, lymphocyte recirculation follows some patterns: B cells rarely recirculate, γδ T cells tend to exist in skin, and most other T lymphocytes recirculate preferentially through their lymph node of origin. HEV-like changes may also be induced in non-lymphoid endothelium at sites of inflammation (e.g. in retinal vessels during the active phase of retinal vasculitis; see Ch. 9, p. 478) and presumably represent sites for preferential adhesion and migration of inflammatory cells. Receptors for specific adhesion molecules are reciprocally expressed on activated lymphocytes (and indeed on all classes of inflammatory cells during acute inflammation; see above), which assist in directing them to sites of tissue injury.

Specific adhesion molecules are expressed on HEV in lymph nodes, where they are involved in physiological lymphocyte recirculation. These molecules are therefore sometimes referred to as 'addressins' (one address only). For each addressin there is a corresponding lymphocyte 'homing receptor'. Circulation through typical lymph nodes is mediated by L selectin on lymphocytes, which binds to GlyCAM-1 on the HEV. In Peyer's patch lymph nodes, HEVs express MAdCAM and VCAM-1 (see Table 7.3), which are the ligands for $\alpha_4\beta_7$ and $\alpha_4\beta_1$ integrins of lymphocytic microvilli. It is likely that each tissue has specific addressins that direct the circulation of surveillance lymphocytes through that tissue; in particular, most mucosal lymphoid tissue (MALT, CALT; see above) has addressins that ensure adequate trafficking of lymphocytes through that tissue during health and disease.

Some cytokines facilitate the interaction of T cells with activated endothelium, such as macrophage inflammatory protein-1β, which has been shown, for instance, to be particularly effective in mediating CD8+ T-cell adhesion to the endothelium (see section on cytokines above). In addition, certain adhesion molecules are involved not only in endothelial cell interactions but also in mediating the close cell–cell contact required during antigen presentation (see below), particularly ICAM-1/LFA-1, ICAM-1/LFA-3, CD44 and its ligand cell surface hyaluronate plus several others (see Table 7.3). In addition, chemokines and their receptors are intimately involved in the recirculation and trafficking of T and B lymphocytes and of APCs. In general, however, it is now clear that adhesion of leucocytes, either to each other or to the endothelium, during normal recirculation or as part of inflammation, is a complex molecular and tissue-specific process.

What turns a lymphocyte on?

Most circulating lymphocytes are resting. Some are 'naïve' cells, which have recently been released from the thymus, or in the adult from peripheral tissues, and have not yet been exposed to antigen. Others are memory T and B cells that can be very long lived. The main stimulus that activates T cells is antigen presented in the form of peptide by professional APCs in the lymphoid tissue. Activation of the T cell induces it to release cytokines, particularly IL-2, which initiates the process of clonal expansion. Depending on the local conditions and the cocktail or 'panel' of cytokines produced by the T cells and by stromal cells in the lymph nodes, further functional diversification is achieved by driving T-cell clonal expansion usually towards one of two T-cell subsets, Th1 or Th2. In addition, there may be expansion of T regulatory cells (Tregs) to try to regulate the response or if IL-bβ is present as well as TGFβ, there may be induction of Th17 cells (see Fig. 7.14).

Th1 cells, expanded by IL-2 and IFN-γ, induce a delayed-type hypersensitivity response (type IV hypersensitivity in the classic nomenclature; see

Table 7.5 Immunopathology of tissue reactions

Hypersensitivity response type	Immune effector process in tissue	Type of mechanism
I	Allergic reaction	Humoral (IgE)
II	Cytotoxicity	Humoral (IgG/M)*
III	Complement	Humoral (Ag/Ig)
IV	Macrophages	Cellular (T cells)†

*Cytotoxicity in this process is antibody dependent.
†Type IV hypersensitivity is the classically described delayed hypersensitivity response, mediated by macrophages and memory T cells.

Table 7.5), which involves considerable macrophage activation, granuloma formation and tissue damage. It should be noted, however, that memory T cells do not release IFN-γ, while release of the chemokine RANTES by tissue cells appears to be important in the recruitment of memory T cells and macrophages to the site of granuloma formation. IL-12, IL-23 and IL-27 produced by macrophages and dendritic cells also play a major role in directing Th1/Th17 T-cell responses.

In contrast, Th2 cells, expanded by IL-2 and IL-4, provide B-cell 'help' and lead to the production of antibodies. In addition, IL-4 inhibits Th1 cell activation and the delayed-type hypersensitivity reaction. IL-10 and IL-13 produced locally in tissues and lymph nodes may condition APCs to induce a Th2 response.

Th1 and Th2 cells and their particular type of cytokines are therefore involved in determining the nature of the pathological event. Classically four types are described (types I, II, III and IV hypersensitivity; see Table 7.5) but mixed responses also occur. Th1 and Th2 cells may initiate reciprocal downregulation of the response via regulated cytokine release or anti-idiotypic mechanisms (see section on tolerance below). Chemokines and chemokine receptor expression have a major part to play in determining whether a Th1 or a Th2 response is induced (see p. 376).

Where are memory cells found?

T effector cells that exit the lymph node lose their expression of L selectin and cannot therefore recirculate through the lymph node. Most of them home to the site of inflammation to promote removal of the antigen and then die *in situ*; a small number of

these cells have the potential to survive as memory cells which can re-enter the lymph–blood circuit and repeatedly home to the peripheral tissue where they first encountered antigen. In contrast, memory B cells do not recirculate but continue to produce antibody of different isotype and with increasing affinity for the antigen and release it into the blood via the efferent lymphatics. Memory cells for the mucosal lymphoid tissues have been shown to express a specific addressin, LPAM-1 (lymphocyte Peyer's patch adhesion molecule-1), or $\alpha_4\beta_7$ integrin which binds to MAdCAM-1 in the GALT (see above). IL-7, an essential cytokine for ontogeny of T cells in mice, is also required for induction of memory cells.

What turns a lymphocyte off?

Most immune reactions do not persist, and it has been presumed that this is the result of effective removal of antigen. Indeed, the corollary is also probably true: that most chronic immunological diseases are the result of persistence of antigen in the tissues in a form that activates lymphocytes, i.e. on the surface of APCs.

T regulatory cells

It can be seen therefore that lymphocytes that are not exposed to antigen in the appropriate form (i.e. on the surface of APCs and in the presence of costimulatory support mechanisms) enter a state of anergy and eventually die out. The process of cell death or apoptosis during lymphocyte ontogeny is well established and is associated with the expression of specific 'suicide' or 'death' genes in the cell (see Box 4.4, p. 395).

As indicated above, however, there may also be specific antigen-driven mechanisms that lead to 'switching off' the immune response, and involving special types of T cells, T regulatory cells (see below under immunotolerance).

The number of T-cell subsets now recognized has increased since the initial discovery of Th1 and Th2 cells in the early 1990s. For instance, the recent recognition of Th17 cells (T cells which preferentially secrete IL-17), which are Th1-like cells with pathogenic properties in mice, has revealed an increasing complexity to the problem of immune-mediated damage (Fig. 7.14). Whether or not a naïve T-cell differentiates into a Th1 cell or a Th17 cell depends greatly on the cytokine milieu in which it finds itself and particularly so with regard to IL-27 (Fig. 7.14).

In addition, a subset of T cells that might have suppressive properties was long considered but generally denied until Sakaguchi in Japan identified a set of CD4 T cells (see Fig. 7.14) that expressed high levels of the IL-2 receptor (CD25) and were also identified by utilizing the transcription factor FoxP3. These cells have been shown to occur endogenously and also to be inducible for instance by tolerizing antigen-loaded dendritic cells. They are generated in the thymus and certain aspects of their function are antigen specific but they are generally non-specific in their effects.

They are present in mice and humans and currently there is considerable interest in developing methods to induce them to high levels so as to prevent a range of autoimmune diseases.

$CD4^+$ $CD25^+$ T regulatory cells are only one set of 'suppressive' T cells exist; there are also cells that produce high levels of IL-10 (Tr1 cells), cells that produce TGF-β (Th3) cells and even some CD8 T regulatory cells, which may be involved in aspects of ocular immune privilege and require NK T cells to mediate their activity.

ANTIGEN RECOGNITION

The immune system recognizes antigen through molecular interaction with specific molecules, three of which are antibody (B-cell receptor, sIg), the TCR, and the MHC molecule. MHC molecules are highly polymorphic, i.e. although basically similar there are many different types (alleles) that occur in each individual. Each TCR, antibody and MHC molecule has varying degrees of ligand-binding specificity, the MHC molecule being required to bind to a large variety of antigens, while antibody is specific for only one antigen. The interactions between antigen and antibody, and antigen and the TCR, have, however, many similarities.

The great majority of immune responses are T-cell-dependent in that the final effector response, including B-cell responses, is achieved through an initial interaction between a resting T cell and an APC (see Fig. 7.10).

THE APC MAKES THE ANTIGEN RECOGNIZABLE

The function of the APC is to capture antigen and to process it into a form that can be recognized by the T cell. The immature (veiled) dendritic cell with its numerous cell surface receptors is ideally designed for this (Fig. 7.21). This it does by partially digesting the antigen into short peptides and com-

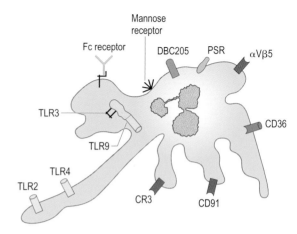

Fig. 7.21 Diagram of immature dendritic cell showing some cell surface receptors for innate immune responses. DBC205 (CD205); PSR, phosphatidylserine receptor; $\alpha_V\beta_5$ integrin; TLR, Toll-like receptor.

plexing the peptide with MHC molecules. Intracellular antigens are complexed with MHC class I molecules for presentation to cytotoxic ($CD8^+$) T cells, while extracellular antigens are complexed with MHC class II molecules for presentation to helper ($CD4^+$) T cells. Each APC can present hundreds of thousands of MHC–peptide complexes on its surface. In addition, some non-protein lipid antigens, such as those in mycobacterial cell walls, can be presented atypically on MHC class I-like molecules, the CD1 receptor. Most of the antigens expressed on an APC surface are self antigens, which promote tolerance (see later). Immunogenic peptides occur at a level of 10–100 copies per cell.

Processing by APCs is under tight cellular control

Intracellular antigens that are likely to be processed and bound to MHC class I mostly comprise host cytoplasmic and nuclear proteins which do not normally induce immunogenic responses, but also include translation products of intracellular 'foreign' antigen such as viruses in infected cells. Proteins are degraded in an ATP-dependent structure (the proteasome; see Box 7.14) and are bound to the MHC class I molecule in the endoplasmic reticulum. The proteasome is a constituent of all cells and accepts ubiquinated peptides and proteins for degradation (see Ch. 3, Box 3.11, p. 160) as part of normal housekeeping duties. The immunoproteasome is specialized in APC to degrade antigens into a set of overlapping peptides. For this purpose it contains two MHC-related proteins, LMP-1 and LMP-2. The

Box 7.14 Processing of antigen for presentation of peptides

Transport of peptide into the endoplasmic reticulum is under the control of two transporter genes, *TAP1* and *TAP2* (TAP = transporter of antigenic peptide) (**A**). MHC class I molecules are also continually cycled through the endoplasmic reticulum but are unstable until they bind peptide. Binding of the peptide to the MHC molecule renders the complex much less susceptible to proteolysis. Binding of the peptide is also guided by calnexin, a chaperonin present in the endoplasmic reticulum, which starts folding the MHC molecule into a shape that can receive the peptide. Calnexin binds to the MHC molecule until a 'good fit' is obtained with an appropriate peptide, at which point it detaches from the complex. MHC–peptide complexes are then rapidly transported to the plasma membrane where they are oriented in such a way that the peptide is exposed to the extracellular compartment for interaction with specific T cells.

Extracellular antigens are processed in a different system, the endosomal compartment. This they do by, first, being taken up into coated pits from which they are transferred to phagosomes to undergo partial proteolysis and then to late endosomes. At this stage they are complexed with MHC class II molecules, which have also been transported to the late endosome from their site of synthesis in the endoplasmic reticulum (**B**). During this process the MHC class II dimer sheds a protein chain, known as the invariant chain, with which it is associated in the endoplasmic reticulum to prevent proteolysis of the MHC molecule. Peptide–MHC class II molecules are then transported to the plasma membrane in the same way as the peptide–class I molecules.

Antigen processing: (**A**) processing of intracellular antigen via MHC class I antigens involves proteasome and TAP genes; (**B**) processing of extracellular antigen via the endosome route involves invariant chain loss.

(Figure courtesy of N Jeffjes.)

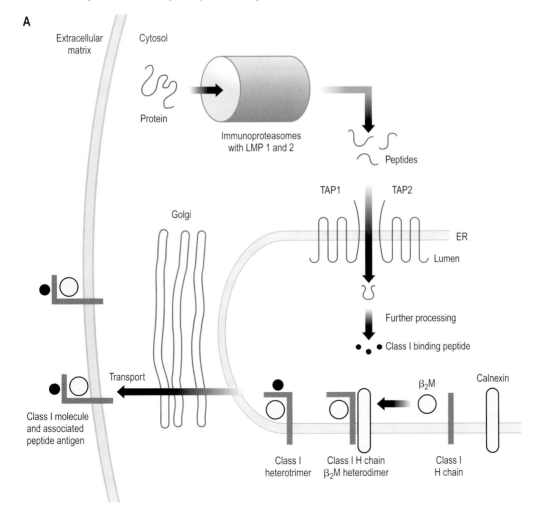

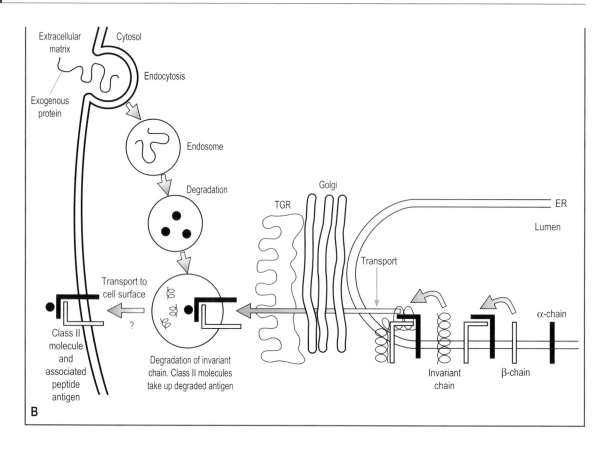

B

peptide is bound specifically to a groove formed by the α_1 and α_2 helical domains of the MHC class I molecule, and is anchored at specific sites to the β-pleated sheets that form the floor of the groove (Fig. 7.22).

Defects in antigen processing can be associated with disease, for instance uveitis in certain patients with the joint disease ankylosing spondylitis and severe rheumatoid arthritis is linked to abnormality in the genes coding for the proteasome and in *LMP-2* genes involved in MHC class I processing. This illustrates how each step in the antigen-processing pathway is essential in ensuring correct presentation of 'normal' non-immunogenic host peptides rather than peptides that may induce inflammatory disease. This also applies to the other genes that regulate the transport of peptides during their intracellular pathway, such as *TAP1* and *TAP2* (see Box 7.14). Loading of peptides via TAP on to the MHC class I molecule is regulated by a further membrane protein, tapasin, while loading of peptide on to the MHC class II molecule is 'chaperoned' by the invariant chains (see Box 7.14).

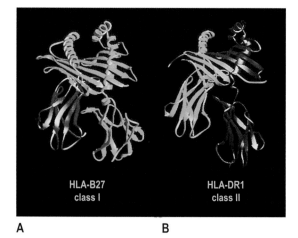

A   **B**

Fig. 7.22 Structure of the MHC molecule. MHC class I is composed of a single-chain molecule with three immunoglobulin domains, combined to β₂-microglobulin (**A**, structure of HLA-B27 molecule). MHC class II is an αβ dimer with close conformational similarity to the MHC class I β₂-microglobulin dimer molecule (**B**, structure of HLA-DR molecule). (Courtesy of Macmillan Magazines.)

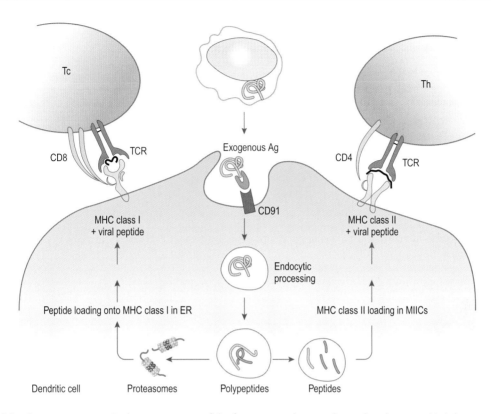

Fig. 7.23 Crosspresentation. In the upper centre of the figure an endogenously produced antigen (Ag) that eventually ends up in cellular debris has been captured by a scavenger receptor (CD91) on a dendritic cell. The antigen is internalized into the endocytic system and polypeptide fragments are produced. Some of these fragments remain in the exogenous processing pathway (right) and are degraded to peptides that are loaded on to MHC class II in MIICs. These peptides are presented to CD4+ T cells. However, some of the polypeptide fragments are released from the endosomes into the cytosol (left), where they are taken up by proteasomes and enter the endogenous processing pathway. These peptides are loaded on to MHC class I in the endoplasmic reticulum (ER) and are crosspresented to CD8+ T cells. (From Mak and Saunders 2006, with permission from Elsevier.)

Although the processing and presentation of intracellular and extracellular antigens have many similarities in detail, there are some fundamental differences. For instance, the term APC refers to cells that express high levels of MHC class II antigen and 'professionally' process extracellular antigen. The term is thus restricted to a few cell types such as macrophages, B cells and dendritic cells. In contrast, the presentation of intracellular antigen to CD8+ T cells on MHC class I has until recently been more difficult to explain. Most cells of the body express low levels of MHC class I and this can be upregulated in cells exposed to cytokines such as IL-1 and IFN-γ. However, effective antigen presentation requires costimulatory molecules, which are not normally present on parenchymal cells. When antigen is presented in the absence of these molecules, the effect is to tolerize the T cell to the antigen.

This is fine for self-antigens but defeats the purpose when intracellular foreign antigen has to be dealt with. Recently the phenomenon of crosspresentation has been shown. In this process dendritic cells phagocytose dead or dying infected tissue cells and the viral or bacterial antigens are then processed within the dendritic cells for presentation on dendritic cell MHC class I antigen in the presence of costimulation. Receptors involved in uptake of dead and dying cells (apoptotic cells) include $\alpha_v\beta_5$ integrin, CD91 and CD36 (scavenger receptors), CR3 (if coated with complement) and phosphatidyl serine (see Box 4.4, p. 395). Crosspresentation involves degradation of polypeptides in the proteasome (Fig. 7.23) and may be a major route for activation of CD8 T cells, as well as activation of CD4 T cells on MHC class II antigens. In this way CD8+ cytotoxic T cells can be directly activated without requiring T-cell help and are therefore armed to induce killing in other infected tissue cells. Thus dendritic cells deal with both extracellular and intracellular foreign antigen while the response to self antigen is minimized.

Making the antigen presentable: the MHC molecule as gift wrapper

Presentation of the peptide by the MHC molecule to the TCR requires binding of the peptide to the groove in the MHC molecule and has some degree of specificity. Thus, only certain peptides will bind to each MHC allotype, of which there are many (see below). The specificity of the interaction between the MHC molecule and the peptide, however, is orders of magnitude less than that for the TCR, which is in turn considerably less specific than antigen–antibody binding. Preferential binding of certain peptides to different MHC molecules, however, is well established both for peptide length and sequence.

The size of the peptide is much more restrictive for MHC class I than for MHC class II. Class I molecules will only bind peptides that are nine or 10 amino acids long, while class II molecules will bind those of any size, but usually between 16mer and 30mer. Class I peptides are anchored to a deep pocket in the groove at the second residue. The C-terminal end of the peptide is also bound to a shallower pocket, normally at the ninth residue. This leaves the peptide essentially free in the middle, apart from some less strong side-pocket binding; as a result the peptide is usually arched in the middle with its amino acid residues projecting outwards to the TCR (Fig. 7.24). It is these exposed residues that determine the specificity of the reaction with the TCR.

In contrast peptides in the class II groove overlie the sides of the molecule. Binding to the class II molecule, however, is restricted to the same number of residues as for class I (i.e. nine or ten) except that they occupy the central portion of the peptide. Anchoring at the second peptide is the strongest, frequently mediated by the non-polar residue proline. A further difference is that anchoring of the peptide to the class II molecule occurs at positions 2, 4, 6 and 9, with greater side-pocket interaction. This has the effect of straightening the peptide to take up a twisted, linear conformation (Fig. 7.24).

These differences in class I and II peptide binding can be accounted for by specific amino acid sequences. In addition, the affinity of a peptide for

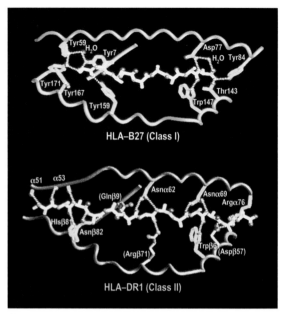

A

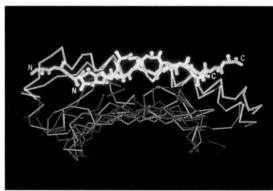

B

Fig. 7.24 Structure of the MHC molecule with bound peptide. Peptides combine in the respective grooves in the molecules (**A**, as viewed from above; **B**, as viewed from the side with peptides in the class II molecule fitting less neatly than in the class I groove and 'hanging' over the end of the groove).

a particular MHC allele is dependent on this sequence and is determined by how well each peptide fits into the pocket in the groove. Clearly, peptides composed of amino acids with large or highly charged side chains will have different requirements for binding than those with smaller amino acids, which might fit easily into the pocket.

Other differences occur in binding of the TCR to MHC class I and II molecules. For instance, crystallization studies have shown that only a single MHC class I complex is required to present peptide to the CD8+ T cell but that two or more class II–peptide complexes combine with two or more TCRs to activate CD4+ T cells. Binding of peptide to the TCR has many resemblances to antigen–antibody binding, although the immunochemistry is not so well established (see section on T-cell activation, p. 414). On the other hand, some believe that repeated sequential binding of antigenic peptide–MHC to the TCR is required before signalling can take place; recent two-photon movie images of the T-cell–dendritic cell interactions *in vivo* in the draining lymph node support this theory.

Other considerations are also important. For instance, immunodominance within a set of peptides is a well-established phenomenon. For any given antigen, only one in 2000 peptides is likely to have sufficient binding affinity to initiate an immune response and it is unclear what represents optimal affinity of the peptide for the receptor: both too little and too much can prevent T-cell activation. In addition, an essential feature of the TCR is a high level of crossreactivity for many different peptides: thus specificity is much less rigorous for the T cell than the B cell. These many factors, i.e. immunodominance of peptides, TCR degeneracy with regard to specificity and the probable need for repeated TCR activation and for crosslinking more than one TCR before cell signalling can occur, all play a part in determining whether an immune response takes place and indeed what type of T-cell priming occurs.

TCRs may occur as αβ dimers or γδ dimers

All T cells have receptors for peptide–MHC complexes. However, a subset of T cells that populates mucosal epithelium has been identified in which the TCRs have similar but distinct structures (γδ T cells; see p. 356 and Fig. 7.30). The function and role of γδ T cells is not clear but they appear to be an evolutionarily primitive type with a tropism for epithelium; they appear to be involved in innate immune responses.

Recent studies have suggested that γδ T cells may not require MHC molecules to recognize antigen but that they can respond to unprocessed peptide. γδ T cells expand 2–10% in response to alkylamines derived from microbes and edible plants and may represent a link between innate and acquired immunity.

γδ T cells are also implicated in autoimmunity; they appear to recognize heat-shock proteins (proteins expressed in 'stressed cells' and highly conserved across species), which have been suggested to play a role in autoimmune diseases such as rheumatoid arthritis and uveitis associated with Behçet's disease. High levels of γδ T cells have also been cultured from the vitreous in a case of sympathetic ophthalmia. As part of the immune response to tumours, γδ T cells have been associated with better survival from choroidal malignant melanoma.

Superantigens

Some diseases induced by organisms are so rapid in their onset and catastrophic in their manifestations that it is difficult to explain their pathogenesis in terms of an adequate innate or acquired immune response. Examples include the endotoxic shock syndrome, meningococcal meningitis and leptospirosis. These disorders are caused by superantigens derived from bacteria (staphylococci, streptococci, mycobacteria and *Clostridia* release superantigens), viruses (e.g. rabies virus) and retroviruses (e.g. mouse mammary tumour virus and human immunodeficiency virus).

Staphylococcal enterotoxins (SE) are a good example of superantigens and are the commonest cause of food poisoning. There are five SEs, SEA–SEE. They have to bind to the MHC class II antigen to be presented to the T cell but they can bind many polymorphic MHC class II molecules. Superantigens do not require processing by APCs because they activate the T cell by binding to the side of the TCR β chain. They are, therefore, quite promiscuous in that they can polyclonally activate several species of T cell. In superantigen infection it is customary to find approximately 10% of the T cells activated, whereas in immune responses to regular antigens very few antigen-specific T cells can be detected either in the circulation or even in the lesion.

Polyclonal activation in superantigen infection may involve autoreactive T cells and thereby initiate an autoimmune disease, which may persist even if recovery from the infection occurs (see below). Studies of preferential Vβ TCR gene usage by lymphocytes infiltrating the tissues may shed light on the nature of the autoantigens in conditions such as uveitis and rheumatoid arthritis and help to identify sequence similarities between autoantigens and superantigens.

Antigens can be presented by other MHC and MHC-like molecules

Antigens presented through the canonical MHC class I and II routes are exclusively small peptides. However, it is well known that other molecules such

A

CD1	Lipid antigen		Source
Cd1b	Ganglioside GM1	Gal—GalNAc—Gal—Gcl (NAN), β, (18–24)	Self
	Glucose monomycolates	Gcl—O, OH, (13–20)	Mycobacteria
Cd1c	Hexosyl-1-phosphoisoprenoids	Hex—O–P–O, (30–32)	Mycobacteria
Cd1d	α galactosyl ceramide	Gal—O, α, N, OH, OH, (2–26), (11–18)	Marine sponge

B

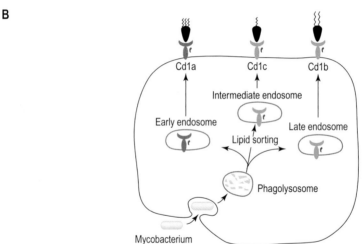

Fig. 7.25 Lipid antigen presentation by CD1 molecules. (**A**) Structures of lipid antigens presented by CD1 molecules. The precise structure of the CD1a antigen is unknown. (**B**) Sorting of mycobacterial lipids. At the bottom left of the figure a mycobacterium has been phagocytosed and degraded. The mycobacterial lipids are sorted by structure into different endosomal compartments where they are loaded on to different CD1 molecules for presentation to T cells. (From Mak and Saunders 2006, with permission from Elsevier.)

as sugars and lipids can evoke T-cell and antibody responses. MHC class Ib molecules include human leucocyte antigen (HLA) -E, -F, -G and in the mouse molecules such as Qa-1. Although these molecules have some diversity, the range of peptides they can present is restricted, e.g. Qa-1 presents only a small set of microbial peptides, while HLA-G is involved in maternofetal antigen presentation.

The MHC-like molecule CD1, which does not contain an α_2-microglobulin protein, has a highly hydrophobic groove with two deep pockets that neatly binds the fatty acid chains of glycolipid antigens while the sugar moieties bind the TCR (Fig. 7.25). CD1d binds NK T cells via αGal-ceramide while CD1c binds γδ T cells via an unknown antigen.

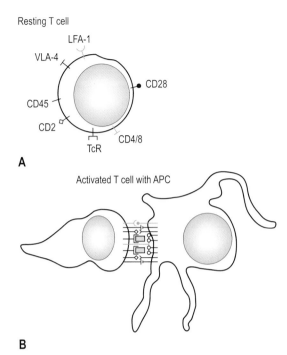

Fig. 7.26 (**A**) Random distribution and low expression of surface molecules on resting T cells; (**B**) clustering of accessory and adhesion molecules on APC and activated T cell during antigen presentation (see Table 7.6).

COSTIMULATION: PRESENTATION OF ANTIGEN REQUIRES 'HELP' FROM OTHER MOLECULES

Although much is known concerning the mechanism of antigen stimulation of T cells at a quantitative level, many questions remain. For instance, it seems inconceivable that a single peptide, even when correctly presented, would be sufficient to activate a T cell. Indeed much more than this is required, not only with regard to the number of TCRs that have to be engaged to activate a T cell but also the range of additional molecules that are bound. Both cell-specific accessory molecules and non-specific adhesion molecules are involved.

Accessory molecules

Activation of the T cell is achieved by the clustering of several cell–cell ligands between it and the APC. Clustering of these ligands at the point of contact between the cells helps to strengthen and prolong the contact between the cells and thus facilitate the presentation of peptide to the TCR (Fig. 7.26). Mobilization of the various sets of molecules to the site of TCR–pMHC interaction occurs with localized membranous patches (lipid rafts, see Ch. 4, p. 175)

and the various ligand receptor pairs participate in the formation of the immunological synapse (see below; T-cell activation). Molecules involved in the formation of the synapse are more directly involved in signalling while the accessory molecules (Table 7.6) provide costimulation.

Two important ligand receptor pairs during CD4$^+$ T-cell activation are the B7 : CD28 interaction and CD40 : CD40 ligand (CD40L). Interaction between these molecules is a prerequisite for T-cell activation and, indeed, in the absence of this 'second signal' presentation of peptide to the TCR is likely to lead to anergy rather than stimulation. B7 is a 45-kDa to 60-kDa cell surface glycoprotein expressed on activated B cells, dendritic cells and macrophages, which binds to CD28, a 44-kDa homodimeric molecule on the T cell, and leads to the proliferation of, and IL-2 secretion by, T cells. B7 can also bind to a second, less well-defined, receptor cytotoxic T-lymphocyte antigen 4 (CTLA-4), whose function is not clear but may be involved in IL-2 production plus promotion of T–B interaction via CD40. CTLA-4 is expressed on T regulatory cells (see later) and is considered to have an immunoregulatory role.

CD40–CD40L interactions are also very important in T-cell activation, and in reciprocal dendritic cell conditioning there is a two-way signalling interaction via this ligand pair. CD40 is present on APCs and can be upregulated. In addition, it is present on many non-APCs such as endothelial cells. CD40L is only present on activated T cells and even then transiently so that the time of CD40L expression in part regulates the overall duration of the immune response. CD40L and a further molecule Lag3 (CD223) may be involved in the concept of APC 'licensing', in relation to activation of cytotoxic T cells (see later, T-cell activation).

Several other accessory molecules are involved in the T-cell/APC interaction synapse to maximize the T-cell/APC contact. Activation of the T cell leads to the expression of integrin adhesion molecules on the cell surface, including LFA-1 and VLA-4 ($\alpha_4\beta_1$) (see Table 7.3). Reciprocal expression on cells promotes binding. VLA-4 also binds to extracellular matrix molecules, as does CD44 – the hyaluronate receptor (see Table 7.3). Some molecules provide costimulation for specific T-cell activities, such as OX40 and ICOS (see Table 7.3) while others such as PD1–PD1L are negative regulators of T-cell activation.

The process of antigen presentation for the generation of an active immune response (immunity)

Table 7.6 Molecules affecting T-cell costimulation

Receptor	Receptor present on	Receptor expression	Ligand	Ligand present on	Functions
CD28	T cells	Upregulated	B7-1, B7-2	B cells, DCs, monocytes, macrophages	IL-2 and IL-2R transcription, cell survival, proliferation, blocks anergy, prevents T-cell apoptosis
CTLA-4	T cells	Segregated*	B7-1, B7-2	B cells, DCs, monocytes, macrophages	Negative regulator of T-cell activation due to dephosphorylation of signalling molecules, downregulates IL-2 transcription, blocks T-cell proliferation
ICOS	T cells	Inducible	ICOSL	B cells, DCs, monocytes, macrophages	Germinal center formation, isotype switching, IL-4 and IL-13 transcription, Th2 responses, prevents T-cell apoptosis
PD-1	Activated T and B cells, myeloid cells	Inducible	PDL1 PDL2	Non-lymphoid cells; inducible on DCs and macrophages	Negative regulator of T cell activation due to dephosphorylation of signalling molecules, downregulates IL-2 transcription, blocks T-cell proliferation
???	Activated T cells?	Inducible?	B7-H3	Induced on APCs	Promotes T-cell proliferation, IFNγ production, regulates Th1 responses
CD40L	T cells NK cells	Upregulated	CD40	B cells, DCs, monocytes	Promotes APC activation, primary T-cell responses, germinal centre formation, isotype switching
4-1BB	T cells	Upregulated	4-1BBL	B cells, macrophages	Promotes CD8$^+$ T cell proliferation and IFNγ (CD137) production
OX40	T cells B cells	Inducible	OX40L	Activated T and B cells, DCs, endothelial cells	Promotes adhesion of activated T cells to endothelium, T-cell proliferation, cytokine production, B-cell antibody secretion
CD27	T cells B cells NK cells	Transiently upregulated	CD70	Activated T and B cells	Enhances T-cell proliferation (but not effector cell generation), required for IgG synthesis and generation of T-cell memory
LFA-1	T cells	Constitutive	ICAM-1,2,3	APCs, activated T and B cells	Mild costimulatory effect on T-cell proliferation, does not activate NF-κB, induce IL-2 transcription or prevent anergy
CD2	T cells	Constitutive	LFA-3 (Hu) CD48 (Mu)	Most hematopoietic cells, APCs	Mild costimulatory effect on T-cell proliferation, does not activate NF-κB, induce IL-2 transcription or prevent anergy
CD47 (IAP)	T cells, epithelial and endothelial cells, fibroblasts	Upregulated	?	APCs?	Mild costimulatory effect on T-cell proliferation

*'Segregated' in this context means that pre-formed CTLA-4 is held in vesicles inside the T cell until activation is under way.

therefore involves multiple molecular interactions and requires costimulatory activity if presentation is to be effective. It is not clear, however, whether all of the above interactions are required to initiate T-cell clonal expansion or whether immunogenicity is a function not just of peptide/TCR specificity but also depends on which and how many of the accessory interactions are entrained.

Getting the message across: cell signalling through the immunological synapse

Cells are stimulated to respond by receptor–ligand interactions at the cell surface which are linked to second messenger systems in the cytoplasm. These are likewise linked to events in the nucleus that mediate protein transcription and ultimately to changes in cell function (see cell signalling; Ch. 4 and Ch. 6). The immunological synapse (also known as the supramolecular activation complex) provides this function for the T cell. The initial contact between the T cell and the APC mediated through reciprocal LFA-1 and ICAM-1 interactions and also probably by CD45, induces changes in the actin cytoskeleton that draw several molecules on both sides in lipid rafts into a stable adhesive complex. The effect is dependent on a signalling molecule Vav. In the centre of the synapse lies the CD3/CD4 (or CD8)/CD45 complex/TCR–pMHC complex surrounded by an inner ring composed of CD2–LFA-3 paired molecules, itself surrounded by an outer ring of ICAM-1–LFA-1 molecules linked to talin and thus to the cytoskeleton (Figs 7.27 and 7.28). The TCR is linked to its second messenger system through a complex of transmembrane dimeric proteins, the CD3 complex which links intracellularly to a signal transduction complex p59^{fyn} (Fig. 7.29). These are collectively known as ITAMs: immunoreceptor tyrosine-based activation motifs. The p59^{fyn} molecule acts in conjunction with the p56^{lck} molecule as the tyrosine phosphorylating mechanism in T cells.

The four TCR–CD3 complexes may each initiate discrete signalling events, the summation of which produces an effective stimulus for T-cell activation (similar to events in neural cells; see Ch. 4). A progressive accumulation of signal thus develops through the sustained presentation of antigen mediated by recruitment of costimulatory and accessory molecules into the membrane surrounding the immunological synapse. In contrast, short-lived con-

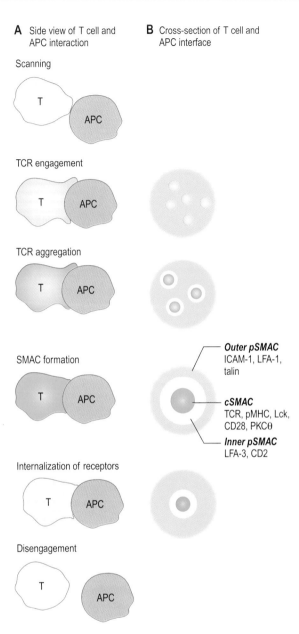

A Side view of T cell and APC interaction

Scanning

TCR engagement

TCR aggregation

SMAC formation

Internalization of receptors

Disengagement

B Cross-section of T cell and APC interface

Outer pSMAC
ICAM-1, LFA-1, talin

cSMAC
TCR, pMHC, Lck, CD28, PKCθ

Inner pSMAC
LFA-3, CD2

Fig. 7.27 T-cell–APC contact interactions. (**A**) Side view and (**B**) cross-section of immunological synapse. T cell first scans the APC surface and if sufficient TCRs like what they see firm engagement takes place with formation of the synapse (SMAC), aided by the other accessory molecules (LFA-1 etc.) TCR internalization then takes place and the activated T cell disengages and migrates off to find its target. (From Mak and Saunders 2006, with permission from Elsevier.)

407

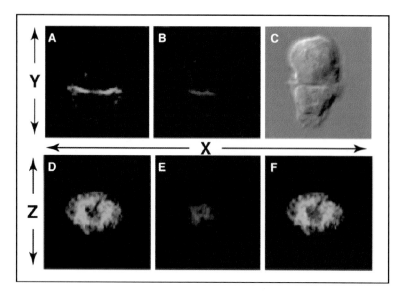

Fig. 7.28 Direct visualization using immunofluorescence (A,B,D,E) and phase-contrast imaging (C) with three-dimensional reconstruction of the SMAC(D → F) and T/APC contact region. (From Mak and Saunders 2006, with permission from Elsevier.)

tacts between APCs and T cells may fail to initiate responses in the T cells and probably do not even involve the TCR. Downstream signalling from the src family of tyrosine kinases is another set of protein tyrosine kinases with docking sites that bind SH-2 molecules. One of these is a protein known as ZAP-70 (associated with the ζ protein of CD3), which plays a major role in sustained TCR signalling. In fact, the interactions between the various signalling molecules through the TCR are a good example of how signalling networks function.

Action of drugs on cell activation

Certain immunosuppressive drugs, used clinically in transplantation and autoimmune diseases, are known to act at various stages in T-cell activation. These include steroids, cyclosporin A, FK506, rapamycin and mycophenolate mofetil. Cyclosporin is particularly relevant to ophthalmology because it is now used in a variety of conditions such as sight-threatening uveitis, advancing scleritis and corneal graft rejection. FK506 and mycophenolate are newer drugs that are under clinical evaluation.

Cyclosporin and FK506 specifically inhibit the transcription of the IL-2 gene in CD4 T cells by binding to intracellular proteins (immunophilins) that subsequently bind a Ca^{2+}-regulated phosphatase, calcineurin. This enzyme is activated by Ca^{2+} influx during T-cell activation and is required for assembly of the nuclear transcription factor (NF-AT, see Fig. 7.29) involved in IL-2 secretion. Cyclosporin may also act via induction of TGF-β release, a cytokine involved both in T regulatory cell function and in induction of Th17 cells.

THE MAJOR HISTOCOMPATIBILITY SYSTEM

Antigen presentation occurs in the context of the MHC antigens. Although our understanding of this process is now quite advanced, much has still to be learned concerning the role of antigens, MHC alleles and TCR usage in specific disease entities.

WHAT ARE MHC ANTIGENS AND WHERE ARE THEY FOUND?

The MHC gene cluster is a region of highly polymorphic genes whose products are expressed on a variety of cells. Class I genes are termed HLA-A, -B and -C, while those of class II are known as HLA-D. Class III genes lie between the centromeric class II genes and the telomeric class I genes (see Box 7.15). MHC genes differ from typical germline genes because they are polymorphic and responsible for some of the traits that distinguish one individual from another. Most germline genes are by definition non-polymorphic (i.e. identical) within a species.

MHC class I genes were discovered during studies in inbred mice of the genetic control of transplantation rejection phenomena. Several other members of HLA-class I have now been discovered but their precise function is not known, for instance HLA-G genes are expressed in the placenta and may have a role in protecting the fetus from attack by maternal NK cells. MHC class II genes were discovered later in analysis of mixed leucocyte reactions, a test that is the basis of tissue typing. MHC gene products

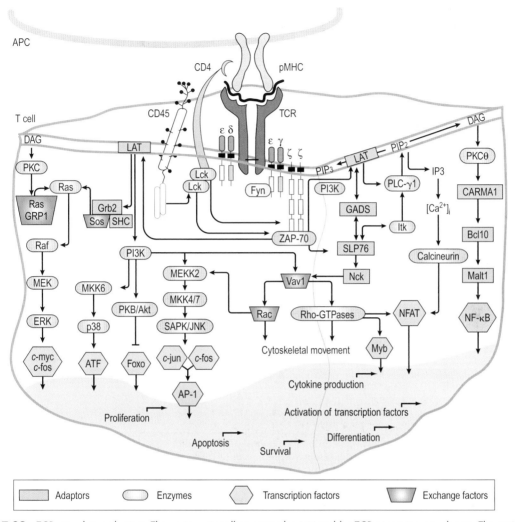

Fig. 7.29 TCR signal transduction. The various signalling cascades initiated by TCR triggering are shown. The major pathways include the Ras/MAPK pathway (far left) leading to c-fos and c-myc activation of the transcription factor c-jun; the activation of ZAP-70 and Vav1, which leads to cytoskeletal movement; the PLC-γ1 pathway, which leads to activation of the transcription factor NF-AT; and PKC activation leading to the activation of the transcriptional factor NF-κB. PI3K has numerous roles in facilitating signal transduction by these major pathways. The transcription factors activated by these pathways lead to new gene transcription that stimulates survival, proliferation, cytokine production and effector cell differentiation, among other outcomes. Details of the players in each pathway and the interactions between them are given in the text. (From Mak and Saunders 2006, with permission from Elsevier.)

were found to be the antigens responsible for inducing graft rejection because of their polymorphism. Studies of pregnancy sera and blood transfusion samples in humans revealed a similar organization of the MHC genes, and many of the allotypes were determined by careful documentation of antibody responses. More than 50 alleles in certain haplotypes have been described by serological techniques and it is likely that more will be discovered. More recently, direct gene sequencing techniques have been used to identify specific alleles and have led to subtype identification within alleles. For instance, on the basis of single amino acid differences in sequence, the HLA-B27 haplotype has been subtyped into seven (HLA B2701–07). This has led to the identification of many more alleles, some of which may differ by a single amino acid only. Correlations between 'molecular' and 'serological'

Box 7.15 Map of the MHC genes

The map of the MHC genes is constantly being revised as new information is added. The HLA-D genes are located towards the centromere and are separated from the class I genes by the complement protein genes (class III). Each of these regions is known to contain multiple genes, which are variably present within each haplotype. For instance the DR4 haplotype contains DRB1, DRB7, DRB8, DRB4 and DRB9; in contrast the DR1 haplotype contains DRB1, DRB6 and DRB9.

Several associated genes are located close to the MHC genes. These include the TAP1 and TAP2 genes, the DMA and DMB genes, and the LMP2 and LMP7 proteasome genes, all of which are involved in antigen processing (see p. 399). The TNF genes are also located in the class III region, as are the RAGE (receptor for advanced glycation end products) genes.

Several genes of unknown function have been identified (as well as pseudogenes) in this region.

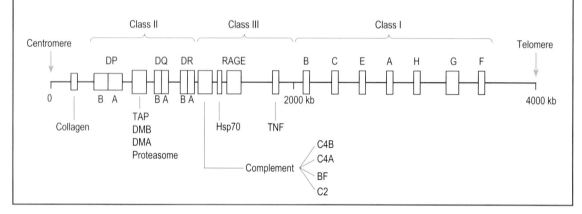

typing are important reference points (Table 7.7). Currently, nearly 300 alleles have been identified for HLA-A, 550 for HLA-B and 150 for HLA-C.

MHC genes control the adaptive immune response, class I regulating CD8 and class II regulating CD4 responses. Different alleles differ in their ability to bind and present different antigenic determinants, and this is probably the basis of each individual's susceptibility to disease.

Studies of the association of disease susceptibility and specific HLA alleles have revealed many interesting linkages. For instance the HLA-DR4 allele is associated with many putative autoimmune diseases such as diabetes mellitus, while protection from diabetes has been linked to the possession of a specific single amino acid (Asp57) at position 57 of the HLA-DQβ chain. 'Molecular' typing indicates that the DR4 locus contains many alleles (~19) located at the DRB1 site and designated DRB1–0401 to DRB1–0419. An association between different forms of HLA-DR4 and clinical types of Vogt–Koyanagi–Harada (VKH) disease has been demonstrated. VKH disease is considered to be an autoimmune disease to melanin, in which there is severe uveitis. In one clinical type the disease runs its course for about 6 months and does not recur. In the second type the

disease may adopt a protracted course or recur frequently over many years. The latter clinical course is associated with HLA-DRB*0405 and/or HLA-DRB*0410, both subtypes of HLA-DRB1, itself a subdivision of HLA-DR4 (see below, Organization of the MHC genes); in contrast the self-limiting form of VKH disease is not linked to either of these genetic types.

Most disease associations have, however, been detected in the class I genes. In particular, the HLA-B27/ankylosing spondylitis/enteric infection/uveitis link is long established. In addition the HLA-B51, but not B52, is linked with Behçet's disease in the Middle East and Japan.

Perhaps the strongest known association or any human disease (> 90%) is between HLA-A29 and a rare form of endogenous posterior uveitis, birdshot retinochoroidopathy.

Organization of the MHC genes in the genome

The MHC genes are located on chromosome 6 (see Box 7.15) while the non-polymorphic component of the class I molecule, β2-microglobulin, is on chromosome 15. The MHC region is very large, occupy-

Table 7.7 Extracted from data by Bodmer et al. (1984) to illustrate the range of molecular and serological diversity in MHC polymorphisms: Allele ≡ molecular typing; Specificity ≡ serological typing

Allele		(N)	Specificity	Allele		(N)	Specificity
DPA1	DPA 0101 ↓ 0401	(9)		DRB5	DRB5 0101 ↓ 0202	(4)	DR51
DPB1	DPB 01011c ↓ 5501	(>80)	DPwl	DRB6	DRB6 0101 ↓ 0201	(3)	
DQA1	DQA 0101 ↓ 0601	(>30)		DRB7	DRB7 01011 ↓ 01012	(2)	
DQB1	DQB1 0501 ↓ 0402	(>40)	DQ5	B	B 0701 ↓ 7801	(>140)	B7 B27 B7801
DMA	DMA 0101 ↓ 0104	(4)		C	Cw 0101 ↓ 1701	(>30)	Cwl
DMB	DMB 0101 ↓ 0104	(4)		E	E 0101 ↓ 0104	(4)	
DRA	DRA 0101 ↓ 0102	(2)		G	G 01011 ↓ 0103	(4)	
DRB1	DRB1 0101 ↓ 10	(>100)	DR1	A	A 0101 ↓ 8001	(>80)	A1
DRB3	DRB3 0101 ↓ 030	(4)		TAP1	TAP1 0101 ↓ 0401	(6)	
DRB4	DRB4 01f ↓ 0103	(5)		TAP2	TAP2 0101 ↓ 0201	(3)	

ing about 4000 kilobases – as large as the entire genome of certain bacteria.

The class II genes, placed near the centromere, are commonly involved in crossing over during meiosis. Unlike non-polymorphic genes both alleles are expressed. Furthermore there are two or three functioning β chain genes in class II, each of which can combine with the α chain. This allows some class II alleles to be expressed in more than one allelic form on the same cell. Thus a heterozygous individual expresses six different class I alleles (two HLA-A, HLA-B and HLA-C from each parent) on separate molecules on each cell. In contrast, for class II many more than six heterodimers can be inherited (commonly there are 10–20 different class II genes per cell) and this permits a large range of peptides to be bound on each cell. Furthermore, each MHC molecule can bind many different peptides with differing affinities (see above).

As for other immune genes that involve recombination events such as the immunoglobulin and TCR genes, there is coordinate expression of the HLA genes, e.g. class I on chromosome 6 and β2-microglobulin on chromosome 13 must be simultaneously activated, and similarly the class II genes during transcription of HLA-DP, -DQ and -DR.

Regulation and transcription of the MHC genes

Regulatory elements that lie 5′ upstream of the MHC class I β_2-microglobulin and class II genes, plus other essential genes like the invariant chain, coordinate the expression of MHC genes. These elements incude the S, X, Y box and the complex on it known as the class II transactivator (CIITA), which regulates MHC class I and II. Mutations in these genes can cause immunodeficiency syndromes.

Cytokines modulate the rate of constitutive transcription of MHC genes. Class I expression is increased by α, β and γ interferons, and induction varies with cell type. IFN-γ also alters transcription of class II: in macrophages, endothelial cells and some parenchymal cells the change is upwards, but in B cells it is decreased. In contrast, IL-4 has the opposite effect on class II expression of B cells. Some cells, such as neuronal cells, do not respond at all to IFN-γ. The interactive responses of immune and tissue cells profoundly affect the final nature and character of the immune response and can convert a tissue-destructive process to a protective response or, depending on the tissue, to an allergic response (see below).

The genetic control of MHC expression and function is also controlled by other genes such as the *TAP1* and *TAP2* genes, which regulate the entry of peptides into the endoplasmic reticulum, the invariant chain gene that regulates stability of the class II complex, and the calnexin gene that regulates the binding of peptide to class I (see p. 399).

T-CELL ACTIVATION

Any molecule, large or small, can act as an antigen but only macromolecules can activate lymphocytes and act as immunogenes. Small molecules may activate lymphocytes if they are bound to a larger molecule; in this situation the small molecule is called a hapten.

Therefore, although peptides may initiate an immune response, there are several constraints on the induction of a response. For instance, there is a minimum size of peptide for an effective response, which in the case of MHC class I responses is precisely nine amino acids, and between 12 and 30 for class II responses (see p. 401). More importantly, the precise interaction between the TCR and the MHC–peptide complex is under the control of genes regulating both sides of this interaction. The TCR genes

have a greater role in determining the specificity of the response than the MHC genes.

THE TCR AND ANTIGEN BINDING

Processing of antigens to peptides in the APC may potentially yield a large number of immunogenic peptides. However, only a small number of these peptides will activate lymphocytes and only one will be specific for a particular cell. This is determined partly by the nature of the antigen but more importantly by the 'TCR repertoire', i.e. the potential range of different TCRs that exist to deal with very large numbers of possible antigens. The immune system has developed a mechanism to deal with this problem, which involves the use of multiple germline genes, each of which undergoes somatic rearrangement on challenge with antigen. The same basic mechanism is used by B cells in their production of antigen-specific antibodies (see below).

TCRs are members of the immunoglobulin gene superfamily (see Box 7.16) and are dimeric proteins composed of an α and a β chain which possess V (variable), D (diverse) and C (constant) regions as for immunoglobulin molecules (Figs 7.30 and 7.31). The V region contains the antigen-binding site and interacts with the peptide–MHC complex. At least 20 families of Vα chains are recognized and a similar number of Vβ families are also known. Several V genes (2–10) exist within each family. A single antigen binds to a single TCR and stimulates antigen-specific clonal expansion. However, as indicated above, several antigens have the potential to bind to the same TCR, each with different affinities, unlike antigen–antibody interactions.

Databases holding germline gene sequences as a reference resource have been set up, such as IMGT (ImmunoGenetics, http://imgt.cnusc.fr.8104). Sequence accession numbers are listed in germline gene tables. At present there are many allelic variations in all four gene segments, C, D, J and V, for each of the α, β, γ and δ TCR chains, totalling over 200 genes. It has been estimated that there are from 1000 to more than 4000 possible combinations of the V, J and C genes, which increases the diversity of TCR$\alpha\beta$-binding capacity enormously. A single V gene encodes a sequence in the TCR, a 'complementarity determining region' (CDR) (Fig. 7.30), which binds to that region on the antigenic protein corresponding to the peptide–MHC complex that binds to the TCR. This region of the antigenic protein is known as an epitope. Each

Box 7.16 Immunoglobulin superfamily of proteins

The immunoglobulin superfamily is characterized by the common structural motif, the immunoglobulin domain. This domain may occur singly in small molecules such as Thy-1 or multiply in both chains of dimers such as the T-cell receptor.

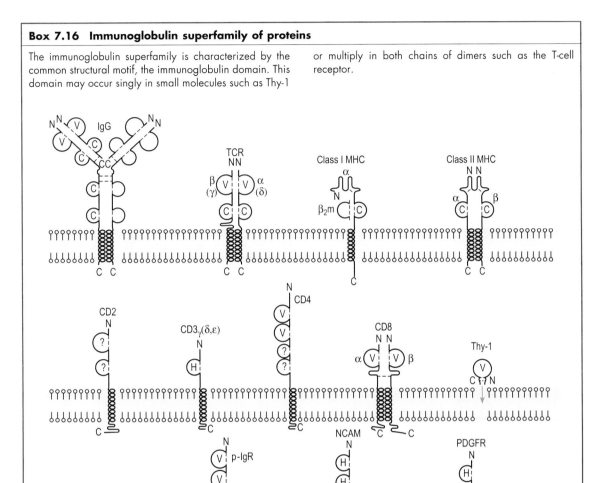

protein may contain several epitopes that interact with different TCRs and produce different responses *in vivo* (similar epitopes exist for CDRs on antibodies; see below). Some epitopes may even induce anergy in a specific clone of T cells.

Immunization with a multideterminant antigen (i.e. an antigen that has several epitopes, which holds true for most protein antigens) will therefore lead to a polyclonal T-cell response in which several T-cell clones are variably activated by each determinant depending on its immunogenicity. Usually one or two epitopes on a molecule are immunodominant.

Epitope mapping of proteins is therefore possible. It has been shown that only about 30% of most proteins contain sequences that are recognized by lymphocytes. For certain autoantigens, such as retinal S antigen (implicated in the pathogenesis of uveitis, see below), various parts of the molecule have been

413

mapped as antibody binding, immunogenic (stimulates T cells *in vitro*), or pathogenic (induces autoimmune uveoretinitis in experimental animals) (peptide band on amino acids from 280 to 364). These sites are different from the rhodopsin-binding

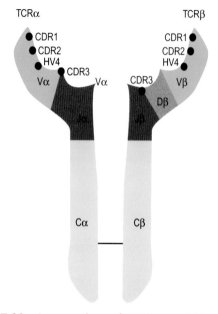

Fig. 7.30 Correspondence of TCR hypervariable regions to TCR gene segments. In this schematic example, the areas of the TCRα and TCRβ proteins derived from the indicated gene segments are shown in different colours. The CDR1, CDR2 and HV4 hypervariable regions are clustered in the variable domains of each chain while the CDR3 region encompasses the VJ joint in the TCRα chain and the DJ joint in theTCRβ chain. (From Mak and Saunders 2006, with permission from Elsevier.)

sites on S antigen, also known as arrestin, (Fig. 7.32) and may represent cryptic epitopes, i.e. epitopes that are revealed only when the molecule is partly degraded.

Conversely, preferential usage of certain clones of T cells with particular Vα and/or Vβ sequences is recognized in certain diseases, such as rheumatoid arthritis and multiple sclerosis, and has also been described in endogenous uveitis, where the (?auto)antigen is suspected but not known. Investigation of the TCR sequences on these cells may provide clues about the nature of the antigen.

Regulation of TCR gene expression is under the control of several 'gene enhancers' such as activating transcription factor (ATF), cAMP-responsive element binding protein (CREB), T-cell factor (Tcf-1) and lymphoid enhancer factor (Lef-1). GATA-3 is a factor that is also important (named for its DNA binding sequence).

The right time and the right place for T-cell activation

One of the long-standing conundrums in T cell activation has been how to explain the logistics of the interaction between a T cell and an APC. As discussed above, antigen traffics either as soluble antigen in the lymph or cell-bound in dendritic cells to the draining lymph node. Recent *in vivo* two-photon studies have shown that T cells entering the lymph node make repeated short interactions with several APCs, and when a T cell meets cognate antigen, it engages in sustained contact (several hours to 2 days) until, when sufficiently activated (as determined by expression of activation markers

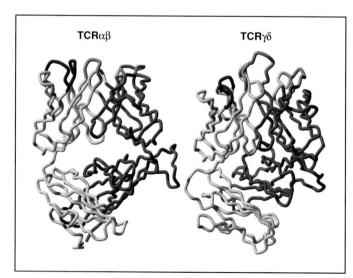

Fig. 7.31 Structures of TCRαβ and TCRγδ. Crystal structures showing the carbon backbone of TCRαβ and TCRγδ. TCRα and δ chains are light grey, TCRβ and γ chains are dark grey. For the α and δ chains, CDR1 is dark blue, CD2 is magenta and CDR3 is green. For the β and γ chains CDR1 is turquoise, CDR2 is pink, CDR3 is yellow and HV4 is orange. (From Mak and Saunders 2006, with permission from Elsevier.)

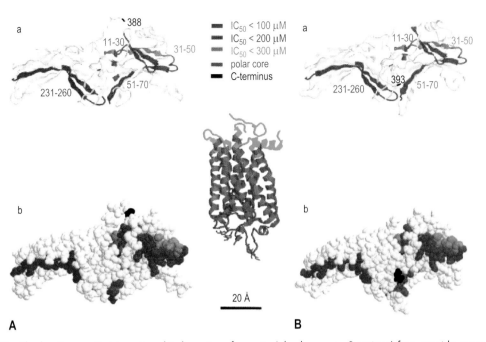

Fig. 7.32 Rhodopsin–arrestin interaction: binding sites of arrestin (also known as S antigen) from peptide competition. In each case, molecule B of the unit cell is shown in (a) ribbon drawing and (b) space-filling model. The picture in the centre represents the rhodopsin structure in the ground state with the cytoplasmic loops in green and the retinal in purple. (From Pulvermüller *et al.* 2000, with permission from the American Society for Biochemistry and Molecular Biology.)

such as CD69), it detaches from the APC. At this point it may undergo a proliferative response or it may emigrate from the lymph node as an effector cell in the search for target antigen.

While T-cell activation in the lymph node can be thus understood, T-cell activation at the site of target antigen (i.e. in the tissues) is more difficult to explain. This is particularly so for cytotoxic T cells, the activation and effector functions of which require *in situ* processes. It has been suggested that APC activation at the site of target antigen could be initiated by a tissue homing-activated T cell emigrating from the draining lymph node. In this scenario the APC in the tissue, usually recently recruited from the bone marrow and in an immature state, would be activated non-specifically by the Th1 cell, through CD40L or other molecules such as LAG (CD223), and this newly 'licensed' APC would then be able to present antigen on MHC class I to a CD8 T cell in the tissues. This three (or more) cell cluster would then be in a position to induce lysis of the target (e.g. virus-infected) cell.

This trafficking process of various cells to the tissues has not been formally shown *in vivo* as yet, but it is an attractive hypothesis to explain not simply how T cells traffic to the target tissue but how they can enact their role. Similar mechanisms probably operate for antigen-specific Th cell activation *in situ*, particularly in the case of sequestered antigens such as those that occur in the eye.

B-CELL ACTIVATION

Until now we have considered only cellular interactions with antigens. However, the first evidence for the existence of an adaptive immune system came through the discovery of antibodies, circulating proteins in the globulin fraction of the serum. Free antibodies are produced by plasma cells, the fully differentiated version of the B cell. B cells are derived from stem cell precursors in the bone marrow and are released into the circulation where they comprise 5–10% of the circulating lymphocyte pool before trafficking to sites of inflammation and to the lymphoid organs. B cells are important not only as antibody producers but also as APCs in their own right.

7 IMMUNOLOGY

ANTIGENS, B CELLS, AND T CELLS: WHICH DOES WHAT?

Antigen recognition by B cells

The rules governing the size of peptide antigen required to induce an immune response apply to T and B cells. However, most T cells are restricted in that they can respond only to peptides. B cells can also respond to carbohydrate and glycolipid antigens producing T-independent B-cell responses. This occurs for instance with blood group antigens.

As indicated above (see Fig 7.9, p. 376) B-cell responses to peptide antigens require T-cell help, usually provided by cytokines such as IL-2, IL-4, IL-5 and IL-6 released from activated Th2 cells. However, B cells also recognize antigen; they do this directly through their surface immunoglobulin (sIg). Here they present antigen on MHC class II molecules to Th cells and in return receive T-cell help, mediated via CD40–CD40L interactions, and undergo differentiation (antigen-specific) and development into plasma blasts. This form of T-cell and B-cell recognition of the same peptide antigen is known as mature B-cell (plasma cell) -linked recognition. Other coreceptor molecules are involved in the formation of the contact site of the B–T-cell interface, e.g. CD30 : CD30L and B-lymphocyte stimulator (Bly5) and its receptor TAC1.

B cells arriving from the bone marrow to the secondary lymphoid tissues traverse the T-cell area on their way to the B-cell follicles. However, if they meet an antigen-specific Th cell, they become trapped in the marginal T-cell zone and start proliferating and producing antibody (a primary lymphoid focus). Some of these B cells mature to antibody-producing plasma cells, which leave the T-cell area and return to the bloodstream and ultimately the bone marrow. In contrast, the majority enter the B-cell area where they form a B-cell follicle, and undergo further maturation on exposure to antigen on follicular dendritic cells in the presence of T-cell help to form the B-cell germinal centre, an antibody-producing mini-factory, with extensive isotype switching taking place.

They then migrate to the medulla and out into the circulation where they home to the bone marrow and differentiate into mature antibody-secreting plasma cells. They may also populate sites of inflammation and develop into plasma cells. Three checkpoints exist therefore for B-cell expansion: the first is at the stage of T-cell help, regulated by CD40L; the second is at the stage of selection in the germinal centre by the follicular dendritic cell delivering anti-apoptosis signals; and the third is at the stage of migration of the mature B cell (plasma cell) to bone marrow and tissues generally. However, most B cells remain in the follicle/germinal centre and secrete antibody directly into the bloodstream via the efferent lymphatics and thoracic duct.

B cells as antigen-presenting cells

Endocytosis of antigen via its sIg receptor activates the B cell to process and present peptide fragments in association with MHC class II on its surface (see above). B cells are efficient APCs but can be activated to present antigen only via the sIg receptor. Therefore, in this regard they act as memory cells.

Although B cells are activated in an antigen-specific manner and their effector molecules (antibodies) are also antigen specific, they induce their effects in an antigen-non-specific way, predominantly via complement. B-cell responses are also greatly enhanced by activation of the B-cell coreceptor complex (CD19 : CD21 : CD81; Fig. 7.33). CD21 is the receptor for complement component C3D thus permitting antibody–antigen–complement interaction.

B-CELL DIFFERENTIATION

B cells are derived from stem cell precursors in the bone marrow (Fig. 7.34). Immature B cells are released into the peripheral lymphoid tissue where they develop into mature B cells. If they do not encounter specific antigen, they undergo apoptosis and are removed within 3–4 days. However, when activated they develop into lymphoblasts and ultimately plasma cells (see above). Some activated cells develop into long-lived memory cells.

Pre-B cells lack membrane-bound IgM and immature B cells may fail to respond to antigen despite the presence of sIgM, owing to lack of accessory molecules. Anergy or tolerance may instead be induced under these conditions. Immature and mature B cells express surface IgM and IgD, whereas activated B cells express IgG after heavy-chain isotype switching. At this stage most of the immunoglobulin is still membrane bound. After some rounds of activation, the cell switches to high secretion of antibody and becomes a plasma cell.

Antibody generation during B-cell ontogeny

The immune system utilizes the same general mechanism to generate an almost infinite range of

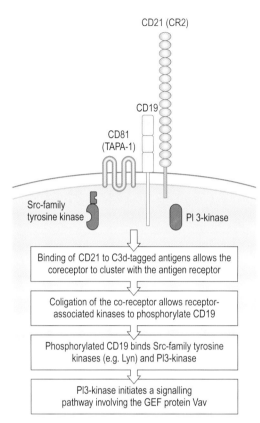

CD21 (CR2)

CD19

CD81
(TAPA-1)

Src-family
tyrosine kinase

PI 3-kinase

Binding of CD21 to C3d-tagged antigens allows the coreceptor to cluster with the antigen receptor

Coligation of the co-receptor allows receptor-associated kinases to phosphorylate CD19

Phosphorylated CD19 binds Src-family tyrosine kinases (e.g. Lyn) and PI3-kinase

PI3-kinase initiates a signalling pathway involving the GEF protein Vav

Fig. 7.33 B-cell antigen receptor signalling is modulated by a coreceptor complex of at least three cell surface molecules, CD19, CD21 and CD81. Binding of the cleaved complement fragment C3D to antigen allows the tagged antigen to bind to both the B-cell receptor and the complement cell surface protein CD21 (complement receptor 2, CR2), a component of the B-cell coreceptor complex. (From Janeway *et al.* 2001, with permission from Elsevier.)

specific antibodies as it does for TCRs, via recombinations of the heavy and light chains of the C (constant) regions, and somatic mutations in the V (variable) regions of the respective antibody and TCR molecules. The genes encoding antibody structure are located on chromosomes 14, 2 and 22 in humans (Fig. 7.35).

In memory B cells particularly, somatic mutations that occur during progression of the B cell through isotype switching to the plasma cells permit the antibody to be 'shaped' to fit the antigen better. This is known as 'affinity maturation' of the B cell and its immunoglobulin molecules, a process that describes the stronger affinity of antibodies for an antigen on repeated exposure. Thus antibodies produced after repeated exposure to the antigen have a much higher

binding capacity for the antigen and are more effective in dealing with its removal. This is the basis of various immunization protocols. Isotype switching is under the control of cytokines and varies for different immunoglobulins; thus IL-4 induces switching to IgG1 and IgE while IFN-γ induces IgG3 and IgG2a and TGF-β induces IgG2b and IgA switching.

Under normal bone marrow conditions of continual cell proliferation and maturation, with unique mutations being produced in each cell at each cell division, a very large range of possible permutations of antigen specificity is met within a short time but initially with low affinity. When the correct match between a particular antigen and receptor occurs, antigen-specific clonal expansion ensues. However, this happens only rarely; most cells expressing a particular sIg do not meet the corresponding antigen and are eliminated.

Somatic mutations occur in the CDR of the V genes

Antigen binding sites are located in the complementarity determining regions (CDRs) of the V segments of the H and L chains (see Fig. 7.7A), particularly in the hypervariable region. However, some overlapping binding to the conserved regions of these proteins may also occur. Mutations that increase the affinity of the antigen–antibody reaction occur in the hypervariable regions and become increasingly important with each exposure to the antigen (affinity maturation). Mutations occur in all three CDRs in both chains and may also occur in some intervening regions of the encoded sequence. Antibody diversity is therefore due to several factors (see Box 7.17).

Box 7.17 Factors controlling antibody diversity

- Multiple germline genes
- Somatic combinatorial diversity
- Junctional diversity
- H and L chains contributing to the antibody combining site
- Somatic mutations

In the mouse it has been estimated that the potential antibody repertoire due to recombination mechanisms is 10^9–10^{11} (i.e. before antigen has initiated a response).

417

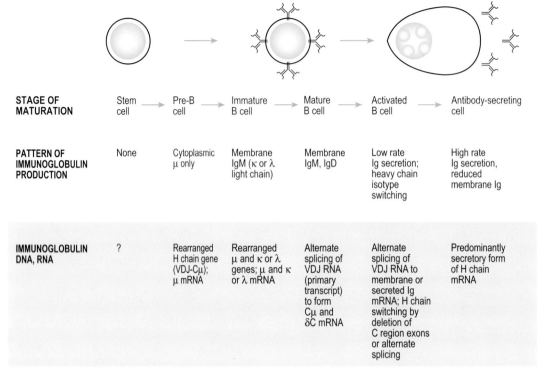

STAGE OF MATURATION	Stem cell	→	Pre-B cell	→	Immature B cell	→	Mature B cell	→	Activated B cell	→	Antibody-secreting cell
PATTERN OF IMMUNOGLOBULIN PRODUCTION	None		Cytoplasmic μ only		Membrane IgM (κ or λ light chain)		Membrane IgM, IgD		Low rate Ig secretion; heavy chain isotype switching		High rate Ig secretion, reduced membrane Ig
IMMUNOGLOBULIN DNA, RNA	?		Rearranged H chain gene (VDJ-Cμ); μ mRNA		Rearranged μ and κ or λ genes; μ and κ or λ mRNA		Alternate splicing of VDJ RNA (primary transcript) to form Cμ and δC mRNA		Alternate splicing of VDJ RNA to membrane or secreted Ig mRNA; H chain switching by deletion of C region exons or alternate splicing		Predominantly secretory form of H chain mRNA

Fig. 7.34 B-cell maturation. (Courtesy of A Abbas.)

Some microbial antigens (superantigens) have the ability to induce a polyclonal response in B cells in the absence of T cells, similar to T-cell superantigens (see p. 405). Superantigens bind to the majority of VH gene families especially VH3⁺ IgM. They also bind to conserved regions of the antibody outside the CDR at FR3 (framework region 3). Antibodies are very important to immunity and protection from microorganisms especially for memory responses to viruses. In such situations the paracrystalline repeated structural epitopes on the virus surface may induce a B-cell response without T-cell help.

Genetic control of antibody production

In addition to the normal TATA boxes of V region promoters (see Ch. 3), immunoglobulin genes contain regions modulated by trans-acting nuclear factors that regulate the promoters and enhancers. Trans-acting nuclear factors are DNA-binding proteins, some of which are specific to B cells. Others occur in a number of cells that have to respond rapidly and quantitatively, e.g. NF-κB (also involved in IL-2 transcription) and NF-AT (the target for cyclosporin and FK506).

IMMUNOLOGICAL TOLERANCE AND AUTOIMMUNITY

Many diseases involve the immune system in the absence of clear evidence for a direct causation by a foreign infective organism. In many of these diseases, antibodies and T-cell-mediated immune responses to 'self antigens' can be demonstrated and these disorders are considered to be 'autoimmune diseases'. The notion that immune responses to self antigens are unusual implies that immunological non-responsiveness to self antigens is the normal situation; this state is known as tolerance. Therefore, autoimmune diseases may be considered to be the result of defects in maintaining tolerance that are associated with actual tissue damage.

In a broader sense, the immune system has evolved mechanisms that downregulate (switch off) the immune response after it has been activated because it would clearly be autodestructive to have a continuing inflammatory response. The mechanisms that invoke tolerance and those that switch off immune responses may be the same.

H chain locus (chromosome 14)

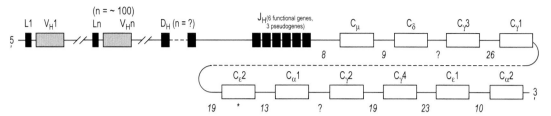

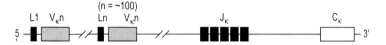

κ chain locus (chromosome 2)

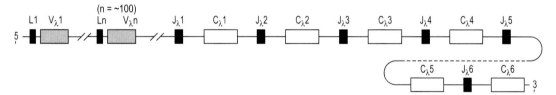

λ chain locus (chromosome 22)

Fig. 7.35 The heavy (H) and light (L) chain genes are located in the sequence in which they are transcribed. There are over 100 V genes, each of around 300 base pairs in length and grouped in six or seven families on the basis of > 80% homology. Each V gene is preceded by a leader sequence characteristic of secreted and transmembrane proteins. There are an unknown number of D genes and five or six J genes. The J and D genes code for the C-terminal region of the V gene including the third complementarity-determining region (CDR) (see below). Each C gene is composed of several exons represented by the single box. The D_H gene is the main genetic determinant of D–H–J diversity. The amino acid composition of the IgH CD3 region is the driving force for selection. Hydrophilic/aromatic amino acid groups are more likely to be selected than hydrophobic groups.

Recombination of the gene segments to generate a mature immunoglobulin is achieved by excision of the intervening DNA and ligation of the immunoglobulin genes. This 'looping out' is facilitated by specific enzymes (recombinases) that act during the earliest stages of B cell maturation. Segments of DNA, 3′ of each V gene and 5′ of each J gene in the noncoding intervening DNA of the light chain and similarly in the VDJ genes of the heavy chain, are excised and reannealed. Recombinases themselves are under genetic control via recombination activation genes (RAG genes).

Recombination occurs in a precise sequence. V_H genes join to the DJ gene, at which point the cell is committed to becoming a B cell. The VDJ sequence then binds to $C\mu$ and a poly-AAA tail is added. The L chain follows the same sequence and the expressed L chain then assembles with the 'm only' H chain in the endoplasmic reticulum. When this pre-B cell expresses the IgM on its cell surface, it becomes an immature B cell.

The μ chain regulates somatic rearrangement by allelic exclusion (activation of genes on one set of chromosomes suppresses activation of the other chromosome) and by initiating L chain rearrangement (the κ chain is activated first; if this is non-productive, λ chain genes are activated). (Courtesy of A Abbas.)

WHAT IS TOLERANCE?

Tolerance may be defined as antigen-induced inhibition of the development, growth, or differentiation of antigen-specific lymphocytes. Tolerance has the following properties.

- It is antigen-specific – individuals who are tolerant to one antigen are not necessarily tolerant to all antigens or even a second antigen.
- Tolerance to autoantigen is acquired during development – immature lymphocytes develop tolerance more easily than adult ones.
- Maintenance of tolerance requires persistence of (auto)antigen throughout the life of the individual.
- Tolerance to foreign antigens can be induced if the conditions are right.

MECHANISMS OF TOLERANCE INDUCTION

Tolerance (better described as immunological non-responsiveness, although this is rather unwieldy) is considered under various forms, e.g. neonatal versus adult, central versus peripheral, innate versus acquired, etc. In fact, tolerance is always acquired; the differences arise when the acquisition of tolerance occurs in the thymus during development (central) or in the peripheral lymphoid tissues during adulthood (peripheral).

Several mechanisms of tolerance have been suggested.

Clonal deletion

This mechanism was originally proposed by Burnet to explain the antigen-induced destruction of self-reactive lymphocytes that occurs in the thymus during development (negative selection). This is a form of activation-induced cell death that is a characteristic of peripheral tolerance as well as central tolerance. However, this does not account for the induction of tolerance to the large numbers of non-thymic antigens that are clearly not present in the thymus during development.

Anergy

Anergy describes T- and B-cell non-responsiveness to specific antigens but in cells with the capability to respond to non-specific mitogenic stimuli, i.e. the cells are in a sort of 'suspended animation'. Anergy in lymphocytes is thought to arise via lack of accessory signals required for antigen presentation (the B7 : CD28 and the CD40 : CD40L interactions are considered particularly important; see above) and has been proposed to account for the non-responsiveness of lymphocytes to peripheral autoantigens. It is therefore considered to be a major mechanism of tolerance induction in the adult.

However, it is likely that clonal deletion and anergy involve the same processes. Thymic education of lymphocytes involves a discrete series of events in arming the T cell to develop towards a CD4$^+$ or a CD8$^+$ phenotype (see Fig. 7.18) and antigen specificity. Each of these steps requires more than one signal and, at any point, lack of a particular signal might induce anergy. If anergy persists, the cell is driven down a pathway towards apoptosis (i.e. deletion). Similar mechanisms exist in the bone marrow and in the germinal centres of lymph nodes and spleen. Apoptotic B cells are removed from germinal centres by the well-recognized 'tingible body' macrophages.

Thus the same mechanisms for removal of autoreactive cells, involving anergy and cell death, probably occur in the periphery and the central lymphoid tissues, although there is a fine balance between deletion and anergy in the induction of tolerance. It has also been postulated that removal of all autoreactive cells occurs in the thymus, both for the large pool of thymic antigens and for tissue-specific antigens, which are transported to the thymus on circulating dendritic cells. This has been shown for certain brain (myelin basic protein) and retinal (interphotoreceptor binding protein and retinal S antigen) proteins. This appears to be under the control of a specific gene expressed in thymic medullary epithelial cells, the autoimmune regulator (*AIRE*) gene.

Active suppression by specific lymphocytes: T regulatory cells

Experimental studies in animals have shown that tolerance, which can be induced to autoantigens and foreign antigens alike using specific techniques (see below), can be transferred via lymphocytes to naïve animals that have not previously been exposed to the antigen. This suggests that at least certain forms of tolerance are achieved by cells that inhibit or regulate the immune response, probably at the level of antigen presentation ('suppressor or regulatory cells') (Fig. 7.36). Regulatory cells have been difficult to identify, mainly because of their lack of responsiveness to specific antigen *in vitro* (anergy). However, recent studies have confirmed that there are several types of Tregs, the most fashionable of which are the CD4$^+$ CD25$^+$ T cells. CD25 is the IL-2

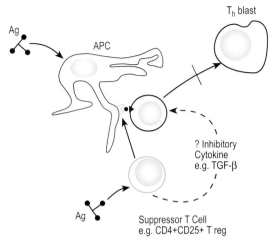

Fig. 7.36 Mode of action of regulatory cells.

receptor and is upregulated on activated T cells. However, it has also been found to be present on a population of natural and induced T cells which are not only unresponsive to antigen *in vitro* but also inhibit the responsive of other antigen-specific T cells when co-cultured. Importantly, when this population of cells is missing from the organism, there is a marked susceptibility to autoimmunity. CD4$^+$ CD25$^+$ Tregs are also defined by the transcription factor FoxP3. Other Tregs are also recognized, such as the IL-10-producing Tr1 cells, the TGF-β-producing Th3 cells, CD8$^+$ suppressor T cells which mediate their action through macrophages and NKT cells, and γδ T cells. It is not clear how Tregs induce the suppression of T effector cells but the effect is believed to be via dendritic cells and not directly through Treg : T effector interactions (Fig. 7.36) (see also p. 397 and Fig. 7.14).

Idiotype regulation

In 1973 Jerne (see Jerne, 1984 for review) proposed a network theory for regulation of the immune response whereby each immune response induces a secondary response that might have an enhancing or inhibitory effect on the primary response (see Box 7.18). This would have the effect of maintaining a balanced state of immunological responsiveness that would clearly be disturbed in the presence of an inciting antigen, but would allow a rapid counter-regulatory response to restore the balanced state. Autoantigens would invoke minimal or no effect on this balance but autoimmune disease might occur if these mechanisms were bypassed. While this system has many intrinsic attractions, evidence for its role in autoimmune disease remains speculative.

Box 7.18 Idiotype regulation

Antibodies and TCRs, being proteins in their own right, can act as antigens when inoculated into allogeneic individuals. They can also induce responses in syngeneic individuals and on this basis it was proposed that all antibody and TCR responses induce an immune response in the same way that tumour cells induce immune responses by virtue of expressing new mutations. This response to antibody or TCR is called an idiotypic response, and the site on the antibody or TCR that induces the response is an idiotope (i.e. an idiotypic epitope). Each idiotypic response in turn induces its own response, which may be inhibitory or stimulatory to the overall immune reaction. Jerne suggested that this 'network' may be a means of diluting out the original immune response and thus switching it off.

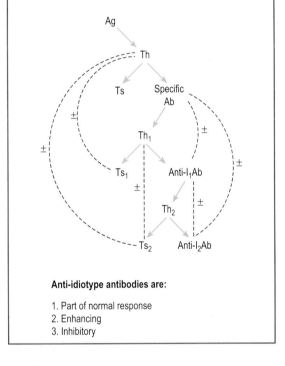

Anti-idiotype antibodies are:

1. Part of normal response
2. Enhancing
3. Inhibitory

Inhibitory cytokines

Several other mechanisms exist whereby immune responses could be switched off. Immune responses may be 'switched off' or downregulated by inhibitory cytokines. Thus, TGF-β has been shown to be a potent immunosuppressive molecule. IL-4, IL-6 and IL-10 inhibit delayed-type hypersensitivity T-cell-mediated responses, while IFN-γ inhibits B-cell responses (see section on cytokines). These responses are not antigen specific and are probably not directly relevant to the mechanism of tolerance induction but may act as the final common mediators in the effector phase of the response (see above, Tregs).

421

In this regard, antibody itself may have an antigen-specific immunosuppressive effect; this may be achieved by several means such as elimination of persisting antigen as immune complexes; direct inhibition of B cells by binding to Fc receptors; regulation of T-cell responses by immune complexes or by peptide blockade; and many others.

T-CELL TOLERANCE IS DIFFERENT FROM B-CELL TOLERANCE

The Th cell is the critical control element for adaptive immune responses. Therefore inhibition of Th responses should lead to inhibition of all self-reactivity. T cells can be rendered unresponsive by very low doses of antigen, while B cells usually require larger doses. Most T-cell tolerance is induced in the thymus by clonal anergy/deletion and is therefore antigen specific and MHC restricted. In the periphery, T-cell tolerance may be induced by aberrant expression of MHC class II antigen on parenchymal cells that lack costimulatory signals. However, in the presence of immunocompetent MHC class II-bearing cells, an autoimmune response may be induced.

B-cell tolerance occurs particularly to antigens that are 'T-independent'. This includes carbohydrate and glycolipid antigens such as the ABO blood groups, and thus has direct clinical relevance. Tolerance is induced by anergy/deletion of antigen-specific B cells in the marrow by mechanisms similar to those described for the thymus. Studies using transgenic mice in which genes for neoantigens and the corresponding antibody were inserted into the genome have elegantly demonstrated that B-cell anergy in the marrow occurs by maturation arrest and failure of these autoreactive B cells to enter the peripheral lymphoid organs. After some time these cells underwent apoptosis (i.e. were deleted). Interestingly, some of these B cells could render the autoantigen non-anergy-inducing by switching the κ/λ chain. B cells that had undergone 'receptor editing' of this nature appeared in the periphery (i.e. were not deleted).

FAILED TOLERANCE

A failure to develop or maintain tolerance to autoantigens leads to the development of autoimmune disease. To some degree, tolerance is incomplete and 'natural autoimmunity' to autoantigens is the norm. This has been shown for most autoantigens including retinal S antigen. However, there are immunological mechanisms in place that inhibit excessive expression of natural autoimmunity.

Autoimmune disease is the dysfunction or damage of tissue caused by immune responses to autoantigens

Autoimmune diseases take many forms, from organ and even cell-specific antibody-mediated diseases such as myasthenia gravis (where the antigens are located at the neuromuscular junction) to widespread systemic diseases such as systemic lupus erythematosus, where the antigen is distributed in all tissues (DNA).

Tissue damage in autoimmune disease can be induced by any of the accepted forms of immunopathological mechanisms (types I–IV; Table 7.5). However, as for most immune mechanisms, autoimmune diseases are usually initiated by CD4$^+$ T cells. Several mechanisms have been proposed to account for this process:

- Molecular mimicry between foreign and autoantigen – as might be expected with the wide range of antigenic peptides occurring in infective organisms – sequence homologies occur with predictable frequency. Processing of foreign antigenic peptide might thus lead to activation of autoreactive T cells if the foreign antigen is 'mistaken' for self. This has been shown for several retinal antigens that have amino acid sequences similar to bacterial and viral antigens, including Gram-negative bacteria such as *Escherichia coli* and parasites such as *Onchocerca*, which causes endemic blindness in certain regions of Africa ('river blindness').
- Bystander activation – the initiation of autoimmune disease may also occur by bystander activation, for instance during infection. Upregulation of costimulatory molecules on APCs in the lymphoid tissues in the vicinity of anergized but not deleted autoreactive T and/or B cells may lead to autoimmune disease. Anergy may require expression of CTLA-4 which if absent may also allow self-autoreactivity.
- Failure of deletion (activation induced self-death) – T-cell deletion and apoptosis is mediated by cell surface molecules such as Fas–FasL. Failure of the apoptotic machinery might lead to autoimmunity.
- Idiotype dysregulation – an idiotypic response to a foreign antigen may reveal an idiotype on an antibody or TCR that has sequence similarity to an autoantigen and thus lead to activation of the autoreactive T cells.
- Polyclonal B-cell activation – certain compounds such as endotoxin and bacterial glycolipids can activate B cells directly, either to produce cytotoxic

antibody or to act as APCs and thus present auto-antigen to responding T cells.

- Failure of suppressor cell activity – evidence exists that tolerance is mediated by regulatory T cells (see above) that homeostatically inhibit autoreactive T cells, possibly by direct cell contact or release of cytokine. Failure of suppressor cell activity would thus permit an autoimmune response to be induced.

- Superantigen – simultaneous activation of several subsets of T cell by superantigens, which do not require processing because they link the T cell and MHC antigen directly, may also lead to activation of autoreactive T cells. Preferential usage of certain TCRs by superantigens may enhance the risk of autoimmune responses.

Parasitic infections persist by giving false signals to the immune system

Diseases caused by parasites are of major medical and economic importance worldwide. Parasites invade the tissues and enter into a symbiotic relationship, sometimes within the cytoplasm of the cell, particularly macrophages. Extracellular parasitic infections are even more frequent, such as those involving nematodes. Examples include filariasis, schistosomiasis and toxocariasis, the first and last of which can infect the eye. Ocular toxocariasis causes blindness in children, presenting as one cause of the white (cat's eye) pupillary reflex.

Parasites present the immune system with enormous problems, partly because they go through a life cycle in which they present different antigens at different times; the host therefore has difficulty in generating an adequate response and may enter a chronic state of inflammation. The parasite achieves this by manipulating or diverting the immune system. Although initially a Th1 response may be induced after infection by the parasite, the response is later diverted to become Th2-mediated with secretion of IL-2, IL-4 and IL-10. Several explanations have been proposed for this change, including defects in the presentation of parasite antigen, inappropriate production of regulatory cytokines such as IL-10 and IL-13, or the induction of a form of tolerance via prolonged binding of the antigen to the TCR. However, rather than being an anergic or impaired type of immune response, the switch from Th1 to Th2 may be quite pronounced. In some respects it is similar to the response in allergic disease because the Th1/Th2 immune response system becomes similarly dysregulated and can lead to excessive mast cell infiltration and eosinophilia, particularly with

helminth infestations. Cytokines play a significant role in protection from parasites. In many infections, induction of a Th1 response using IL-12, IL-23 and IL-27 can help to get rid of parasites. In toxoplasma infection, IL-5 also appears to be important and may regulate production of IL-12. Parasites may also derail the innate immune system by producing inhibition of macrophage activation, blocking complement, preventing apoptosis of the infected macrophage and molecular mimicry techniques.

In other circumstances, however, an anergic type of response is elicited by the parasite until it dies and its contents are released into the tissues. Toxoplasma retinochoroiditis is thought to occur by this mechanism. This condition is a relatively common cause of posterior uveitis, characterized by one or more large chorioretinal scars that undergo spontaneous reactivation, producing recurrent attacks of uveitis as the organisms spread. This disease may be controlled *in utero* or in adulthood/childhood, and attacks the central nervous system and the eye. Experimental studies have shown that while the toxoplasma cysts persist as discrete viable entities in the retina, little or no inflammation is induced, i.e. an apparent state of 'immunological ignorance' exists, at least with regard to the live parasite. However, inflammatory change is observed in areas of retina where no parasite appears to occur, suggesting either that the dead parasite is rapidly destroyed *in situ* or that secondary autoimmune reactions are occurring in response to release of host antigens from damaged retina.

ALLERGY AND IMMEDIATE HYPERSENSITIVITY

The immune system's attempts to rid itself of harmful foreign elements can sometimes be so exaggerated or inappropriate that the host is damaged in the process. Such a situation arises in type I hypersensitivity involving IgE responses to foreign antigens, thereby causing allergy. However, not all allergic responses are IgE mediated.

ATOPY, ASTHMA AND ALLERGIC EYE DISEASE

The prototype allergic disease is asthma, in which reversible obstruction of the airways occurs. This is, however, the outward acute manifestation of a chronic inflammatory process in the mucous membranes and skin of affected individuals. Asthma frequently coincides with chronic dermatitis (eczema), rhinitis and sinusitis, and conjunctivitis. The genetic

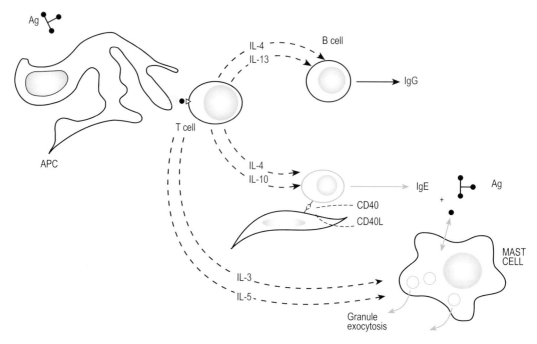

Fig. 7.37 Mast cell activation is dependent on antigen-specific activation of T cells (Ag) which, in concert with concomitant engagement of the CD40 membrane protein by the CD40 ligand (CD40L), induces an isotype switch in the presence of Th2-type cytokines to direct the B cell to produce IgE. IgE–antigen complexes are then available to activate the mast cell.

predisposition to synthesize IgE specific for certain external antigens is known as atopy, but all patients with asthma are not necessarily atopic. Other forms of asthma in non-atopic individuals are recognized (intrinsic versus extrinsic asthma). Similarly all patients with severe allergic conjunctivitis are not always atopic. These concepts are being confirmed clinically by the selective efficacy of monoclonal antibody anti-IgE therapy in the treatment of refractory asthma.

Allergic conjunctivitis induced by specific antigens such as pollens or housedust mite may be chronic (perennial allergic conjunctivitis) or intermittent (seasonal allergic conjunctivitis), and usually produces mild symptoms. Chronic conjunctivitis in severe atopy is more damaging, often with involvement of the cornea (atopic keratoconjunctivitis; see next section). A distinct clinical entity with massive follicular conjunctivitis and corneal opacification is known as vernal keratoconjunctivitis. In addition, contact lens wear is associated with a significant amount of allergic eye disease, producing giant papillary conjunctivitis.

In spite of the clinical differentiation between various forms of allergy it is likely that the underlying mechanisms are similar. Mast cells have long been recognized as effector cells in allergic disease. However, mast cells are dependent on IL-3 and IL-5 production by T cells, which is ultimately induced by antigen presentation to T cells (Fig. 7.37). In this regard, conjunctival dendritic cells have been considered to be major contributors to allergen capture and presentation to T cells locally in the tissues. In addition, other cells such as eosinophils are important in tissue damage.

Mast cell degranulation

The allergic response is characterized by mast cell degranulation, mediated either by IgE or by non-IgE mechanisms (see below). The role of antigen-specific IgE in this response can be demonstrated *in vivo* experimentally by the passive cutaneous anaphylaxis test. However, it should be realized that IgE is neither sufficient nor essential to induce mast cell-related allergic disease. Also involved are chemokines, mediating not only leucocyte recruitment but also mast cell activation through mediators such as eotaxin 1 (CCR3) and MIP-1α.

Mast cell degranulation leads to the release of preformed mediators including histamine and serotonin, which bind to a variety of receptors and induce second signalling events with release of a great variety of secondary agents depending on the cell type. This includes NO˙, prostacyclin, smooth muscle relaxants and many others. Several receptors exist for histamine (H_1, H_2, H_3, etc.), which can be distinguished by pharmacological agents.

Mast cells also synthesize and release newly formed materials after stimulation. These include prostaglandin D_2 (vasodilator and bronchoconstrictor), leukotrienes (LTC_4, LTD_4, LTE_4, previously known as slow-releasing substance A; cause prolonged bronchoconstriction), and platelet activating factor (PAF).

Recently cytokine release by mast cells has been recognized as a major inflammatory pathway. TNF-α, IL-1, IL-4, IL-5, IL-6, IL-13 and several colony-stimulating factors are released and help to recruit cells to the site of antigen exposure on the mucous membrane.

THERE ARE TWO TYPES OF MAST CELL

Mast cells are derived from precursors in the marrow and mature into one of two phenotypes depending on the microenvironment in which they reside. Stem (c-kit) cell factor is an important mast cell growth factor. In humans, mucosal mast cells contain tryptase (M_T), histamine and heparin in their secretory granules, while connective tissue mast cells contain chymase in addition (M_{TC}). In the normal conjunctiva and choroid, M_{TC} cells predominate (Fig. 7.38). However, in allergic conjunctivitis M_T cells appear to increase in number in association with the expression of adhesion molecules such as E selectin and ICAM-1. These changes are likely to be important in the pathogenesis of disease (see below). The significance of mast cell heterogeneity is not yet clear but it would appear that M_T are involved in the active stages of inflammation.

Mast cells may also have a role in the initiation of the immune response. Mast cells express MHC class I and class II antigens, and presentation of exogenous antigen to T cells leads to activation reciprocally of the mast cell with release of chemokines and cytokines. These direct the overall response towards a Th2-type response.

IgE AND HELPER T CELLS

There are two types of IgE receptor: FcεRI, which is present in mast cells, basophils and activated eosin-

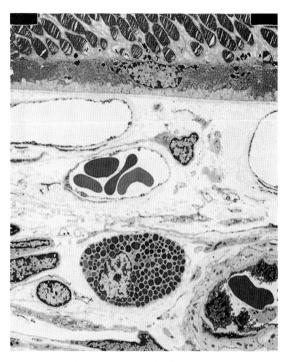

Fig. 7.38 Electron micrograph of a mast cell in the rat choroid containing numerous α granules.

ophils, and FcεRII (CD23), a low-affinity receptor present on many cell types including B, T and dendritic cells, monocytes and some thymic epithelial cells. FcεRII is important for initial antigen capture by dendritic cells.

IgE-mediated degranulation of mast cells occurs via high-affinity receptors (FcεRI). Signalling via the IgE receptor is inducible only by IgE–antigen complexes and requires local production of IgE by infiltrating B cells.

Isotype switching in B cells from IgG to IgE requires binding of the cell surface antigen CD40 on the B cell to a ligand on the T cell (gp39). This can also be induced by mast cells that express the CD40 ligand and promote local production of IgE in the tissue under cytokine stimulation (Fig. 7.39). Thus the disease can be perpetuated locally and enter a phase of chronicity, as occurs in asthma.

MECHANISM OF DISEASE PRODUCTION IN ALLERGIC DISEASE

Exposure of atopic individuals to allergen is accompanied by an immediate response mediated by mast cell degranulation and a later response occurring after 4–6 hours. Recent studies have shown that this

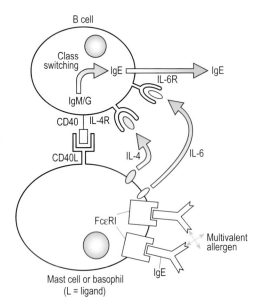

Fig. 7.39 Mast cells can themselves initiate isotype switching via CD40 because they express the CD40L antigen when they combine with allergen–IgE complexes. In this way the allergic response is amplified and perpetuated.

later response is induced by cytokine release from mast cells, which causes recruitment of M_T cells and basophils to the tissue and expression of adhesion molecules which promote eosinophil accumulation. In addition, release of the chemokine eotaxin by mast cells is probably the main stimulus for eosinophil recruitment. Basophils are circulating granulocytes that are similar in many respects to tissue mast cells in their expression of FcεRI and release of cytokines. However, they are considered to be of a different lineage in the bone marrow. T cells are not involved in this stage of the disease.

Eosinophils are strictly regulated because of their potential toxicity. In the absence of infection, very few eosinophils are produced. Even in the presence of an eosinophil, entry to the tissues is tightly controlled by eotaxins (via CCR3) and by other chemokines such as MCP-3, MCP-4 and RANTES.

Release of granule content by eosinophils, particularly erythropoietin (EPO), eosinophil major basic protein (MBP) and eosinophil cationic protein (ECP), causes much of the tissue damage. Eosinophils are attracted to the site of inflammation by specific adhesion molecules, particularly VCAM-1, on the endothelial cells. Induction of VCAM expression on endothelial cells is mediated by cytokine release from other inflammatory cells such as macrophages

and T cells, and it is now becoming clear that T cells are intricately involved in destructive tissue damage in allergic disease. In addition, neutrophils are attracted to the site as a result of upregulated adhesion molecule expression, particularly of E selectin and ICAM-1 in the acute stage. Neutrophils are themselves responsible for considerable tissue injury in certain forms of allergic disease and may even describe a subtype of refractory asthma. The risk of superadded infection in these cases is unclear.

In the later stages of the disease, increased numbers of T cells may be recruited as part of the continuing inflammatory response because of persistent adhesion molecule expression on endothelial cells, especially VCAM. T cells are then available to interact with APCs, particularly activated B cells, causing further release of IL-3, IL-5 and GM-CSF, which perpetuates the disease.

ORGAN AND TISSUE TRANSPLANTATION

Transplants or grafts are described as syngeneic when they are between genetically identical individuals, allogeneic when they are between individuals of the same species and xenogeneic when they are between individuals of different species. Allogeneic and xenogeneic grafts are normally not accepted and rejection is described as acute, chronic or accelerated.

The discovery of HLA antigens came about as a result of studies that attempted to explain how organ and tissue grafts, especially skin grafts, between members of the same species were rejected. Only in the case of genetically identical individuals were grafts accepted. For instance, in skin grafts not only was there rejection of the initial graft between two non-identical individuals but also subsequent attempts to graft donor skin between the same two individuals led to an even more rapid rate of rejection, indicating that there was some sort of memory response to the antigens in the original graft. Rejection of grafts was considered to be the result of the presence of alloantigens on 'passenger leucocytes' (leucocytes present in the donor tissue which will express different MHC antigens from the host), which permitted presentation of a wide range of peptides to the host, thus leading to a polyclonal T-cell expansion. Damage is believed to be the result of alloantigen-specific CD8+ cytotoxic T cells recognizing MHC antigens on the donor tissue. The number of mismatches on the MHC antigens between the donor and host determines the rapidity and acuteness of the graft rejection. Mismatching at the minor alloantigen loci is considered to be the cause of chronic rejection, while accelerated rejection occurs predominantly between xenogeneic grafts or in individuals who have been sensitized to the donor, e.g. via previous blood transfusion. Disparities and MHC loci are determined by the mixed leucocyte response, an *in vitro* test in which leucocytes derived from one individual (donor) are mixed with those from another individual (host) and the proliferation of the leucocytes determined by incorporation of radioactive thymidine. The donor leucocytes may be irradiated to prevent them from proliferating so that any response is the result of antigen presentation to host T cells. If the number of MHC disparities between the host and the donor is large there is a correspondingly high proliferative response.

Thus, in most types of organ transplantation, donor leucocytes, particularly dendritic cells, are considered to play a part in the recognition of alloantigen via the 'direct' route of allosensitization as described above. However, in recent years the possible contribution of sensitization to alloantigens via the indirect route has assumed greater importance and involvement of CD4+ T cells in tissue damage in addition to or separately from CD8+ T cells has been recognized. The indirect route of allosensitization involves host MHC class II on antigen-presenting cells, which present donor peptides to the host T cells, i.e. donor antigen-presenting cells (leucocytes) are not involved in the process. More recently it has been recognized that many types of chronic rejection are the result of the indirect route of antigen presentation. It is important to remember that donor MHC molecules can also act as antigens and so donor peptides may actually be MHC antigens which have been processed and presented by host APCs via the indirect pathway.

Corneal transplantation differs from other forms of skin and solid organ transplantation in that donor leucocytes from the grafted tissue are few in number and are generally not equipped to activate the host T cells directly. The indirect route of allosensitization must therefore operate at least in the initiation of the response, although theoretically it is possible that the direct route may play a part in later events if antigen presentation on non-professional cells is a realistic possibility.

Corneal transplantation differs from other types of transplants in several other important respects.

Acute rejection in human corneal grafts is reputedly less frequent than in other solid organ grafts even when no attempt has been made to match the grafts at MHC loci, unless the host site is 'high risk' (this usually correlates with the level of original damage to the host cornea, e.g. herpetic infection). There is also a significant incidence of late 'graft failure' in which the endothelium decompensates and is replaced by a fibrous retrocorneal membrane; this has similarities to chronic graft rejection in other tissues. Hyperacute corneal graft rejection is not normally recognized as an entity.

The role of other cells in graft rejection is also increasingly being recognized. Th cells, especially Th1 cells, almost certainly have a role via CD40–CD40L interactions and may perhaps involve cross-presentation of antigen. In addition, non-specific factors activating cells of the innate immune system such as macrophages are likely to play a significant role. Clinically, in corneal graft rejection it is well recognized that rejection can be triggered by an unrelated event such as herpes simplex virus infection in the graft or even by a simple procedure such as corneal suture removal. Presumably, non-specific activation of macrophages and dendritic cells via CD40 upregulation is sufficient to lead to activation of previously primed or memory T cells leading to rejection.

Finally, rejection of xenografts (initially performed in cornea) is mediated by preformed antibody and generates hyperacute rejection, induced through failure of complement regulatory protein over species barriers.

TUMOURS INDUCE IMMUNE RESPONSES

Clinicopathological studies have long indicated that tumours induce some form of immune response in the host. This is based mainly on observations of T-cell, macrophage and NK cell infiltration of tumours independent of whether there is any inflammatory response or tissue necrosis. Experimental studies of chemically induced tumours have also shown that transplantation of resected tumours to the original host, or to a host previously sensitized to tumour antigens, leads to rapid rejection of the tumour, but not when the tumour is transplanted to a syngeneic naïve host. Rejection is tumour specific. Thus tumours possess specific antigens and these induce an MHC class I-restricted T-cell cytotoxic response.

Tumour antigens may be tumour specific, i.e. only expressed on that tumour, or they may be tumour associated in which case they are also expressed on normal cells. Most tumour antigens are identified in transplantation-type experiments such as that described above in which cloned cytotoxic T cells are generated. This allows identification of the tumour-derived peptides and the genes that regulate their expression in the tumour. Tumour antigens are believed to be recognizable by cytotoxic T cells in this manner owing to antigenic mutation that converts the normal self protein, which would induce tolerance, to a non-self protein, which is recognized as foreign and induces immunity. Thus some tumour antigens are products of normal cells such as tyrosinase in melanoma cells. However, many tumour antigens are produced by oncogenes, genes which are implicated in the cell cycle and in cell differentiation, These include *p21 ras*, *HER-2/neu*, the very important *p53* gene and others not normally expressed on cells, such as the MAGE series of proteins expressed by melanoma cells including cells of the choroid. Several viral genes may also be expressed in tumours including those for the SV40 T antigen, the human papillomavirus E6 gene and the EBV antigen. Certain B-cell tumours are indirectly linked to EBV genes particularly in the presence of immunodeficiency and appear to involve the translocation of the *myc* oncogene to the immunoglobulin locus. Retroviruses also have the potential to induce malignant transformation of normal cells including the *src*, the *myc* and the *k-ras* gene. The human T-cell lymphotropic virus-I gene is also implicated in certain aggressive T-cell tumours and interestingly is also involved in some forms of intraocular inflammation (uveitis).

Certain tumour antigens are recognized by antibodies as well as by cytotoxic T-cell lines. These include the oncofetal antigens, carcinoembryonic antigen and α-fetoprotein. Other tumour-associated antigens are linked to tumours such as the surface glycoprotein MUC-1 in breast cancer, S-100 in neural crest cell tumours and malignant melanoma, and cytokeratins in epithelial cell tumours.

Immune cells infiltrating tumour are considered to be effector cells against the tumour at least in some instances. Indeed the process of immune surveillance in which T cells and antigen-presenting cells migrate through the tissues detecting altered self antigens applies particularly to tumours and is necessary for the initiation of the antitumour response. Tumour-infiltrating lymphocytes (TIL) include both CD4+ and CD8+ cytotoxic cells and the former probably supply essential cytokines to the latter to promote tumour-killing ability. Some tumours aberrantly express MHC class II antigens plus costimulatory molecules; they may directly present tumour antigens to CD4+ T cells and initiate the immune response *in situ*.

NK cells may also be important in killing tumours, particularly those that have been induced by viruses. IL-2-activated NK (lymphokine-activated killer, LAK) cells have a markedly enhanced ability to lyse tumour cells and they are in trials as immunotherapeutic agents. Macrophages are also important in tumour killing usually via release of TNF-α, a cytokine that was first identified by its ability to induce necrosis in tumours. Tumour cells appear to be unable to synthesize superoxide dismutase which is required to protect cells from the TNF-α-induced release of cytotoxic superoxide free radical.

Despite the variety of mechanisms for tumour killing, many tumours evade death. Tumours utilize a variety of strategies, e.g. they downregulate MHC class I thus inhibiting cytotoxic T-cell killing; they may not express costimulatory molecules necessary for T-cell activation; they may secrete immunosuppressive cytokines such as TGF-β; tolerance to tumour cells may occur if the tumour antigen is expressed during the neonatal period; antigenic modulation of the tumour may occur if the antigen binds non-complement binding antibody; or the tumour antigen may be prevented from gaining access to the immune system by a dense glycocalyx on the cell surface. The immune response to tumours is more likely to be modulated by any or some of these mechanisms, thus explaining why tumour immunity is imperfect and cancer remains a major cause of death.

The recent explosion of knowledge concerning antigen presentation has led to the suggestion that tumours evade the immune system by promoting tolerance rather than immunity. Accordingly, intensive research is now ongoing in attempts to induce antitumour immunity by 'vaccinating' patients with mature dendritic cells loaded with tumour-specific antigens. The main difficulty with this approach is identifying peptides specific for the tumour that are sufficiently immunogenic.

THE EYE AND THE IMMUNE SYSTEM

The eye participates in all aspects of immune responses like any other tissue, but the immune response is modulated by the cells and tissues of the eye. In this respect the eye (and the brain) are regarded as immunologically privileged (see Introduction). Both the innate and acquired immune systems function in ocular defence mechanisms.

THE INNATE IMMUNE SYSTEM AND THE EYE

Reference has already been made to the several physical and chemical barriers to ocular infection included in the blink reflex, the lids, and the components in the tears such as lysozyme, lactoferrin and complement (see also Ch. 4). Lysozyme is effective against Gram-negative bacteria and certain fungi but is ineffective against Gram-positive organisms such as *Staphylococcus aureus*. Lactoferrin and transferrin, however, are more effective in defence against Gram-positive bacteria because they bind iron, an essential cofactor for eukaryotic as well as prokaryotic cell growth. In addition, tears have specific anti-adhesive properties for bacteria and therefore inhibit bacterial attachment and invasion of the ocular surface, and are incidentally important for prevention of contact lens contamination.

Tears also contain polymorphonuclear leucocytes (PMNs), which increase in number when the lids are closed for prolonged periods, e.g. during sleep. The anti-adhesive properties of tears extend to these cells, ensuring that they pass through the lacrimal passages and do not penetrate the corneal surface. Many of these leucocytes pass directly from the conjunctival vessels through the epithelial layers into the tear film. PMNs contain numerous antibacterial protein enzymes, including proteinase 3, myeloperoxidase (which generates free radicals), calprotectin, β-lysin and the cathepsins.

Tear lipid also has an antibacterial effect. This applies to both short- and long-chain fatty acids, the former affecting surface properties of the bacterial cell membrane and the latter having a direct effect on metabolism.

THE ACQUIRED IMMUNE SYSTEM AND THE FIRST LINE OF DEFENCE IN THE EYE

Tears contain immunoglobulins such as IgA (see Ch. 4) and occasional specific immune cells such as lymphocytes. IgA is produced by B cells in the lacrimal gland and secreted as sIgA in the tears. In addition, the lacrimal gland produces other immunosuppressive cytokines such as TGF-β. The TGF-β knockout mouse exhibits extensive ocular surface

pathology, indicating the importance of this cytokine in tears. The conjunctiva forms part of the mucosal immune system through which tolerance to environmental antigens may be induced (see p. 418). More importantly, the conjunctiva contains numerous dendritic cells (similar to Langerhans' cells in the skin) which act as APCs in the draining lymph nodes in the afferent limb of the immune response. It is thus possible to become sensitized to environmental antigens and allergens via the conjunctiva.

Conjunctival sensitization to environmental antigens is best demonstrated by the allergic response. The common antigens are pollens, housedust mite and animal dander (particularly cat dander). Although the effect is produced locally, the initial sensitization is a systemic one via mechanisms described previously (see pp. 393 and 423). This results in local conjunctival mast cells becoming loaded with antigen-specific IgE, which renders these cells acutely sensitive to re-exposure to antigen. In addition, the sensitization is long lived and can lead to chronic inflammation if repeated frequent degranulation episodes occur (see above). Thus seasonal allergic conjunctivitis can progress to perennial conjunctivitis and, in atopic individuals, may manifest as severe atopic conjunctivitis and/or vernal keratoconjunctivitis. Much of the damage in vernal keratoconjunctivitis is thought to be induced by eosinophils, because eosinophil cationic protein levels in tears are greatly increased in both atopic and vernal keratoconjunctivitis. In addition, different types of allergic conjunctivitis are associated with different patterns of cytokine production and Th cell patterns. Th2-like profiles are linked to vernal keratoconjunctivitis, while Th1 is associated with atopic keratoconjunctivitis. There may also be a defect in histaminase function in allergic eye disease causing prolonged histamine effects after mast cell degranulation.

The corneal surface also contains populations of intraepithelial and stromal leucocytes, some of which have the characteristics of dendritic APCs (Fig. 7.40). The role of these cells in protective immune responses is not clear but there is evidence that like the conjunctival cells they can capture antigen and transport it to the draining lymph node. In addition, they are likely to respond to cytokines produced by surrounding epithelial cells in response to Toll receptor engagement by common invading microorganisms such as herpes viruses and bacterial pathogens. This may be a direct effect of the pathogen; for instance, the obligate intracellular

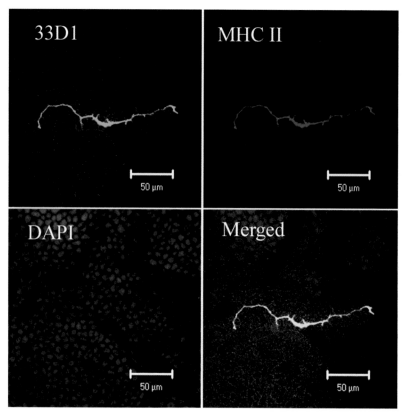

Fig. 7.40 Confocal microscope images of mouse corneal epithelium showing dendritic cells stained for MHC class II antigen with two different antibodies (MHC class II, red and 33DI green). The epithelial cells are stained blue (Dapy). The bottom right-hand image is a merged image of the other three panels.

parasite *Chlamydia*, which is the cause of the worldwide blinding disease trachoma, signals through TLR2 inside epithelial cells (Fig. 7.41). Indeed the possibility of regulating host : pathogen interactions has been tested in an experimental model of *Pseudomonas* keratitis in which 'silencing' of expression of TLR9 was achieved using small interfering RNA for this receptor.

PROGRESSIVE OCULAR SURFACE DISEASE

Certain other ocular surface diseases occur that do not appear to be allergic in nature but are considered to be immune mediated if not autoimmune in their pathogenesis. These include cicatrizing conjunctival disorders, various forms of 'melting' corneal disorders and a number of scleral and orbital inflammations.

Cicatrizing disease of the conjunctiva

Subconjunctival fibrosis occurs in certain rare disorders such as benign mucous membrane pemphigoid and the Stevens–Johnson syndrome. Both are considered to be autoimmune in nature by virtue of the detection of antibodies to basement membrane components. Pemphigoid is characterized by progressive cicatrization of the conjunctival stroma

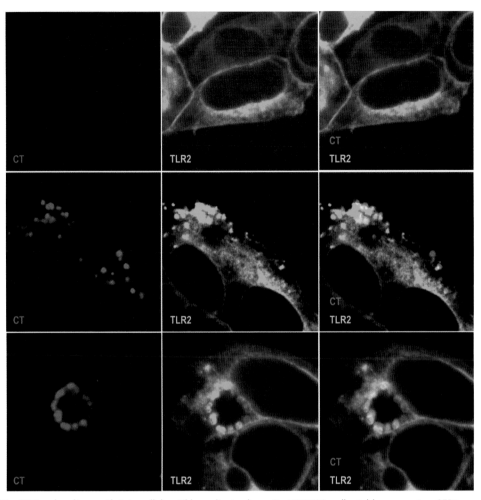

Fig. 7.41 TLR2 colocalizes with intracellular *Chlamydia trachomatis*. HEK293 cells stably expressing CFP-tagged TLR2 (green) were infected with *C. trachomatis*. Uninfected cells (top row) and infected cells at 16 hours (middle row) and 24 hours (bottom row) postinfection were stained using a monoclonal antibody against *Chlamydia* lipopolysaccharide. (From O'Connell *et al.* 2006, with permission from the American Society for Biochemistry and Molecular Biology.)

leading to severe shallowing of the fornices (see Ch. 9). In this condition, specific autoantibodies against conjunctival epithelial β_4 integrin, a component of the hemidesmosome (see Box 4.5, p. 186) have been identified. This is in contrast to bullous pemphigus, a skin disorder that does not affect the conjunctiva but is characterized by widespread areas of epithelial detachment, and in which antibodies against other proteins such as desmoglein and plectin may be detected. Dysregulation of TGF-β in conjunctival cells has been reported in ocular pemphigoid.

The Stevens–Johnson syndrome has similar appearances but is much more acute, although less progressive. This condition is normally associated with drug administration in which the drug is considered to act as a hapten. The severity of the condition is

431

limited in its effects by the degree and duration of exposure to the drug.

Keratitis and 'melting' corneal ulcers

Many forms of keratitis are considered to be immune mediated, including postherpetic disciform keratitis (see Ch. 9) in which residual herpes simplex virus antigen may play a role. In addition, certain debilitating corneal diseases characterized by peripheral corneal thinning and ulceration, sometimes leading to perforation, are possible candidates for classification as autoimmune disorders mainly because of their association with 'classic' autoimmune diseases such as rheumatoid arthritis and their lack of association with infective agents. In this condition reductions in T 'suppressor' cells have been reported as well as increases in B cells and anticorneal epithelial antibodies. Some forms of peripheral ulcer such as Mooren's ulcer (see Ch. 9) have been linked to a cornea-associated antigen, calgranulin, also found in peripheral blood neutrophils and filarial nematodes. These disorders occur just distal to the source of corneal epithelial stem cells at the limbus, which suggests a defect at this level.

Inflammatory disorders of the orbit and sclera

While many inflammatory conditions of the sclera (scleritis) are considered to be autoimmune, or at least immune mediated, it is important to consider infectious aetiologies such as syphilis and other bacterial causes. Spontaneous (autoimmune) inflammatory disorders of the episcleral tissue and the sclera (episcleritis and scleritis) represent a type IV immunopathological disease with close association with rheumatoid arthritis and a similar pathogenesis. Rare histological studies have shown activated CD4+ T cells in the lesion in a perivascular location, in addition to macrophages. CD8+ T cells have also been demonstrated, but in fewer numbers. There is also a prominent vasculitic component to the disease with extensive necrosis of the scleral layers. Typical granulomatous lesions are a feature of this condition (nodular scleritis). However, not all of these lesions are T-cell-dominated because B-cell 'follicles' have been identified in some cases. In addition, increased matrix metalloproteinase activity has been detected in these lesions (e.g. collagenase and stromelysin).

Although the antigen for scleral inflammation has not been identified, it is presumed to be a component of the extracellular matrix such as dermatan sulphate proteoglycan or type 1 collagen. Scleritis

most commonly affects the anterior sclera but if it affects the posterior sclera it is more difficult to diagnose. In addition, it may be mistaken for a less well-defined group of orbital inflammatory disorders known as pseudotumour of the orbit, for which the aetiology remains obscure but which responds to systemic steroid therapy.

A specific form of pseudotumour known as orbital myositis, in which an acute inflammatory swelling of a single ocular muscle occurs, is particularly responsive to steroid therapy. The autoantigen in this disorder is assumed to be a component of the ocular muscle.

Swelling of the orbital muscles also occurs in dysthyroid eye disease, causing proptosis and exophthalmos, but in this condition all four muscles are involved. This disorder is closely linked to Graves' disease of the thyroid in which thyroid autoantigens such as thyroglobulin are implicated. Patients with dysthyroid eye disease have circulating lymphocytes that react with ocular muscle cell membrane antigens. However, thyroglobulin does not appear to be the important antigen for ocular muscle damage, and some other antigen such as the thyroid stimulating hormone receptor may be involved. Models of thyroid ophthalmyopathy using T cells sensitized to the thyroid stimulating hormone receptor have been reported. Immunological studies have shown that the T-cell infiltrate is almost exclusively Th1 in type with secretion of IL-2 and IFN-γ.

Inflammatory disease of the lacrimal gland may be primary (autoimmune) as in Sjögren syndrome or secondary as in sarcoidosis in which the aetiology is unknown. In both disorders there is a deficiency of tear secretion that produces a secondary keratoconjunctivitis (keratoconjunctivitis sicca or the dry eye syndrome), common in the elderly. Primary Sjögren syndrome involves other secretory glands such as the salivary glands and is characterized by specific autoantibodies against ribonucleoproteins (antiRo and antiLa) whose role in the pathogenesis of the condition is not clear. Biopsies of salivary gland tissue have shown a predominant T-cell infiltrate but with little evidence of T-cell activation (as evidenced by the lack of IL-2 receptors). In contrast, recent studies of conjunctival biopsies from patients with Sjögren syndrome have shown significant T-cell infiltrates with activation markers. In addition, extensive adhesion molecule expression has been detected in the lacrimal gland, not only on endothelial cells but also on the acinar epithelial cells. Both VCAM-1 and E selectin are upregulated on the endothelium, indicating that this chronic disease is in a state of persistent activation. Eventually these glands undergo involutionary atrophy.

The eye as a privileged site and corneal graft

The eye has been considered atypical immunologically since the first corneal graft in a human was attempted more than 100 years ago and was shown to survive longer than expected. However, the eye as an immunologically privileged site was not formally recognized until 1945 when the eminent immunologist Peter Medawar demonstrated tolerance to foreign antigens by the brain and eye. The basis for this phenomenon was attributed to the avascularity of the cornea and/or to the lack of lymphatic drainage for intraocular structures. However, it has been shown experimentally that, shortly after corneal grafting, cytotoxic T cells specific for corneal antigens can be detected in the circulation and appear to be generated in the secondary lymphoid tissues. The lack of ocular lymphatics therefore does not seem to militate against the development of antigen-specific immunity to antigens placed in the eye.

Despite this, immunological 'privilege' is a demonstrable phenomenon and a property of the intraocular compartments, because antigens and cells including some xenogeneic tumour cells appear to be well tolerated in the anterior chamber of the eye, and heterotopic grafts at other sites from the same donor are not rejected as might be expected. This has been termed anterior chamber-associated immune deviation (ACAID) and is a form of tolerance which itself requires an intact eye–spleen axis. The teleological significance of ACAID is unclear, unless it might be supposed that ocular antigens are not 'seen' by the thymus during development; T cells reactive against ocular antigens would not be deleted and escape of antigen from the eye in adulthood would induce a foreign (severe) -type antigen response. ACAID may reduce this risk. However, the discovery of the autoimmune regulator (AIRE) gene in the thymus, which also modulates ocular immune responses, would suggest that this explanation is untenable. ACAID appears to be mediated during the efferent arm of the immune response and has been attributed to cytokine release by cells within the eye, particularly the immunosuppressive cytokine TGF-β. Other possible mediators of ACAID include α melanocyte-stimulating hormone and vasoactive intestinal peptide. Similar immunosuppressive properties exist in the vitreous and subretinal space. In addition the RPE can be stimulated to release immunosuppressive or immunopotentiating cytokines, depending on the conditions. More recently, 'immunological privilege' in the eye has been attributed to the constitutive expression of FasL for instance on the endothelium of the cornea and on RPE cells, and may promote apoptosis of activated Fas-expressing T lymphocytes infiltrating the eye during inflammatory reaction. Fas–FasL interactions in the eye appear to involve IL-10. However, Fas–FasL interactions may also be pro-inflammatory.

ACAID-like mechanisms may extend to innate immunity and have implications for the ability of the eye to counteract microorganisms. Thus the eye appears to be the preferred site for certain parasites such as *Toxoplasma* and *Toxocara* (see Ch. 8) and intravenously injected fungi such as *Candida* may find a 'tolerant' environment within the retina and vitreous with disastrous effects on vision. In addition, certain viruses such as cytomegalovirus and herpes simplex can proliferate unchecked within the retina. While there is no direct evidence that this is a result of the less than optimal immune microenvironment within the eye, it is a possibility that remains to be tested.

Despite these properties of the intraocular compartments, bacterial infection during intraocular surgery is remarkably infrequent. This has been attributed in part to the direct bacteriostatic properties of the aqueous, which have been shown to inhibit bacterial growth *in vitro*. The nature of this activity is not known but several antibacterial proteins are present in the aqueous, including complement, immunoglobulin, defensins and β-lysin. In addition it is dependent on the size of the bacterial inoculum and the virulence of the organism (see Ch. 8).

Intraocular inflammation

A common cause of visual impairment is intraocular inflammation. This may be exogenous, in which the organism is clearly evident such as in bacterial endophthalmitis (see Ch. 9) or cytomegalovirus retinitis, or it may be endogenous, in which no causative organism can be found. Endogenous intraocular inflammation is termed uveitis and may affect the anterior segment (iridocyclitis, inflammation of the iris and ciliary body) or posterior segment (posterior uveitis). Posterior uveitis may take many clinical forms, such as multifocal choroiditis and retinal vasculitis.

Intraocular inflammation is thought to be immune mediated. Acute anterior uveitis has a strong

IMMUNOLOGY

association with HLA-B27 alloantigen in over 50% of cases and is linked to ankylosing spondylitis and low-grade enteric infection with organisms such as *Yersinia* and *Klebsiella*. Posterior uveitis is much less closely linked to MHC class I antigens, except for certain well-defined syndromes such as birdshot retinochoroidopathy (HLA-A29) and Behçet's retinal vasculitis (HLA-B51 in oriental and middle eastern races). Vogt–Koyanagi–Harada disease has been closely linked to HLA-DR4 (subtype DRB1 0405; see Box 7.15 and p. 4.11) and more recent studies suggest a similar association with sympathetic ophthalmia.

Posterior uveitis, however, has close similarity to certain experimental CD4+ T-cell-mediated uveoretinal inflammations (experimental autoimmune uveoretinitis) in which the autoantigens have been well defined. Most of these are derived from the outer retinal layers and include the visual protein rhodopsin. The relationship between EAU and clinical endogenous posterior uveitis is, however, tantalizingly tenuous because patients with these diseases do not have significantly raised levels of antibodies to retinal antigens, although they do manifest T-cell responses to these antigens. Most tests are insufficiently sensitive to demonstrate these effects. Clinical studies of aqueous and vitreous samples have also been relatively uninformative to date, although in certain diseases such as Fuch's heterochromic cyclitis high levels of CD8 T cells have been found. In addition, high concentrations of IL-6 and IL-8 have been detected in ocular fluid samples from patients with uveitis, and Fas–FasL interactions have been shown to be active in patients with acute anterior uveitis.

A major indicator that posterior uveitis is immune mediated is its clinical response to immunosuppressive agents such as cyclosporin A and, currently, several immunological approaches including anti-CD4 humanized monoclonal antibodies and oral tolerization schedules are being evaluated for their efficacy in this condition. Other immunosuppressive agents are now being used in a range of ocular inflammatory diseases including mycophenolate mofetil and FK506.

CONCLUSION

The eye and its several tissues may be involved in any of the immune responses described in this chapter, either as a primary target of attack (e.g. in disciform herpetic keratitis or toxoplasmic choroiditis) or as part of a generalized immune disorder such as in Wegener's granulomatosis or sarcoidosis. The pathological processes and the mechanisms of initiation of immune responses are fundamentally similar from tissue to tissue. However, as stated in the Introduction, each tissue has its unique micro-environment and this undoubtedly plays a part in the final expression of the immune response.

FURTHER READING

Abbas AK, Lichtman AH. Basic Immunology, updated edn 2006–2007: with student consult access. Philadelphia: W. B. Saunders Co. Ltd; 2006.

Abbas AK, Lichtman AH, Pillai, S. Cellular and molecular immunology: with student consult online access, 6th edn. Philadelphia: W. B. Saunders Co. Ltd; 2006.

Baeuerle PA. Pro-inflammatory signaling: last pieces in the NF-kappaB puzzle? Curr Biol 1998; 8:R19–R22.

Colgan J, Rothman P. All in the family: IL-27 suppression of Th17 cells. Nature Immunol 2006; 7:899.

Forrester JV, Lumsden L, Duncan L, Dick AD. Choroidal dendritic cells require activation to present antigen and resident choroidal macrophages potentiate this response. Br J Ophthalmol 2005; 89:369–377.

Hancock WW, Gao W, Faia KL, Csizmadia V. Chemokines and their receptors in allograft rejection. Curr Opin Immunol 2002; 12:511–516.

Janeway CA Jr, Medzhito R. Innate immune recognition. Annu Rev Immunol 2002; 20:197–216.

Jerne NK. Idiotype networks and other preconceived ideas. Immunol Rev 1984; 79:5–24.

Kawai T, Akira S. Innate immune recognition of viral infection. Nature Immunol 2006; 7:131–137.

Mak TW, Saunders M. The immune response: basic and clinical principles. Amsterdam: Elsevier Academic Press; 2006.

Matsuda JL, Kronenberg M. Presentation of self and microbial lipids by CD1 molecules. Curr Opin Immunol 2001; 13:19–25

O'Connell CM, Ionova IA, Quayle AJ, Visintin A, Ingalls RR. Localization of TLR2 and MyD88 to *Chlamydia trachomatis* inclusions. J Biol Chem 2006; 281:1652–1659.

Pulvermüller A, Schröder K, Fischer T, Hofmann KP. Interactions of metarhodopsin II: arrestin peptides compete with arrestin and transducin. J Biol Chem 2000; 275:37679–37685.

Ramana CV, Gil MP, Schreiber RD, Stark GR. Stat1-dependent and -independent pathways in IFN-gamma-dependent signaling. Trends Immunol 2002; 23:96–101.

Roitt IM, Martin SJ, Delves PJ, Burton D. Roitt's essential immunology (Essentials). Oxford: Blackwell Publishing; 2006.

Rudolph MG, Wilson IA. The specificity of TCR/pMHC interaction. Curr Opin Immunol 2002; 14:52–65.

Yeung RS, Ohashi P, Mak TW. T cell development. In: Ochs HD, Edward-Smith CI, Puck JM, eds. Primary immunodeficiency diseases: a molecular and cellular approach. Oxford: Oxford University Press; 2006.

8 MICROBIOLOGY AND INFECTION

INTRODUCTION

In humans a pathogen is a microorganism that causes disease. Encounters between potential pathogens are frequent but in general we do not succumb to these insults easily. As to whether the invading pathogen is successful depends largely on the virulence of the microorganism, the dose of the infecting agent, and the ability of the host to combat such invasion.

The skin and mucous membranes always harbour a variety of microorganisms, which make up the resident flora. Their presence is not essential for the life of the host but they play an important role in maintaining normal health. This is certainly true of the organisms of the intestinal flora, which are required to synthesize vitamin K and aid the absorption of other nutrients (fat-soluble vitamins). Their presence also prevents colonization of mucous membranes and skin by pathogenic bacteria. In their normal site microorganisms do not produce disease but if introduced to a foreign site they may become pathogenic. Under what conditions and with what factors microbial virulence increases is still largely unknown. Ocular pathogens produce disease after gaining access to the otherwise healthy eye. On the other hand if ocular resistance is impaired then certain organisms, which under healthy conditions do not cause disease, for example opportunistic bacteria and fungi, will produce severe infection.

This chapter considers the basic biological, biochemical and pathogenic characteristics of pathogenic organisms. In addition, a brief overview of methods of diagnosis and a brief summary of agents used to combat infectious disease are given.

HOST DEFENCE MECHANISMS AND BACTERIAL PATHOGENICITY

The degree of inflammation evoked by infection is dependent not only on the pathogenicity and virulence of the invading organism but also on the host systemic and local tissue responses (which include both acute and chronic inflammatory changes and the immune response). Defence against invasion entrains both the *innate* and *acquired* immune responses (see Ch. 7) and the eye itself has a range of innate defence mechanisms.

BARRIER DEFENCES AND THE FIRST LINE OF ATTACK

Blinking
Blinking is a very effective cleansing mechanism. The lashes are also able to trap microbes, preventing access on to the globe. In addition, the lids contain sebaceous glands that secrete lactic acid and fatty acids in a low pH environment, which has a direct inhibitory effect on bacterial replication.

Tears contain many antimicrobial compounds
The tear film is at neutral pH and constant blinking acts as a mechanical barrier against infection. Lactoferrin, lysozyme, β-lysin, secretory immunoglobulin A (IgA), IgG and complement are all present within the tear film, protecting against bacterial invasion (see Ch. 7). Protection is also afforded by tear leucocytes, which in particular increase in numbers when the eyelids are closed.

The integument–cornea and conjunctiva act like the 'skin of the eye'
The conjunctiva normally has a commensal population of bacteria preventing colonization with pathogenic bacteria. These include, diphtheroids, *Moraxella* spp., staphylococci and streptococci. However, once colonization with pathogens occurs an acute inflammatory response ensues with hyperaemia and infiltration of the conjunctiva with leucocytes. Leucocytic infiltration and vascular ingrowth of the cornea may also occur (see Ch. 9). The bacteria/organisms gain access to this layer.

HOST IMMUNITY TO INFECTION

The concentration of several serum proteins, known as *acute-phase proteins*, increases during infection. *C-reactive protein* is an acute-phase protein, so called because of its ability to bind to the C-protein of pneumococci. The binding of C-reactive protein to bacterial cell walls promotes binding of complement and thus further enhances phagocytosis. Complement (see Ch. 7) is a group of about 20 serum proteins, some of which are also classified as acute-phase proteins. Bacterial lipopolysaccharides (derived from their cell wall) can activate the properdin system and alternative complement pathway. The consequence of complement activation includes increased phagocytosis, chemotaxis (activating further phagocytes), increasing both blood flow and vascular permeability, and finally lysis of infected cells, viruses and bacteria. Interferons α, β and γ are a group of proteins produced by a variety of cells that increase in infection and induce a state of antiviral resistance to uninfected tissue cells. They are produced early in infection and are the first line of resistance against viral infection.

Bacteria
The cell walls of most bacteria have adjuvant properties (an adjuvant being a substance that enhances the immune response to an antigen), and are able to activate complement, macrophages, polyclonal B cells and T cells, and also facilitate the processing of antigen by professional antigen-presenting cells (see Ch. 7). Hence, in response to an antigenic load of bacteria, both humoral and cell-mediated immune responses are initiated.

Role of antibody
Antibodies have many antibacterial roles. They can trigger complement-mediated damage to the outer lipid layers of the cell wall of Gram-negative bacteria, bind to capsular proteins (acting as opsonins), thus facilitating phagocytosis, and bind to toxins released by bacteria, neutralizing their toxic effect and preventing bacterial invasion through the tissues. For example, group A streptococci have receptors for epithelial surfaces that can be blocked by an antibody, and the streptococcal M proteins or the capsular proteins of *Meningococcus* spp., which inhibit phagocytosis, can also be neutralized by antibody.

Killing mechanisms
A number of microbial products cause activation of phagocytosis (monocytes and macrophages). These products are generally derived from bacterial cell walls and include endotoxin (lipopolysaccharide) from Gram-negative bacteria and muramyl dipeptide from bacterial peptidoglycans in the cell wall (see p. 438). Ultimately almost all bacteria are killed

by phagocytes as a result of chemotaxis; this attracts the phagocytes, the bacteria become attached to the phagocyte cell surface (lectin adhesion binding; see Ch. 7) and then are internalized into the cell. Principally there are two major pathways to kill bacteria – oxygen-dependent and non-oxygen-dependent. The former requires the production of oxygen intermediates, generated by enzymes, for example myeloperoxidases and cytochrome oxidase enzymes (see Ch. 4). Non-oxygen-dependent mechanisms are generated within the lysosome in an acidic environment. Examples include lactoferrin-mediated (neutrophil) killing. Lactoferrin is released by neutrophils and its activity is blocked in the presence of iron, which binds the lactoferrin rendering it unavailable to bacteria even at an acidic pH. Macrophages are also activated by lymphokine secretion from activated T cells, particularly interferon-γ, granulocyte–macrophage colony-stimulating factor, and tumour necrosis factor.

Viruses

A typical viral infection starts with local invasion of epithelial surfaces, followed by a viraemic phase and infection of the target organ. Both humoral and cell-mediated responses to viruses occur through recognition of specific antigens on the virus or virally infected cell. Viral antigens (coded for by the viral genome) are glycoproteins, usually glycosylated by the host cell during budding (see p. 444). Antigens expressed on the virion or infected cell surface may be potential targets for the immune response.

Role of antibody

Antibodies may prevent virus–cell interactions that lead to absorption and penetration of the host cell and viral replication. However, antibodies neutralize some components of viral surfaces more effectively than others (e.g. the haemagglutinin and neuraminidase components of influenza virus). Also the additional effect of complement assists neutralization and lysis of virus-infected cells. Antibodies that coat the virus-infected cells may induce antibody-dependent cell-mediated cytotoxicity by the binding of phagocytes to the Fc part of the antibody (see Ch. 7).

Cell-mediated immunity and lymphokines

Although viruses can induce specific T-cell responses (both CD4$^+$ and CD8$^+$ T lymphocytes), this does not necessarily confer protective immunity to the virus. Certainly, interferons have pronounced antiviral effects, which are also seen with other cytokines (see Box 8.2).

Although all of these mechanisms exist to enhance immunity to microorganisms, they also serve to increase both the pathogenicity and virulence of the invading organism. For example, the consequence of complement activation and the subsequent liberation of vasoactive amines and infiltration of the tissue with phagocytic cells may be destruction of the tissues before any protective immune response is mounted. Also, in an attempt to combat the infection the potential reparative local and systemic responses of the host tissue may serve only to cause considerable ocular damage and visual loss. This is particularly seen with bacterial endophthalmitis, which develops rapidly because of the virulence of the infecting microbe and the immune response elicited. On the other hand, tissue damage may be directly related to the cytopathic effect of the organism, for example toxoplasmosis and herpes viral retinitis (see Ch. 9).

BACTERIAL PATHOGENICITY

The human body has an abundant commensal population of bacteria that live in symbiosis with the host. All bacteria are potentially pathogenic, and pathogenicity is a relative term that depends on the integrity of host defences. Host resistance may be impaired systemically or locally, for example when access is gained to the eye and adnexae, in an otherwise healthy individual. Such infections are referred to as opportunistic and are becoming increasingly important with the spread of diseases such as acquired immune deficiency syndrome (AIDS) in which the immune system is defective. In contrast, true pathogens are organisms that can produce disease in the healthy individual and within normal environmental conditions.

How do bacteria cause disease?

Pathogenicity denotes the ability of microorganisms to cause disease, whereas *virulence* of the organism denotes the degree of pathogenicity of each individual organism. The pathogenicity of bacteria depends on several factors, including their capability to withstand unsuitable environmental conditions and whether the organism is transmissible to the human host. Bacteria display considerable variability in their ability to breach the natural defence mechanisms of the body and invade the tissues. Tissue invasion may occur via the direct cytotoxic action of the microbial activity or, more commonly, via the release of toxins. Toxins released by bacteria are usually subdivided into exotoxins and endotoxins. In addition, certain bacteria produce substances that are not directly toxic but that do facilitate spread of the organism through the host tissues at the site of

inoculation. These include, for example, the following group of enzymes:

- *Collagenase* – usually released by bacilli; allows spread by disruption of collagen in connective tissue.
- *Coagulase* – facilitates the deposition of fibrin and coagulates plasma. Fibrin coats the bacteria and thus defends against the host response.
- *Hyaluronidase* – this enzyme hydrolyses hyaluronate in the extracellular matrix of connective tissue. This in turn aids the spread of the organism through the tissue. (This property is used by ophthalmologists when administering local anaesthesia.)
- *Streptokinase* – this enzyme activates fibrinolysin, converting plasminogen to plasmin, which dissolves fibrin clots and facilitates spread through tissues (enzyme produced most frequently by haemolytic streptococci).
- *Leukocidins* – bacteria (e.g. group A haemolytic streptococci) can produce enzymes that *lyse* red blood cells and tissue cells. Such enzymes include streptolysin O.

Toxins

Exotoxin

Exotoxins (Fig. 8.1) are proteins liberated from bacteria (usually Gram-positive bacteria) and may produce specific effects at sites distant from the primary inflammatory response (e.g. *Clostridium botulinum*). They are antigenic and readily destroyed by heat. These proteinaceous toxins have molecular weights from 50 to 150 000 kDa, and can be converted to non-toxic products that may alternatively be used to confer immunity against the pathogenic bacteria (e.g. *Tetanus* toxoid). Exotoxins are extremely potent, and their effect is usually measured in terms of the minimum lethal dose – the smallest amount of toxin required to kill a guinea-pig within 4 days of subcutaneous inoculation.

Endotoxins

Endotoxins are lipopolysaccharides derived from the cell wall component of lysed or dead Gram-negative bacteria upon autolysis. Unlike exotoxins they are heat stable. The molecular weight of these molecules ranges between 100 and 900 kDa. Although antigenically distinct, all endotoxins have a similar core structure, which is reflected in their similar effects (Fig. 8.1). Systemic and immunological effects of endotoxin include:

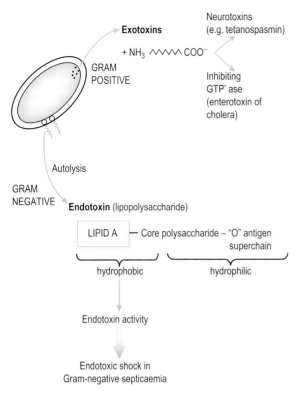

Fig. 8.1 Bacterial toxins.

Box 8.3 Exotoxins and endotoxins	
Exotoxins	**Endotoxins**
Excreted proteins	Lipopolysaccharide liberated after autolysis
Highly toxic	Need large doses to be toxic
Antigenic/promote	Non-antigenic antibody production
Heat labile	Relatively stable

- *Fever* – injection of endotoxin in humans produces fever after 30 minutes. A second more prolonged fever occurs secondary to the release of endogenous pyrogen.
- *Tolerance* – repeated daily doses of toxin result in a cessation of the febrile response. This occurs as a result of antibody production and active removal of antibody/endotoxin complexes by the reticuloendothelial system.
- *Lethal shock* – endotoxic shock occurs after large doses of toxin and is similar to, if not compounded by, profound septicaemia.
- *Schwartzman phenomenon* – 24 hours after endotoxin is injected intradermally, a second-day intravenous injection of endotoxin produces profound haemorrhagic necrosis at the injection site, with endothelial cell damage, platelet aggregation and thrombosis. This reaction is accompanied by similar systemic pathological changes causing widespread intravascular coagulation, particularly in the lungs and kidneys.
- *Induction of complement* – endotoxin may itself activate the alternative (properdin) complement pathway (see Ch. 7), causing direct cell damage and activating a further inflammatory response.

In Gram-negative septicaemia, the major effect and morbidity is the result of endotoxaemia. Besides attempted eradication of the bacterium with sensitive antimicrobial therapy, newer therapies that include using genetically engineered humanized monoclonal antibodies directed against both endotoxin (core determinant) and tumour necrosis factor-α have been investigated clinically with mixed success. *Superantigens* are products of minor lymphocyte-stimulating genes (see Ch. 7) and cause polyclonal stimulation of T cells. They are generally coded for by retroviruses and are mentioned here because of their phenotypic relationship with endotoxins released by pathogenic bacteria, for example *Mycoplasma arthritides* T-cell mitogen. Other types of superantigens are derived from bacteria, e.g. the staphylococcal M protein.

There are many other intrinsic microbial factors that increase the pathogenicity of the organism, and these include bacterial evasion of host-killing mechanisms and the ability of the microbe to survive outside the host environment (e.g. in vectors). For instance, because bacterial proliferation occurs predominantly within the host, survival of the bacterial species outside the host may be dependent on its spore-forming capabilities and these include the production of spores by Gram-positive bacteria, and the ability to weather adverse environmental conditions and increase the spread of these organisms. Bacterial spores contain an outer coat, a cortex and a core with a chromatinic nucleus. When conditions are favourable again, the spore germinates to form a vegetative cell, and replication begins. Some bacteria replicate outside the host, for example *Salmonella* which can multiply in food and *Pseudomonas* which has been found growing in contaminated eye-drop formulations; these bacteria have been implicated in the causation of bacterial keratitis. Other methods of evading host-killing are employed, for instance *Pneumococcus* has a capsular coat that resists phagocytosis and *Bacillus* species and acid-fast tubercle bacilli produce enzymes designed to resist superoxide destruction after ingestion (see

Box 8.4 Pathogenicity of bacteria

Bacteria avoid complement-mediated damage by:

- Having outer capsules preventing complement activation
- Altering their outer surface so that complement receptors on phagocytes cannot gain access
- Producing enzymes that degrade complement
- Preventing the insertion of the membrane attack complex (see Ch. 7)
- Secreting proteins (decoy proteins) that cause complement to be deposited on them and not on the bacterium itself.

Box 8.4). Transmissibility of infectious agents is very much increased when the microbial agent is able to survive in other hosts, often without causing disease, and then inoculation of the primary host may occur by vector transmission of these agents, such as the deer tick (*Ixodes scapularis*) and *Borrelia burgdorferi*, giving rise to Lyme disease. The mechanisms of pathogenicity leading to pyogenic and chronic infections are described in Chapter 9.

BACTERIA

Bacteria form heterogeneous groups of unicellular, prokaryotic (cells without nuclear membranes) organisms. Their diameter is usually around 1 μm and under the light microscope they are morphologically categorized as cocci (round) and bacilli (cylindrical). Further morphological subdivisions into fusiform bacilli (tapered at both ends), filamentous (long threads) and vibrios (spiral) are also made. Other particular features of bacteria, which relate to their degree of pathogenicity, include the presence of a cell wall capsule, which consists of polysaccharide and is a feature of Gram-positive bacteria. Spore formation, as mentioned above, occurs in adverse environmental conditions and is a feature of such genera as *Bacillus* and *Clostridium*. Flagella, which may be single or multiple, and pili (fimbriae) are features of many Gram-negative bacteria. Bacteria can be further classified with respect to their affinity for dyes (staining), culture requirements and bacterial reactions.

STAINING WITH DYES REFLECTS CELL WALL COMPOSITION

Gram stain
The Gram stain method is by far the most widely used stain and differentiates bacteria that resist

decolouration with acetone. The method involves first staining with crystal violet (blue–black), then iodine, followed by decolourizing with acetone, and finally counterstaining with carbol–fuchsin (red). Thus Gram-positive cell walls, which consist of predominantly mucopeptides, comprising *N*-acetylglucosamine and *N*-acetylmuramic acid, teichoic acids and mucopolysaccharides, resist decolouration with acetone and stain blue–black by this method. On the other hand, Gram-negative cell walls consist of three layers – a mucopolypeptide inner layer and outer layers of lipoproteins and lipopolysaccharides – which are susceptible to leaching of the stain with acetone (because of their lipid content) and can thus be counterstained with carbol–fuchsin.

Ziehl–Neelsen stain
This method stains acid-fast and alcohol-fast bacilli (e.g. *Mycobacterium*) that resist decolouration with acid and then alcohol. The bacterium is initially stained with carbol–fuchsin, heated gently, decolourized with acid and/or alcohol, and then counterstained with malachite green or methylene blue (modified or full Ziehl–Neelsen stain to detect *Nocardia* and *Mycobacterium* respectively).

There are several other special staining methods that assist in the differentiation of bacteria on microscopy, such as periodic acid–Schiff (PAS) stain and Gomori's methenamine silver stain, which are selective for fungal elements, such as hyphae. Also, acridine orange may be used to detect fungi and bacteria such as *Nocardia*. Similarly, immunofluorescent antibody techniques are used to detect antigenic determinants, particularly *Chlamydia* and the protozoan *Acanthamoeba*. The use of exfoliative cytology is useful in differentiating between non-infectious and infectious causes, particularly in external eye disease. For example, an eosin–methylene blue mixture (Hansel stain) is used for the rapid detection of eosinophils, whereas Giemsa-stained conjunctival scrapings are used both to detect bacteria and to identify the inflammatory cell component. Exfoliative cytopathology may lead to more information than Gram stains in cases of, for example, conjunctivitis of unknown aetiology.

BACTERIA CAN BE DIFFERENTIATED BY THEIR CULTURE REQUIREMENTS

Bacteria differ in their growth characteristics depending on which nutrient culture is used, the atmospheric (aerobic or anaerobic) conditions, and ambient temperatures. The following media are

Microbiological investigation of bacterial keratitis

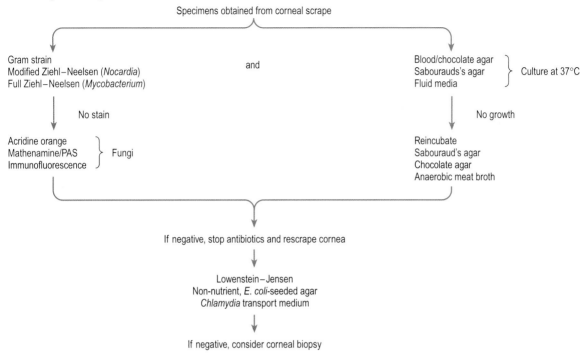

Fig. 8.2 Microbiological investigation of bacterial keratitis.

commonly used for bacterial and fungal culture in ophthalmic practice:

- *Solid media*
  - blood agar (nutrient agar, containing 5–20% horse blood)
  - chocolate agar (heated blood agar)
  - Lowenstein–Jensen medium (contains glycerol, malachite green and whole egg)
  - Sabouraud's agar (a fungal growth plate containing glucose, peptone and agar, enriched with yeast extract and chloramphenicol)
  - Theyer–Martin medium (selective, chemically enriched, chocolate agar)
  - Non-nutrient, *Escherichia coli*-enriched agar (for *Acanthamoeba* identification in cases of bacterial keratitis)
- *Fluid media* – many contain meat extract used to enrich media because of the protein degradation products, carbohydrates, inorganic salts and growth factors; e.g. Robertson's meat broth (nutrient broth with minced meat), brain–heart infusion broth and thioglycolate media.

Other environmental factors affecting growth include hydrogen ion concentration; most organisms have a fairly narrow optimal pH range (usually pH 6–8). On the other hand bacteria do differ as to the optimum temperature for growth, which can vary from 15–20°C to 50–60°C for thermophilic bacteria. Most organisms are mesophilic and grow best at 30–37°C. Figure 8.2 demonstrates a proposed microbiological investigatory algorithm for the isolation of pathogens in a common ophthalmological setting – bacterial keratitis (based on Ficker *et al.*, 1991).

GRAM-POSITIVE BACTERIA

Gram-positive cocci are the major aerobic flora of the outer eye.

Gram-positive cocci include *Staphylococcus* and *Streptococcus* species. *Staphylococcus aureus* and *Staphylococcus epidermidis*, the major aerobic flora of the outer eye, are spherical and occur predominantly as clusters but can also occur as short chains and pairs.

441

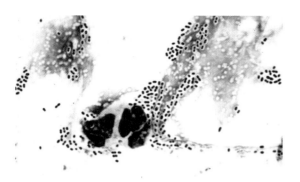

Fig. 8.3 Gram-stained preparation from a swab from a corneal ulcer demonstrating pneumococci and polymorphonuclear leucocytes (original magnification: ×300).

They are aerobic, non-motile and non-spore-forming. Both grow well on blood agar and are differentiated by their respective biochemical reactions, where *Staphylococcus aureus* has coagulase activity (coagulase positive). The virulence of *Staphylococcus aureus* is in part the result of the production of lipase, proteinase and hyaluronidase.

Streptococcus pneumoniae is encapsulated and occurs in pairs or short chains. These bacteria may be further serotyped according to the composition of the capsular polysaccharide. This species is aerobic, non-motile and capable of lysing red blood cells on agar, which is known as α-haemolysis. Because of the capsular coat, *S. pneumoniae* is relatively resistant to phagocytosis, promoting its pathogenicity (Fig. 8.3). *Streptococcus pyogenes* is spherical and occurs in pairs or short chains. Most strains are facultative anaerobes and grow well on enriched media at 37°C with 10% carbon dioxide.

Streptococci can be classified by their action on red blood cells and by biochemical tests, which will differentiate the various subgroups. Partial haemolysis (α-haemolysis) leads to a greenish discolouration on agar (partial lysis of erythrocytes), whereas complete haemolysis (β-haemolysis) leads to a colourless defined zone on agar. Pyogenic streptococci can be further classified by identification of the Lancefield group antigens of the polysaccharide coat. The most common pathogens in this group are Lancefield group A, β-haemolytic streptococci. More than 20 antigenic extracellular products are produced by group A streptococci. These include streptokinase, streptodornase (deoxyribonuclease), hyaluronidase, erythrogenic toxin (responsible for the rash in scarlet fever, and can be identified by intradermal injection

of erythrogenic toxin), diphosphopyridine nucleotidase and haemolysins.

Gram-positive rods

Gram-positive rods include the genera of *Bacillus*, *Clostridium*, *Corynebacterium* and *Propionibacterium*. Bacilli are large, rod-shaped, aerobic and spore forming. Clostridia are also spore forming but are anaerobic. Corynebacteria are aerobic but are not spore forming and exist as commensals on the skin and mucous membranes. Propionibacteria are not spore forming. *Propionibacterium acnes* is anaerobic and resides on the eyelids and within the meibomian glands, and is a recognized cause of chronic low-grade endophthalmitis following routine extracapsular cataract extraction and intraocular lens implantation. Infection with the other Gram-positive rods is very rare within the eye but extremely destructive, as can be seen with *Clostridium perfringens* (gas gangrene), which produces a particularly vicious suppurative panophthalmitis.

Gram-positive filaments

The actinomycetes are members of the order Actinomycetales. They are Gram-positive bacteria that are filamentous and grow in the form of a mycelial network similar to filamentous fungi. Unlike fungi, their hyphae are less than 1 μm in diameter and their cell wall does not contain chitin (a fibrous, tough, water-insoluble homopolysaccharide of β sheets of *N*-acetylglucosamine). The two genera that cause disease in humans are *Actinomyces* and *Nocardia*. *Actinomyces israelii* is a Gram-positive, non-spore-forming anaerobic bacterium producing filaments, diphtheroid and coccoid forms, often referred to as *streptothrix*. This species is a common cause of lacrimal canaliculitis and dacrocystitis. *Nocardia* spp. are branched filamentous aerobic actinomycetes. They are related to mycobacteria in that they are weakly acid-fast. *Nocardia asteroides* is the most frequent cause of nocardial keratitis and endophthalmitis. A full classification of Gram-positive bacteria is shown in Fig. 8.4.

GRAM-NEGATIVE BACTERIA

Gram-negative cocci and ophthalmia neonatorum

Neisseria species are aerobic, non-motile, Gram-negative cocci. They appear as pairs (diplococci) and grow well on enriched culture media with 10% carbon dioxide. *Neisseria gonorrhoeae* and *Neisseria meningitidis* are differentiated by the fermentation of carbohydrates: both organisms ferment glucose but

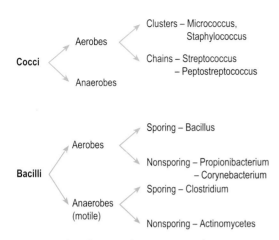

Fig. 8.4 Classification of Gram-positive bacteria.

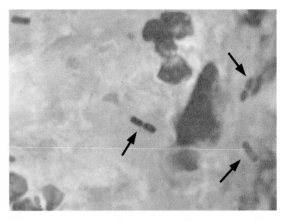

Fig. 8.5 Gram-stained preparation of a conjunctival swab to demonstrate *Moraxella* bacilli (arrows) (original magnification: × 1000).

the meningococci also ferment maltose. Both agglutinins and antibodies to meningococcus can be measured. Growth of *Gonococcus* is optimal on enriched chocolate media, for example Thayer–Martin medium. *Ophthalmia neonatorum* refers to any infection in the newborn (within 28 days of birth). In general this refers to conjunctival infection, chiefly gonococcal and chlamydial, that follows contamination of the eyes of the fetus during vaginal delivery. Rapid diagnosis to prevent blindness from corneal ulceration is obtained from examination of smears of pus from the conjunctiva, conjunctival and cervical scrapings, and cultures. Other causes include silver nitrate prophylaxis of gonococcal infection, staphylococci, pneumococci, *Haemophilus* and herpes simplex type II virus. The time of onset of the conjunctivitis may indicate the cause, as gonococcal disease is said to occur 2–3 days postpartum and chlamydial infection at days 5–7 postpartum. Treatment of both parents and child is with the appropriate sensitive systemic antibiotic: cephalosporin or penicillin for gonococcus; and erythromycin for chlamydial infection.

Gram-negative bacteria produce devastating endophthalmitis

Pseudomonas, Haemophilus, enterobacteria and *Brucella* are all examples of Gram-negative rods. *Pseudomonas aeruginosa* is aerobic, non-motile, and difficult to distinguish from enterobacteria. This group of bacteria produces a water-soluble green pigment, pyocin, that diffuses through medium. Different strains of *Pseudomonas* have been identified by bacteriophage typing and by the different pyocins they produce. This organism is highly viru-

lent because of the copious amounts of enzymes it releases. These not only facilitate tissue destruction, but also act via the production of β-lactamase, negating the effects of most antimicrobial agents. *Haemophilus* is a small, non-motile, non-spore-forming, aerobic bacterium and requires either, or sometimes both, X factor (haematin) and V factor (diphosphopyridine nucleotide) for growth. *Haemophilus influenzae* (Pfeiffer's bacillus) is a small coccus that occurs in small chains and is best cultured on brain–heart infusion agar or chocolate agar. When encapsulated (serotypes A–F) with a polysaccharide coat, *H. influenzae* becomes more virulent and invasive. This bacterium in either its capsulated or non-capsulated form is a common cause of upper respiratory tract infections, particularly in chronic obstructive airway disease. It can also cause sinusitis, and with direct spread through the thin orbital walls may give rise to orbital cellulitis. Haematogenous spread to the globe may give rise to metastatic endophthalmitis if the blood–aqueous barrier has been compromised, for example as a result of intraocular surgery. Non-encapsulated species include *H. egyptius* (Koch–Weeks bacillus) and *H. ducreyi*, the causative organism of chancroid and Parinaud's ocular glandular syndrome. *Moraxella* is a Gram-negative diplobacillus (square-ended coccus–bacillus), similar to *Haemophilus*, which may be grown from purulent conjunctival infections and may also cause corneal ulceration (Fig. 8.5).

Enterobacteria are small aerobic and facultative anaerobic Gram-negative rods found in the flora of the intestine. Within this family are the genera, *Escherichia, Proteus, Shigella, Salmonella, Klebsiella* and *Yersinia.* They are not normally pathogenic (except for *Shigella* and *Salmonella*, which produce dangerous enterotoxins), but are excellent opportunistic pathogens. For instance, *E. coli* is the commonest cause of urinary tract infection and is implicated along with other enterobacteria in both surgical and traumatic wound infections. They are motile with polar flagella, and grow well on MacConkey agar. Colonies may be identified by their biochemical reaction, fermenting glucose or lactose. Further identification can be made by looking for the presence of either somatic (cell wall) or flagellar antigens, or both. Strain identification can also be performed by bacteriophage and bacteriocidin typing. *Serratia marcescens* is an enteric organism that can contaminate contact lens solutions, and has been reported to cause both infective keratitis and endophthalmitis. Endophthalmitis is a devastating complication of intraocular surgery and penetrating trauma (with or without the presence of an intraocular foreign body, see Ch. 9). Inoculation of the eye with the organism may occur directly from the patient's own commensal flora, from hand–eye contact, from the surgery, or from metastatic spread commonly from the bowel or urinary tract (see Ch. 9). A vitreous biopsy must be performed and samples must be taken for cytological examination with Gram and Giemsa stains, and for culture on blood agar, chocolate agar and Sabouraud's agar so that the agent can be identified and its antibiotic sensitivity determined quickly. A similar microbiological approach to the investigation of endophthalmitis may be employed, as described for keratitis but the urgency is greater. Infections with *Klebsiella*, *Campylobacter* and *Yersinia* have been associated with HLA-B27 anterior uveitis, although the significance of this is still unclear (see Chs 7 and 9). Further classification of Gram-negative bacteria is summarized in Fig. 8.6.

SPIROCHAETES

Members of this family of microorganisms, which includes the genera *Borrelia*, *Treponema* and *Leptospira*, share many features in common with Gram-negative bacteria. Spirochaetes have a unique helical structure, with flagellate-type structures permitting a special type of spiral motility. *Borrelia* are large and Gram-negative, but are not easily visualized by light microscopy because they are too slender and too weakly refractile; they are best visualized by dark-ground microscopy. *Borrelia burgdorferi* is transferred through the intermediate host of the tick, *Ixodes ricinus* (the deer tick – endemic in deer populated areas), and causes Lyme disease (arthritis, con-

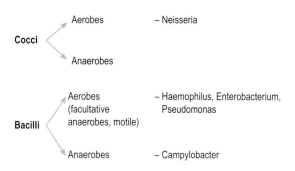

Fig. 8.6 Classification of Gram-negative bacteria.

junctivitis and encephalomyelitis). Lyme borreliosis is detected by immunofluorescent assay or enzyme-linked immunosorbent assay (ELISA) to measure specific IgM and IgG antibodies in the patient's sera. *Borrelia*-specific DNA has also been detected in aqueous or vitreal samples of patients with chronic intraocular inflammation by the polymerase chain reaction, but the relationship to infection is weak.

Treponema pallidum is a strict parasite that cannot survive outside the host. The spirochaetes may be visible under dark-ground microscopy or by silver staining (Levaditi silver method), but serology is the mainstay of diagnosis. Serological tests fall into two groups: the reagin tests (Venereal Diseases Research Laboratory) and complement fixation tests, both of which return to normal months after treatment. However, the tests lack specificity and false-positives do occur. Specific antibody tests, including *T. pallidum* immobilization and fluorescent treponemal antibody absorption (FTA-Abs), are now utilized in cases where the diagnosis is in doubt. The FTA-Abs is the first test to become positive in syphilis and usually remains positive after treatment.

ACID-FAST BACILLI

Mycobacteria are acid and alcohol fast (i.e. resist decolourization with acid or alcohol), aerobic, thin, straight rods. They cannot be stained by the Gram method and so the Ziehl–Neelsen stain is employed. These bacteria do not grow on ordinary media, and are cultured on special media, for example Lowenstein–Jensen medium, for several weeks. The two most important pathogenic species in humans are *Mycobacterium tuberculosis* and *Mycobacterium leprae* (*M. leprae* cannot be grown on artificial media). Some atypical mycobacteria, for example *M.*

avium and *M. fortuitum*, also cause ocular disease, including indolent corneal ulcers and endogenous endophthalmitis, particularly in the immunocompromised host (see section on AIDS, p. 450).

MOLLICUTES

Mollicutes are a class of microorganisms bounded by a membrane. Although they are bacteria, *Mycoplasma*, for example, are unique in that they lack cell walls. They resemble L-forms of bacteria (cell wall-deficient bacteria) but unlike them are independent, naturally occurring, microorganisms. Several pathogenic species exist within this class; these include *Mycoplasma pneumoniae*, *Mycoplasma hominis* and also *Ureaplasma urealytica*, which has been implicated in the aetiology of conjunctivitis and uveitis associated with Reiter syndrome. *Ureaplasma urealytica* is known as a T strain because of the minute colonies it forms on semisolid enriched medium, which grow best at pH 6 and produce urease (i.e. they ferment urea). Other strains of *Mycoplasma* stain poorly with the Gram stain, but may still be classified as Gram-negative. Mycoplasmas differ from bacteria in that their replication can be inhibited with antibody alone without the activation of complement.

SYNERGISTIC INFECTIONS

Synergism is where a combined action gives rise to a significantly greater effect than the sum of the two individual effects. In terms of bacterial pathogenicity, it appears that combinations of microorganisms potentiate the ability of each one to cause infection – *pathogenic synergy*. Under certain circumstances, for example after infection of epithelial surfaces with virus, the normal commensal bacterial population proliferates to a level where it induces inflammation. This synergy is seen in Vincent's ulcerative gingivostomatitis, which results from pathogenic synergy between herpes simplex virus and the normal commensal spirochaetes of the oral mucosa (*fusospirochaetes*) and anaerobic *Bacteroides* species. Such conditions of synergy may also exist in ocular infections. Herpes simplex keratitis may permit the normal commensal flora of the lids and conjunctival sac to infect the virus-laden epithelial cells and underlying corneal stroma, resulting in an associated microbial keratitis.

Different bacteria can also act synergistically. Bacterial synergistic gangrene occurs 1–2 weeks after abdominal or thoracic surgery and is caused by microaerophilic or anaerobic streptococci combined with *Staphylococcus aureus* or aerobic coliform bacilli. The surgical wound becomes swollen and tender, and central necrosis occurs, while the patient becomes systemically toxic. Similarly, Meleney's chronic undermining ulcer is a slowly progressive gangrene that occurs after surgery; the wound develops fissures and sinuses but the patient is not systemically toxic. Again this condition is caused by a synergy of streptococci and staphylococci. A summary of ocular pathogens is shown in Tables 8.1 and 8.2.

VIRUSES

Viruses are obligate intracellular parasites in that they can replicate only inside cells. The intracellular viral genome, which consists of either RNA or DNA, can direct the metabolic activity of the host cell, but outside the host cell viruses are metabolically inert and exist as inert particles of nucleic acid.

Table 8.1 Common ocular bacterial pathogens

Organism	Infection
Gram-positive cocci	
Staphylococcus aureus	Blepharoconjunctivitis
Staphylococcus epidermidis	Corneal abscess and postoperative endophthalmitis
Streptococcus pneumoniae	Corneal abscess/ conjunctivitis
Streptococcus pyogenes	
Gram-positive bacilli	
Propionibacterium	Postoperative endophthalmitis
	Chronic meibomitis
Gram-positive filaments	
Actinomyces	Canaliculitis, dacryocystitis
Nocardia	Corneal abscess/ endophthalmitis
Gram-negative bacteria	
Neisseria	Conjunctivitis/ endophthalmitis
Moraxella (Axenfeld's)	Conjunctivitis
Pseudomonas	Corneal abscess/ endophthalmitis
Haemophilus	Conjunctivitis/orbital cellulitis

445

Table 8.2 Rare ocular bacterial pathogens

Organism	Infection
Enterobacter	Corneal abscess Endophthalmitis
Francisella Yersinia	Ocular–glandular syndrome
Brucella	Uveitis (during recurrence stages of infection)
Spirochaetes	Uveitis, chorioretinitis
Borrelia	Conjunctivitis, uveitis, chorioretinitis, optic neuritis
Mycoplasma	Reiter syndrome

Box 8.5 Useful definitions in virology

Capsid – symmetrical protein shell enclosing genome
Capsomere – morphological unit seen on electron microscopy
Virion – complete infective viral particle (intact)
Envelope – lipoprotein membrane expressing both host and viral antigens

Classification of viruses is based on their constituent nucleic acid and further subdivided according to morphology. Viruses vary in size from 10 to 300 nm in diameter.

MORPHOLOGY

Capsomeres are the structural units (protein) seen on electron microscopy of viral particles (Fig. 8.7), forming the capsid, a symmetrical protein shell enclosing the nucleic acid core. A lipoprotein envelope expresses both host and viral antigen on its surface, and is present usually only on larger viruses. Capsid symmetry is described as cubic or icosahedral, when the sides are of equal length, or helical when the capsomeres are arranged around a spiral of nucleic acid. All these features may be useful in the diagnosis of viral disease when tissues are examined under electron microscopy.

Viruses contain DNA or RNA

Viruses are classified according to their nucleic acid content, which is either DNA (single or double stranded) or RNA. They may be further subdivided according to size and morphology as described

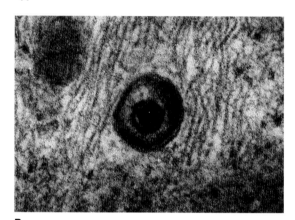

Herpes simplex virion

Fig. 8.7 Electron micrograph of herpes simplex virion.

above, immunogenic properties, methods of transmission, inclusion body formation and symptomatology. These features are discussed for each group of viruses below.

Viral inclusion bodies

Viruses can replicate in the nucleus or cytoplasm of the host cell. Either way, pronounced changes occur in the cell (see Ch. 9). The synthesized particles can occasionally be seen on light microscopy and are referred to as 'inclusion bodies'. Inclusion bodies represent sites of viral synthesis or replication. The site and appearance of these inclusion bodies can be diagnostic of a particular viral family. Examples of inclusion bodies are the intranuclear inclusions produced by DNA viruses. These bodies are surrounded by a clear halo and by the nuclear membrane. RNA viruses generally demonstrate cytoplasmic inclusions, which are smaller than the nuclear inclusions seen with DNA viral contamination. RNA viruses are eosinophilic if they are composed predominantly of viral protein and basophilic if they are composed of a high concentration of nucleic acid. Inclusions are well demonstrated in haematoxylin & eosin-stained tissue preparations. One of the herpes viruses, cytomegalovirus, produces both cytoplasmic and nuclear inclusions. The nuclear inclusions are referred to as 'owl's eye' inclusion bodies, in which enlargement of both the cytoplasm and the nucleus occurs, hence the virus's name (see Ch. 9).

DIAGNOSIS OF VIRAL DISEASE

Diagnosis of viral infection can be made by either direct isolation of the virus or using serological techniques for the detection of antigen or antibody responses. Serological tests of antigen expression in peripheral blood can be determined by immunofluorescence or by haemagglutination inhibition methods. Antibody responses can be detected by a rising titre from illness to convalescence by radioimmunoassay (RIA) or enzyme-linked immunosorbent assay and complement fixation tests. Tissue culture techniques with specific cell lines can permit isolation of the virus after *in vitro* replication. Using electron microscopy and light microscopy of tissue samples, the viral particles or inclusion bodies, which are discussed below, can then be visualized.

DETECTING INFECTIOUS AGENTS IN THE ABSENCE OF SUCCESSFUL CULTURE OR SEROLOGY

A new approach for the detection of infectious agents in ophthalmic disease is via the analysis of intraocular fluids or tissues using polymerase chain reaction (PCR; see Ch. 3). In addition, organism-specific humoral responses can be detected in ocular fluids and both these methods are becoming indispensable tools in the diagnosis of infectious intraocular inflammation. Goldmann and Witmer reported a method to calculate whether specific antimicrobial antibodies are being produced within tissues, which is highly supportive of local infection (see Box 8.6). There have been numerous reports on the detection of infectious agents in ocular fluids (for review see de Boer *et al.*, 1995), which include *Toxoplasma*, herpes virus and treponemal infections. A more sensitive and specific method of detecting infectious agents in cases of uncertain diagnosis may be obtained from tissue/fluid samples processed to determine viral DNA by producing multiple copies of the viral DNA present in the specimen using PCR technology. This technique is now almost routine as

***

Box 8.6 Local antibody production in the diagnosis of infectious intraocular inflammation

Goldmann–Witmer coefficient (C):

$$C = \frac{\dfrac{\text{Antibody tite in}}{\text{ocular fluid}}}{\dfrac{\text{Antibody titre in serum}}{}} \times \frac{\dfrac{\text{Total IgG in}}{\text{ocular fluid}}}{\dfrac{\text{Total IgG in serum}}{}}$$

When $C = 3$ then local antibody production is present. C can be compared between, for example, viruses. When comparing two coefficients C and C_1, the ratio is defined as positive when it is equal to 4.

***

the result of the expanding development of specific oligoprimers of viral DNA. PCR enables the detection of viral DNA in samples of vitreous and retina in cases of possible virus-induced posterior uveitis and retinal necrosis. In addition, with the expanding development of specific primers, particularly for bacterial and fungal pathogens, PCR is now being used as an aid to diagnosis of infective chronic endophthalmitis, such as that caused by *Propionibacterium acnes* following cataract surgery.

VIRUSES CAUSE DISEASE BY SUBTERFUGE

Viruses gain access to the body by infecting epithelium or epidermal cells. After a short incubation period they may cause a pathogenic effect at the initial site of entry (e.g. conjunctivitis). More commonly the initial contact produces no symptoms (i.e. it is subclinical), but after a longer incubation period of a few weeks a distant effect on a target organ via lymphatic, haematogenous, or neural spread of the virus develops. Many viruses then become dormant and never recur. However, such latent infection may become overt, especially in the immunocompromised host, when host defence mechanisms are significantly impaired. This is thought to be the mechanism of infection such as cytomegalovirus retinitis in patients with AIDS.

The host response to viral infection

An overview of the general aspects of host immunity to viral infection has been discussed on p. 438. More specifically, once the virus enters the cell by adhesion to cell surface receptors such as intercellular adhesion molecule 1 (ICAM-1) and integrins (which occur constitutively on retinal pigment epithelial cells; see Ch. 7), it rapidly loses its protein coat and integrates its nucleic acid into the normal DNA and RNA of the cell, which in turn perturbs the metabolism of the cell leading to cell dysfunction and death. Inflammation and tissue damage may be the result not only of direct viral cell damage but also of the host response during recovery from viral infection as a consequence of the host mobilizing antimicrobial immunity. There are many innate mechanisms to inhibit viral colonization, such as structural barriers that prevent the virus from invading the epithelial surface (for example, the stratified squamous epithelium of the skin, cilia in the respiratory tract, and acid in the stomach). Most viruses do not replicate well at the high temperatures present in the febrile patient (there are exceptions such as poliovirus), especially within the central nervous system. The host initiates a humoral response, which includes the production of antibody, complement, and interferon (see p. 436) and a cellular response involving T and B lymphocytes, macrophages and polymorphonuclear leucocytes (see Ch. 7). Viruses that cause local infection at epithelial surfaces, for example viral conjunctivitis, can produce recurrent disease through exogenous re-infection. The frequency and severity of the infection is dependent on the number of virions exposed to the epithelial surface.

Viruses can remain dormant within the host genome: the herpes virus

Latent infections are said to occur when not all virus has been eradicated from the tissues and it persists in a non-replicatory state within the cell. Endogenous re-infections occur typically in the herpes group of viruses. Infection with herpes simplex virus is characterized by a primary infection, which may be subclinical but still induces a cell-mediated and antibody response that can be detected serologically. The virus then becomes latent (not actively replicating) in the dorsal root ganglion cells of the nerve that supplies the site of the primary infection. The virus can at any time be reactivated, giving rise to recurrent clinical disease despite the presence of specific antiviral antibodies. In the presence of a disturbed immune system, such as the immunocompromised host, reactivated herpetic infection can be severe and may lead to death from pneumonia or meningoencephalitis. Ocular infection with herpes simplex type 1 virus can give rise to conjunctivitis, uveitis, uveoretinitis and keratitis. A culture or smear of the conjunctiva or cornea during these episodes demonstrates microscopic intraepithelial vesicles and contains syncytial giant cells and eosi-

Table 8.3 Classification of viruses in ocular disease

Virus	Infection
RNA viruses	
Orthovirus	
Influenza	Conjunctivitis
Paramxyovirus	
Mumps	Conjunctivitis/keratitis
Measles	Keratitis
Picornavirus	
Coxsackie	Conjunctivitis
Togavirus	
Rubella	Keratoconjunctivitis
Retrovirus	
HIV	Keratoconjunctivitis/ retinopathy
DNA viruses	
Herpes virus	
Zoster	Keratoconjunctivitis
Simplex 1 and 2	Uveitis/retinitis
Epstein–Barr	Conjunctivitis
CMV	Uveitis/retinitis
Adenovirus	
Serotype 3	Pharyngeal conjunctival fever
Serotype 8	Endemic keratoconjunctivitis
Serotype 1–11, 14–17	Conjunctivitis
Pox virus	
Vaccinia	Blepharoconjunctivitis
Molluscum contagiosum	Conjunctivitis

nophilic intranuclear inclusions, which assist in the diagnosis. However, corneal scrapings from patients with disciform keratitis (see Ch. 9) rarely yield virus.

OTHER VIRAL DISEASES (see Table 8.3)

Rubella

Rubella is an acute febrile illness characterized by a rash and lymphadenopathy (suboccipital). The virus is a 60-nm diameter RNA virus and forms by budding from the endoplasmic reticulum into intracytoplasmic vesicles. The virus releases haemagglutinin, which agglutinates red blood cells from 5-day-old chicks, thus forming the basis of the test. The virus can also be propagated *in vivo* but has no characteristic cytopathic effects. If rubella is contracted during the first trimester of pregnancy it can have devastating effects, ranging from mental retardation and severe abnormalities in the fetus, including ocular manifestations such as microphthalmos, nuclear cataract and 'salt and pepper' retinitis. The infectious virus may be detectable in ocular structures up to 3 years after birth. At present in the UK the majority of children are immunized with vaccine for rubella, incorporated into the triple vaccine MMR (measles, mumps and rubella) schedule. Also, as part of population screening, both preconceptual and antenatal assessments include testing for rubella antibody status in these women.

Adenovirus

The adenovirus group consists of over 30 antigenic types (serotypes). The virus contains double-stranded DNA, the content of which is specific for each adenovirus type. The infective virus particle is 70–90 nm in diameter and has an icosahedral capsid composed of 352 capsomeres. The virus may be cultured and grown from corneal and conjunctival scrapings on HeLa cell lines, and identified by neutralization tests. As the disease progresses, the viraemia may be identified serologically by a rising titre of neutralizing antibody to the virus. Two main subgroups of ocular adenoviral infection occur, which include: (1) epidemic keratoconjunctivitis (serotypes 3, 7, 8 and 19); and (2) pharyngoconjunctival fever (serotypes 1, 2, 3, 5, 7 and 14).

ONCOGENIC VIRUSES

All families of DNA viruses have members that give rise to tumours either naturally or experimentally. On the other hand only the retroviruses of the RNA family of viruses have this potential. While viruses have not generally been cited as major environmental agents in human cancer, they do play a large and important role. Examples worldwide include hepatocellular carcinoma, cervical cancer and nasopharyngeal carcinoma. In all these cases a transmissible virus appears to be an important primary aetiological factor.

Human papillomavirus (HPV)

HPV represents a set of viruses of over 40 strains. They induce epithelial proliferation (e.g. benign papilloma) and under certain undefined conditions, where synergism between HPV and other cofactor carcinogens exist, malignant conversion may occur. Both HPV-16 and HPV-18 are implicated in the aetiology of cervical carcinoma; 50% of cervical cancer biopsies contain HPV-16 DNA. These papillomaviruses can cause warts that affect the eye, giving rise to both lid and conjunctival papillomas (see Ch. 9). Molluscum contagiosum (pox virus) is thought to have oncogenic properties, particularly with the presence of the classic C particle (budding viral

particle which consists of nucleic acid) in the cytoplasm.

Hepatitis B virus (HBV)

This DNA virus has become firmly associated with primary hepatocellular carcinoma. Gene sequences of HBV persist in cell lines derived from these tumours.

Hepatitis C virus (HCV)

HCV is transmitted via blood contamination and is therefore more frequently seen in intravenous drug abusers. In addition to hepatitis, which becomes chronic leading to cirrhosis, hepatocellular carcinoma occurs in up to 15% of cases.

Epstein–Barr virus (EBV)

EBV is the agent that causes infectious mononucleosis (glandular fever). It is also associated with Burkitt's lymphoma and nasopharyngeal carcinoma. EBV can transform B lymphoblasts in culture to an indefinite growth pattern. In nasopharyngeal carcinoma, an increase in serum IgA levels in response to EBV accompanies the early stages of tumour growth, and it is at this point in the growth pattern that the tumour is more radiosensitive.

Retroviruses

These RNA viruses cause leukaemia and lymphoma, and include the recently discovered viruses, human T-cell lymphotropic viruses (HTLVs), which are associated with T-cell lymphomas, including mycosis fungoides and Sézary syndrome. They also have recently been implicated in the aetiology of uveitis in certain ethnic groups (Japanese). HTLV-1 is endemic in Japan, the West Indies and the central belts of Africa.

Mechanisms of viral oncogenesis

Tumour virus DNA, like all viral DNA, integrates into the host chromosomal DNA. This recombinant event may cause mutations, which occur randomly within the host chromosomal DNA. Integration of the viral genome can alter the expression of neighbouring host genes. Retroviruses and other oncogenic viruses carry signals for gene expression in long terminal repeats sequences, which promote transcription of adjacent host genes that are important in neoplasia (e.g. the *myc* gene). Where different viruses cause similar neoplasms, they promote ectopic expression of some cellular genes, all with oncogenic potential (c-*onc*; cellular oncogenes), which closely resemble viral oncogenes (v-*onc*). In addition, some viruses code for proteins that are

449

required for neoplastic transformation. As such, an infected cell can express cellular proteins that may induce neoplasia, particularly if expressed continuously in an uncontrolled way.

Virus may also enhance tumour formation by indirect mechanisms that cause immunosuppression of the host, allowing other latent oncogenic viruses to stimulate a mitotic state. This may explain the features of virally associated tumours in patients with AIDS (e.g. Kaposi's sarcoma and non-Hodgkin's lymphoma). Tumours may also be secondary to the chronic cytopathic effects of the virus, which in turn stimulates adjacent healthy cells within the tissue to undergo metaplasia and potentially neoplastic change.

HUMAN IMMUNODEFICIENCY VIRUS (HIV)

HIV-1 and HIV-2 form part of a heterogeneous group of retroviruses. Three major retroviruses have a particular tropism for CD4+ lymphocytes. These include the human T-cell lymphotrophic viruses (HTLV-1 and HTLV-2) and HIV-1 and HIV-2. These retroviruses are characterized by the enzyme reverse transcriptase, which enables the viral genome to be integrated into the host genome. Inoculation may lead to a latent infection in which the virus persists and is passed on to the daughter cells during mitosis. Findings of molecular analysis of the HIV genome have demonstrated three gene groups, including genes that code for structural proteins, reverse transcriptase, and regulator genes. HIV gains entry into CD4+ T cells via binding to CD4 antigen and CXC chemokine receptors (CXCRS) on the cell surface. Other cells in addition to CD4+ T cells can be infected with HIV because of their coexpression (albeit at lower frequency) of these receptors, including monocytes and microglial cells of the central nervous system.

AIDS was first described in the USA in 1981, where homosexuals suffered from opportunistic infections in the form of *Pneumocystis carinii* pneumonia and Kaposi's sarcoma. Worldwide epidemiological studies have shown that AIDS is transmitted in three principal ways. Type I is urban spread (USA and Europe) in homosexuals and intravenous drug abusers. Type II is African spread, which is mainly heterosexual. Type III spread is seen in South-east Asia, and is yet to be fully defined. HIV infection can manifest in several ways, from asymptomatic/acute febrile illness during seroconversion to severe immunodeficiency. Seroconversion to anti-

> **Box 8.7 Summary of WHO classification**
>
> *Group I* Asymptomatic or persistent generalized lymphadenopathy
> *Group II* Early: weight loss < 10%, minor mucocutaneous manifestations
> *Group III* Intermediate: weight loss > 10%, chronic diarrhoea, recurrent pneumonia
> *Group IV* Late: AIDS (as defined by CDC)
>
> Each subgroup is divided into A, B or C depending on either the total lymphocyte count or the CD4+ T lymphocyte count.

HIV antibody occurs 4–12 weeks after the acute infection, but there may be longer delays in the formation of antibodies. Another syndrome associated with HIV infection is persistent generalized lymphadenopathy syndrome, defined as persistent lymphadenopathy for more than 3 months in two or more extrainguinal lymph nodes. About 33% of HIV antibody-positive patients fulfil the Center for Disease Control (CDC) definition of persistent generalized lymphadenopathy. The World Health Organization (WHO) grading (see Box 8.7 for summary) incorporates both severity of clinical manifestations and laboratory data, which in turn allows prognostic stratification for further clinical studies.

The diagnosis of AIDS is complex, but AIDS is defined as an illness characterized by one or more of the listed CDC indicator diseases depending also upon the status of laboratory evidence of HIV infection. Some of the more common indicator diseases include oesophageal conditions, *Pneumocystis carinii* pneumonia, cytomegalovirus (CMV) retinitis, *Cryptococcus* and primary lymphoma of the brain. Countries are now incorporating the CDC 1993 revisions of the definition of AIDS (see Box 8.7), which include a further three diseases on the list of indicator diseases defined in 1987, namely pulmonary tuberculosis, recurrent pneumonia within a period of 12 months, and invasive cervical carcinoma. Also, the definition of AIDS has been expanded to include all HIV-positive persons with CD4+ T-lymphocyte counts <200 per µl. Since the advent of newer antiretroviral therapy (see below) and the indication for earlier treatment of patients with HIV infection without other clinical evidence of disease, the incidence of opportunistic infections such as CMV retinitis is changing, at least in the western world.

Laboratory tests in the diagnosis of HIV and AIDS

HIV can be detected in bodily fluids but is more readily obtained from peripheral blood. The virus is isolated *in vivo* by co-culture with normal lymphocytes in the presence of the cytokine, interleukin-2. Multiplication of the virus can then be detected by reverse transcriptase assay or HIV antigen expression in culture. Antibodies to HIV have no natural protective or neutralizing action, but the diagnosis of HIV is based entirely on detection of antibodies to HIV-1 by enzyme-linked immunosorbent assay or Western blotting (serum reacting against HIV proteins recorded on electrophoretic gel). Western blotting demonstrates both IgG and IgM antibodies against envelope protein and structural proteins coded for by the *gag* gene (p55), which breaks down to p24, p18 and p15 proteins (see Box 8.8). The earliest laboratory finding in HIV infection is that of a p24 (core protein) antigenaemia, followed after about 2–3 weeks by an antibody response. Other laboratory indicators of HIV infection include falling CD4+ T lymphocyte counts and anti-p24 antibody titre, and a rising titre of core antigen, which are all indicative of progression to AIDS. These markers may appear up to 12–18 months before the onset of clinical features of AIDS and are thought to indicate an increased replication and load of the virus. More recently viral load can be more accurately assessed (see Box 8.9), and therefore patients on therapy can be monitored by both CD4+ T-cell count and viral HIV load.

Associated ocular infections in AIDS

Before the newer antiretroviral therapy became available (see below), nearly 25% of patients with AIDS presented with an opportunistic ocular infection. The most common infection is CMV retinitis, occurring in 15–46% of patients. Initial treatment with ganciclovir or foscarnet is successful in over 80% of cases, but acute relapse occurs within 3 weeks unless maintenance therapy is given. The rate of relapse on maintenance therapy is directly related to the presence of positive leucocyte CMV cultures. Another common opportunistic ocular infection is *Toxoplasma* chorioretinitis, which can be treated with a combination of pyrimethamine and sulphametopyrazine or clindamycin. Again, maintenance is required because a relapse rate of up to 30% has been reported on cessation of treatment. Fungal endophthalmitis is more frequent in intravenous drug abusers with AIDS. Cryptococcal choroiditis may be seen following an extension of cryptococcal meningitis and disseminated cryptococcus. *Pneumocystis carinii* choroidopathy is a relatively new clinical entity and has been described following the use of aerosolized pentamidine.

Box 8.8   HIV genome

Structural genes
The *gag* gene codes for a precursor protein, p55, which is cleaved into p24, p18 and p15. The envelope gene codes for a glycoprotein enclosing the viral particle. The *env* gene is expressed as a glycoprotein which is cleaved to form two envelope proteins (gp41 and gp120).

Regulatory genes
Viral genome consists of transactivating genes, which do not behave like oncogenes, but act in a positive feedback mechanism on an enhancer sequence on the viral genome, stimulating viral transcription and acting as a mitogen on adjacent healthy cells to proliferate (e.g. B cells and Kaposi's sarcoma).

Polymerase gene
This gene encodes for reverse transcriptase, which transcribes viral RNA into DNA, and can be incorporated into the host genome.

Box 8.9   Tests for HIV infection

- HIV culture
- HIV antigen (p24)
- HIV nucleic acid (PCR)
- HIV antibody (ELISA and Western blot)

Determining viral load
Using PCR technology, viral HIV load can be obtained by amplifying HIV genome RNA. After PCR a modified ELISA estimation detects down to 50 genome numbers/ml blood.

Box 8.10   Ocular infections associated with AIDS

- Cotton wool spots (see Ch. 9)
- CMV retinitis
- *Toxoplasma* chorioretinitis
- Herpetic keratitis (both simplex and zoster)
- Herpetic acute retinal necrosis and retinitis
- Candidal and cryptococcal endophthalmitis
- Tubercle chorioretinitis
- *Histoplasma* retinitis
- *Pneumocystis carinii* choroidopathy

Box 8.11   HIV and highly active antiretroviral therapy (HAART)

Reverse transcriptase inhibitors
Zidovudine is an antiviral agent that is highly active against HIV. It is phosphorylated in both infected and uninfected cells to a monophosphate derivative by thymidine kinase. Further phosphorylation to the triphosphate derivative (zidovudine-TP) inhibits viral reverse transcriptase. Zidovudine-TP is also incorporated into the RNA chain, inducing chain termination.

Proteinase inhibitors and nucleoside analogues
Indinavir inhibits recombinant HIV-1 and HIV-2 proteases, thereby preventing cleavage of viral precursor proteins, resulting in immature non-infectious particles. Indinavir is used in combination with nucleoside analogues. Nucleoside analogues act as chain terminators of HIV reverse transcriptase. Patients can be recurrently tested for proteinase resistance and changes in nucleoside analogues are used to prevent generation of resistant strains.

Box 8.12   Factors predisposing to fungal disease in the eye

Exogenous
- Local trauma
- Contact lens wear
- Topical antibiotics and steroids

Endogenous
- Immunocompromised patients (haematogenous spread)
- Non-ketotic diabetic ketoacidosis (from adjacent air sinuses)
- Contamination of indwelling catheters or intravenous line

Antiretroviral therapy increases CD4⁺ T-cell numbers and restores antigen-specific CD4⁺ T-cell responses

More recently, highly active antiretroviral therapy (HAART) has been employed in the treatment of AIDS and HIV infection. This form of therapy involves using a combination of agents that includes nucleoside analogues and protease inhibitors (see Box 8.11). HAART increases CD4⁺ T-cell numbers and more recently has been shown to restore CMV-specific CD4⁺ T-lymphocyte responses. Indeed there have lately been reports of a series of patients who have discontinued maintenance therapy with anti-CMV agents such as ganciclovir while on HAART without significant recurrence of retinitis.

FUNGI

Fungi are eukaryotic (cells with nuclear membranes) organisms with multiple chromosomes containing both DNA and RNA, and are capable of reproducing sexually. They can be divided broadly into three groups: yeasts, filamentous fungi and dimorphic fungi. Most fungi causing orbital infections are ubiquitous, aerobic and capable of growing on simple media. They are normal commensals of the respiratory, gastrointestinal and female genital tracts, and are also found in up to 25% of conjunctival sacs within the normal population. Despite their ubiquitous nature some fungi are more common in hotter climates, producing a distinct geographical distribution. For example, *Histoplasmosis capsulatum* is endemic in the Mississippi delta. The pathogenesis of fungal infection varies with the site and is also affected by various predisposing factors that play an important role. For example, exogenous mycotic infection may follow a local corneal abrasion with vegetable matter, particularly if an ocular surface or intraocular foreign body is present. Inflammation of the ocular adnexae and ocular surface disease (such as dry eyes or contact lens wear) also predispose to fungal infection. *Candida albicans* is the most frequently encountered cause of endogenous fungal infections, particularly in the immunocompromised host. It must be remembered that most fungi are opportunists and that infection occurs only when favourable conditions prevail (see Box 8.12).

TYPES OF FUNGI AND DISEASES THEY CAUSE

Yeasts

Candida albicans is an oval unicellular fungus that reproduces by budding (Fig. 8.8). It is a common saprophyte of the gastrointestinal tract and is the most frequently reported cause of endogenous fungal endophthalmitis. *Cryptococcus neoformans* is found in pigeon droppings, and in the immunocompromised host can cause meningoencephalitis and chronic endophthalmitis.

Filamentous

The nematophytes are a group of fungi that cause ringworm (tinea). This family includes the genera *Trichophyton*, *Microsporum* and *Epidermatophyton*.

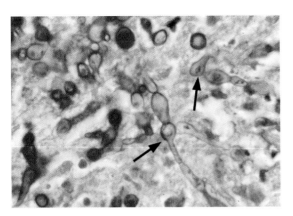

Fig. 8.8 *Candida* sp. can be identified by the presence of septae and budding yeasts (arrows) (PAS; original magnification: × 800).

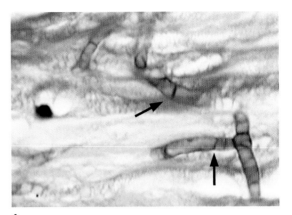

A

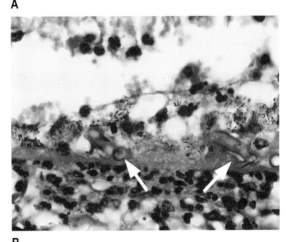

B

Fig. 8.9 (**A**) The hyphae of *Aspergillus* sp. are septate (arrows) and tend to branch at right angles within the stroma of the cornea (methenamine silver stain; original magnification: × 800). (**B**) *Mucor* is the largest of the pathogenic fungi and is of variable diameter (arrows) in this example from the outer retina (PAS; original magnification: × 600.)

Aspergillus fumigatus produces spores that are ubiquitous and can cause superficial infections such as conjunctivitis and keratitis, and a slowly progressive granulomatous orbital inflammation. *Mucor* (Zygomycetes) gives rise to the cerebrorhinoorbital syndrome (mucormycosis). This infection occurs more commonly in non-ketotic diabetic ketoacidosis and in debilitated patients with, for example, metastatic neoplastic disease (Fig. 8.9). Early diagnosis is critical to avoid a fatal outcome.

Dimorphic fungi

This family of fungi can grow as yeasts or filaments. The yeast form is generally found in infected tissues and causes a spectrum of intraocular inflammatory conditions including optic neuritis, chorioretinitis and panuveitis. Within this family are the fungi causing *blastomycoses*, which occur more commonly in the south-eastern USA. *Coccidioides immitis* is endemic in the south-western region of the USA, and, although it leads primarily to a pulmonary infection, choroiditis can occur secondary to dissemination of the fungus into the circulation. *Coccidioides immitis* is pathogenic in the healthy individual, unlike other fungal infections. Finally *Histoplasma*, which is endemic in the Mississippi delta, often gives rise to a mild febrile illness or may be asymptomatic. The organism reaches the choroid by haematogenous dissemination, but active choroiditis is not common. Presumed ocular histoplasmosis syndrome is a multifocal choroiditis associated with the formation of subretinal neovascular membranes, whose true aetiology remains unknown. It is thought to be related to an initial exposure to *Histoplasma*, but active choroiditic lesions do not contain fungus (although *Histoplasma* antigenaemia has been found). Patients may present with a positive histoplasmin skin test (up to 90% of cases), but positive tests are also common in the healthy population of the endemic areas. A clinically identical syndrome occurs elsewhere in Europe and Asia, unassociated with histoplasmin skin test positivity.

DIAGNOSIS OF FUNGAL INFECTIONS: LABORATORY INVESTIGATIONS

Microscopy and cytopathological techniques can help to distinguish the morphology of the fungi which, as previously discussed, may be spherical or filamentous; both forms are Gram positive. Specimens can be grown on Sabouraud's medium (glucose–peptone agar, pH 5.6), which is especially important if microscopy is uninformative. Immunofluorescent techniques can also be used to determine antibody titres for specific fungal infections. More recently, sensitive PCR methods of detecting fungal DNA from vitreous samples are being established to rapidly ascertain the causative organisms in infectious posterior intraocular inflammation.

INTRACELLULAR PARASITES

CHLAMYDIA

Chlamydia are small bacteria which, like viruses, are unable to grow on inanimate media. They are obligate prokaryotic parasites, which contain both DNA and RNA, but require host cells to provide both phosphorylated intermediate metabolites and purine bases to replicate in the cytoplasm of the host cell. They are around 400 nm in diameter and divide by binary fission to produce particles that condense to form smaller bodies (200 nm). They grow well in cell culture (McCoy media). The genus *Chlamydia* comprises three species: *C. psittaci*, *C. trachomatis* and *C. pneumoniae* (see Ch. 9).

Classification

Indirect immunofluorescence has identified 14 individual *trachomatis* subtypes. They include serotypes causing trachoma inclusion conjunctivitis (TRIC) and lymphogranuloma venereum. Some of the common pathogenic subtypes are listed in Box 8.13.

Laboratory diagnosis and treatment

The diagnosis of chlamydial infection is based on cytological analysis of Giemsa-stained conjunctival scrapings, which identifies basophilic intracytoplasmic inclusion bodies, and also the pattern of inflammatory cell response. *Chlamydia* is isolated from swabs transported in sucrose phosphate transport medium and inoculated on to cycloheximide- and idoxuridine-treated McCoy cells. Using fluorescent antibody staining methods, inclusions can be detected within 24 hours. Immunofluorescence of tears or blood is a highly sensitive test for the detection of both IgG and IgM antibodies, which correlates well with the degree of clinical inflammation. *Chlamydia* is highly sensitive to tetracycline, erythromycin and rifampicin. Topical treatment with tetracycline daily for 6 weeks, or systemic treatment with oral tetracycline or erythromycin daily for 3 weeks, is effective in paratrachoma and trachoma.

PROTOZOA

Protozoa are unicellular eukaryotic parasites, and humans are often an accidental intermediate host in their life cycle.

Toxoplasmosis

Toxoplasma gondii is an obligate intracellular protozoon and transmission to humans is by faecal spread of sporocysts from the cat host. Humans acquire the infection from inadequately cooked meat, which may contain cysts of *Toxoplasma*. These cysts are destroyed at temperatures above 70°C. The parasite may become encysted and lie dormant for years, without evoking any clinical host response. The clinical manifestations vary according to the timing of the infection. The proliferative form of the parasite measures about 5 μm in diameter and is crescent shaped. The retinal cysts that develop contain many protozoa, which are thought to break down periodically and cause a reactivation of choroiditis (Fig. 8.10; see Ch. 9). In many areas, it is thought that the adult form of the disease is latent, following a primary infection *in utero*. However, with the

---

Box 8.13   Serotypes of *Chlamydia*

- TRIC subtypes A–C – trachoma (eye–eye contact)
- TRIC subtypes D–K – paratrachoma (sexually transmitted)
- L1, L2, L3 – lymphogranuloma venereum

Box 8.14   *Chlamydia*

- Fifteen serotypes have been identified by radioimmunoassay with monoclonal antibodies.
- Species of *Chlamydia* share a specific membrane glycoprotein similar in structure to the lipopolysaccharide found in the outer membranes of Gram-negative bacteria.
- Major outer membrane proteins (MOMP) constitute 60% of the outer coats of *C. trachomatis*.
- The *MOMP* gene is highly conserved but two variable domains code for serotype-specific epitopes.
- MOMP are immunodominant and when released promote pathogenic responses in the host.

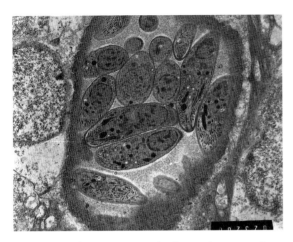

Fig. 8.10 Electron micrograph of *Toxoplasma gondii* bradyzoites within a cyst in the retina (original magnification: ×7500).

> **Box 8.15 Clinical manifestations of toxoplasmosis**
>
> *Transplacental*
> Mothers acquire the parasite during pregnancy, which may result in stillbirth. Intracranial calcification, mental retardation and chorioretinitis are features of the congenital syndrome. Asymptomatic retinal inflammation and cyst formation may occur at this stage, where recrudescence of the chorioretinitis may occur at any time as a result of cyst rupture.
>
> *Infection acquired in childhood*
> This may result in a fatal meningoencephalitis.
>
> *Infection acquired in adulthood*
> This frequently results in a febrile illness with clinical and haematological features similar to those of infectious mononucleosis. In certain geographic locations adult-acquired chorioretinitis occurs. Ocular toxoplasmosis presents as a discrete single lesion in the choroid/retina. Recurrences present as satellite lesions of the original scar.

difference in clinical picture noted in areas of South America between children and adults, it is also postulated that adults may acquire primary chorioretinitis in certain geographic locations. The iritis that often accompanies ocular toxoplasmosis is a hypersensitivity reaction to systemically released protozoal antigens. It is also thought that autoimmunity may also play a role in this disorder by releasing potent autoantigens after retinal damage. However, the evidence for this is not strong. Patients with ocular toxoplasmosis develop immune reactivity, predominantly to specific *Toxoplasma* antigens. Studies of the animal model of toxoplasmosis have shown that removal of both CD4$^+$ and CD8$^+$ T cells will lead to recurrence of the disease.

Toxoplasma are sensitive to various antimicrobial agents, including pyrimethamine, sulphadiazine and clindamycin. Ocular toxoplasmosis is generally treated with a combination of these antimicrobials and adjunctive systemic steroid therapy.

Diagnosis of *Toxoplasma* commonly requires serological assays and tissue sampling

The diagnosis of toxoplasmosis can be made on morphological examination of specimens where crescent-shaped nucleate protozoa (approximately 5 μm in diameter) can be demonstrated both intra- and extracellularly in the infected tissue. Serological analysis can be performed in an attempt to identify active *Toxoplasma* infection. These tests include the Sabin–Feldman dye test, which depends on the ability of antibodies to prevent the uptake of methylene blue by living *Toxoplasma* organisms. The results become positive approximately 2–4 weeks after acquired toxoplasmosis and remain positive for years. Complement fixation tests become positive later, approximately 4–8 weeks after acquired toxoplasmosis, low levels returning after a few months. Immunofluorescence antibody tests where high titres are present denote recent infection, and the presence of specific IgM or IgA antibodies in the newborn suggests congenital infection. The presence of IgG antibodies against *Toxoplasma* in the population can be explained by past infection and thus is not discriminatory for ocular disease and may not even be related to eye lesions. Detection of local antibody synthesis in the eye by intraocular fluid analysis is a valuable diagnostic tool. Paired aqueous and serum antibody analysis gives rise to a ratio (Goldmann–Witmer coefficient), which if raised suggests active ocular toxoplasmosis. In most adult cases of ocular toxoplasmosis, the diagnosis is made from the clinical appearance only (see Box 8.15).

Acanthamoeba

Acanthamoeba polyphaga is a cause of indolent corneal ulceration prominent particularly in contact lens wearers. *Acanthamoeba* is free living and may be recovered in both nasal and pharyngeal swabs but the incidence of clinical disease is low, suggesting that subclinical exposure to infection is the rule and normally the corneal architecture and host

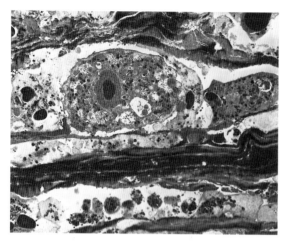

Fig. 8.11 Electron micrograph of *Acanthamoeba* cyst.

immunity are sufficient to prevent overt disease. The amoeba may be grown from specimens of corneal scrapes or contact lens cases when plated on *E. coli* nutrient-deficient agar. The clinical diagnosis can be difficult, and corneal biopsies or corneal button specimens at the time of penetrating keratoplasty may be required to demonstrate the amoeba in culture or by histology (Fig. 8.11). *Acanthamoeba* exists in two forms: trophozoites, which feed on enterobacteria and are proliferative by binary fission, and cysts. Topical treatment for acanthamoebiasis is propamidine isethionate, chlorhexidine digluconate and polyhexamethyl biguanide.

HELMINTHS

A number of helminths responsible for disease are obligate parasites, in that the human is essential for the worm to complete its life cycle. Sometimes, however, infection is accidental, i.e. the hosts for completion of the worm's life cycle belong to other animal groups. The following is a brief classification of the common parasitic helminths:

- Trematodes
  - *Schistosoma*
- Cestodes
  - *Taenia*
  - *Echinococcus*
- Nematodes
  - *Toxocara*
  - *Filaria*
  - *Trichinella*

As mentioned, helminths are parasites and, as such, the worm benefits from the worm–host relationship and the host is harmed. Antibodies are produced against the worm, and act on the blood stage of the worm life cycle by activating complement, antibody-dependent cytotoxicity, or opsonization and enhanced phagocytosis, but in general antibodies appear to be unprotective in many cases. The worm is able to resist the immune response in several ways, either by actively suppressing the host immune response or by modulation of antigenic determinants on the surface of its body so that immune responses are not as easily initiated. Cell-mediated immune responses are also important in the provision of immunity, as is described in more detail below. Worm infestation also provokes a marked type I hypersensitivity reaction with a profound IgE response and eosinophilia and, histologically, eosinophils are seen in tissue lesions in large numbers.

IMMUNOLOGICAL RESPONSE TO PARASITES

Parasite infestations stimulate more than one immunological defence mechanism. Various kinds of effector cells such as macrophages, neutrophils and eosinophils defend the host against invasion by parasites. Cytotoxic T cells have a direct destructive effect against intracellular parasites, for example *trypanosomes*. CD8+ T cells are thought to protect against the tissue stage of parasitic infection, and can act as cytotoxic T cells. CD4+ T cells are responsible for mediating immunity against the blood stages of parasitic infections, and act as helper cells for antibody production. Both these classes of T cells secrete cytokines, which in turn promote an effective immune response, stimulating proliferation of T cells and in some cases, such as interferon γ, directly inhibiting parasite multiplication. Other cells involved in the immune response against parasites include macrophages, which also secrete cell-specific cytokines thereby regulating the inflammatory response, and in addition are directly phagocytic. Neutrophils are phagocytic and can kill a variety of parasites, by both oxygen-dependent and oxygen-independent mechanisms. An increase in eosinophils and the production of high levels of IgE are commonly seen in parasitic infections, particularly by worms. The increase in eosinophils is likely to be T-cell dependent. Although eosinophils are less phagocytic than neutrophils, they kill parasites by similar mechanisms involving degranulation of the cell. The antigens released induce a secondary

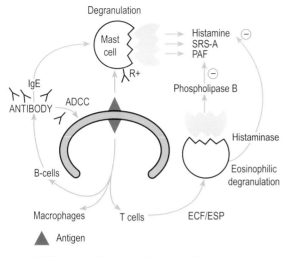

Fig. 8.12 The immune response to helminth infection.

ADCC	Antibody-dependent cytotoxicity
ECF	Eosinophil chemotactic factor
ESP	Eosinophil stimulation promoter
PAF	Platelet aggregation factor
SRS-A	Slow-reacting substance A

Box 8.16   Immunological response to helminth infection

- IgE-mediated allergic response
- Eosinophilia (serologically and histologically)
- Specific IgG and IgM humoral response
- Active cell-mediated immunity

IgE-dependent degranulation of mast cells and further recruitment of eosinophils (Fig. 8.12) (see Box 8.16 and Ch. 7).

TOXOCARIASIS

Toxocara canis and *Toxocara cati* are nematodes involved in human infection. The natural hosts are dogs and cats, respectively, and human infection is not obligatory for completion of the life cycle. Further discussion of the pathology of *Toxocara* is given in Chapter 9. Toxocariasis is caused by infection with larvae of the nematode worms, the adult forms of which are found in the intestine of dogs and cats where they lay eggs which are excreted in the faeces. *Toxocara* mounts a specific IgE response, and a skin test of intradermal injection of worm protein will give rise to an acute inflammatory response in the dermis (Fig. 8.13). Antibodies can be detected in the

---

Box 8.17   Onchocerciasis

- Microfilaria can be identified in skin biopsies, cerebrospinal fluid, urine, blood and ocular tissue samples.
- Dead or dying microfilaria incite an inflammatory immune-mediated response (Mazzotti reaction).
- Diagnosis of presumed ocular involvement can be obtained from biopsies of characteristic skin nodules.
- Treatment with ivermectin causes paralysis of the microfilaria and reduces side effects of treatment related to the death of microfilaria.
- Prevention is by eradicating black fly infestation by DDT spraying of river basins.
- The predilection of *Onchocerca* for the eye may be the result of a crossreaction between filarial and retinal antigens (molecular mimicry; see Ch. 7).

---

peripheral blood of patients by immunofluorescent or enzyme-linked immunosorbent assays. Specific IgM antibodies can be detected in the acute phase with haemagglutination assays. These serological tests are frequently negative and antibodies may be detected in samples of vitreous or aqueous. Treatment of ocular disease is with oral thiabendazole or albendazole, which is better tolerated. Sometimes, especially in granulomatous disease, enhancement of the inflammatory reaction occurs and so systemic steroids are given as well.

FILARIASIS

Filarial nematodes are thread-like worms. Infestation with these genera promotes a marked specific IgG and IgE response and eosinophilia. Immunity is thought to be directed predominantly toward the microfilaria (first-stage larvae).

Onchocerciasis

Onchocerciasis (river blindness) is endemic within the river basins of West and Central Africa, and is the most frequent helminthic ophthalmic infection. Onchocerciasis accounts for over a million cases of blindness worldwide. In Nigeria 43% of recorded blindness is the result of *Onchocerca*. Humans are the natural host of the adult worm and the black fly is the intermediate host, transmitting the disease. Microfilaria reach the cornea from the periorbital skin and conjunctiva, leading to keratitis, iridocyclitis, retinitis and optic atrophy. The microfilaria elicit an IgE response and cause eosinophilia, as with most worm infestations.

457

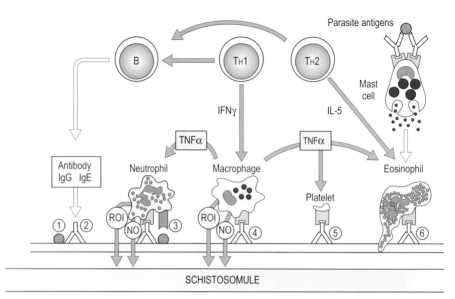

Fig. 8.13 Possible effector responses of schistosomules. This diagram illustrates the various effector mechanisms that have been shown to damage schistosomes *in vitro*. Complement alone damages worms (1) and also does so in combination with antibody (2). Antibody sensitizes neutrophils (3), macrophages (4), platelets (5) and eosinophils (6) for antibody-dependent cell-mediated cytotoxicity. Neutrophils and macrophages probably act by releasing toxic oxygen and nitrogen metabolites, whereas eosinophils damage the worm tegument by release of major basic protein. The response is potentiated by cytokines (e.g. tumour necrosis factor-α). IgE antibody is important in sensitizing both eosinophils and local mast cells, which release a variety of mediators, including those that activate the eosinophils. (Reproduced from Roitt *et al.*, 1996, with permission.)

Both *Wuchereria bancrofti* and *Loa loa* can directly invade the eye during the microfilarial stage, which can lead to a granulomatous uveitis and subretinal inflammatory lesion. Particularly *Loa loa* can be seen to migrate across the subconjunctiva, often accompanied by acute redness and itching. Occasionally the microfilaria can invade the globe and are found in subretinal lesions.

Trichinosis

Trichinella spiralis is a nematode parasite that lives in the gut mucosa. Human infection is usually the result of eating undercooked meat. Larvae can infiltrate the extraocular muscles and the resulting granulomatous reaction presents as a painful and proptosed eye. The inflammatory myositis eventually settles and the larvae often become calcified. Again, very rarely, intraocular spread of the larvae occurs and retinal haemorrhages, subretinal lesions and papilloedema can occur.

Trematodes

Schistosomes are the only trematodes (flukes) that cause ocular disease. The larval stages (cercariae) are released from the snail, penetrate the epidermis and then enter the lymphatic system. Immature worms then enter the lungs and further mature before disseminating into the veins. *Schistosoma haematobium* promotes a granulomatous reaction in the ocular adnexae (lacrimal gland) and may be found in the subconjunctival tissue associated with a profound eosinophilic response.

ANTIMICROBIALS

This section only hopes to serve as a summary of the multitude of agents now available against microbes. Antibiotics are often defined as having a broad or narrow spectrum with respect to the bacteria they are active against. Antibiotic sensitivities of the organism can be determined by antibiotic culture tests in the laboratory, facilitating more specific antimicrobial treatment and overcoming the increasing problem of resistance to antibiotics. The minimal inhibitory concentration (MIC) for a given culture system is that concentration of the agent below which bacterial growth is not inhibited. This is important for systemically administered antibiotics, where, for example, the MIC for gentamicin is close to the plasma concentrations of gentamicin associated with renal toxicity. However, the MIC is determined by *in vivo* culture systems and the concentration within an infected tissue or for intracellular organismal infections may be much lower than that in plasma, and treatment failure may occur.

Antimicrobial therapy must therefore have 'selective toxicity' in that the agent kills or inhibits microorganisms at concentrations that are well tolerated by the host tissues. The best examples of selective toxicity are provided by those antimicrobials that interact with bacterial cell wall synthesis, because host cells do not have such structures. Antimicrobials may be defined as *bactericidal* (fungicidal); these agents kill microorganisms even in the absence of an immune response. Other agents are described as *bacteriostatic*, these inhibit the growth of the microorganisms. Antimicrobials that are bacteriostatic at low concentrations may become bactericidal at higher concentrations, for example erythromycin.

MECHANISM OF ACTION

Broadly, antimicrobial agents exert their effect by interacting with: (1) bacterial cell wall synthesis, (2) cytoplasmic membrane, (3) protein synthesis and (4) nucleic acid synthesis.

Inhibition of cell wall synthesis

Many antibiotics act via the inhibition of bacterial cell wall synthesis. The major antibiotic groups that act by this method include penicillin and cephalosporin (β-lactams), and vancomycin and bacitracin. The structures of the cell walls of Gram-positive and Gram-negative bacteria are different but do in common contain peptidoglycan chains, held together via peptide chains. In the case of penicillins and cephalosporins, which possess β-lactam rings, both bind to proteins in the cell membrane, known as penicillin-binding proteins. The amount and nature of these proteins vary between the genera of bacteria. The end result of antibiotic binding is the inhibition of crosslinking of peptidoglycan strands. The resulting weakened areas within the bacterial cell wall are susceptible to autolytic enzymes normally present, which destroy the cell.

There are many penicillin derivatives which have a wide range of therapeutic advantages over one another, for example the generation of penicillins resistant to staphylococcal penicillinase, such as flu-

cloxacillin. Other β-lactam derivatives include carbapenem, which is a potent antibiotic and β-lactamase inhibitor, and clavulanic acid (a penem derivative), which is also a β-lactamase inhibitor and is usually combined with other penicillins to achieve a bactericidal effect. All β-lactams are bactericidal, have low toxicity and penetrate well into inflamed tissues. Their major limitation is the increasing distribution of β-lactamase-producing bacteria rendering the antibiotic inactive.

Interaction with the cell membrane

The microbial cell membrane is a lipoprotein layer surrounding the cytoplasm. A number of antimicrobials, including polymixins, imidazoles and polyenes (against fungi), interfere directly with the cell membrane.

Imidazoles are a group of synthetic antimycotic agents that have a broad spectrum of activity and act by inhibiting the synthesis of estrol sterols at the cytochrome P_{450} microsomal cellular level (see Ch. 6). The sterols are important for the integrity of the fungal cell wall, which if disrupted ultimately leads to cell lysis. This group of drugs exhibits a broad spectrum of antimycotic action, particularly against *Candida* and *Aspergillus*. Polyenes include amphotericin B and nystatin. Nystatin is an antibiotic isolated from *Streptomyces noursei*. The antifungal activity of nystatin is dependent on it being bound to the sterol component of the membrane of sensitive fungi. The drug is effective against *Candida*, *Cryptococcus* and the *Trichophyton* group of fungi, and can be either fungicidal or fungistatic. Amphotericin is a macrolide antibiotic that binds to cell membranes and interferes with ionic transport and permeability of the fungal cell wall. This ultimately causes cell lysis. However, ocular penetration of this drug is poor via all routes of administration. The drug is also easily inactivated and thus topical treatment has poor efficacy, because of its formulation. It is also painful when used topically on the eye. This drug is active against *Candida*, *Aspergillus*, *Cryptococcus*, *Histoplasma*, *Coccidioides* and *Blastomyces*.

Polymixins are cyclic peptides that adsorb to negatively charged lipids in the cell membrane, disorganizing the membrane and leading to a progressive loss of function. Polymixins are not entirely selective in their action, which results in a high degree of nephrotoxicity and neurotoxicity. They are, however, broad spectrum and are effective against Gramnegative bacteria including *Pseudomonas* but not *Proteus* species. With the advent of antipseudomonal β-lactams (carbenicillin and methicillin) their systemic use has declined, but they are still used in some topical preparations.

Inhibitors of protein synthesis

Antibiotics may inhibit bacterial protein synthesis without toxicity to the host because bacterial ribosomes are sufficiently different from human ribosomes. Human ribosomes have a sedimentation coefficient of 80S (60S and 40S subunits) and bacterial ribosomes have a sedimentation coefficient of 70S (50S and 30S subunits). Antibiotics inhibit ribosomal translocation and thus protein synthesis; for example, tetracyclines act by inhibiting aminoacyltransferase RNA and the messenger RNA–ribosome complex, thus preventing protein synthesis. Tetracyclines have a broad-spectrum activity against both Gram-positive and Gram-negative bacteria and also *Chlamydia*.

Aminoglycosides, which include gentamicin, tobramycin, neomycin and amikacin, prevent the reading of codons on the messenger RNA, resulting in defective proteins. They require aerobic transport mechanisms to enter the bacterial cell and are thus inactive against strict anaerobes and streptococci that do not exhibit oxidative transport mechanisms. All the aminoglycosides are to some extent ototoxic and nephrotoxic, which necessitates drug monitoring in an attempt to reduce their side effects.

Erythromycin is a macrolide that acts by binding to ribosomal subunits and interfering with translocation. The action of erythromycin is predominantly bacteristatic at low concentrations but at higher concentration it is bactericidal.

Chloramphenicol is active against many Gram-positive and Gram-negative bacteria, including the genera of *Mycoplasma*, *Haemophilus*, *Neisseria* and *Salmonella*. It acts by inhibiting peptidyltransferase.

Chloramphenicol is bacteristatic but also has bactericidal activity against *Haemophilus influenzae* and *Neisseria meningitidis*. It is one of the major topical antibiotics used in ophthalmology in the UK but its systemic use is limited because of the rare but potentially fatal aplastic anaemia that may occur very rarely with topical therapy.

Drugs acting on nucleic acid synthesis

Antimicrobials may inhibit nucleic acid synthesis by interfering with the synthesis of purines and pyrimidines. Examples include the antivirals, cytosine arabinoside and trifluorothymidine, and the antifungal agent 5′-fluocytosine. This compound is converted to 5′-fluorouracil, an antimetabolite that inhibits DNA synthesis. It is used in combination with other antifungal agents to restrict host toxicity.

Sulphonamides are active against Gram-positive and Gram-negative organisms. They act by inhibiting the metabolism of para-aminobenzoic acid to folate, which is essential for bacterial metabolism, DNA synthesis and survival. Sulphonamides are bacteristatic and slow acting as it takes several generations to deplete the folate pool and inhibit bacterial growth. Host cells are unable to synthesize folate and are thus not affected by sulphonamides.

Nalidixic acid and the newer 4-quinolones, e.g. ciprofloxacin, inhibit DNA replication by their action on bacterial DNA gyrase (DNA topoisomerase II), and interfere with the tertiary structural formation of DNA. Ciprofloxacin is active against many strains of *Pseudomonas aeruginosa*, *Staphylococcus aureus* and *Haemophilus influenzae*.

ANTIVIRALS

There are very few effective antiviral agents, and these are largely confined to the herpetic and DNA-related viruses. This is of particular importance in ophthalmology because of the high prevalence of herpes zoster ophthalmica and herpes simplex keratitis.

Aciclovir

This drug is a guanine derivative and acts against the herpes group of viruses, but has minimal action against CMV. It acts by inhibiting DNA polymerase after first being activated by the viral enzyme thymidine kinase. It may be used in an ointment formulation for topical treatment of herpes simplex keratitis. Its role in the treatment of herpes zoster keratitis is still questioned, but its systemic use during the active vesicular phase of the illness is said to reduce the incidence of ocular complications.

Idoxuridine

This agent inhibits the replication of DNA after it has been phosphorylated in infected cells. It can be used only topically, and in combination with dimethylsulphoxide (DMSO) can be painted onto active herpetic cutaneous lesions.

Ganciclovir

This agent has good activity against CMV. It acts by inhibiting DNA polymerase. It can be administered only by the intravenous route, and is toxic to both kidney and bone marrow. Intravitreal depots may be given in refractory cases of CMV retinitis. Treatment of CMV retinitis has been discussed in Chapter 6.

MECHANISMS OF ANTIMICROBIAL RESISTANCE

With the increasing use of antibiotics, resistant organisms will appear. Microorganisms may become resistant to antimicrobial agents by either mutation or inheriting new genetic information in the form of resistant plasmids. Enzyme-mediated resistance is the most important form of antimicrobial resistance and is mostly plasmid mediated. In Gram-negative bacteria these plasmids can be transferred between different genera within the bowel, in burns, and in peritoneal dialysis fluid, leading to rapid expansion of antimicrobial resistance. This exchange of genetic material may code for enzymatic inactivation of antibiotic, for example β-lactamase, or inhibition of metabolic pathways (e.g. para-aminobenzoic acid synthesis) and alteration of the permeability of the bacterial cell wall to the drug (see Box 8.19).

It is important to remember that resistance factors are often unstable and may be lost from bacteria, especially if there is no selective pressure from antibiotics to maintain them. A summary of commonly used antibiotics is given in Table 8.4. Development of antibiotic resistance may be secondary to acquisition of the antibiotic resistance genes that exist closely related to plasmids and therefore can be transferred as described above. Recently bacterial gene mutations have been described, conferring resistance to antibiotics such as fluoroquinolone, in *gyr*A and *gyr*B genes (DNA gyrase) and *par*C and *par*E genes (topoisomerase IV).

Box 8.19 Antimicrobial resistance

Microorganisms develop resistance by:

- Alteration of target site (bacterial cell wall or cytoplasmic membrane) against β-lactams or erythromycin
- Preventing transport of drug into microbe (e.g. aminoglycosides)
- Bypassing antimicrobial-induced metabolic block (e.g. sulphonamides)
- Producing enzymes that inactivate the antimicrobial: β-lactamase (β-lactams), acetyltransferases (aminoglycosides)

Table 8.4 Bacterial sensitivities of commonly used antibiotics

Antibiotic	Bacterial sensitivity
Penicillins	
Penicillin G	Gram-positive cocci
Penicillin V	Gonococcus
Ampicillin	Haemophilus
Carbenicillin	Pseudomonas, Proteus
Methicillin (penicillinase resistant)	Staphylococcus
Cephalosporins	
Cephalexin	Gram-positive cocci
Cephadrine	Penicillin resistant
Cefuroxime	Staphylococcus
Aminoglycosides	
Streptomycin	Mycobacterium
Neomycin	Gram-positive cocci
Gentamicin	Escherichia coli
Tobramycin	Proteus/Pseudomonas
Kanamycin	
Macrolides	
Erythromycin	Staphylococcus aureus
	Streptococci
	Neisseria, Mycoplasma, Moraxella
Miscellaneous	
Chloramphenicol	Haemophilus, Neisseria Bordetella, Bacteroides, streptococci, Proteus, Pseudomonas
Sulphonamides	Streptococci, Haemophilus, Chlamydia, E. coli, Moraxella
Ciprofloxacin (4-aminoquinolone)	Proteus, Pseudomonas, Moraxella

STERILIZATION AND DISINFECTANTS

Sterilization is the destruction of all microbial life, so that none can reproduce. This is required for surgical instruments, dressings, intravenous and intraocular fluids, and topical eye medications. Disinfection means the destruction of microbial pathogens, and also some other organisms. The skin, for example, can be disinfected but never made sterile.

STERILIZATION

Wet heat is the most effective form of sterilization. Autoclaves are designed so that articles are exposed to steam at high pressures. All air must be evacuated from the autoclave so that only saturated steam is inside, and the pressure must be raised to ensure penetration and to increase temperatures. When a pressure of 100 kPa is applied to steam, the temperature increases to 121°C. After 120 minutes all bacteria, spores, fungi and viruses are killed. The materials are dried after the steam has been evacuated in a vacuum pump. High-pressure vacuum pumps are available, providing higher temperatures and pressures and thus reducing the sterilization time. Tests to ensure that adequate sterilization has occurred must be carried out routinely. Highly resistant organisms are placed in packs, or a spore strip of, for example, *Bacillus stearothermophilus* is used, where a temperature of 121°C for 12 minutes is required to kill 1×10^5 spores.

Powders, oils, greases and cutting instruments that may lose their sharp edge cannot withstand steam sterilization. Such items are sterilized with dry heat in a fan-assisted large drying oven capable of producing heat to 160°C. Dry heat at 160°C takes several hours to sterilize, although heat up to 190°C (which is more difficult to achieve) is quicker.

Ethylene oxide is a gas that mixes completely with air at low pressures. It acts as a sterilizing agent at much lower temperatures than air and thus can be used, for example in sterilizing electrical equipment, plastics and rubber, which are sensitive to heat. Aeration of the equipment is required to rid it of this potentially explosive gas, which can take 24–48 hours to achieve. This form of sterilization acts by denaturing bacterial proteins.

Gamma-radiation is highly effective but costly. As such, its general use is mainly large-scale industrial sterilization of disposable medical items, for example syringes, catheters and surgical dressing packs.

DISINFECTANTS

Many chemicals are available as disinfectants but none guarantees sterility. The simplest disinfectants are sanitizers, such as phenol-based solutions, because they reduce bacterial flora, but have little action against Gram-negative bacteria and do not destroy spores. A 20% solution of formalin in ethanol kills bacteria, spores, fungi and many viruses, but takes many hours to do so. Glutaraldehyde is an alkaline solution that kills vegetative bacteria and some fungi quickly and is viricidal but it also takes many hours to kill spores. Glutaraldehyde can be used for metal instruments and glass lenses, for example Goldmann tonometer prisms, provided they are clean, because the disinfectant is not active in the presence of organic matter. A solution of 70% ethyl alcohol in water kills non-sporing organisms in seconds, but not in the presence of blood or pus. Ethyl alcohol is also active against viruses, but not adenovirus, and therefore cannot be recommended for lens disinfection in ophthalmology. Iodine in alcohol is very useful against bacteria but not spores. Its main disadvantage is that it stains and is irritant. Chlorhexidine and hexachlorophene are used as skin disinfectants. They are able to remove most pathogens on the skin but it should be emphasized that hexachlorophene used over a large area can lead to toxic absorption. The use of disinfectants and sterilization of topical eye-drop formularies were discussed in Chapter 6.

FURTHER READING

Adler MV, ed. ABC of AIDS. London: British Medical Association; 1987.

Autran B, Carcelain G, Li TS, Blanc C, Mathez D, Tubiana R, Katlama C, Debre P, Leibowitch J. Positive effects of combined antiretroviral therapy on CD4+ T cell homeostasis and function in advanced HIV disease. Science 1997; 277:112–116.

Bartlett JD, Jaanus SD. Clinical ocular pharmacology, 3rd edn. Boston: Butterworth; 1995.

de Boer JH, Luyendijk L, Rothova A, Kijlstra A. Analysis of ocular fluids for local antibody production in uveitis. Br J Ophthalmol 1995; 79:610–616.

Ficker L, Kirkness C, McCartney A, Seal D. Microbial keratitis – the false negative. Eye 1991; 5:549–555.

Forrester JV, Okada AA, Ben Ezra D, Ohno S. Posterior segment intraocular inflammation guidelines. The Hague: Kugler Publications; 1998.

Garner A, Klintworth GK. Pathobiology of ocular disease: a dynamic approach. New York: Marcel Dekker; 1993.

Goldmann H, Witmer R. Antibodies in the aqueous humour. Opthalmologica 1954;127:323–330.

Holliman R. Uncommon infections. Prescribers Journal 1992; 32:127–133.

Janeway CA Jr, Travers P. Immunobiology: the immune system in health and disease. London: Blackwell Scientific Publications; 1994.

Jawetz E. Review of medical microbiology, 17th edn. Norwalk: Lange; 1987.

Komandurin KV, Viswanathan MN, Wieder ED, Schmidt DK, Bredt BM, Jacobson MA, McCune JM. Restoration of CMV-specific CD4+ T-lymphocyte responses after ganciclovir and highly active retroviral therapy in individuals infected with HIV-1. Nat Med 1998; 44:953–956.

Luzzi G, Peto TEA, Weiss RA. HIV and AIDS. In: Warrell DA, Cox TM, Firth JD, Benz EJ eds. Oxford textbook of medicine, 4th edn. Oxford: University Press 2007.

Roitt I, Brostoff J, Male D. Immunology, 4th edn. St Louis: Mosby; 1996.

Rothova A. Ocular involvement in toxoplasmosis. Br J Ophthalmol 1993; 77:371–378.

Seal DV, Bron AJ, Hay J. Ocular infections: investigation and treatment in practice. London: Martin-Dunitz; 1998.

Varmus HE. Retroviruses. Science 1988; 240:1427–1435.

Weller IVD. Clinical immunology and AIDS, Vol. 21, parts 1 and 2. Oxford: Medicine International, The Medicine Group, Medical Education International; 1993.

9 PATHOLOGY

INTRODUCTION

This chapter describes basic aspects of disease processes with reference to specific entities relevant in ophthalmology.

INFLAMMATION

Inflammation is the dynamic process by which living tissues react to injury. The injurious agent may be physical, chemical, infective or immunological. The classical signs of acute inflammation are redness, heat, swelling, pain and loss of function. The initial three signs are demonstrated by the 'triple response' induced in the skin after surface injury (see Box 9.1). Following the triple response leucocytes (neutrophils and monocytes) migrate to the site of injury. They may be attracted by chemotaxins released from other leucocytes, complement components or pathogenic bacteria. Once within the tissues, leucocytes clear the injurious agent by phagocytosis. This process involves opsonization of bacteria by complement components before engulfment within the leucocyte. Once within the leucocytes the lysosomes fuse with the phagosome and bacteria may be killed by oxygen-dependent formation of free radical or by activation of lysosomal enzymes. Various chemical mediators are also released from inflammatory cells or are present within plasma. Those released from inflammatory cells include histamine, serotonin, prostaglandins and leukotrienes as well as a range of cytokines. These mediators may result in vasodilatation (serotonin, prostaglandins), increased vascular permeability (histamine, leukotrienes) and lymphocyte proliferation and macrophage activation (cytokines). Those present in plasma are interrelated cascade systems including the clotting cascade, fibrinolysis, complement system and bradykinin system. The outcome of acute inflammation depends on various

465

Box 9.1 The triple response

The first stage in the inflammatory reaction occurs in blood vessels in damaged tissue. If a blunt instrument is pressed and pulled across the skin, the following changes occur:

- The blood vessels constrict and a white line appears.
- The capillaries dilate and a dull red line appears (flush).
- Arteriolar dilation occurs and there is a larger expanding zone (flare).
- Fluid leaks from the capillaries and causes the tissue to swell (wheal).

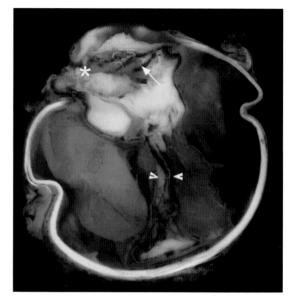

Fig. 9.1 Enucleation was required after a cataract operation with an intraocular lens implant (arrow) was complicated by a dehiscence of the wound (*). Gram-positive cocci were found in the vitreous abscess. The retina (arrowheads) was detached by haemorrhage.

factors including the infecting organism and the extent of tissue necrosis. Inflammation may resolve, suppurate, repair with organization and scarring, or progress to chronic inflammation. These potential outcomes may be demonstrated in the cornea where a small traumatic erosion may resolve without scarring. Bacterial keratitis may lead to formation of a corneal abscess that may ultimately heal with extensive scarring. Ongoing chronic inflammation may occur with herpes simplex stromal keratitis.

INFLAMMATORY DISEASE DUE TO INFECTION

Bacterial infections

Intraocular bacterial infections are rare but highly destructive. The pathogenicity of bacteria varies according to the species (see Ch. 8) and this is reflected in the nature of the immune response to the organism.

Pyogenic infection

Pyogenic bacterial infection of the intraocular compartment is termed endophthalmitis and may be exogenous or metastatic. Panophthalmitis (in which the infection involves the whole of the ocular and periocular tissues) describes a rapid and devastating tissue destruction, which may be complete by 48 hours (Fig. 9.1). Irrespective of the Gram-stain reaction, bacteria can be equally virulent, particularly in an immunocompromised host, and they have a similar pattern of tissue dissolution. Gram-positive cocci are among the commoner organisms that produce a purulent infection when introduced into the eye either by accidental or surgical trauma or by blood spread. The vitreous is an ideal medium for bacterial proliferation, in that the sites for ingress

of inflammatory cells (e.g. retinal vessels, the optic disk and pars plana) are some distance from the proliferating pathogens. (Therapy may also be less than optimal because the barrier imposed by the endothelium of the retinal blood vessels impedes the diffusion of antibiotics; see Ch. 6.)

Neutrophils are the predominant cell type in metastatic endophthalmitis, i.e. when bacteria enter the eye via the bloodstream, as in bacterial endocarditis or after contamination of an indwelling intravenous catheter. During bacterial killing neutrophils may release lytic enzymes that can lead to the total destruction of all layers of the retina.

The ocular coats normally provide an excellent barrier to invasion by bacteria. However, if the cornea is in some way compromised, as for instance during the inappropriate use of steroids in corneal ulceration, the prolonged and incorrect use of contact lenses or inadequate wound closure after intraocular surgery, direct bacterial entry through the cornea may occur.

Pyogenic infection requires urgent attention, a primary aim of which is to identify the causative organisms. This depends critically on obtaining good-quality diagnostic material. Scrapings of a corneal ulcer must be thorough and good microbiological plating and culture procedures must be followed. Vitrectomy fluids should be centrifuged carefully so that rapid culture and bacterial sensitivities can be used to initiate correct antibacterial chemotherapy. Several factors increase the risk of endophthalmitis (see Box 9.2).

Chronic infection: granulomatous reactions

The mycobacteria (tuberculosis, leprosy), the actinomycetes (skin and lung infection) and the spirochaetes (syphilis, yaws) are responsible for chronic destruction of tissue. *Borrelia burgdorferi*, a spirochaete transmitted by ticks, may cause arthritis, neurological disease and conjunctivitis (Lyme disease). *Bartonella* spp., which causes cat scratch disease, has also been implicated as a cause of neuroretinitis. Pathogens that produce a chronic infection induce humoral and cell-mediated responses in the host (see Ch. 7); the latter is characterized by macrophages, lymphocytes and plasma cells. Many of the pathogenic organisms, such as *Mycobacterium tuberculosis*, have the capacity to survive within the host macrophage. In the case of *M. tuberculosis*, macrophages attempt to limit the spread of the organism by accumulating around the dead and dying (necrotic) cells killed by the organism. The macrophages then become more elongated taking on an epithelium-like morphology (epithelioid macrophages). This collection of epithelioid macrophages is known as a granuloma. Fusion with neighbouring macrophages forms a characteristic multinucleate giant cell (Langhans' cell). The central mass of dead tissue within the granuloma appears cheese-like macroscopically, hence the terms 'caseous necrosis,' 'caseating' and 'caseation.'

The response of macrophages to form multinucleate giant cells and granulomas around a focus of tissue destruction is a non-specific and commonly observed response to living or dead pathogenic organisms or their products. It is also a feature of a number of diseases in which granulomatous reactions are found, but in which the aetiology is unknown, e.g. sympathetic ophthalmitis (see Ch. 7) and sarcoidosis (see Boxes 9.3 and 9.4). It is important to appreciate that this reaction is seen in most low-grade inflammations, such as foreign-body reactions to suture material, wood or endogenous materials such as degenerate fat or lysed blood (Fig. 9.2).

Immunologically, these reactions represent a delayed-type hypersensitivity response (DTH response; see Ch. 7) mediated by T helper type 1 cells in which macrophages represent the effector cell.

Viral infections

The following viruses most commonly cause ocular disease: herpes simplex virus, herpes zoster virus (varicella group) and cytomegalovirus.

Herpes simplex keratitis (Box 9.5)

In the past this was a common and important disease, but the availability of effective antiviral therapy has resulted in a dramatic reduction in the

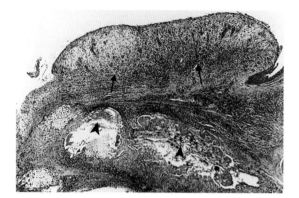

Fig. 9.2 A pyogenic granuloma in the conjunctiva consists of a mound of proliferating capillaries and fibroblasts surrounded by inflammatory cells (arrows). In this case the granuloma arose over suture material (arrowheads).

Box 9.4 A sarcoid granuloma around a blood vessel in the retina

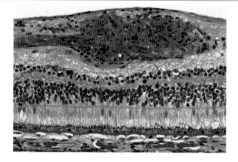

Note that a granulomatous reaction is a response principally by macrophages to a wide variety of stimuli [living and dead microbiological pathogens, endogenous host breakdown products, and foreign (exogenous) material]. This is not to be confused with 'granulation tissue', an exuberant proliferation of capillaries, fibroblasts and inflammatory cells over a defect in the epithelium (Fig. 9.2). In ophthalmic practice, granulation tissue formation occurs most commonly over chalazia and the sutures used for strabismus surgery; the term 'pyogenic granuloma' is used when this forms a polypoid lesion (see Fig. 9.2).

Box 9.5 Herpes simplex in the eye

Type 1 herpes simplex virus causes superficial corneal ulceration which is finger-like or dendritic within the epithelium. Primary herpes simplex infection usually occurs through the oral mucosa, the lips or the skin of the face. This is followed by transneural and subsequently latent viral infection in the neurones of the trigeminal ganglion and the sympathetic ganglia. The virus is morphologically detectable by ultrastructural investigation within the corneal cells (keratocytes and epithelial cells) and nerves (see figures below). A variety of possible triggers (ultraviolet light, cold) reactivate the virus, which migrates along the sensory nerves to the corneal epithelium. The virus then invades, replicates and spreads within the epithelium.

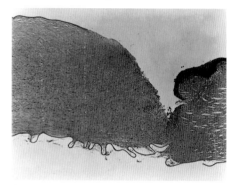

A

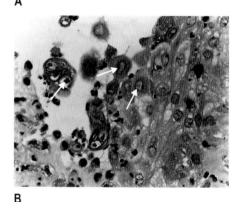

B

(**A**) Herpes simplex ulceration of the cornea at the host–graft junction after keratoplasty.

(**B**) The epithelial cells contain intranuclear inclusion of herpes viral particles (arrows).

number of complications that arose previously. These included chronic fibrosis and scarring (disciform keratitis) with stromal vascularization and persisting chronic inflammation: leakage of lipid-rich plasma into the corneal stroma leads to pale yellow deposits (secondary lipid keratopathy).

Herpes zoster ophthalmicus

Herpes zoster virus infects the ganglia and branches of sensory nerves such as the trigeminal nerve, producing vesicle formation in the skin in the distribution of the affected nerve or its branches. The eyelids, conjunctiva, cornea and uveal tract are involved in the inflammatory process. A lymphocytic infiltrate appears around the long and short ciliary nerves and is present in the choroid and ciliary body.

Acute retinal necrosis

Acute retinal necrosis has only been recognized as a disorder in the past three decades. The condition can be unilateral or bilateral and usually occurs in immunocompetent individuals. Acute retinal necrosis is usually caused by infection with herpes simplex or varicella–zoster virus. Morphological distinction of these viruses can be difficult in retinal biopsies and polymerase chain reaction or in situ hybridization may be more helpful in providing an accurate diagnosis. Enucleation specimens show sectorial or massive haemorrhagic retinal necrosis, associated with vitreous exudation and choroidal inflammatory cell infiltration. Intranuclear viral inclusion bodies can be seen by light microscopy. Ultrastructural examination reveals viral particles within retinal neurones and within the retinal pigment epithelium (RPE) and vascular endothelium. The virion appears as a central electron-dense core with a surrounding layer (the capsomere) and an outer envelope. The dimension of the infective viral particle is 190–220 nm (see Ch. 8).

Progressive outer retinal necrosis

In immunocompromised individuals, herpes simplex and herpes zoster viruses may cause destruction of the outer retina without the accompanying vitritis, retinal vasculitis or papillitis usually associated with acute retinal necrosis.

Cytomegalovirus retinitis

Before antiretroviral therapy became available cytomegalovirus retinitis was a common ocular infection in individuals with acquired immunodeficiency syndrome (AIDS). It is characterized by progressive areas of retinal necrosis, usually without

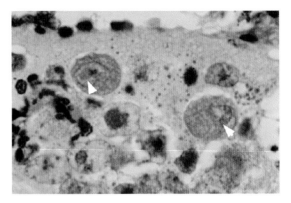

Fig. 9.3 In cytomegalovirus infection the necrotic retina contains enlarged cells in which characteristic owl-eye intranuclear inclusions are present (arrowheads) (phloxine tartrazine stain).

haemorrhage. Infected cells are often enlarged with a characteristic owl-eye inclusion body (Fig. 9.3).

Chlamydial infection

On a global scale, ocular infection by Chlamydia trachomatis (see Ch. 8) is the commonest cause of human blindness. The organism is spread by direct contact and is also insect-borne. In an environment with poor hygiene the disease flourishes but the Chlamydiaceae respond to broad-spectrum antibiotics, particularly tetracyclines, and as living standards improve the incidence of blindness as the result of trachoma should decline (see Box 9.6). Chlamydial conjunctival infection in developed countries, for instance, is much less sight threatening than in less developed nations and is associated with genitourinary infection.

Fungal infection (see Ch. 8)

In Europe the most important fungal pathogens include:

- Candida spp.
- Aspergillus spp.
- Mucor spp.

Aspergillus and Candida spp. may directly invade the cornea, iris and lens in postoperative infections or can be blood-borne, particularly in drug addicts. In the latter individuals the infection may present as a vitreous abscess.

Mucormycosis is the result of a blood-borne infection and occurs in patients with poorly controlled diabetes or who are immunocompromised. The

469

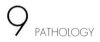

Box 9.6 Trachoma

Trachoma is described in four stages:

- In stage I there is epithelial infection with early lymphoid hyperplasia and polymorphs within the conjunctival stroma, which is oedematous.
- Stage II is often subgrouped into type A, in which the lymphoid follicular reaction predominates, or type B, in which there is fibrosis with the formation of papillae. The latter reaction probably represents the effect of secondary bacterial infection. The papillae are formed by fibrovascular proliferation within the thickened and inflamed stroma. The cornea is involved at this stage with ingrowth of a fibrovascular pannus onto the superior corneal periphery.
- Stage III is characterized by fibrous replacement of the inflammatory tissue.
- In stage IV there is contraction within the palpebral conjunctival stroma so that there is internal deformation of the lids (entropion) and trichiasis, which leads to abrasion of the cornea by the lashes. Suppression of tear production is the result of inflammation and fibrosis within the lacrimal gland and its ductular system. Secondary changes occur in the conjunctival epithelium, e.g. stratification and loss of goblet cells, and these also impair tear film stability.

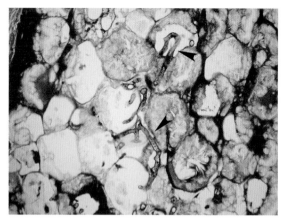

Fig. 9.4 *Mucor* is the largest of the pathogenic fungi and consists of broad, non-septate branching hyphae (arrows). In this case the hyphae are present within infracted orbital fat.

fungus has a predilection for the lumen of blood vessels, which are occluded by secondary thrombosis: the organism parasitizes the ophthalmic artery and its branches leading to necrosis of the orbital tissues, the nose and the eye (Fig. 9.4).

The following fungal infections are more prevalent in the USA: coccidioidomycosis, cryptococcosis, histoplasmosis and blastomycosis.

Protozoal and metazoal infections
(see Ch. 8)

Toxoplasma gondii
This is the commonest protozoal parasite to infect the eye. Congenital infection may occur when a woman becomes infected for the first time during pregnancy. Infection causes a classical tetrad of symptoms (meningoencephalitis, hydrocephalus, intracranial calcification and retinochoroiditis). Disease severity depends on in which trimester the infection occurs. Congenital ocular toxoplasmosis is a recurring and progressive disease because of the persistence of the parasite as bradyzoites within tissue cysts, which can reactivate. Foci of reactivation can be seen as an irregular area with associated vitreous haze at the border of a retinochoroidal scar.

Acquired infection is usually from cysts in undercooked meat or from oocysts in soil contaminated with cat faeces. Acquired infection is commonly asymptomatic although some individuals will develop a flu-like illness with lymphadenopathy. Retinochoroiditis may occur as a result of acute acquired infection but in contrast with congenital infection there is no pre-existing scar. *Toxoplasma* retinochoroiditis is less common in immunocompromised patients than cytomegalovirus retinitis but can cause extensive retinal necrosis. Individual parasites (tachyzoites) and cysts (containing bradyzoites) can be identified in paraffin sections (Fig. 9.5).

Acanthamoeba spp.
The incidence of acanthamoebal keratitis initially increased with greater use of soft contact lenses, but this form of keratitis it is now less common because of increased realization of the importance of hygiene of the contact lenses. This is a free-living protozoal parasite and the main source of contamination is the fluid in the contact lens case and scales on taps. These loci often contain bacteria that provide nutrition for the protozoa. In the cornea, the acanthamoebae phagocytose remnants of dying keratocytes and polymorphs (Fig. 9.6). The organism can be difficult to identify without the use of immunohistochemistry. Acanthamoebal keratitis is painful and responds only slowly to appropriate therapy.

Toxocara canis
The adult worm of *Toxocara canis* lives in the intestinal tract of the puppy and the eggs are passed out

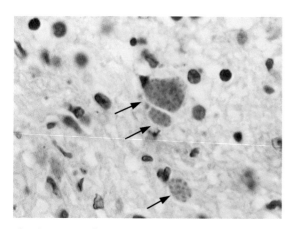

Fig. 9.5 *Toxoplasma* cysts (arrows) in a retina in which the normal architecture has been destroyed.

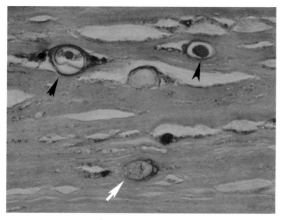

Fig. 9.6 *Acanthamoeba* cysts (black arrowhead) and a trophozoite (white arrow) lying between the corneal stromal lamellae in a soft contact lens wearer (PAS stain).

with the faeces. Infants may ingest the eggs, which release second-stage larvae in the stomach. The larvae of *Toxocara* can pass easily through the body tissues and the living organisms do not elicit an inflammatory response. However, should the organisms die, the immune system is activated and there are three possible outcomes:

- At the posterior pole, a slowly developing low-grade fibrous reaction within the retina can produce a tumour that resembles a retinoblastoma.
- In the midperiphery, a more rapid active inflammatory reaction, which is characterized by the presence of numerous eosinophils, is followed by

exudation into the retina and subretinal space, and then secondary retinal detachment.
- Inflammation and fibrosis occur in the vitreous base over the pars plana, and can induce a specific form of pars planitis.

Other parasites
In equatorial climates, infection by helminths such as *Wuchereria* sp. causes blindness when microfilariae migrate into the retina and vitreous.

NON-INFECTIOUS INFLAMMATORY DISEASE

Granulomatous reactions
Granulomatous reactions, similar to host responses in chronic infections, can occur in non-infectious reactions to endogenous and exogenous material.

Reactions to endogenous materials
Products of plasma, blood or cell breakdown can induce a giant cell granulomatous reaction when released into tissue. The commonest eyelid granuloma is the chalazion, which is a reaction to a blocked meibomian gland duct (see Box 9.7). Rupture of a cyst derived from a blocked pilosebaceous follicle in the eyelid skin (epidermal inclusion cyst) releases keratin into the adjacent epidermis. In children 'dermoid' cysts occur at the points of fusion of the facial processes and are characterized by a content of keratin and hairs and a wall, which incorporates hair follicles. Rupture of a dermoid cyst can occur spontaneously or at surgery with spillage of keratin and hair into the orbit, which carries the risk of chronic and painful orbital inflammation.

Red cells and plasma in the extracellular matrix provoke an inflammatory reaction and the cellular response depends on the presence of fibrinolysins (plasmin and plasminogen activator) in the tissue fluids. In the anterior chamber, fibrin is diluted by the aqueous and is rapidly dissolved by fibrinolysins present in the aqueous. The cellular response to red cells is restricted to migration of macrophages from the iris vessels into the anterior chamber. The haemomacrophagic reaction in the vitreous after bleeding from a tear in the retina or from torn preretinal vessels in vasoproliferative retinopathy is similar (Fig. 9.7). Similar haemogranulomas also occur within the orbit after trauma followed by bleeding (traumatic blood cysts).

Reactions to exogenous non-biological materials
Implantation in tissue of vegetable or organic matter such as wood excites a similar cellular response to

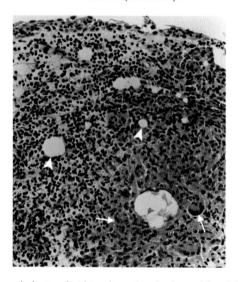
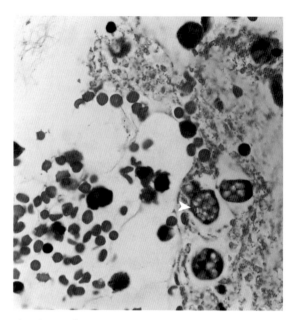

Fig. 9.7 After a vitreous haemorrhage, the red cells are phagocytosed by macrophages, which contain intact cells and lysed red cells (arrowhead). The granular material is haemoglobin released from the red cells.

copper and tin, and the reaction to copper ions is pyogenic for reasons that are as yet unknown. Similar reactions may be seen on occasions to materials used in ophthalmic surgery (see Box 9.8).

NON-GRANULOMATOUS INFLAMMATORY REACTIONS

Lymphocytes and plasma cells are found in a number of conditions in which the aetiology and pathogenesis are unknown. Many clinical forms of anterior and posterior uveitis, e.g. Behçet's disease, are characterized by diffuse and intense lymphocytic and plasma cell infiltration. Lymphocytic perivasculitis is a feature of demyelinating disease (multiple sclerosis) in the optic nerve and of retinal vasculitis. In endocrine exophthalmos there may be focal clusters of lymphocytes (lymphorrhages) within the extraocular muscles (Fig. 9.8).

AUTOIMMUNE DISEASE

The basic mechanisms of autoimmune disease pathophysiology have been dealt with elsewhere (see Ch. 5). In the eye and orbit many examples of autoimmune disease provide valuable pathological information. Many inflammatory diseases of the

that of sutures derived from cotton or synthetic materials (see Fig. 9.2). Synthetic fibres or fragments of plant are seen in polarized light as birefringent particles surrounded by macrophages and lymphocytes. Metallic fragments are slowly dissolved in tissue fluids, but elements such as iron are toxic to the retina, which undergoes neuronal loss, so that metallic foreign bodies in the vitreous or retina are especially dangerous. Brass contains

Box 9.8 Materials used in ophthalmic surgery

Plastic encircling bands made from silicone are used to indent the sclera in detachment surgery, in part because they produce little inflammatory reaction. However, there is always a surrounding fibrous capsule. In contrast a giant cell granulomatous reaction occurs around sutures (see Fig. 9.2). Particles of glass or the plastic used for intraocular lenses (polymethylmethacrylate; PMMA) do not stimulate a marked inflammatory reaction: the membranes on the posterior lens capsule are derived from metaplastic lens epithelial cells, not inflammatory cells. The silicone plastic plates and tubes (Molteno tubes and setons) that are designed to drain aqueous in advanced neovascular glaucoma do not excite an inflammatory response, although like the encircling bands the drainage orifices can be blocked by a fibrous capsule. Of the viscous fluids instilled to replace ocular fluids, hyaluronic acid (Healon) is inert, while silicon oil employed in retinal detachment surgery stimulates a low-grade macrophagic reaction after the oil becomes emulsified (see figure).

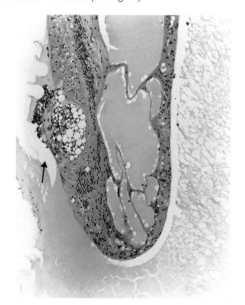

This is the edge of a retinal hole in an eye in which a retinal detachment was treated by intravitreal silicon oil. On the inner surface of the retina there is a clump of macrophages that have phagocytosed emulsified oil globules (arrow). Cysts are present within the detached retina, which exhibits long-standing photoreceptor atrophy.

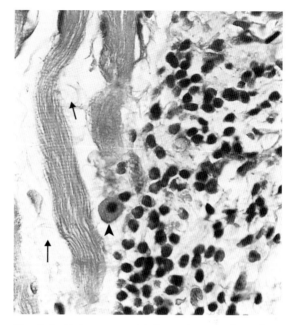

Fig. 9.8 Endocrine exophthalmos. The striated muscle fibres in the extraocular muscle are separated by lipid and mucopolysaccharide (arrows). Adjacent to the muscle fibres there are collections of lymphocytes and a mast cell (arrowhead).

eye and adnexae occur in the absence of identifiable causative organisms. Some are associated with generalized connective tissue disease or diseases with a recognized autoimmune aetiology. Others are restricted to the eye and periocular tissues. The following section describes some of these disorders.

Sjögren syndrome
Sjögren syndrome is a disorder of the acinar glands of the conjunctival and oral mucosa. In addition, the secretory acinar tissue of the lacrimal gland is destroyed by a lymphocytic infiltrate with formation of lymphoepithelial lesions. Impaired secretion of saliva and tears leads to a dry mouth and dry eyes, respectively, and there is an associated loss of goblet cells in the conjunctival epithelium with stratification of the surface epithelium.

Rheumatoid eye disease
Destruction of ocular tissue in rheumatoid arthritis is T-cell-mediated but also includes an immune complex-mediated vasculitis. Impairment of blood flow to the anterior segment causes a necrotizing scleritis and peripheral corneal ulceration, which are

473

serious complications of rheumatoid arthritis. Spontaneous central corneal ulceration (often without an inflammatory cell infiltration) occurs in rheumatoid disease (corneal melt), a phenomenon that is promoted by release of metalloproteinases but is poorly understood. If the destruction of collagen in the sclera is severe, the tissue undergoes fibrinoid necrosis with a granulomatous reaction around the necrotic sclera. Thinning of the sclera leads to exposure of the underlying uveal tract (scleromalacia perforans) but ciliary body prolapse and perforation are uncommon because of secondary fibrosis. In some patients the inflammatory process is slower and is accompanied by a reactive fibrosis with massive thickening of the sclera (brawny scleritis). A localized inflammatory reaction at the posterior pole of the eye causes macular oedema and the mass may simulate a malignant melanoma (posterior scleritis).

Other ocular surface disease

Autoimmune disease is seen in the skin of the eyelid in bullous diseases such as pemphigus. In the conjunctiva, autoimmune responses against basement membrane components and the attachments of the epithelium lead to severe stromal fibrosis (ocular mucous membrane pemphigoid). Immunofluorescence studies performed on tissue submitted in Michel's transport medium shows linear deposition of immunoglobulin G and sometimes C3 along the basement membrane. Detachment of epithelium from the basement membrane leads to inadequate protection and predisposes to secondary inflammation and the exudation of fibrin. In the fornix, a fibrinous exudate provides a scaffold for fibroblastic migration; the subsequent scarring process leads to adhesions between the eyelids and the globe (symblepharon).

Lens-induced uveitis

Autoimmunity to degenerate lens protein is well recognized. A cataractous lens contains proteins that are the breakdown products of the primary soluble crystallins and other proteins (see Ch. 5). Leakage of lens protein into the anterior chamber, either spontaneously or as a result of trauma, may induce a massive giant cell granulomatous reaction. Macrophages and lymphocytes enter the anterior chamber from dilated blood vessels in the iris and ciliary body, and may enter the lens cortex itself directly through a rupture in the lens capsule. There are commonly significant numbers of neutrophils and eosinophils in the inflammatory infiltrate. The

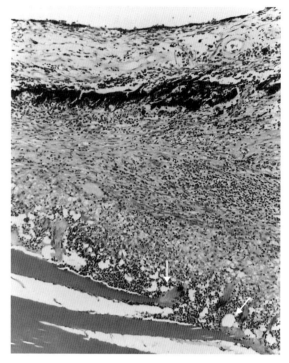

Fig. 9.9 In lens-induced uveitis, lens cortical matter is attacked by a giant cell granulomatous reaction (arrows) and fibrovascular tissue proliferates from the posterior surface of the iris.

inflammatory cells then pass directly through the epithelium of the pars plana during the associated cyclitis (Fig. 9.9).

Leakage of lens protein into the anterior chamber does not automatically induce a prominent inflammatory response. Sometimes lens protein is relatively inert and induces an uncomplicated macrophage response. This may be associated with a rise in pressure caused by outflow obstruction by engorged macrophages (phakolytic glaucoma). If the rupture is acute, the outflow system is blocked by lens matter (lens particle glaucoma).

Sympathetic ophthalmitis

A bilateral granulomatous inflammation of the choroid, ciliary body and iris (panuveitis) can occur after injury to one eye; the injury usually includes uveal incarceration within the sclera. The uveal tract becomes considerably thickened and the inflammatory infiltrate is characterized by the presence of lymphocytes, plasma cells, eosinophils and macrophages, which contain a fine dusting of melanin

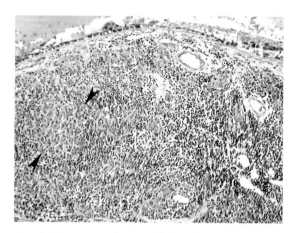

Fig. 9.10 In sympathetic ophthalmia there is expansion of the choroid by a chronic inflammatory infiltrate including granulomas (arrowhead). A fine dusting of melanin pigment within macrophages is characteristic. The choriocapillaris is spared and the retinal pigment epithelium contains infiltrating macrophages.

granules and fuse to form multinucleate cells (Fig. 9.10). The inflammatory process involves the retinal pigment epithelium with the accumulation of macrophages at this site (Dalen–Fuchs nodules). Sympathetic ophthalmitis is considered an autoimmune disease, possibly induced by retinal autoantigens. The posterior ciliary nerves are also involved in the inflammatory reaction and there is often evidence of lens-induced uveitis.

Severe inflammation in the uveal tract may lead to leakage of plasma into the subretinal space. This detaches the retina and causes blindness. Aqueous production by the ciliary epithelium may also be reduced by the inflammatory processes, with a fall in intraocular pressure. Prolonged ocular hypotonia results in shrinkage of the eye and an apparent thickening of the sclera. The process is referred to as phthisis bulbi (phthisis means wasting or shrinkage) and a series of complex but non-specific changes ensues. The detached retina becomes gliotic, a term used to indicate replacement of dying neurones by proliferating glial cells. The RPE proliferates on the inner surface of Bruch's membrane and undergoes metaplasia to form fibroblasts. At the end-stage the fibrous tissue undergoes further metaplasia to compact and cancellous bone (phthisis bulbi with ossification) (see p. 489).

TRAUMA

Although rapid closure of the lids is frequently effective in protecting the eye, the commonest forms of trauma to the eye are of a mechanical nature, and can vary from a minor scratch on the corneal surface to complete perforation by a sharp object or missile. The former type of injury is described as penetrating if only the outer part of the corneoscleral coat is damaged, and as perforating if the wound passes into and through the eye.

PHYSICAL TRAUMA

Physical injuries encompass mechanical (surgical, accidental and criminal trauma), ionizing radiation and exposure to extremes of temperature.

Mechanical trauma
Mechanical (non-surgical) trauma is the commonest form of ocular injury.

Blunt trauma
Blunt trauma describes mechanical injury in which the globe remains intact. Many of the effects are predictable. Anteroposterior deformation separates the delicate attachments between the intraocular structures, e.g. the zonular fibres, rupture of which causes lens dislocation. Separation of the attachment of the ciliary muscle to the scleral spur leads to collapse of the trabecular meshwork and secondary glaucoma (angle recession glaucoma).

The least well understood complication of blunt trauma is widespread retinal oedema (commotio retinae), which may be caused by transient spasm of the retinal vessels producing ischaemia and damage to endothelial cells with leakage into the tissue. However, it is equally likely to result from transient interruption of axoplasmic flow in the ganglion cell processes. Blunt trauma may also cause shearing of photoreceptors, leading to atrophy of the photoreceptors and focal reactive proliferation of the RPE into the retina (pseudoretinitis pigmentosa).

Trauma (accidental or non-accidental) in infants can lead to a number of findings, most commonly bilateral retinal haemorrhages associated with subdural haematoma. The mechanism of these retinal haemorrhages is unclear although the action of shearing forces at the vitreoretinal interface is currently favoured.

Perforating/penetrating injuries

Penetrating and perforating injuries are caused by a wide variety of weapons, tools, sporting equipment and domestic utensils, and almost inevitably lead to severe disorganization within the ocular structures.

Thermal damage to eye and adnexae

Cryotherapy is used surgically to induce an adhesive scar by freezing and thawing (cryotherapy) in the peripheral retina during the prophylaxis or treatment of retinal detachment. Cryoablation is also used to destroy the ciliary body in cases of intractable glaucoma, the aim being to suppress aqueous formation.

Ocular damage due to radiant energy

Light in the visible wavelengths, at normal levels of intensity, does not have acute harmful effects on the cornea, lens or retinal photoreceptors, because the cornea and lens absorb the ultraviolet and blue wavelengths. However, the production of free radicals by photons (e.g. hydrogen peroxide, superoxides) and the presence of free radical scavengers (e.g. vitamin A, superoxide dismutase and glutathione transferase) are finely balanced and may be overcome in conditions of excess exposure to ultraviolet light (as in snow blindness, in which the corneal epithelium is damaged).

Photic damage to photoreceptors

The delicate interrelationships between the rod and cone photoreceptors have been described in previous chapters. Photon bombardment of the photoreceptors at the macula over six or more decades has been suggested as a contributing factor in age-related macular degeneration.

Damage to the eye by laser (light amplification by stimulated emission of radiation)

The damage caused by laser energy is dependent on the wavelength, the site of absorption and the quantity of energy released. In panretinal photocoagulation, which is used to treat diabetic vasoproliferative retinopathy, the outer third of the retina and the underlying RPE cells are destroyed. Reactive proliferation of RPE at the edge of the burn leads to clinically visible pigmentation around a white circle, which is the result of a 'scar' formed by glial cells. Transpupillary thermotherapy (TTT) uses infrared light to heat (to 40°C) choroidal melanomas and bring about tumour cell necrosis.

Several types of laser are used in ophthalmology to treat various disorders of ocular function (see Table 9.1).

Table 9.1 Lasers used in ophthalmology		
Type of laser	Wavelength (nm)	Application
Argon (CW)	Green (457, 488, 514, 610)	Ablation of RPE/ outer retina (in diabetic retinopathy)
YAG/Nd	Pulse 1064	Disruption of lens capsular membranes; destruction of ciliary body (glaucoma)
Excimer (CW)	193	Radial keratometry Remodelling of corneal surface; refractive keratometry

CW, continuous wave; YAG/Nd, yttrium–aluminium–garnet/neodymium

Ionizing radiation

Each of the three types of ionizing radiation in common use in medical practice has applications in ophthalmology:

- charged particles (electrons and α-particles)
- uncharged particles (neutrons)
- electromagnetic radiation (X-rays and γ-rays).

Proton beam therapy is now an accepted choice for the external treatment of ocular melanomas, while γ-emitters such as ^{106}Ru and ^{60}Co can be applied topically to the sclera over a melanoma in the form of a radioactive plaque. X-rays and γ-rays are used for the external beam treatment of retinoblastoma.

The unit (gray; Gy) is a measure of the amount of energy absorbed in the target tissue. For melanomas, a dose of up to 110 Gy is required at the base of the tumour if a ^{106}Ru plaque is applied, while 40–60 Gy external radiation is required for the treatment of a retinoblastoma. With such high doses, cataract is inevitable if the lens is not shielded. Radiotherapy in and around the eye and orbit can have short- and long-term side effects (see Box 9.9).

CHEMICAL INJURY

Toxic chemicals of any sort will damage the delicate ocular tissue when applied externally. Acid and alkali burns are encountered most commonly in clinical practice, but detergents can also cause significant damage.

Box 9.9 Complications of irradiation therapy: effects on cells and tissues

Radiation from any source has a profound effect on nuclear DNA, with fracture of chromosomes, dislocation and translocations. In the short term the consequence is tissue destruction and suppression of cell division, which is essential for the ablation of tumour tissue. In the long term, the consequences are:

- Endarteritis – infiltration of the vessel wall by inflammatory cells and proliferation of spindle cells (myofibroblasts, intimal fibroplasia) within the internal elastic lamina. Narrowing of the vessel lumen contributes to tumour destruction by ischaemic necrosis (see figure). A long-term secondary complication of radiation arteritis is dilation of the capillary bed (telangiectasia). (Radiation vasculopathy in the retina is discussed on p. 478.)
- Loss of hair, teeth and glandular tissue. Irradiation of the orbit damages lacrimal gland tissue and leads to a dry eye.
- Massive necrosis of normal tissue when the radiation dose is excessive.
- An increased risk of mutations, with malformation in offspring and the induction of a second malignant tumour.

Irradiation causes an endarteritis with endothelial cell swelling, fibrin deposition and inflammatory cell infiltration.

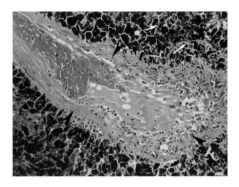

This is an irradiated melanoma with radiation endarteritis (black arrowheads) and surrounding pigment laden melanophages resulting from tumour necrosis (white arrows).

Acid burns

Acids (hydrochloric, nitric and sulphuric) and acidic fluids coagulate proteins, so that diffusion through the cornea and the sclera into the eye may be limited. Necrosis of epithelial and stromal cells leads to reactive fibrosis in the conjunctiva with eyelid distortion (entropion and ectropion). Corneal scarring requires keratoplasty to restore vision.

Alkali burns

Alkalis, such as ammonia and sodium hydroxide, pass through tissue easily and the high pH is sufficient to destroy the cells of the lens, uveal tract and retina as the alkaline fluid diffuses through the vitreous as far as the optic nerve.

TISSUE RESPONSE TO TRAUMA: REPAIR IN OCULAR TISSUES

The eye, like any other tissue, responds to injury by an initial acute inflammatory response followed by vascularization and wound closure in a fibroblastic scarring response. These responses may fundamentally alter the architecture and specific function in the tissue and can have serious effects on vision. For example, the wound response of the retina to retinal hole formation and detachment is to stimulate glial proliferation, termed proliferative vitreoretinopathy. This proliferation does not, however, restore retinal and choroidal integrity but has the opposite effect by contracting and shortening the retina, to the point that retinal reattachment may be surgically impossible. Similar serious consequences result from scarring in other ocular tissues.

Cornea

The corneal epithelium regenerates at the limbus and spreads rapidly across the cornea. Bowman's layer does not regenerate. Stromal keratocytes transform into fibroblasts to heal stromal wounds. Desçemet's membrane does not regenerate. The corneal endothelium fills in defects by sliding and in so doing deposits secondary layers in Desçemet's membrane: the membrane is elastic and there is often recoil at the edge of a deficit.

Iris

The presence of fibrinolysins in the aqueous inhibits fibrin clot formation, and scar tissue does not appear in the iris stroma; hence the persisting patency of defects made by iridectomy and iridotomy procedures. Reactive proliferation of the iris pigment epithelium may occur in response to trauma.

Lens

The lens epithelium responds to some forms of trauma by undergoing fibrous metaplasia.

Retina

Damaged nerve cells are replaced by glial cells, which are derived from perivascular astrocytes and Müller cells. In the RPE there is proliferation and metaplasia to fibrous tissue. A combination of glial cells and metaplastic RPE cells is found in preretinal membranes, particularly when such cells migrate via a retinal hole.

Choroid
The melanocytes of the choroid do not proliferate in response to trauma; scar tissue in the choroid is derived from scleral fibroblasts.

Sclera
Scars are formed by proliferation of episcleral fibroblasts.

Optic nerve
Trauma is followed by axonal loss and demyelination with reactive proliferation of glial cells and connective tissue cells.

Radiation vasculopathy
Ionizing radiation impairs the low-level replicative capacity of the endothelium of blood vessels; in many organs this accounts for the long-term ischaemic effects (see p. 480). In the retinal vessels there is extensive leakage of plasma constituents into the vessel wall and surrounding tissues. Irradiation of malignant melanoma has a similar effect on tumour blood vessels.

VASCULAR DISEASE

Vascular disease may be inflammatory or degenerative (see below). Primary inflammatory vascular disease (vasculitis) is frequently linked to autoimmune mechanisms, while degenerative vascular disease may be age related and/or metabolic (see below).

INFLAMMATORY VASCULAR DISEASE

Inflammatory vascular disease may be diagnosed clinically by the detection of antibodies to endothelial or inflammatory cells (e.g. antineutrophil cytoplasmic antibodies).

Vasculitis
The common feature of vasculitis is inflammation of a vessel wall often accompanied by necrosis. The two most common mechanisms are direct injury to the vessel wall by infectious agents and immune-mediated inflammation. The vasculitides are commonly classified according to the size of the vessel principally affected. Temporal arteritis and Taka-

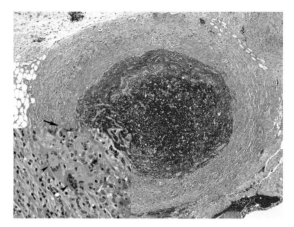

Fig. 9.11 In temporal arteritis the lumen may be occluded by thrombus. There is intimal proliferation and inflammatory cell infiltration of the media with multinucleated giant cells (black arrows and inset) in relation to the internal elastic lamina.

yasu arteritis are the principal large vessel vasculitides. Those involving medium sized vessels include classical polyarteritis nodosa and Kawasaki disease. The small vessel vasculitides include Wegener granulomatosis, Churg–Strauss syndrome, microscopic polyarteritis and Henoch–Schönlein purpura.

Temporal (giant cell) arteritis
Because it is treatable, the diagnosis of this blinding (and sometimes lethal) polysymptomatic disease is a matter of urgency. Any patient over 50 years of age, who develops the symptoms of unilateral or bilateral visual disturbance or blindness, facial pain, jaw claudication and signs such as a thickened tender temporal artery and optic disk swelling, requires immediate immunosuppressive therapy. A biopsy of the artery with several transverse cuts will reveal obliteration of the lumen; the disease is patchy and therefore may be discovered in only one of the six to 10 blocks taken. Microscopic examination shows extensive inflammatory cell infiltration, with lymphocytes, plasma cells, eosinophils and macrophages in the media (Fig. 9.11). Multinucleate giant cells are usually located near to the fragmented internal elastic lamina. The lumen is obliterated by a fibrin thrombus, which becomes organized and recanalized. The adventitia and the small periarterial vessels are often involved in the chronic inflammatory process.

Three points are noteworthy:

- Temporal arteritis is a systemic but patchy disease; negative histology does not exclude the diagnosis.
- Steroid therapy does not always totally suppress the inflammatory process and prevent occlusion of the arteries with subsequent blindness in the contralateral eye.
- A raised erythrocyte sedimentation rate is not essential for the diagnosis.

Temporal arteritis involves the cerebral arteries, the ophthalmic arteries, the posterior ciliary branches and the central retinal arteries. Thrombotic occlusion of the central retinal artery will cause infarction of the inner two-thirds of the retina. The intraretinal arterioles are not directly involved because these vessels do not possess an elastic layer. For this reason, elastic tissue has been suspected as the antigenic stimulus for this autoimmune reaction.

Ischaemic optic neuropathy, an outcome of degenerative arteriopathy, can mimic temporal arteritis particularly in elderly patients with a moderately raised erythrocyte sedimentation rate.

Takayasu disease
This condition resembles temporal arteritis but the major vessels arising from the arch of the aorta are involved. Unlike temporal arteritis, Takayasu disease usually occurs in patients under 50 years of age.

Polyarteritis nodosa
In polyarteritis nodosa medium- and small-sized arteries are focally involved in an inflammatory process, which leads to fibrinoid necrosis of the vessel wall and thrombosis. This leads to ischaemia and focal infarction in the heart, central nervous system, kidney and muscle. Polyarteritis nodosa may involve the ophthalmic artery, the central retinal artery and, in addition, the retinal and choroidal blood vessels; subretinal exudation of plasma leads to retinal detachment in this condition.

Wegener granulomatosis
The classical histological picture of Wegener granulomatosis is of a small vessel vasculitis with necrosis and granulomatous inflammation. This classic triad is not present in all biopsies and suspected cases should be interpreted in conjunction with the clinical signs and symptoms. Ocular manifestations include scleritis, corneoscleral ulceration or an orbital mass. These ocular findings may be part of the generalized systemic disease or its limited form. Generalized disease classically presents with renal, lung, upper respiratory tract and paranasal sinus involvement. The limited form manifests upper respiratory and lung disease without kidney involvement. Serology for circulating antineutrophil cytoplasmic antibodies (c-ANCA) is positive in over 90% of patients with generalized Wegener granulomatosis but in only 60% of those with the limited form.

Systemic lupus erythematosus
In this multisystem autoimmune disease, antibodies to blood constituents such as leucocyte DNA are responsible for anaemia, thrombocytopaenia and leukopaenia. Phospholipid antibody levels are raised and the consequent disturbances of coagulation explain the occlusive vasculopathy and haemorrhagic diathesis. In addition DNA–antiDNA antibody complexes are formed in response to the release of DNA from dying cells, and these initiate a type III hypersensitivity reaction. Small vessel vasculitis may occur in association with systemic lupus erythematosus and is responsible for tissue damage in the heart, lungs, kidney, brain and skin.

Ocular disease is rare but appears as a 'lupus retinopathy' characterized by the presence of retinal microinfarcts; in rarer, more severe, forms there is occlusive disease of the central retinal artery and vein with haemorrhagic infarction. Choroidopathy is uncommon as a clinical manifestation, but may be apparent on fluorescein angiography.

DEGENERATIVE VASCULAR DISEASE

Degenerative vascular disease (atheroma, atherosclerosis) is a major cause of morbidity and mortality in industrialized nations, and is also increased in metabolic disease such as diabetes.

Hyalinization
In ageing, hypertension and diabetes, the walls of arterioles and venules become thickened by deposition of collagen (hyalinization) with a loss of the normal smooth muscle layer (Fig. 9.12). Consequently there is a reduced capacity to respond to metabolic demand while narrowing of the lumen reduces the overall perfusion of the tissues. Hypertension can be superimposed on both diabetic and senile degenerative vasculopathy, adding a contractile (vasospastic) component to the disease.

Vasoocclusive disease
Retinal vasoocclusive disease may be macro- or microvascular. Macrovascular occlusions involve the central retinal artery or vein, or its major branches.

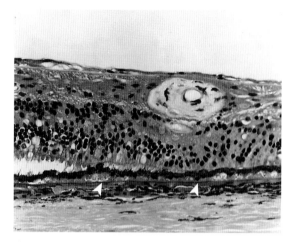

Fig. 9.12 A hyalinized retinal vessel with a thickened wall and narrowed lumen lies within an atrophic retina in which the normal neurones are replaced by glial cells. The photoreceptor layer is atrophic over the pigment epithelium, which is separated from Bruch's membrane by basal linear deposit (arrowheads).

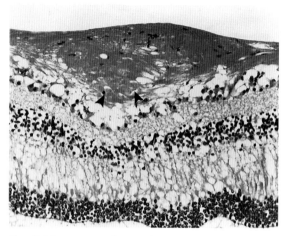

Fig. 9.13 A microinfarct in the retina is seen as a swollen sector of disrupted axons. Smudgy eosinophilic structures (cytoid bodies) represent the swollen ends of axons (arrowheads). The infarct mainly involves the nerve fibre layer.

Microvascular occlusion occurs at the precapillary vessel level, causing capillary non-perfusion and tissue ischaemia.

Microvascular occlusion

The following abnormalities may be found in conditions in which focal precapillary occlusion causes patchy interference with blood flow within the retina such as hypertension, diabetes, AIDS, radiation vasculopathy and the vasculitides:

- *Microinfarction* – fluffy white swellings (cotton-wool spots) in the retina on ophthalmoscopy are representations of the swollen ends of interrupted axons. Build-up of axoplasmic flow occurs at the edge of the area previously supplied by the occluded vessel (Fig. 9.13).
- *Hard exudates* – underperfusion of the vascular bed and damage to the endothelium of the deep capillaries leads to plasma leakage into the outer plexiform layer. Clinically this exudation is yellow and well circumscribed. Histologically 'hard' exudates are eosinophilic masses, and these contain foamy macrophages with lipid in the cytoplasm (Fig. 9.14).
- *Microaneurysms* – another effect of ischaemia on the capillary is weakening of the wall by necrosis of the supporting cell (the pericyte) in diabetes and the endothelial cell in central retinal vein occlusion. The ensuing small bulges or blowouts in the capillary wall are referred to as micro-

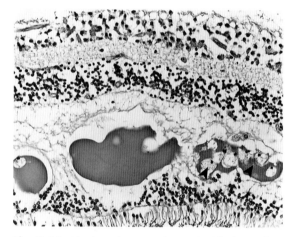

Fig. 9.14 Hard exudates are the result of leakage of plasma through the capillary endothelium. The exudates occur in the outer plexiform layer and foamy macrophages (arrowheads) are attracted to the deposit in an attempt to remove it.

aneurysms. With time, microaneurysms become filled by basement membrane deposits and consequently may disappear on fluorescein angiography.

- *Haemorrhage* – breakdown of the vessel wall leads to leakage of red cells and can take several forms in the retina:

Box 9.10 Vasoproliferative retinopathy

Proliferation of new blood vessels within and on the inner surface of the retina (intraretinal and preretinal neovascularization) is the most serious complication of diabetic retinopathy and is also a feature of central retinal vein occlusion. The precise mechanisms that initiate this process are under intense investigation. Ischaemic areas of the retina may release vasoformative factors (both stimulating and inhibiting) which diffuse into the retina and vitreous and stimulate endothelial cells to proliferate at the edge of the ischaemic area. However, it is possible that bloodborne vasoformative factors and changes in blood flow and/or blood viscosity may also contribute. The new vessels arise in the prevenular capillaries and in the walls of hyalinized venules, and proliferate within and on the surface of the retina. If the vitreous is detached, the fibrovascular tissue grows on the inner surface of the retina; the membrane contracts, leading to retinal detachment. Fibrovascular proliferation within the attached vitreous leads to haemorrhage and further formation of traction bands. The diffusion of vasoformative factors from the vitreous through the posterior and anterior chambers induces blood vessel formation on the iris surface (rubeosis iridis) and the inner surface of the trabecular meshwork, sealing off the angle and causing secondary (neovascular) glaucoma. In sickle cell disease, preretinal neovascularization takes the form of fanlike structures in the vitreous.

Box 9.11 Retinopathy of prematurity

In the premature infant vascularization of the retina is incomplete. Normally the blood vessels grow from the disk toward the periphery during intrauterine life, and the process is not complete until term, particularly at the temporal periphery, furthest from the disk. The extension of the normal vascular bed appears to be a response to the relative hypoxia of the proliferating neural cells. Migration of blood vessels does not occur while the premature infant is maintained in an atmosphere of high oxygen tension, possibly because the neural tissue is adequately oxygenated and the drive for normal vascularization is lost. Excessive proliferation of blood vessels (retinopathy of prematurity) occurs when the infant is returned to an atmosphere containing a normal partial pressure of oxygen. The peripheral non-vascularized retina is now ischaemic and the neovascular outgrowths from the peripheral vessels proliferate rapidly and in a disorganized manner within the retina and vitreous. The process may result in bilateral retinal detachment in the worst cases, but many cases of retinopathy of prematurity regress without permanent damage. Non-invasive techniques for the measurement of blood oxygen levels and careful control of the oxygen levels in the incubator can reduce the incidence of retinopathy of prematurity. Where necessary, retinopathy of prematurity can be treated by laser photocoagulation of the peripheral non-vascularized retina.

- Flame haemorrhages follow rupture of a small arteriole so that blood tracks into the nerve fibre layer.
- Dot haemorrhages follow rupture of capillaries in the outer plexiform layer; these are smaller and more circumscribed than flame haemorrhages.
- Blot haemorrhages are larger than dot haemorrhages, and represent bleeding from capillaries with tracking between the photoreceptors and the RPE
- *Neovascularization* – newly formed vessels grow from the venous side of the capillary bed within an area of arteriolar non-perfusion; this change represents a response to ischaemia within the retina. These vessels leak on fluorescein angiography and they occur in an eye, which will progress to vasoproliferative retinopathy (see Box 9.10). Vasoproliferation also occurs in retinopathy of prematurity (see Box 9.11), which is also intricately associated with relative retinal ischaemia.

Macrovascular occlusion

Macrovascular occlusion refers to obstruction of vessels of diameters equal to or greater than a medium-sized arteriole. It includes thrombotic occlusion of the central retinal artery, in association with systemic conditions such as hypertension and atherosclerosis.

- *Hypertension* – the classic textbook appearances of the retina in accelerated (malignant) hypertension, i.e. haemorrhage, exudates and papilloedema, are not normally seen with contemporary antihypertensive therapy. In the earlier literature, retinal vessels in mild cases of hypertensive retinopathy were described as being of 'copper-wire' or 'silver-wire' appearance, as a result of hyalinization. In more advanced disease, narrowing of the blood column followed spasm of the vessels, producing ischaemic damage to the endothelium distal to the constriction. Swelling and degeneration of the endothelium was followed by leakage of fibrin into the vessel wall and further narrowing of the lumen. Fibrinoid necrosis, such as is characteristic of hypertensive renal vasculopathy, may be found in the walls of choroidal and retinal vessels in uncontrolled hypertension. If the choriocapillaris is occluded by fibrinoid necrosis there is exudation beneath a necrotic retinal pigment

epithelium, leaving small areas of depigmentation (Elschnig's spots).

- *Central retinal artery occlusion* – the central retinal artery is an end-artery, and obstruction of flow leads immediately to blindness. The normally transparent retina becomes opaque, preventing transmission of the red reflex created by the choroidal vasculature except at the macula where the choriocapillaris is visible (the classic cherry-red spot). Central retinal artery occlusion may be the result of thrombosis in a degenerate central retinal artery but is more often the result of an embolus, typically from a mural thrombus on the endocardium after a myocardial infarction, an atheromatous plaque in the carotid artery, or the heart valves in subacute bacterial endocarditis. After total infarction, none of the inner retinal tissue survives and vasoformative factors are not released; thus rubeotic (neovascular) glaucoma occurs as a complication in fewer than 5% of cases, unlike central retinal vein occlusion in which up to 50% of cases may progress to glaucoma. Emboli may originate from many sources (see Box 9.12).

- *Central retinal vein occlusion* – the characteristic difference between central retinal artery and vein occlusion on fundoscopy is the presence of extensive haemorrhages within the retina in the latter. There may also be some recovery of vision in venous occlusion, unlike retinal occlusion, but in a significant number of patients rubeotic (neovascular) glaucoma develops within 3 months. Pre-retinal neovascularization and glaucoma are most frequent where there is extensive retinal ischaemia and may be prevented by peripheral retinal photoablation if the ischaemia is identified by fluorescein angiography. Frank neovascular glaucoma is usually not amenable to treatment, which is usually aimed at palliation of symptoms. It is often necessary to reduce intraocular pressure by inserting a plastic drainage tube into the eye (Molteno implant or setons). Enucleation of the eye may be necessary ultimately, to relieve intractable pain. Central retinal vein occlusion is also seen in a younger age group, where it may be extremely difficult to differentiate from retinal vasculitis (see above); in some women blood hyperviscosity as a result of oral contraception may be implicated. This form of central retinal vein occlusion has a better prognosis if it is the result of retinal vasculitis, and steroids or cyclosporin A will prevent its progression to neovascular glaucoma.

Box 9.12 Embolism

An embolus is any abnormal mass of matter carried in the bloodstream and large enough to occlude a vessel. The various types of embolism are listed below:

- *Thrombotic* – thrombus formation in the leg and pelvic veins is the principal cause of pulmonary embolism and intraoperative and postoperative death. In the retinal or choroidal vessels an embolus can originate from a thrombus on the mitral and aortic valves or from ulcerating atheromatous plaques in the aorta or carotid arteries. Another source may be a mural thrombus in the left ventricle.

- *Air embolism* occurs when negative pressure in the neck veins follows thyroid surgery or when fluid or air is forced into the venous circulation during a blood transfusion. Frothing of the blood in the right ventricle interferes with ventricular pumping and is fatal.

- *Tumour emboli* are usually small and not visible in the retinal circulation; larger metastases occur in the choroid.

- *Fat and marrow embolization* occurring after severe trauma to the limbs and trunk is accompanied by multiple fractures. Purpuric spots are seen on the upper thorax, and small haemorrhages are found in the retina. A severe form may rarely occur as Purtscher retinopathy in which florid embolization of multiple small vessels occurs.

- *Emboli from atheromatous aortic or carotid plaques* may consist of cholesterol/calcified tissue/fibrin/platelets, and can be seen migrating through the retinal circulation by ophthalmoscopy or videofluorescein angiography.

- *Septic emboli* were described in the retina by Roth in 1905, when subacute bacterial endocarditis was common. The typical Roth's spot has a white centre and red surround, and is thought to be the result of vascular damage from an impacted mass of white cells and bacteria in a retinal arteriole. The similarity between this appearance and the deposit of leukaemic cells or a simple infarct surrounded by red cells in a thrombocytopaenic immunosuppressed patient has broadened the definition of Roth's spots in contemporary ophthalmology.

- *Amniotic fluid embolism* is a complication of parturition particularly when manipulation of the fetus is required. Release of amniotic fluid, vernix, hairs and fetal squames into the maternal circulation is commonly fatal.

On clinical and pathological examination, a haemorrhagic retinopathy is striking with dot, blot and flame haemorrhages. The haemorrhages later resolve, leaving an atrophic retina containing prominent white sclerotic vessels in enucleated eyes. Transverse serial sections through the optic disk

Box 9.13 Pathogenesis of central retinal vein occlusion

The radius of the central vein in the lamina cribrosa of the optic disk is about 50% of that in the prelaminar part of the disk and smaller than that in the retrolaminar region. Furthermore, this narrowing of the vein within the lamina cribrosa becomes more variable with age. This is an unusual configuration (in most venous drainage systems the tributaries have a smaller radius than trunk vessels) and it can be explained by the necessity to maintain a high pressure in the retinal capillary bed against an intraocular pressure of 10–20 mmHg. The resistance provided by venous narrowing in the lamina cribrosa is disadvantageous in that flow is markedly increased in the narrowed segment and the resultant turbulence predisposes to thrombosis, particularly if there is an increase in blood viscosity (e.g. hyperglobulinaemia, polycythaemia) or in intraocular pressure. While systemic factors are important, an anatomical explanation has attractions because central retinal vein occlusion is almost always unilateral.

Other important systemic factors in central retinal vein thrombosis include abrupt falls in systemic blood pressure and hence the pressure in the central artery. If these are coupled with a diseased retinal vasculature (which predisposes to underperfusion and stasis in the vascular bed) the criteria for Virchow's triad are fulfilled.

usually reveal evidence of recanalization of the central retinal vein and non-occlusive degenerative disease of the central retinal artery. A thrombus, fresh or undergoing organization, in the vein is a histological rarity, but its occasional presence justifies the clinical term of 'central retinal vein thrombosis' or 'thrombotic' glaucoma. The pathogenesis is not entirely clear (see Box 9.13). Neovascularization occurs on the cupped disk, which is often distorted, as well as on the inner surface of the retina.

Vasculopathy: Coats disease

Loss of integrity in the vascular bed with leakage of plasma and red cells into the vessel wall can occur in the absence of inflammation or systemic disease. Coats disease is a good example of a congenital and unilateral primary retinal vasculopathy occurring within one sector of the retina, Children, commonly males, are normally affected within their first 4 years. The vascular abnormality is a result of an abnormal endothelium in both arterioles and venules, which leads to massive leakage of lipid-rich plasma into the retina and the subretinal space (see Fig. 9.35A,

p. 508). The clinical appearance may resemble a retinoblastoma.

METABOLIC DISEASE

The eyes and extraocular tissues are involved in a number of systemic metabolic diseases and the ophthalmic complications may often be the most serious complication from the patient's viewpoint.

DIABETES

Diabetic retinopathy is predominantly a microvascular disease in which capillary occlusion and retinal ischaemia are the major features (see above). The fundamental abnormality in the smaller vessels is multilayering of the basement membrane and degeneration of the endothelial cells and the pericytes.

Diabetes may affect other tissues in the eye; histological features include:

- vacuolation of the iris pigment epithelium
- thickening of the basement membranes of the ciliary processes
- cataract (there are no specific features).

EYE DISEASE ASSOCIATED WITH THYROID DYSFUNCTION

Endocrine exophthalmos may present with unilateral (15%) or bilateral proptosis and limitation of ocular movement in the absence of other clinical signs of hyperthyroidism. In addition to the clinical signs, the diagnosis is usually made by abnormally high values of triiodothyronine (T_3) and thyroxine (T_4), and low values of thyroid-stimulating hormone. The demonstration of uniform swelling of the extraocular muscles on computed tomography or orbital ultrasonography confirms endocrine exophthalmos, and is present in a high proportion of cases (up to 85%) in the absence of overt proptosis.

Histological examination of the extraocular muscle demonstrates perivascular lymphocytic infiltration (lymphorrhage) with mast cells and glycosaminoglycan accumulation within and around muscle fibres (see Fig. 9.8). As the disease progresses there is replacement fibrosis between the muscle fibres. Study of the nerves at the orbital apex reveals loss of larger axons in the motor nerves; this is attributed to compression by the swollen muscle and explains the limitation of movement (ophthalmoplegia).

DISORDERS OF AMINO ACID METABOLISM

Homocystinuria

The biochemical abnormality in this disease is a reduction in levels of cystathione β-synthetase. Patients suffering from this condition are at surgical and anaesthetic risk because of a tendency to thromboembolic disease, which can be fatal. Dislocation of the lens (inferiorly and somewhat posteriorly) is the result of an acquired metabolic abnormality of the zonular fibres. Histological examination of the zonular fibres reveals deposition of a thick band of periodic acid–Schiff-positive material on the inner surface of the ciliary processes and the pars plana.

Cystinosis

The biochemical disturbance occurs in the lysosomal membrane transport of cystine, which is continuously released in the lysosomes in the degradation of protein. In cystinosis the amino acid is trapped within the lysosome because of a defect in the transport system. The ocular manifestations – the accumulation of birefringent cystine crystals in conjunctiva, cornea, choroid, pigment epithelium and retina – have long been recognized. Alcohol fixation (100%) is necessary for histological verification of the presence of cystine crystals in a conjunctival biopsy.

MITOCHONDRIAL DISORDERS

Mitochondria contain DNA in chromosomes, which are self-replicating and encode enzymes involved in oxidative phosphorylation. When mutations occur in mitochondrial chromosomes, the defect is passed on via the ovum because the sperm does not have cytoplasmic constituents; thus mitochondrial disorders are maternally transmitted (see Ch. 3).

Leber's hereditary optic atrophy

Leber's hereditary optic atrophy is the result of point mutations in mitochondrial chromosomal DNA; this interferes with ATPase 6. Young males lose vision because of demyelination in the optic nerve in this disease: the papillomacular bundle is most severely affected.

Mitochondrial cytopathy

Mitochondrial cytopathies (e.g. Kearns–Sayre syndrome) are a group of disorders in which abnormal mitochondrial metabolism is manifest as skeletal and extraocular muscle weakness. The central nervous system is involved and the abnormalities in the RPE lead to photoreceptor atrophy. Death is caused by myocardial arrhythmias.

DYSTROPHIES

Dystrophies are disorders in which functional and morphological abnormalities appear in cells at various stages in life.

RETINAL DYSTROPHIES

There are many disorders in which visual loss is the result of photoreceptor degeneration associated with patchy atrophy and proliferation in the RPE; the term 'retinal pigment epitheliopathy' is appropriate. A detailed account is outwith the scope of this chapter and the reader is referred to the recommended reading list. A dystrophy may initially involve only the peripheral retina and progress later toward the macula, or may primarily involve the macula–the heredomacular degenerations. In many disorders, it is now possible to demonstrate genetic abnormalities (see Ch. 3).

An updated list of the genetic abnormalities can be obtained on the Internet (www.ncbi.nlm.nih.gov/omim).

Three examples of retinal dystrophies are provided here.

Retinitis pigmentosa

This group of diseases affects individuals in early adult life (for details of the genetic aspects see Ch. 3). The first symptoms are night blindness and a progressive reduction in visual field from the periphery toward the posterior pole. At the end-stage, retinal function is restricted to the central macular region ('tunnel vision'). Cataract is a common late complication. Fundoscopy reveals retinal atrophy, opacification and narrowing (hyalinization) of the retinal vessels, and mixed fine and coarse strands of pigmentation ('bone spicules'): the macular region is spared until the final stages.

On microscopy of advanced disease, the outer nuclear layer at the fovea appears as a single layer of cells with markedly stunted photoreceptors. Towards the periphery, the outer nuclear layer vanishes and is replaced by Müller cells, which fuse with the RPE. The RPE cells react by proliferation and migration into the retina to become distributed around the hyalinized vessels (Fig. 9.15), hence the 'bone spicules' seen on fundoscopy.

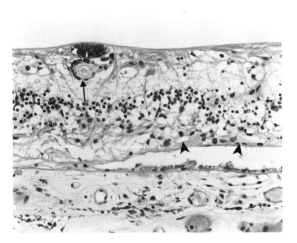

Fig. 9.15 In retinitis pigmentosa there is extensive atrophy of the photoreceptor layer, which is replaced by glial cells (arrowheads). The retinal pigment epithelium migrates into the retina and forms clusters around hyalinized blood vessels (arrow).

Recent reports have shown that autosomal dominant forms of retinitis pigmentosa are associated with mutations in the gene coding for rhodopsin, the rod photoreceptor pigment, which is located on the long arm of chromosome 3q and in the peripherin gene on chromosome 6p; other abnormalities which may implicate a single abnormal amino acid have been found on chromosomes 7p, 7q, 8 and 19q. If the rhodopsin molecule is abnormal, it is not difficult to appreciate that the normal process of disk replacement will be disturbed and that this will lead to photoreceptor atrophy. Other dominantly inherited forms have been associated with genes mapping to the long arm of chromosome 8 and mutations were shown in the peripherin gene (photoreceptor cell-specific glycoprotein), which is located on the short arm of chromosome 6. The loci for the X-linked forms of retinitis pigmentosa have also been identified on the short arm of the X chromosome (Xp11 and Xp21). The availability of genetic probes for the investigation of retinal degenerations has led to a massive increase in the volume of information in these disorders.

Vitelliform dystrophy (Best disease)
This is an autosomal dominant heredomacular degeneration in which there is loss of central visual acuity associated with a disk of yellow tissue at the macula. Histologically there is a massive accumulation of lipofuscin in the RPE cells in association with atrophy of the photoreceptor layer of the retina.

Stargardt disease (fundus flavimaculatus)
In this condition there is atrophy of the macula in association with the appearance of small yellow flecks. At the end-stage the outer layer of the retina is lost and the pigment epithelium is absent, so the gliotic retina fuses with Bruch's membrane. At the earliest stages the RPE is enlarged by accumulation of lipofuscin and melanin.

CORNEAL DYSTROPHIES

This term includes a large group of inherited conditions that cause bilateral, slowly progressive, corneal opacification and occur in the second, third and fourth decades of life. The conditions are conveniently classified as epithelial, stromal or endothelial, although the stromal diseases may involve the other layers. Unfortunately eponymous titles abound in this group of diseases.

Epithelial dystrophies
Superficial dystrophies involve the epithelium, which is unable to maintain normal replication and adhesion to Bowman's layer. Degeneration of cells with cyst formation leads to an unstable epithelium in Cogan's microcystic dystrophy. Separation of cells with invagination of neighbouring cells leads to the formation of loops of basement membrane; this is a diagnostic feature of Meesman's dystrophy. These changes may also be non-specific and the diagnosis often depends on a strong family history and the clinical appearance in bilateral symmetrical disease.

Corneal dystrophies of Bowman's layer
Reis–Buckler dystrophy is an autosomal dominant dystrophy that results in fine reticular opacities in the superficial cornea in early adult life. The histological features are not specific with nodules of fibrous tissue between Bowman's layer and the epithelium. Electron microscopy shows characteristic electron-dense rods. Thiel–Behnke dystrophy is a histologically identical Bowman's layer dystrophy that has a honeycomb pattern on clinical examination and presents in older patients. In Thiel–Behnke dystrophy electron microscopy shows curly fibres within the superficial fibrous nodules.

Stromal dystrophies
Although the opacities are the result of deposits of abnormal material in the stroma, there may be extensions into Bowman's layer and the endothelium may be involved. Many of the stromal

485

Box 9.14 Transforming growth factor-β-induced associated corneal dystrophies

Many of the corneal dystrophies are associated with mutations in the transforming growth factor-β-induced gene (*BIGH1*) situated on chromosome 5q31. This encodes a protein that is expressed on the cell membrane of corneal epithelium and stromal keratocytes and plays a role in adhesion and wound healing. Mutations in this gene result in abnormal folding for the resulting proteins. Accumulation of these proteins forms amyloid or other non-fibrillar deposits. The transforming growth factor-β-induced associated corneal dystrophies include the dystrophies involving Bowman's layer (Reis–Buckler, Thiel–Behnke) and the stromal dystrophies (granular, lattice and Avellino). All transforming growth factor-β-induced associated corneal dystrophies show autosomal dominant inheritance with complete penetrance.

dystrophies share a common genetic abnormality (see Box 9.14).

Lattice dystrophy

Inherited in an autosomal dominant manner, this dystrophy is characterized clinically by fine lines crisscrossing the stroma. Microscopy shows the deposits to consist of amyloid (Fig. 9.16). Secondary non-specific amyloid deposition is sometimes seen in the cornea at the end-stage of postinflammatory scarring and fibrosis. Lattice dystrophy commonly recurs in a graft.

Macular dystrophy

In this autosomal recessive disorder, the corneal opacities take the form of smudgy 'snowflake'-like areas; these are predominant in the axial region and cause severe visual impairment. This disease is a localized form of mucopolysaccharidosis. Mucopolysaccharide (acidic glycosaminoglycans) granules accumulate in the cytoplasm of the keratocytes and in the adjacent interlamellar spaces when the cells rupture. The corneal endothelial cells are involved and the material also accumulates within Descemet's membrane and beneath the epithelium (Fig. 9.17). Macular dystrophy rarely recurs in a graft. An identical histological appearance can occur in patients with a systemic mucopolysaccharidosis e.g. Morquio syndrome.

Granular corneal dystrophy

This is an autosomal dominant inherited disorder in which the anterior corneal stroma contains discrete opaque granules within transparent tissue.

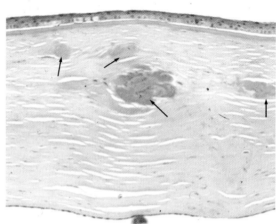
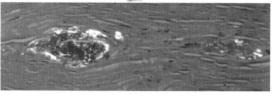

Fig. 9.16 Upper panel: in lattice dystrophy of the cornea, stromal deposits (arrows) have the staining characteristics of amyloid and exhibit apple green birefringence when a Congo red-stained section is observed in polarized light (lower panel).

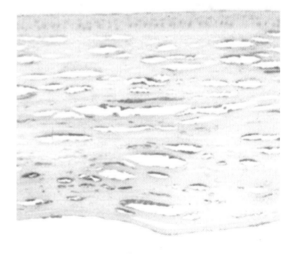

Fig. 9.17 In macular dystrophy of the cornea, mucopolysaccharide is deposited within the keratocytes and the endothelium (colloidal iron stain).

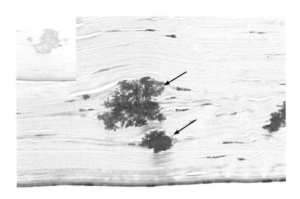

Fig. 9.18 In granular dystrophy of the cornea the hyaline amorphous deposits (keratinoid) stain strongly with the Masson stain and weakly in a haematoxylin & eosin-stained section (see inset).

Histologically the mid and anterior stroma and Bowman's layer contain non-birefringent hyaline bodies (Fig. 9.18) with positive staining for a keratin-like substance (so-called 'keratinoid'). The endothelium and Desçemet's membrane are not involved and the biochemical constituents of the hyaline material are unknown. Granular dystrophy occasionally recurs in a graft.

Combined granular–lattice dystrophy (Avellino dystrophy)

In the original reports, the combination of stromal amyloid deposits and the classic stromal granular deposits in the superficial cornea was thought to be a feature of individuals of Italian origin. Subsequently the disease has been found to be more widespread and the spectrum of the disease process more diverse than was originally thought.

Labrador keratopathy

Exposure to excessive sunlight, as in the desert or icebound climates (e.g. Labrador), causes deposition of golden yellow 'keratinoid' particles of protein (as yet unidentified) beneath the epithelium, in Bowman's layer, and in the superficial stroma.

Endothelial dystrophies

This is a group of disorders characterized by corneal oedema with opacification, occurring relatively early in life in the absence of pre-existing inflammation, glaucoma or identifiable systemic metabolic disorders. The clinical patterns are more important in the

classification than the pathological findings, which often overlap.

Congenital hereditary endothelial dystrophy

A cloudy cornea in childhood or early adult life may occur in this dystrophy, which can be autosomal recessive or autosomal dominant. The endothelium is abnormal and may be attenuated and vacuolated, but the characteristic feature is seen in Desçemet's membrane, which shows fine lamination because of the deposit of an abnormal layer of collagen at the ultrastructural level.

Iridocorneal endothelial syndrome

This disorder is non-familial, unilateral and occurs in adults. The corneal endothelium, as studied by *in vivo* specular microscopy, reveals areas of degenerate endothelial cells, which have a bright halo around a dark spot; these areas may be surrounded by endothelial cells of normal appearance. The late outcome in the so-called iridocorneal endothelial syndrome is corneal decompensation and oedema and/or glaucoma. This corneal endothelial abnormality is seen in association with several conditions:

- progressive atrophy of the iris stroma (essential iris atrophy)
- glaucoma due to endothelial sliding across the trabecular meshwork in the presence of a normal iris (Chandler syndrome)
- the presence of an iris naevus (the iris naevus syndrome).

In this syndrome the affected endothelial cells undergo marked changes at the ultrastructural level, such as bleb formation and the acquisition of numerous surface microvilli on the posterior surface.

Posterior polymorphous dystrophy

In this rare familial bilateral non-progressive disease, circumscribed or diffuse opacities are not usually severe enough to require keratoplasty until after the second decade. Morphologically, in the severe diffuse form of the disease, the posterior corneal surface is lined by stratified cells with prominent desmosomal attachments resembling corneal epithelial cells (Fig. 9.19).

Fuchs' endothelial dystrophy

In this common dystrophy, elderly patients are affected, females more than males. The clinical presentation includes bilateral diffuse oedema with cloudiness of the stroma. The abnormalities are restricted to epithelial oedema and thickening of

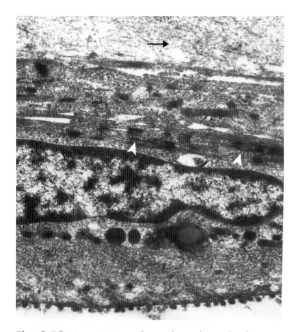

Fig. 9.19 In posterior polymorphous dystrophy the cornea is lined on its posterior surface by cells that, by electron microscopy, exhibit all the features of epithelial cells with intracytoplasmic filaments and desmosomal attachments (arrowheads). An abnormal collagenous layer (arrow) is deposited on the posterior surface of the original Descemet's membrane.

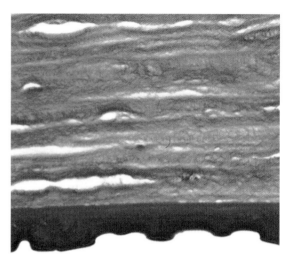

Fig. 9.20 In Fuchs' dystrophy Descemet's membrane is thickened and large excrescences project from the posterior surface (PAS stain).

Descemet's membrane with an obvious reduction in the endothelial cell population. Large nodular excrescences are present on the posterior surface of Descemet's membrane (Fig. 9.20), and the endothelial cells are of widely varying size. When excrescences (Hassall–Henle warts) are confined to the far periphery of the normal cornea, the effect on corneal transparency is minimal.

DEGENERATIVE DISEASE

Many ocular diseases are manifestations of the effects of ageing on the eye and orbit. Ageing involves a decline in the tissue cellularity, compounded in many individuals by a reduction in blood flow caused by degenerative vascular disease (see above). At the histological level the normal tissue constituents become atrophic and are replaced by an acellular collagenous matrix. Degenerative disease of tissues commonly involves connective tissue components such as collagen, elastin and proteoglycans. In contrast, dystrophies may occur at any age because they represent a disturbance of normal cellular functions (*dys* – altered; *trophy* – nutrition). Dystrophies may involve a single matrix constituent.

HYALINIZATION

This vague term is derived from the Greek word *hyalos*, which implies a glassy appearance. In histopathology it is used to describe the replacement of normal cells by an acellular, almost transparent, matrix (which in fact consists of collagens and glycoproteins). Hyalinization is typically seen in the eye and kidney in the walls of small blood vessels in ageing, benign hypertension and diabetes (see p. 483). Leakage of plasma into the vessel wall, owing to breakdown of the normal endothelial barrier, is thought to be one cause of hyalinization.

ELASTIC FIBRE DEGENERATION

Elastic fibres can be visualized with special stains (such as orcein). They appear as fine strands in tissues such as skin and blood vessels. The constituent protein, elastin, is arranged in coils, imparting elasticity to the strand (see Ch. 4). 'Elastotic degeneration' in skin is frequently the result of chronic sun exposure, which induces defective fibroblast

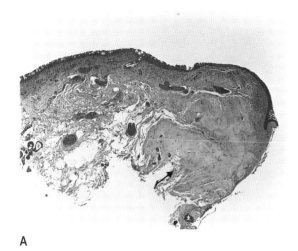

A

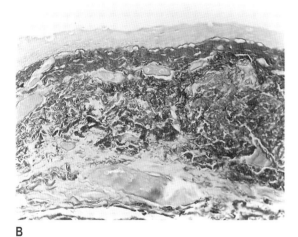

B

Fig. 9.21 (**A**) In an excised pterygium, the stroma is hyalinized and thickened by deposition of degenerating elastin (arrow). (**B**) The degenerate elastin can be demonstrated using a special stain (orcein).

function and an altered elastic matrix, which has poor elasticity. Reduced skin elasticity is also seen in pseudoxanthoma elasticum. In this condition ruptures in Bruch's membrane expose the choroid (angioid streaks).

Pinguecula and pterygium
In the conjunctiva, deposition of elastic-like material causes thickening and formation of nodules on the bulbar conjunctiva (pinguecula). In individuals exposed to a hot, dry, dusty environment, foci of elastotic degeneration form at the limbus in the interpalpebral fissure and encroach on the cornea as a wing-shaped wedge (pterygium) (Fig. 9.21). Various changes including dysplasia and carcinoma

Box 9.15 Calcification and ossification in ocular tissues

In the cornea a variety of conditions are associated with calcification of Bowman's layer and the superficial stroma. Deposits of calcium form a band across the cornea in the interpalpebral space and this is usually a non-specific response. Band keratopathy also occurs in hyperparathyroidism, hypervitaminosis D, and sarcoidosis (see p. 467). Calcification occurs in the fibrous tissue and in the degenerate cortex of a cataractous lens. In the calcified fibrotic lens substance, strips of lamellar and woven bone are laid down in trabeculae so that the lens takes on the appearance of a transverse section of a small bone such as rib (cataracta ossea). Bruch's membrane may be calcified in Paget disease of bone and as part of the ageing process.

Ossification may also occur in phthisis bulbi (see p. 471), usually in the metaplastic fibrous tissue derived from proliferation of the RPE in a hypotonic eye. Bone formation in this situation is of immature (woven) and mature (lamellar) type, and is located on the inner surface of Bruch's membrane. The ossification may extend into the vitreous and choroid, and an enucleated phthisical eye may be so hard that it is impossible to cut into the specimen without prior immersion in decalcifying fluid.

may occur in the epithelium overlying the elastotic tissue.

CALCIFICATION

Calcium is deposited in both normal and diseased tissue as hydroxyapatite crystals $[Ca_{10}(PO_4)_6(OH)_2)]$ In hypercalcaemic states such as hyperparathyroidism, hypervitaminosis D and excessive bone resorption from skeletal metastases, calcium is deposited in normal tissue such as the kidney and the conjunctiva; this process is called metastatic calcification.

By contrast, calcium can be deposited in hyalinized connective tissue (blood vessels) or necrotic tissue (such as posttuberculous scars in lung, atheromatous plaques, necrotic tumour tissue in a retinoblastoma) in a normocalcaemic state; this is referred to as dystrophic calcification. Calcification of ocular tissues also occurs in the end-stage phthisical eye (see Box 9.15).

AMYLOID

Amyloid is an insoluble protein deposited in tissues particularly around blood vessels and in basement

> **Box 9.16 Amyloid in ocular tissues**
>
> Amyloid may be observed as a solitary nodule within the eyelid, the orbit, or in the conjunctiva in the absence of systemic disease. Amyloid is deposited in the choroid and vitreous in systemic amyloidosis. In the cornea, amyloid deposition (see Fig. 9.16) is the characteristic feature of lattice dystrophy.

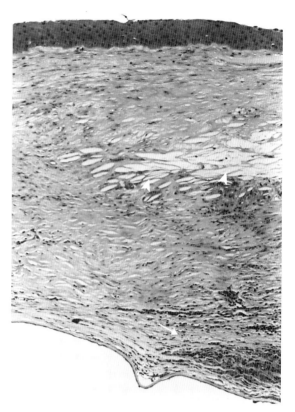

Fig. 9.22 At the end-stage of corneal inflammatory disease the stroma is invaded by blood vessels that leak lipid in the form of cholesterol crystals (arrowheads). There is an intense inflammatory infiltrate (arrow).

membranes. In haematoxylin & eosin-stained sections amyloid has a homogeneous pink appearance; staining with Congo red followed by examination in polarized light reveals apple green birefringence (Fig. 9.16). Amyloid was previously classified into two main groups primary and secondary. Knowledge of the mechanisms of amyloid deposition has made this classification obsolete and amyloid is now classified as systemic or localized.

Systemic

- Associated with monoclonal plasma cell proliferation, e.g. myeloma, Waldenstrom macroglobulinaemia. The amyloid is light-chain-derived (AL) from fragments of immunoglobulin.
- Associated with chronic inflammation, e.g. rheumatoid arthritis; genetically inherited familial Mediterranean fever. The amyloid is derived from serum AA protein (AA), an acute-phase reactant in many inflammatory conditions.

Localized

- Amyloid derived from polypeptide hormones may be deposited in endocrine tumours, e.g. medullary carcinoma of thyroid.
- Amyloid derived from prealbumin may be deposited in the heart, brain and joints in the elderly. Cerebral deposits of amyloid are important in Alzheimer's disease.

Amyloid also affects the eye (see Box 9.16).

The exfoliation syndrome (pseudoexfoliation syndrome)

Previously this disorder was considered to be confined to the eye, where it was seen as fluffy white deposits on the surface of the lens, the ciliary processes, the iris surface and the inner surface of the trabecular meshwork. Involvement of the outflow system leads to secondary open-angle glaucoma or 'exfoliation glaucoma'. Microscopy reveals an amorphous eosinophilic substance with a characteristic fibrillar structure when examined by electron microscopy. It is now known that the disorder is systemic and exfoliation deposits can be identified in the skin and viscera of individuals with ocular disease. The true pathogenesis of the exfoliation syndrome is not fully understood. Immunohistochemical studies have demonstrated the presence of elastic-related substances (elastin, fibrillin, amyloid P and vitronectin) and basement membrane proteins, e.g. laminin, fibronectin, nidogen, entactin and glycosaminoglycans within the exfoliation substance.

FATTY DEGENERATION

The most innocuous form of fatty infiltration in tissue is seen in the peripheral corneal stroma as part of the normal ageing process and is described as arcus senilis. After prolonged inflammation followed by corneal vascularization, plasma lipids leak from the blood vessels and are deposited in the stroma (Fig. 9.22).

Deposition of fat (neutral lipids and cholesterol) in the intima of medium and large muscular arteries (atheroma) is followed by thrombosis (see above under vascular disease). Lipids within clumps of macrophages in the dermis of the eyelid (xanthelasma) are usually a feature of ageing, but hypercholesterolaemia must be excluded.

CATARACT

Cataract is almost a normal part of the ageing process but also occurs after any insult to the lens (see Ch. 4).

Cataract associated with ageing

The lens crystallins (see Chs 1 and 4) break down to albuminoids, partly as an age-related process and partly in response to exposure to light, particularly of ultraviolet/blue wavelength. The amino acids (e.g. tyrosine) that are released are converted to epinephrine and melanin, so that lens pigmentation progresses from yellow to brown (brunescent cataract) to black (cataracta nigra) (see Ch. 4).

Secondary cataract

The biochemical requirements for the maintenance of transparency of the tissue are discussed in Chapter 4. Any metabolic disturbance, such as diabetes or hypocalcaemia, may potentially alter this microenvironment and can lead to lens opacification. The epithelial cells in the lens are also particularly sensitive to ionizing radiation and mechanical trauma; breakdown of transport mechanisms in the membranes of the lens fibre cells and the epithelium promotes ionic imbalance and fluid inflow, causing disorganization of the lens proteins and loss of transparency.

GLAUCOMA

Although malformation of the outflow system can lead to congenital or juvenile glaucoma (see Ch. 2), the most common forms of glaucoma are the result of degenerative disease and may be subclassified into primary or secondary types.

Primary open-angle glaucoma

Primary open-angle glaucoma (POAG) is a disease, which increases in incidence with age. The disease has a genetic basis – mutations have been identified in the *GLCA1* (chromosome 1 open angle glaucoma gene) in both early and late onset glaucoma. This gene encodes a 57-kDa protein known as the TIGR (trabecular meshwork inducible glucocorticoid

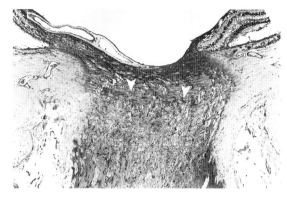

Fig. 9.23 The optic nerve is atrophic in advanced primary open-angle glaucoma and the lamina cribrosa (arrowheads) is bowed posteriorly so that the optic disk is cupped.

response) or MYOC (myocillin). Linkages to other genes on chromosome 3p have also been identified.

In POAG the raised intraocular pressure is attributable to abnormal resistance of the outflow system; however, to date no significant morphological abnormality has been demonstrated within the outflow system. Nonetheless in POAG obstruction to aqueous outflow develops progressively and the intraocular pressure gradually rises from the normal value of 18–23 mmHg to 25–35 mmHg.

The slow, progressive rise in intraocular pressure may be accompanied by occlusive disease in the posterior ciliary arteries, so that ischaemic optic atrophy may contribute to visual loss. Damage to the prelaminar optic nerve fibres may therefore be compounded by pressure-induced ischaemia in the capillary bed of the optic disk or to direct mechanical pressure preventing axoplasmic flow (see Ch. 4) in the axons passing through the lamina cribrosa. Nerve fibre bundles passing into the optic nerve head above or below the horizontal line on the temporal side of the disk are selectively damaged and the prelaminar part of the nerve becomes atrophic (Fig. 9.23). Clinically, defects occur in the visual field (arcuate scotoma), but fibres from the macula, the papillomacular bundle, are spared. As the atrophy progresses, the cup in the optic nerve head is enlarged more extensively in the vertical plane than in the horizontal.

Primary closed-angle glaucoma

Primary closed-angle glaucoma is also the result of degenerative disease. With age the globe becomes

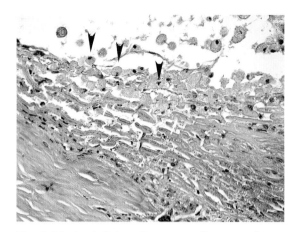

Fig. 9.24 In phakolytic glaucoma swollen macrophages that have phagocytosed lens matter (black arrowheads) clog the trabecular meshwork (white arrows).

smaller and the lens enlarges. The anterior surface of the lens displaces the pupillary part of the iris anteriorly and the anterior chamber becomes shallow; as the angles become narrower, pressure builds up behind the iris and pushes the peripheral iris towards the trabecular meshwork. This initiates a vicious circle and pressure rises in the posterior chamber to reach levels of 40–80 mmHg. Because the pressure increase is acute, the effect on the prelaminar nerve fibres is to block axoplasmic flow so that the optic disk swells (papilloedema).

Secondary glaucoma
Secondary glaucoma is also of two types: secondary open-angle and secondary closed-angle. In secondary open-angle glaucoma the angle is obstructed by cells in inflammation (uveitis), haemorrhage or tumour cell infiltration, or by lens matter when a degenerate lens capsule ruptures, flooding the anterior chamber with cortical lens matter and macrophages which have phagocytosed the lens cell fragments (phakolytic glaucoma; p. 471) (Fig. 9.24).

In secondary closed-angle glaucoma, the chamber angle may be closed mechanically by anterior displacement of the lens, for instance by an intraocular tumour (e.g. uveal melanoma or retinoblastoma). A more common form of secondary closed-angle glaucoma occurs in uveitis, in which fibrin initiates adhesion formation between the peripheral iris and the trabecular meshwork (anterior synechiae), or the pupillary iris and the lens (posterior synechiae). Both can produce a rise in pressure because of

obstruction to flow at the pupil (iris bombé) or in the angle. A special form of secondary glaucoma is neovascular (rubeotic) glaucoma caused by fibrovascular proliferation in the chamber angle; this is most commonly secondary to retinal ischaemia (diabetes and central retinal vein occlusion; p. 477). Rubeotic fibrovascular proliferation produces adhesions between the iris and the trabecular meshwork, which lead to a painful high-pressure glaucoma that is particularly resistant to therapy.

Congenital glaucoma in infants and children is the result of malformation of the chamber angle and failure of development in the trabecular meshwork.

DEGENERATION IN THE VITREOUS
Degeneration of the vitreous in humans commences in the late teens. Age-related degeneration takes the form of liquefaction of the collagen gel so that the collagen fibrils come out of suspension and form a precipitate. Clumped vitreous collagen fibrils are opaque and can interfere with vision in the form of 'floaters.' Vitreous gel liquefaction continues progressively over many years, a process known as syneresis. Vitreous syneresis and posterior vitreous detachment may occur as an acute event. Eventually a point is reached when the entire gel collapses and the loose attachments to the posterior retina and optic nerve give way. This is known as posterior vitreous detachment and, if the process is sufficiently forceful, may cause retinal hole formation particularly at points where vitreoretinal adhesion was firmest, e.g. the peripheral retina. The retinal hole or tear allows fluid to pass beneath the retina, which separates from the RPE. Rupture of a blood vessel may cause vitreous haemorrhage.

Asteroid hyalosis
One rather unusual degeneration that occurs in the vitreous is the formation of small particles containing calcium soaps (palmitate and stearate). This resembles a starlit sky, hence the descriptive terminology; the aetiology is unknown.

AGE-RELATED MACULAR DEGENERATION AND DISCIFORM DEGENERATION OF THE MACULA
Some 5% of the population over the age of 70 years have some degree of visual disturbance in one or both eyes that on examination manifests as minor patches of depigmentation in the macular region.

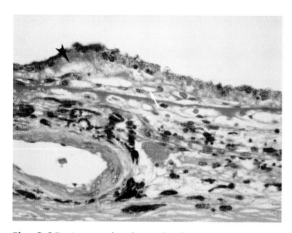

Fig. 9.25 In age-related macular degeneration the retinal pigment epithelium overlies a basal linear deposit (arrowhead), which attracts blood vessels (arrow); this precedes the florid fibrovascular proliferation seen in disciform degeneration of the macula. The overlying retina is detached by artefact.

These tiny yellow spots are referred to as drusen, and may be discrete (hard) or more diffuse and confluent (soft). The demonstration *in vivo* of submacular deposits by fluorescein angiography and indocyanin green permits a more accurate classification and identification of 'soft' drusen. Histological examination of the macula reveals atrophy of the photoreceptors over well-defined eosinophilic mounds beneath the RPE in the case of hard drusen and more linear granular bands in diffuse drusen. These deposits are situated between the cell basement membrane and Bruch's membrane. The term 'basal linear deposit' refers to a third type of deposit between the RPE cell membrane and its basement membrane. This deposit cannot be recognized clinically, although the abnormality can initiate neovascularization beneath the RPE (choroidal neovascularization) (Figs 9.12 and 9.25). Bruch's membrane is sometimes thickened or calcified, although the choriocapillaris only rarely shows degenerative replacement fibrosis.

At the cellular level, first macrophages and later endothelial cells proliferate in the deposits (soft drusen and basal linear deposit) beneath the RPE (Fig. 9.25). In a proportion of cases newly formed capillaries develop and the disease at this stage of choroidal or subRPE neovascularization is treatable by laser. Rupture of the vessels leads to oedema and haemorrhage, and this attracts more macrophages and further neovascularization. The RPE undergoes

fibrous metaplasia with deposition of collagen, contributing to the disk-shaped mass beneath the macula (disciform degeneration). A massive haemorrhage within the disciform focus may extend to the equator of the globe (Fig. 9.32A, p. 504) and sometimes ruptures through the retina into the vitreous. This causes severe visual loss. The haemorrhage then becomes organized, producing a grey subretinal mass that may be mistaken clinically for a tumour such as a malignant melanoma (see below).

Subretinal neovascularization may also occur in other disorders such as inflammatory disease. However, in pathological specimens, focal inflammatory disease in the choroid is not commonly observed because such eyes are rarely examined in the acute state.

Classically the 'presumed ocular histoplasmosis' syndrome is an inflammatory disorder associated with subretinal neovascularization. This syndrome is characterized by a triad of signs: scars and haemorrhagic detachment of the macula, peripheral punched-out areas of chorioretinal atrophy, and peripapillary chorioretinal scarring. Histological examination of the lesions has shown that the subretinal lesions contain RPE cells, fibroblasts and capillaries, but it is noteworthy that histoplasmosis is confined to North America.

PERIPHERAL DEGENERATION IN THE RETINA

The application of indirect ophthalmoscopy has revealed a wide variety of abnormal features in the peripheral retina; the majority are not of significance, but the following are important in terms of their complications.

Peripheral microcystoid degeneration

Microcystoid degeneration occurs within the outer plexiform layer and appears as a honeycomb on clinical and macroscopic examination. Tears in the inner and outer leaves can lead to retinal detachment. A rare complication of this degeneration is haemorrhage within a large cyst formed by coalescence of microcysts; the altered blood simulates a malignant melanoma (Fig. 9.32B, p. 504).

Lattice degeneration

This bilateral disease is important as a predisposing factor in rhegmatogenous detachment, i.e. due to fluid movement from the vitreous to the subretinal space through a retinal hole. On macroscopic

493

examination, lattice degeneration appears as an oval circumferential zone, 1–3 mm in diameter, traversed by white hyalinized blood vessels and speckled by foci of proliferating pigment epithelial cells. Histology reveals occluded vessels in the centre of a strip of retina, which is atrophic and fused with Bruch's membrane. In the overlying vitreous there are condensations of the collagen matrix and liquefaction of the gel. A tear (usually horseshoe-shaped) may occur at the junction between the anterior part of the atrophic strip and the adjacent normal retina as a result of the simple mechanical forces exerted on the vitreous base by ocular movement. In some but not all cases, fluid passes through the hole into the subretinal space and detaches the retina.

PHAKOMATOSES, MALFORMATIONS AND CHROMOSOMAL ABNORMALITIES

PHAKOMATOUS MALFORMATIONS

A group of hamartomatous malformations of the neural or vascular tissues of the eye are associated with involvement of other organs or tissues. In general hamartomas, which are tumour-like malformations derived from tissues normally present at that site, are benign, but there may be progression to malignancy such as the progression of skin or conjunctival naevi to malignant melanoma or sarcomatous changes occurring in neurofibromas.

Neurofibromatosis (type 1; von Recklinghausen disease)

This autosomal dominant condition, the result of a mutation in the *NF-1* gene on chromosome 17, is characterized by café-au-lait spots and neurofibromas of the skin. Other features are variably present. Ocular abnormalities include:

- melanocytic proliferations on the anterior surface of the iris (Lisch nodules)
- malformation of the chamber angle: goniodysgenesis (see Ch. 2)
- thickening of the posterior uvea by proliferation of melanocytes and other neural crest cells, more specifically large cells that resemble cells of sympathetic ganglia and Schwann cells
- retinal glial hamartomatous tumours
- optic nerve glioma.

Von Hippel–Lindau syndrome

This is a dominantly inherited familial cancer syndrome caused by mutation in the *VHL* gene on chromosome 3p. The cardinal features of von Hippel–Lindau syndrome are angiomata of the retina and haemangioblastoma of the cerebellum. Renal cell carcinoma also occurs in some patients. The ocular disease is characterized by capillary haemangiomas developing in the periphery of the retina throughout life; leakage from the abnormal vessels causes deposition of lipid exudates in the retina followed by an exudative detachment. Indirect ophthalmoscopy and fluorescein angiography permit identification of the vascular malformations and laser treatment may be effective at an early stage. Histologically, nests of proliferating capillaries within the retina are surrounded by glial cells and lipid-laden macrophages.

Sturge–Weber syndrome

This syndrome, also known as encephalotrigeminal angiomatosis, is characterized by naevus flammeus, a vascular malformation of the facial skin and angioma of the meninges. There is no clear evidence that the disease is hereditary. The main ocular finding is of choroidal haemangioma (Fig. 9.32C, p. 504). Glaucoma occurs in Sturge–Weber syndrome and is the result of vascular proliferation in the anterior segment.

Tuberose sclerosis

This is an autosomal dominant condition caused by a mutation on one of three genes on chromosomes 16, 12 and 9. The condition is characterized by hamartomas in multiple organ systems. In the eye these astrocytic hamartomas form small yellow tumours within the retina and may be misdiagnosed as retinoblastoma (Fig. 9.35B, p. 504). In the central nervous system, tumours derived from astrocytes are multiple and located in the walls of the ventricles. Associated neoplasms are angiomyolipomas in the renal cortex and rhabdomyomas in the myocardium.

MALFORMATIONS AND SYNDROMES ASSOCIATED WITH CHROMOSOMAL ABNORMALITIES

Intrauterine malformations of the eye can occur as a result of intrauterine exposure to teratogenic agents such as toxic chemicals (alcohol), drugs (thalidomide) and ionizing radiation, or may represent the effects of a detectable genetic abnormality. In many cases the cause of a malformation is unknown. Knowledge of the normal development of the eye (see Ch. 2) is essential for an understanding of ocular malformations (see Box 9.17).

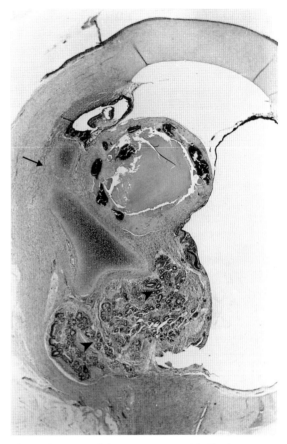

Fig. 9.26 Part of the eye in trisomy 13. The lens is displaced towards a fibrous ingrowth (arrow), which contains cartilage. The retina is folded and contains numerous circular rosette-like structures (arrowheads).

The current literature abounds with studies on the ocular pathology associated with chromosomal abnormalities of various types such as trisomies, deletions, translocations, point mutations, etc. (see Ch. 3). Two of the more comprehensively studied entities will be described to illustrate the range of malformations that may occur.

Trisomy 13 (Patau syndrome)

The ocular pathology in trisomy 13 illustrates various forms of malformation. The cornea and chamber angle are malformed and a persistent hyperplastic primary vitreous is common. The latter appears as a mass of fibrous tissue around the posterior surface of the lens and is the result of a failure of regression of the tunica vasculosa lentis. An anterior coloboma is present and is characterized by a fibrous ingrowth that contains nodules of cartilage. The coloboma occurs as a result of failure of fusion of the anterior edges of the inferonasal optic fissure. Retinal dysplasia is extensive with a failure of the primitive retinal cells to form into the normal layers. Optic nerve malformation is limited to hypoplasia (Fig. 9.26).

The systemic malformations are not compatible with survival as they are extreme examples of brain malformations (arrhinencephaly) along with cardiac and renal malformation. Malformations of this nature are now only rarely seen in the laboratory because of early screening.

Trisomy 21 (Down syndrome)

The systemic disturbances in this disorder are well known. In the eye, the important components are a high incidence of axial thinning of the cornea (keratoconus) and cataract. Small nodules are formed by spindle cells on the iris (Brushfield's spots); myopia and the attendant complication of retinal detachment may require surgical intervention.

NEOPLASIA

A neoplasm is a proliferation of cells the growth of which is progressive, purposeless, regardless of surrounding tissue, not related to the needs of the body and persists after the stimulus that initiated it has been withdrawn.

Table 9.2 Histological classification of tumours

Histological origin	Benign	Malignant
Epithelial cells		
Surface	Papilloma	Carcinoma (squamous, basal cell, etc.)
Glandular	Adenoma	Adenocarcinoma
Mesenchymal cells		
Adipose	Lipoma	Liposarcoma
Fibrous	Fibroma	Fibrosarcoma
Cartilage	Chondroma	Chondrosarcoma
Bone	Osteoma	Osteosarcoma
Smooth muscle	Leiomyoma	Leiomyosarcoma
Striated muscle	Rhabdomyoma	Rhabdomyosarcoma
Neuroectodermal cells		
Glial cells	Nerve	Glioma
	Ganglioneuroma	Neuroblastoma
Retinal cells		Retinoblastoma
Melanocytes		Melanoma
Meninges	Meningioma	Malignant meningioma
Schwann cells	Neurofibroma	Malignant peripheral nerve sheath tumour
Haemopoietic/Lymphoreticular		Leukaemia
		Lymphoma
Germ cells	Benign teratoma	Malignant teratoma
		Dysgerminoma
		Seminoma

Tumours may arise from any tissue in the body but for convenience these are divided into five groups. Not all malignant tumours have a benign counterpart and similarly there are some types of benign tumour for which malignant counterparts are extremely rare.

Neoplasms may be classified clinically, as benign or malignant or according to their histological tissue of origin (see Table 9.2). A benign tumour is usually well circumscribed and may be encapsulated. They grow slowly and remain localized at the site of origin. They may affect the host by producing pressure on adjacent structures (e.g. proptosis secondary to pleomorphic adenoma of lacrimal gland). Malignant tumours have an irregular, ill-defined boundary and are non-encapsulated. They grow rapidly with local and distant spread and produce effects by destroying adjacent structures (e.g. liver metastases from uveal melanoma)

PATHOGENESIS OF NEOPLASIA

Premalignancy

A number of pathological conditions are associated with the development of malignancy. The main categories include malignant transformation of benign tumours, chronic inflammatory conditions and intraepithelial neoplasia.

Benign tumours may undergo malignant transformation. A good example of this is colonic cancer arising from a benign adenoma. This is thought to occur by progressive acquisition of genetic changes. Malignant transformation of benign tumours is less common in ophthalmic pathology. Adenocarcinoma arising in a longstanding pleomorphic adenoma of the lacrimal gland is one example. Certain chronic inflammatory conditions, particularly if they are very longstanding, may undergo transformation to cancer. In Sjögren syndrome there is lymphocytic infiltration of the lacrimal gland with acinar atrophy later leading to the clinical symptoms of dry eye. Evolution to lymphoma occurs in a significant number of patients with Sjögren syndrome possibly by the development of monoclonal lymphocytic populations within the lacrimal gland. Intraepithelial neoplasia represents an intermediate stage in the production of cancer. In the skin, excessive exposure to ultraviolet light may lead to development of an actinic or solar keratosis. Clinically these appear as hyperkeratotic lesions on the face and histological examination reveals premalignant changes in the epidermis. This is seen as an increased mitotic rate, a loss of the normal polarity of maturation from basal cells to squamous cells, and a marked variation in the size and shape of nuclei (pleomorphism) within the epithelium (dysplasia). These histological changes precede invasion through the basement membrane of the epithelium into the underlying tissue, and are therefore designated carcinoma *in situ*.

Carcinogenesis

Both environmental and genetic factors contribute to a cell undergoing malignant change. This should be regarded as a multistep process. The three major environmental factors that induce tumours are chemicals, radiation and viruses. In chemical carcinogenesis the first step, initiation, involves a short exposure of the cell to a carcinogen. This is followed by promotion, the long-term exposure to a substance that is usually not mutagenic but acts by stimulating cell proliferation (although some compounds can act as both initiators and promoters, so-called complete carcinogens). Ionizing radiation directly damages DNA, especially during cell proliferation, and can result in a range of changes from single gene mutations to major chromosome deletions. Ultraviolet radiation mainly affects the skin-forming pyridimine dimers that can usually be excised by DNA repair mechanisms. In xeroderma pigmentosum these are deficient and multiple skin tumours occur. Viruses may contribute to the development of some human cancers (see Ch. 8). Oncogenic viruses may contribute to several conditions in the eye. Conjunctival papillomas and papillomas of the lacrimal passages may be caused by human papilloma virus types 16 and 11 respectively. Epstein–Barr virus contributes to the development of orbital Burkitt's lymphoma and to intraocular diffuse large B-cell lymphoma occurring in the immunosuppressed.

A genetic influence in cancer is now well recognized. Certain syndromes inherited in a Mendelian fashion show a high risk of cancer. Examples of these include xeroderma pigmentosum, an autosomal recessive trait where failure of DNA repair leads to skin cancer; and neurofibromatosis, an autosomal dominant trait characterized by multiple neurofibromas and increased risk of sarcoma, that is the result of a defect of the *NF-1* gene on chromosome 17. In Li–Fraumeni syndrome there is a high risk of several types of cancer, such as childhood sarcomas and breast cancer in young women. This is the result of a germ-line mutation of the *p53* gene.

Oncogenes and tumour suppressor genes

Cellular proto-oncogenes are normal genes that stimulate cell division. Tumour suppressor genes are normal genes that inhibit cell division. Proto-oncogenes and tumour suppressor genes are active during somatic growth, regeneration and repair and the balance between stimulation and inhibition of cell growth is strictly controlled. This balance is permanently lost in cancer cells.

Cellular proto-oncogenes code for a number of proteins involved in cell proliferation, including growth factors, growth factor receptors, signal transducers within the cell cytoplasm and nuclear-regulating proteins. In cancer these normal genes are permanently changed to oncogenes and proliferation is uncontrolled. Proto-oncogenes may become oncogenes by mutation, resulting in the production of a functionally abnormal protein or overexpression.

Tumour suppressor genes are normal genes that switch off cell proliferation. Loss of both copies of a tumour suppressor gene is required for cancer to develop. Loss of the *Rb* gene is important in the development of retinoblastoma (Ch. 3).

Tumour spread and metastases

Malignant tumours spread by several routes:

- Local invasion of normal tissue (e.g. basal cell carcinoma)
- Lymphatic spread (e.g. squamous carcinoma of the eyelid) or haematogenous spread (e.g. malignant melanoma of the choroid)
- Intraepithelial spread (e.g. Pagetoid spread of sebaceous carcinoma of the eyelid)
- Dissemination along natural passages (e.g. retinoblastoma extending to subarachnoid space; bronchial carcinoma spreading to pleura; ovarian carcinoma involving peritoneum).

The basic mechanisms of tumour cell invasion involve several mechanisms:

- Tumour cells secrete lytic enzymes to breach the basement membrane
- There is a loss of cell–cell adhesion molecules, often accompanied by an increase in cell–matrix adhesion molecules
- Increased cell movement allows tumour cells to penetrate further and spread.

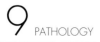

HAMARTOMAS

A hamartoma is a tumour-like but non-neoplastic malformation consisting of a mixture of tissues normally found at a particular site. The commonest forms of hamartoma are those composed of blood vessels and those involving melanocytes of the skin.

Haemangiomas

Capillary haemangiomas are a proliferation of small calibre vascular channels with a lobulated growth pattern. Cavernous haemangiomas consist of large calibre thick-walled vascular channels with intervening fibrous septae. Both capillary and cavernous haemangiomas may occur in the eyelid, orbit or choroid. Extensive haemangiomas may occur as part of encephalo-trigeminal angiomatosis (Sturge–Weber syndrome). Capillary haemangiomas may regress spontaneously during childhood but cavernous haemangiomas show no tendency for spontaneous regression.

Naevi

The word 'naevus' means a birthmark, but most naevi are acquired during childhood and adolescence. Melanocytes are of neural crest origin and migrate through the dermis to reach epithelial cells. A naevus is the result of abnormal migration, proliferation and maturation of these neuroectodermal cells. Initially the melanocytes form clumps at the junction between the epidermis and dermis. Clinically this appears as a brown macule, referred to as a junctional naevus. With age the proliferating melanocytes begin to detach from the epithelium and migrate into the dermis forming a brown papule. When proliferation is found in the dermis as well as the junctional area the naevus is classified as compound. At a later stage the proliferation is wholly in the dermis and is classified as an intradermal naevus.

Naevi, similar to their cutaneous counterpart, occur in the conjunctiva. In the iris and choroid, naevi are seen as static flat brown or black areas. Naevi in any site may occasionally progress to malignant melanoma.

CHORISTOMAS

In contrast with hamartoma a choristoma is a tumour-like but non-neoplastic malformation consisting of a mixture of tissues not normally present at a particular site.

Dermoid

Epibulbar dermoids are relatively common choristomas. They occur as a nodule (smooth white swellings from which hairs project) on the bulbar conjunctiva in children or at the outer angle of the bony orbit on the skin. Histological examination reveals a mixture of fat, fibrous tissue, hair follicles and sweat glands.

Phakomatous choristoma

This is a rare lesion presenting as a nodule in the eyelid. It is composed of epithelial cells and basement membrane, resembling lens capsular material, set in a dense fibrous stroma.

TERATOMA

This is a tumour derived from totipotent germ cells. They can occur at any site in the mid-line where germ cells have stopped on their migration to the gonads. Orbital teratomas are rare and occur in neonates. An orbital teratoma causes proptosis and histological examination of the large cystic retroocular mass will reveal tissue derived from the three embryonic germ cell layers such as respiratory or gastrointestinal epithelium, stroma containing fat, cartilage and bone, and neuroectodermal tissues. Most orbital teratomas are benign and surgical removal is curative.

BENIGN EPITHELIAL TUMOUR

Benign tumours of surface epithelium

A papilloma is a benign tumour originating from an epithelial surface. In the eyelid the commonest tumours are basal cell papilloma (seborrhoeic keratosis) and squamous cell papillomas. The former retains the basaloid appearance of the basal cells of the normal epidermis whereas the latter shows features of squamous differentiation. Benign squamous proliferations may be associated with poxvirus (molluscum contagiosum) or human papillomavirus (viral wart). Conjunctival papillomas can be pedunculated or sessile. The pedunculated papillomas are usually covered by conjunctival epithelium whereas sessile papillomas commonly show squamous differentiation. Conjunctival papillomas are also commonly associated with human papillomavirus.

Benign tumours of adnexal glands

An adenoma is derived from the ducts and acini of glands. In the eyelid and caruncle these may be derived from sweat glands, pilosebaceous hair follicles and sebaceous glands, the largest being the meibomian gland in the tarsal plate. Sweat gland adenomas are subclassified according to the degree of differentiation towards acinar or ductular structures. Similarly tumours of hair follicles are classified according to differentiation towards different components of the hair follicle. For example, a pilomatrixoma shows differentiation towards hair matrix. Sebaceous adenomas are proliferations of lipid-laden sebaceous cells and most commonly occur as a yellow mass at the caruncle.

MALIGNANT EPITHELIAL TUMOURS

Basal cell carcinoma

Basal cell carcinoma is the most common malignant tumour in clinical ophthalmology accounting for more than 90% of malignant eyelid tumours. It usually occurs in Caucasians over 50 years of age and is associated sunlight exposure. It may also occur in younger patients in association with the Gorlin–Goltz syndrome (basal cell naevus syndrome). Clinically these tumours may present as nodular lesions, which later may develop a central ulcer with a rolled edge. Morpheiform types present as a scirrhous plaque. Occasionally basal cell carcinomas are pigmented because of melanin deposition and clinically may be confused with malignant melanoma. Basal cell carcinoma is locally aggressive and adequate surgical excision is the treatment of choice to prevent recurrence and orbital invasion. Orbital invasion may necessitate exenteration.

Four main histological subtypes should be recognized:

- *Nodular/Solid basal cell carcinoma* – consists of well-circumscribed and relatively large islands of proliferating basal cells (Fig. 9.27A). Mitotic figures are usually plentiful. At the periphery of the tumour cell islands the cells are arranged as a palisade. Cystic degeneration may occur in this subtype (nodulocystic). Surgical excision should not present problems
- *Superficial basal cell carcinoma* – is less common than the nodular subtype and presents as a scaly plaque. Histology shows small nests of tumour cells budding from the undersurface of the epidermis only as far as the superficial dermis. There may be substantial gaps between the nests of tumour cells such that complete surgical excision may be difficult.
- *The infiltrative/morpheic subtype* – is a more aggressive form of basal cell carcinoma where the tumour cells grow in small strands rather than

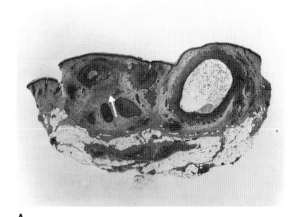

A

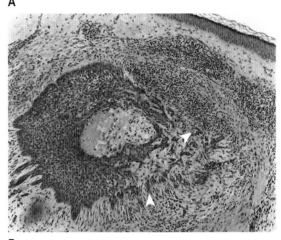

B

Fig. 9.27 (**A**) This basal cell carcinoma is of predominantly nodulocystic type. There is an area transforming to the infiltrative subtype (arrowhead). (**B**) In the infiltrative subtype the tumour infiltrates as cords of cells in a dense fibrous stroma (arrowheads).

nests and are embedded in a dense fibrous stroma (Fig. 9.27B). Peripheral palisading is much less pronounced than in the other subtypes. Infiltrative basal cell carcinoma does not have a distinct border making adequate surgical excision difficult.
- *The micronodular subtype* – is also a more aggressive form. The tumour forms small nodular aggregates of basaloid cells and, similar to the infiltrative subtype, subclinical involvement is often significant.

Squamous cell carcinoma

Compared with basal cell carcinoma the incidence of this form of malignancy is low, representing   499 between 1 and 5% of all eyelid cancers. Risk factors for squamous cell carcinoma include sunlight exposure and immunosuppression. Clinically, squamous cell carcinoma presents as a rapidly growing nodular ulcer or as a papillomatous growth, which in some cases has an overlying keratinous horn. Inadequate primary local excision may be followed by recurrence and orbital invasion. Lymphatic spread may occur to preauricular and submandibular lymph nodes according to the site of origin – upper and lower lid respectively.

Histologically, squamous cell carcinoma may be classified as well, moderate or poorly differentiated. In a well-differentiated tumour the cells have glassy, pink cytoplasm and intercellular bridges and keratin pearls may be present (Fig. 9.28). Some of these features are lost in more poorly differentiated tumours but intercellular bridges can usually still be identified. Rarely, squamous cell carcinoma will adopt a spindle cell morphology and this variant is more aggressive.

In situ and invasive squamous cell carcinoma may also involve the conjunctiva and cornea. The morphology of these tumours is identical to that of the eyelid tumours and they are also associated with sunlight exposure and immunosuppression, particularly AIDS.

Sebaceous gland carcinoma

Sebaceous gland carcinoma accounts for 1 to 5% of all eyelid cancers. These tumours usually originate in the meibomian gland but may also arise from the gland of Zeiss or sebaceous glands of the eyelid skin. Sebaceous gland carcinoma commonly occurs in elderly patients and shows a female preponderance. The clinical appearance of sebaceous gland carcinoma is variable and it may be indistinguishable from squamous cell carcinoma or basal cell carcinoma or may mimic a range of benign conditions including chalazion and blepharoconjunctivitis.

The variable clinical appearance is related to the different histological growth patterns of this tumour. These tumours may show a nodular or diffuse pattern of growth and may be well, moderate or poorly differentiated. The nodular pattern consists of lobules of tumour cells with foamy or vacuolated cytoplasm (Fig. 9.29A). Diffuse tumours show individual tumour cells spreading within the surface epithelium (Pagetoid spread) and adnexal structures. Lipid within the tumour cells may be demonstrated in unprocessed tissue using conventional fat stains such as Oil Red O (Fig. 9.29B). Immunohis-

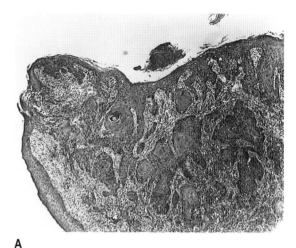

A

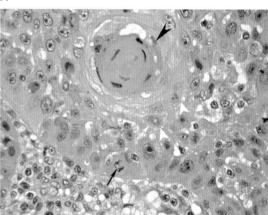

B

Fig. 9.28 (**A**) Squamous cell carcinoma of the eyelid infiltrates extensively through the underlying tissue. (**B**) The cells show keratinization (black arrowhead) and intracellular bridges (white arrowhead). There is a mitotic figure (black arrow).

tochemistry may also be helpful in the diagnosis. The prognosis is poor compared with most other malignant eyelid tumours but is significantly improved with early diagnosis and surgery.

MALIGNANT MELANOMA

Conjunctiva

Malignant melanoma may arise from primary acquired melanosis, a pre-existing naevus or *de novo*. Primary acquired melanosis appears as unilateral or bilateral, diffuse flat areas of conjunctival pigmentation in middle-aged to elderly patients. Two main subtypes are recognized:

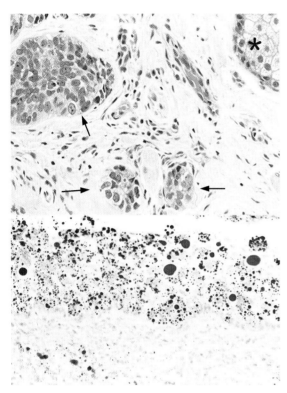

Fig. 9.29 (**A**) The islands (arrows) of infiltrating sebaceous gland carcinoma contain cells with pale cytoplasm that bear some resemblance to normal sebaceous gland cells (*). (**B**) A stain for fat (Oil Red O) reveals malignant cells infiltrating the conjunctival epithelium in Pagetoid spread of a sebaceous carcinoma.

- *Primary acquired melanosis without atypia* – there are an excess number of basally located melanocytes without cytological atypia. These lesions are similar to cutaneous senile lentigo and are not premalignant.
- *Primary acquired melanosis with atypia* – this can be graded mild to severe. In mild cases atypical melanocytes are confined to the basal layers. There is progressive involvement of the whole epithelium with moderate and severe atypia. Primary acquired melanosis is a premalignant condition.

Conjunctival melanoma presents as a raised, pigmented or fleshy conjunctival lesion. It has a definite tendency to metastasize to regional lymph nodes but may also spread to brain and other organs. The prognosis is worse for tumours thicker than 5 mm and located in the fornix. Complete excision is the treatment of choice. Those arising on a background of primary acquired melanosis may be multifocal and topical chemotherapy with mitomycin C can be helpful.

Uveal melanoma

Malignant melanoma of the uveal tract arises from melanocytes in the iris, ciliary body and choroid and the relative incidence is roughly in proportion to the volume of tissue in each compartment – 8, 12 and 80% respectively. These tumours are almost always unilateral and grow initially as pigmented or non-pigmented plaque-like lesions; the macroscopic appearances are shown in Figure 9.30(A–D).

Iris melanomas

Iris melanomas are usually slow growing nodular tumours that may be present for many years. On histology, iris melanomas may consist of small, rather bland, spindle-shaped cells and the diagnosis depends on the identification of surface or stromal invasion. Recurrent iris melanomas often transform into pleomorphic epithelioid tumours. Although they often remain localized for a long period of time, iris melanomas can spread diffusely on the iris surface and around the chamber angle, resulting in secondary glaucoma as a result of infiltration of the trabecular meshwork.

Ciliary body and choroidal melanomas

Ciliary body and choroidal melanomas can grow to a large size (10–20 mm) before recognition. The macroscopic appearances can vary considerably. The tumours may be ovoid or nodular and the classical mushroom shape, caused by tumour spread in the subretinal space after breaching Bruch's membrane, is rare. Tumours may be amelanotic, light grey/brown or, rarely, heavily pigmented. Extraocular extension may be identified in relation to collector channels (anteriorly), vortex veins (in the mid periphery) or short ciliary vessels (posteriorly). Larger tumours may undergo spontaneous necrosis.

On histology, the tumours are classified according to cell type as spindle, epithelioid and mixed (Fig. 9.31). In practice the majority of tumours are of mixed cell type. Vascular patterns may be assessed in melanomas in a periodic acid–Schiff (PAS) stain. There are nine recognized patterns including parallel, parallel with cross-linking and a network of closed vascular loops. The presence of microscopic intrascleral spread or extraocular extension is also important for staging uveal melanoma. Metastatic spread (most commonly to the liver) usually occurs within 2–3 years but has also been recorded up to 40 years later. Immunohistochemistry, which is usually positive for S100, HMB45 and Melan A, can

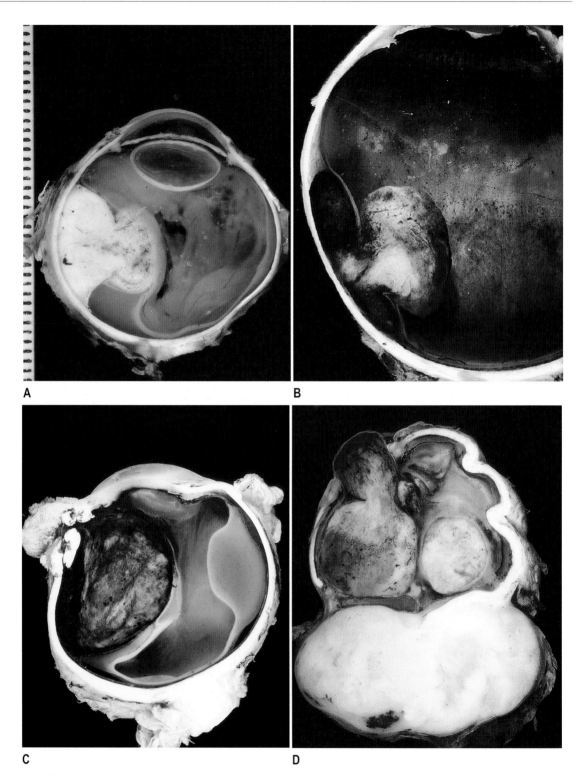

Fig. 9.30 Various macroscopic appearances of uveal melanoma. (**A**) The majority of tumours are amelanotic and have a mushroom shape. (**B**) A partially pigmented melanoma that has perforated the retina. (**C**) This ovoid black melanoma has leaked fluid into the subretinal space causing an exudative retinal detachment. An attempt to remove the tumour surgically was abandoned. (**D**) An advanced melanoma perforating the anterior and posterior sclera.

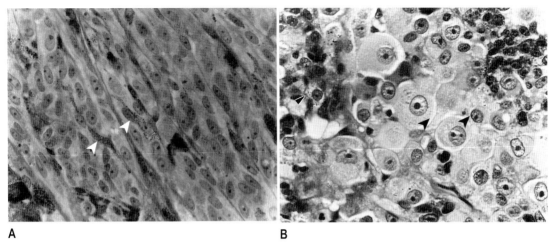

Fig. 9.31 **(A)** In this malignant uveal melanoma of spindle B type the cytoplasm of the cells contains melanin granules (arrowheads). **(B)** Epithelioid melanoma cells are much larger than spindle B cells and are separated from each other by prominent intercellular spaces (arrowheads).

be a useful ancillary technique, particularly in meta-static melanoma.

Enucleation may be the treatment of choice at the time of diagnosis or may follow failure of other forms. Enucleation following local or 'endo-' resection will show a large coloboma at the surgery site. Recurrent tumour may be evident at the edge of the coloboma. Ionizing radiation may be used in the form of plaque brachytherapy or proton beam. Enucleation following irradiation may show results from no apparent effect on the tumour to complete necrosis or infarction. Alternatively enucleation may be performed for recurrent tumour. Additional histological evidence of irradiation includes neovascular glaucoma, cataract and radiation retinopathy.

Prognostic parameters in uveal melanoma include:

- *Age of patient* – the prognosis is worse for older patients
- *Tumour size* – larger tumours carry a worse prognosis
- *Tumour location* – ciliary body location carries a worse prognosis compared with choroid
- *Cell type* – tumours containing an epithelioid cell component carry a poorer prognosis than those composed only of spindle cells
- *Vascular patterns* – tumours with a closed loop vascular pattern on PAS stain carry a poorer prognosis
- *Cytogenetics* – loss of heterozygosity of chromosome 3 (monosomy 3), particularly when com-

bined with additional copies of chromosome 8q is strongly associated with death from metastases. Whereas aberrations, particularly numerical gain, of chromosome 6p are associated with a more favourable prognosis.

Uveal melanoma can be simulated clinically by various other entities. Some typical examples are shown in Figure 9.32(A–D).

NEURAL TUMOURS

Neurofibroma and schwannoma

These tumours arise within the orbit and are derived from peripheral nerves. Neurofibroma is derived from the endoneurium and schwannomas from the Schwann cells intimately surrounding axons. On histological examination neurofibromas consist of spindle cells with wavy nuclei and collagen with occasional axons running through the tumour. Neurofibromas, particularly the plexiform and diffuse subtypes, may be associated with neurofibromatosis type 1. Schwannomas show a palisaded arrangement of spindle cells (Antoni A) and myxoid (Antoni B) areas and, in contrast to neurofibromas, there are occasional axons in the peripheral part of the tumour. Degenerative changes, with thick-walled blood vessels with evidence of previous haemorrhage and atypical nuclei, are relatively common. Occasionally a schwannoma may contain melanin pigment and the differential diagnosis of extraocular extension of a spindle cell melanoma should be considered.

503

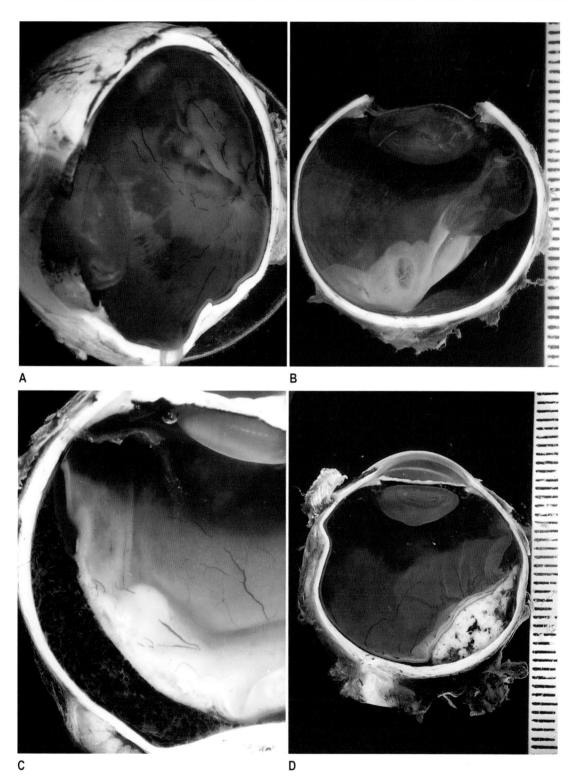

Fig. 9.32 Diseases simulating uveal melanomas. (**A**) Blood arising from disciform degeneration of the macula. (**B**) Bleeding into a macrocyst arising from a peripheral microcystoid degeneration of the retina. (**C**) Angioma of the choroid. (**D**) Metastatic tumours from breast or lung.

Malignant peripheral nerve sheath tumours

Malignant peripheral nerve sheath tumours are rare in the orbit. Most arise *de novo* without previous evidence of a neurofibroma or schwannoma. They may be associated with neurofibromatosis type 1.

Retinoblastoma

Retinoblastoma is a malignant tumour of infancy which is lethal if untreated; the incidence is 1 in 20 000 live births. The tumour arises from embryonal retinal cells and can be unilateral or bilateral. The macroscopic appearances are of a smooth-surfaced white mass that may show endophytic growth, into the vitreous or exophytic growth into the subretinal space (Fig. 9.33A–D). Yellowish areas of necrosis or bright white flecks of calcification may be evident within the tumour. On histology the tumour consists of small blue cells with scanty cytoplasm. There is usually a high mitotic rate with prominent apoptosis and areas of necrosis within the tumour indicating high cell turnover. DNA from necrotic tumour may precipitate on blood vessel walls or as basophilic lakes. Differentiation may be seen in the form of:

- Homer–Wright rosettes – a multilayered circle of nuclei surrounding eosinophilic fibrillar material
- Flexner–Wintersteiner rosettes – a circle of cells limited internally by a continuous membrane (Fig. 9.34)
- Fleurettes – primitive photoreceptor bodies arranged in 'fleur de lys' shape. These structures are most commonly found in irradiated tumours

Features of prognostic importance in retinoblastoma include tumour size, degree of differentiation, choroidal invasion and optic nerve invasion. With early diagnosis and modern treatment, including irradiation and chemotherapy, cure rates are in excess of 90%. In untreated cases death is caused by tumour spread to the brain through the optic nerve or along the meninges; metastatic dissemination is via the bloodstream to the viscera and skeleton.

The genetics of retinoblastoma are discussed in Chapter 3, but it is noteworthy that the abnormal gene carries the risk of a pineal tumour in childhood (trilateral retinoblastoma), soft tissue and osteogenic sarcoma in early adult life and carcinomas in later life.

The differential diagnosis of retinoblastoma includes:

- Coats disease (Fig. 9.35A)
- Astrocytic hamartoma (Fig. 9.35B)
- Retinopathy of prematurity
- Persistent hyperplastic primary vitreous (Fig. 9.35C)
- Endophthalmitis (Fig. 9.35D)
- *Toxocara* retinitis

Astrocytic hamartoma

Benign astrocytic tumours occur in the retina as part of the tuberous sclerosis syndrome or as an isolated feature. They consist of astrocytes, which form a matrix conducive to the deposition of calcospherites. The presence of calcification may lead to an erroneous diagnosis of retinoblastoma.

Glioma

Juvenile and adult forms of optic nerve glioma are recognized, the former carrying a good prognosis; the latter are very rare and invariably lethal, being associated with extensive intracranial extension.

Around 50% of gliomas involve the orbital portion of the nerve but the intracranial or chiasmal portions may also be involved. In the orbital portion the tumour may cause proptosis in addition to optic disc swelling and visual loss. Computed tomography or magnetic resonance imaging may be helpful in delineating the location, configuration and extent of the tumour. In over 50% of patients the tumour does not grow but in the remaining cases the tumour does grow and may require surgical intervention. The affected region of the nerve may be excised or if there is extensive tumour with secondary complications, such as exposure keratitis, then the eye may be removed along with the affected segment of the nerve. Optic nerve gliomas have an excellent prognosis following complete surgical excision although vision is usually sacrificed.

Excised tumours show a fusiform swelling of the nerve and the residual nerve may be barely visible within the tumour mass. The histology of these tumours is identical to that of intracranial astrocytomas and the majority are pilocytic, often containing areas of myxoid degeneration and Rosenthal fibres (Fig. 9.36). A potential diagnostic pitfall is that these tumours can induce proliferation of the overlying arachnoid. This hyperplastic tissue may be misdiagnosed as meningioma if the biopsy contains only perineural tissue.

Meningioma

Meningioma of the optic nerve may be primary, arising from the meninges of the optic nerve, or

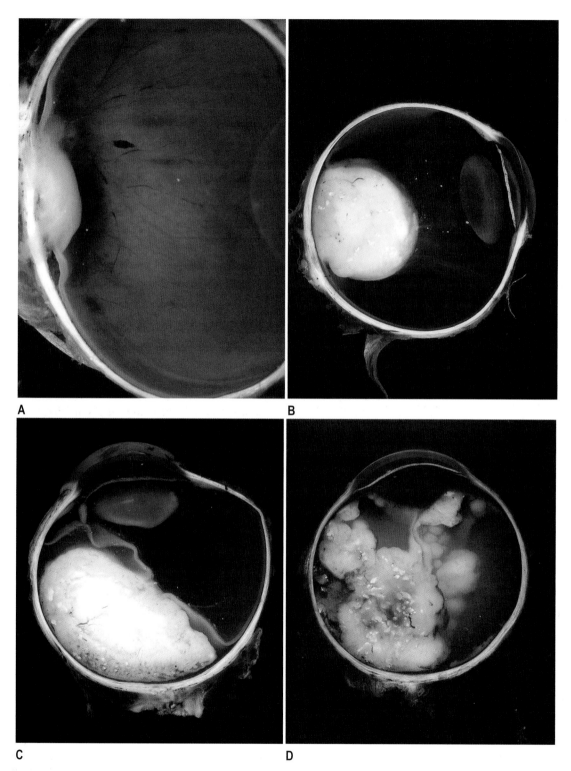

Fig. 9.33 Macroscopic appearances of retinoblastoma. (**A**) A small retinoblastoma overlying the optic nerve head contains few flecks of calcium. (**B**) A large retinoblastoma with seedlings in the vitreous. (**C**) An exophytic retinoblastoma detaching the retina. (**D**) A large exophytic retinoblastoma with prominent calcification and funnel-shaped retinal detachment.

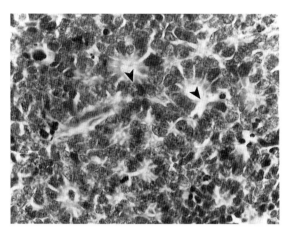

Fig. 9.34 A retinoblastoma is characterized by Flexner–Wintersteiner rosettes, which are lined internally by a membrane similar to the outer limiting membrane of the normal retina (arrowheads). Mitotic figures are plentiful in these tumours.

secondary, as the result of extension of an intracranial meningioma. In adults meningiomas of the optic nerve characteristically show indolent growth but in children they may be more aggressive. The tumour ensheaths the optic nerve, which may become atrophic. The histology is similar to intracranial meningioma with a transitional pattern, sometimes with psammoma bodies, predominating.

TUMOURS DERIVED FROM MUSCLE

Leiomyoma/leiomyosarcoma
A leiomyoma occasionally arises from the smooth muscle of the iris and ciliary body. The malignant counterpart, leiomyosarcoma, is extremely rare.

Rhabdomyoma/rhabdomyosarcoma
Benign tumours of striated muscle are virtually unknown in the eyelid and orbit.

Rhabdomyosarcoma is the most common orbital malignancy of childhood. It generally occurs in the first two decades of life and usually presents with rapidly progressive proptosis and displacement of the eye. If clinical suspicions are high then a prompt biopsy should be performed to confirm the diagnosis and the patient should be treated with a combination of chemotherapy and radiotherapy. With this regimen the survival of children with rhabdomyosarcoma has dramatically improved. On macro-

scopic examination these tumours consist of tan-coloured fleshy tissue. On histopathological examination rhabdomyosarcoma can be divided into three subtypes (embryonal, alveolar and pleomorphic). The embryonal subtype is the most common type in the orbit, consisting of sheets of small ovoid to spindle-shaped cells (Fig. 9.37). Cytoplasmic cross striations can be seen, with difficulty in a small number of cases. Immunohistochemistry for *MyoD1*, a muscle regulatory gene, may be helpful in confirming the diagnosis. Alveolar rhabdomyosarcoma is more common in older children; pleomorphic rhabdomyosarcoma is rare in the orbit and usually occurs in adults.

VASCULAR TUMOURS

Haemangiomas
These are described under hamartomas.

Epithelioid haemangioma
Epithelioid haemangioma, previously named angiolymphoid hyperplasia with eosinophilia, is a benign vascular lesion that may occur on the eyelid skin or occasionally in the orbit. It consists of blood vessels with prominent endothelial cells and accompanying inflammatory cells including lymphoid follicles and prominent eosinophils.

Kaposi sarcoma
This is a tumour of endothelial cells that may occur as a rapidly growing tumour on the eyelid and conjunctiva. It most commonly occurs in immunocompromised patients, especially those with AIDS, and is caused by infection with herpes virus type 8. Histologically these tumours consist of malignant spindle cells lining a network of sieve-like spaces containing extravasated red cells.

OTHER CONNECTIVE TISSUE TUMOURS

Tumours can be derived from any of the cellular constituents of connective tissue including adipose tissue, cartilage and bone. Orbital lipomas are considered to be relatively rare but this may reflect under-diagnosis because of the difficulty of distinguishing a lipoma from excised orbital fat. Primary liposarcoma rarely involves the orbit. Similarly, cartilaginous neoplasms of the orbit are extremely rare. Orbital osteosarcoma is also rare but well recognized as a second primary neoplasm following successfully treated retinoblastoma.

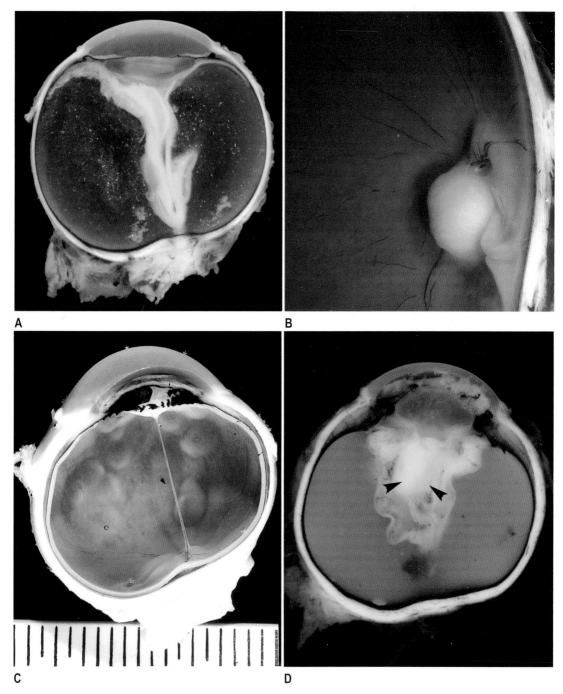

Fig. 9.35 Diseases simulating retinoblastoma. (**A**) In Coats disease the abnormal vasculature leaks lipid-rich plasma, and cholesterol crystals are present in the subretinal exudate. (**B**) Astrocytic hamartoma appears as a static round nodule projecting from the retina into the vitreous. (**C**) Persistent hyperplastic vitreous forms a white mass behind the lens and the persistent hyaloid artery passes back to the optic nerve head. (**D**) In metastatic endophthalmitis an abscess fills the vitreous cavity forming a white mass (arrowheads) and the retina is detached.

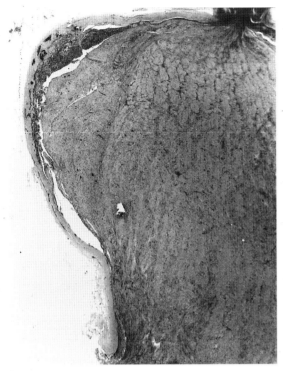

A

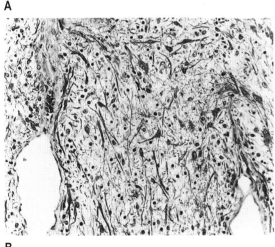

B

Fig. 9.36 (**A**) Low-power view of an optic glioma that has infiltrated the nerve columns but has preserved some recognizable architecture. (**B**) At higher magnification the tumour consists of irregularly arranged proliferating astrocytes with elongated cytoplasmic processes (phosphotungstic acid hydrochloride stain).

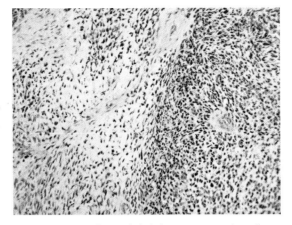

Fig. 9.37 In embryonal rhabdomyosarcoma the cells are ovoid to spindle shaped and there are alternating cellular and myxoid areas.

Solitary fibrous tumour, haemangiopericytoma and giant cell angiofibroma are a group of related neoplasms that, compared with other connective tissue tumours, are relatively common in the orbit. Histologically they all consist of spindle cells and have in common the presence of a thin-walled branching vascular pattern. Haemangiopericytoma is more cellular than solitary fibrous tumour, which frequently contains collagenous areas. Giant cell angiofibroma contains multinucleated stromal giant cells. Solitary fibrous tumour and giant cell angiofibroma usually pursue a benign course. The behaviour of haemangiopericytoma is variable and metastases may occur.

LYMPHOID TUMOURS

The tissues behind the orbital septum contain neither lymphatics nor lymphoid tissue. Lymphocytes may however be found in the conjunctiva, the lacrimal gland and the lacrimal drainage system.

Lymphomas of the ocular adnexa include lesions of the conjunctiva, eyelids, lacrimal gland and orbit. Those situated in the conjunctiva are associated with a lower incidence of systemic disease (20%) compared with those of the orbit (35%), lacrimal gland (40%) or eyelid (67%). Ocular lymphomas may be the first manifestation of disseminated disease and it is essential to undertake a full systemic and haematological examination of all patients presenting with ocular lymphoma. Before the widespread availability of immunohistochemistry and molecular techniques the classification of ocular lymphoid neoplasms was confusing and controversial. It is now accepted that the majority of lymphoid proliferations can be classified as benign (reactive lymphoid hyperplasia) or malignant (lymphoma) and terms such as 'pseudolymphoma' should be avoided.

The most common ocular lymphoproliferative lesions include:

- Benign lymphoid hyperplasia, a similar process to reactive follicular hyperplasia of lymph nodes may form a tumour mass within the conjunctiva or orbit.
- Extranodal marginal zone lymphoma (EMZL) is the most common type of ocular lymphoma and is a low grade B-cell lymphoma derived from the mucosal associated lymphoid tissue. EMZL usually follows an indolent course but it may recur at other extranodal sites or rarely undergo transformation to high-grade lymphoma.
- Follicular lymphoma is identical to its nodal counterpart and in the majority of cases represents part of a systemic disease.
- Diffuse large B-cell lymphoma is less common and around 40% of cases are associated with systemic disease. These lymphomas tend to pursue an aggressive clinical course.
- Primary intraocular lymphoma involves the retina, subretinal space, vitreous and optic nerve. It can occur in conjunction with or independent of primary central nervous system lymphoma. These are rare lymphomas but there has been a dramatic increase in incidence in recent years. The majority are diffuse large B-cell lymphomas. They usually occur in elderly patients but can also be associated with AIDS.

Many other lymphomas may uncommonly involve the ocular region including mantle cell lymphoma, B-cell chronic lymphocytic leukaemia, Burkitt's lymphoma, peripheral T-cell lymphoma and natural killer cell lymphoma. Ocular Hodgkin's disease is very rare. Leukaemic infiltration of the eye or orbit may also occur. In particular, granulocytic sarcoma can present as an isolated orbital mass in an otherwise healthy child.

LACRIMAL GLAND TUMOURS

Pleomorphic adenoma (benign mixed tumour)

Pleomorphic adenoma is the most common epithelial tumour of the lacrimal gland. It usually occurs in late to middle age but may occur at any age. This

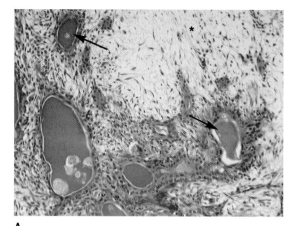

A

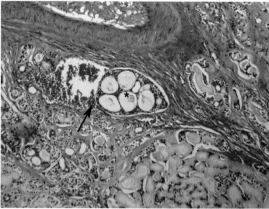

B

Fig. 9.38 (**A**) Pleomorphic adenoma consists of benign branching glands (arrows) lying within a myxoid stroma (*). (**B**) Adenoid cystic carcinoma has a Swiss-cheese pattern (*) and may show vascular (arrow) and perineural invasion.

tumour is slow-growing and pseudoencapsulated with surface bosselations. Histologically it consists of a mixture of epithelial and mesenchymal elements including myxoid tissue, cartilage, fat and, rarely, bone (Fig. 9.38A). It is important to completely excise these tumours because if they are 'shelled out' they can recur and there is a small but significant risk of surviving residual tumour undergoing malignant change to a pleomorphic carcinoma (malignant mixed tumour).

Adenoid cystic carcinoma

This is the second most common epithelial neoplasm of the lacrimal gland after pleomorphic adenoma. Although it is usually diagnosed in middle-aged or older patients, it frequently occurs in younger patients as well. The history is shorter than for pleomorphic adenoma and the patient may present with proptosis, numbness, pain and diplopia because invasion of nerves and extraocular muscles may occur early in tumour development. Histologically these tumours can assume a range of patterns the most common of which is a cribriform or 'Swiss-cheese' pattern (Fig. 9.38B). These are aggressive neoplasms that require radical surgery with supplemental radiotherapy or chemotherapy.

Other malignant epithelial tumours

A small number of epithelial tumours of the lacrimal gland are adenocarcinomas arising *de novo* with no evidence of a pre-existing benign mixed tumour. Mucoepidermoid carcinoma is another rare form of carcinoma that may arise in the lacrimal gland.

Lacrimal sac tumours

Tumours of the lacrimal sac are uncommon and are usually of epithelial origin. Papillomas may show an exophytic, inverted or mixed growth pattern and the epithelium may be of squamous or transitional cell type. Carcinoma of the lacrimal sac may develop within a papilloma or arise *de novo*. These are locally aggressive tumours and if neglected can invade surrounding structures.

METASTATIC TUMOURS

In adults metastatic tumours most commonly involve the uveal tract (Fig. 9.32D). Orbital involvement occurs about one-tenth as often and metastases to the eyelid and conjunctiva are rare. Most metastatic tumours are carcinomas and the most common primary sites are usually the breast, prostate, lung or gastrointestinal tract but metastases from a wide range of primary carcinomas has been described. In children metastatic disease is usually orbital and uveal involvement is rare. Orbital involvement by neuroblastoma, Ewing sarcoma, Wilms tumour and rhabdomyosarcoma may occur.

DISORDERS MISDIAGNOSED AS NEOPLASMS

Cysts

Eyelid
Simple cysts are common in the eyelid. These include:

- *Sudoriferous cysts* or sweat gland cysts (hidrocystomas) are derived from the ducts of the glands of Moll. The cysts are thin-walled and appear as translucent or bluish swellings at the lid margin. Histologically they are lined by a double layer of epithelium with an inner layer of cuboidal cells and an outer later of myoepithelial cells.
- *Epidermoid cysts* may occur secondary to obstruction of the duct of a pilosebaceous follicle or as the result of epithelial inclusion following trauma or surgery. Epidermoid cysts are lined by keratinizing squamous epithelium and are filled with keratin. A foreign body giant cell reaction may be seen in relation to cyst rupture.
- *Dermoid cysts* occur in children as a result of the incarceration of ectoderm between the frontal and maxillary process during embryogenesis. Dermoid cysts contain hairs and pilosebaceous follicles.

Conjunctiva
Cystic lesions are also common in the conjunctiva. Epithelial inclusion cysts are the result of previous trauma with incarceration of conjunctival epithelial nests in the stroma. Lymphatic cysts occur when ectactic lymphatics coalesce. This lymphangiectasia may occur as a hamartomatous malformation or secondary to inflammation.

Orbit
Cysts may also occur in the orbit and computed tomography scans may be helpful in identifying some lesions. Dermoid cysts may also occur in the orbit and should be excised intact because leaked contents may induce a granulomatous inflammatory reaction. A mucocoele is an expansion of the paranasal space secondary to drainage obstruction from chronic sinusitis. It consists of a cystic cavity lined with epithelium, which sometimes contains goblet cells. Haematic cyst is an organizing haematoma, which can occur spontaneously, or following blunt trauma.

Pseudoepitheliomatous hyperplasia

Surface epithelium overlying an inflamed stroma or tumour can be stimulated by various released growth factors. This may result in an exuberant proliferation of the epithelium that can be mistaken for squamous carcinoma by the unwary. This benign reactive process has been termed pseudoepitheliomatous hyperplasia.

Idiopathic orbital inflammation

Idiopathic orbital inflammation (formerly inflammatory pseudotumour) is a non-granulomatous

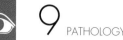
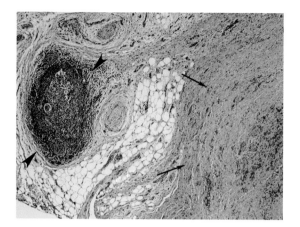

Fig. 9.39 In idiopathic orbital inflammation the orbital fatty tissue is replaced by fibrous tissue (arrows). There is an accompanying inflammatory cell infiltrate that may include lymphoid follicles (arrowheads).

inflammatory process within the orbit for which there is no recognized local cause or any underlying systemic disease. The disease presents as a unilateral or bilateral mass, which clinically may be mistaken for tumour. In biopsy specimens an early lesion shows oedema of orbital tissues and an inflammatory infiltrate composed predominantly of lymphocytes and plasma cells and lymphoid follicles may be present. As the disease progresses collagen is laid down and the collections of inflammatory cells may be separated by fibrous tissue (Fig. 9.39). Most cases show a dramatic response to corticosteroid therapy unless the lesion has extensive fibrosis. Other immunosuppressive agents, such as azathioprine, or low-dose radiotherapy may be used in patients who fail to respond to steroids. Idiopathic sclerosing inflammation is a distinct form of orbital inflammation characterized by a slow and relentless fibrosing process with progressive involvement of orbital structures. It may be part of a multisystem disease with progressive fibrosis at other sites.

RECENT TECHNOLOGICAL ADVANCES

CYTOLOGY

Cytology involves the study of individual cells removed from a lesion. Cytological preparations lack the architectural clues used for diagnosis in tissue sections and diagnosis relies on nuclear and cytoplasmic features. The diagnosis of malignancy is the major objective of cytopathology. Cytological preparations may be obtained from ocular lesions in two ways:

- *Impression cytology* – this is a useful technique for studying the cells of the conjunctival surface. Discs of cellulose acetate paper are pressed against the bulbar conjunctiva and then stained with different stains for examination under the microscope. This is a useful technique for assessing dry eye where reduction in goblet cells may be seen on a PAS stain and surface keratinization can be identified with Papanicolaou stains. This technique is also useful for diagnosing and mapping conjunctival intraepithelial neoplasia and primary acquired melanosis with atypia. For primary acquired melanosis, a Masson–Fontana stain is useful to identify melanin pigment.
- *Fine-needle aspiration* – this technique is increasingly being used for the preoperative diagnosis of intraocular malignancy. It is particularly useful when the clinician is faced with an isolated amelanotic mass, which could be melanoma or metastatic carcinoma. Intraocular lesions are best accessed via the pars plana and up to two passes can be made with a fine needle. Cells obtained may be placed directly onto a glass slide or suspended in saline for cytospin preparations and then stained with Giemsa or Papanicolaou stains for examination under the microscope. Immunohistochemistry may be a useful ancillary technique for subtyping cells from tumours. Fine-needle aspiration may also be useful for the preoperative diagnosis of orbital, lacrimal gland and eyelid tumours.

IMMUNOHISTOCHEMISTRY

Immunohistochemistry is a method of detecting the presence of specific proteins in cells or tissues and consists of the following steps:

- A primary antibody binds to a specific antigen.
- A secondary enzyme-conjugated antibody is then bound to this primary antibody–antigen complex.
- An appropriate substrate and chromagen are added and the enzyme catalyses the formation of a coloured deposit at the sites of antibody–antigen binding. The resulting staining is usually brown in colour but red or purple chromagens may be used in heavily pigmented lesions such as melanoma.

The introduction of antigen retrieval techniques including proteolytic digestion and more recently

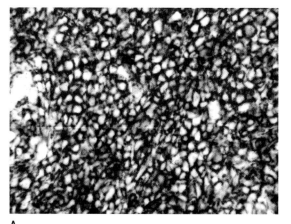

A

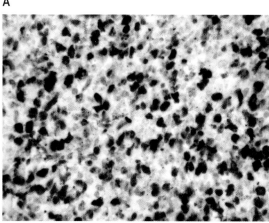

B

Fig. 9.40 **(A)** Immunohistochemistry for CD20 shows membranous staining of the cells in this B-cell lymphoma. **(B)** Immunohistochemistry for MIB 1(proliferating cell nuclear antigen) shows widespread nuclear staining indicating a high proliferation fraction.

microwave antigen retrieval has vastly improved the range of antibodies that can be used on formalin-fixed, paraffin-embedded tissue sections. With the dramatic expansion in this technique it is now automated in the majority of large pathology departments.

Immunohistochemistry has an important role in the diagnosis of many tumours. This is particularly the case for lymphomas and soft tissue tumours, for which a panel of antibodies is usually required for accurate diagnosis and subtyping (Fig. 9.40A). Other markers are important in providing prognostic information. For example, the association of high MIB1 (a cell proliferation marker) labelling indices is a poor prognostic indicator in lymphomas (Fig.

9.40B). Certain markers may also indicate the likely response to treatment. Positive oestrogen and progesterone receptors in breast cancer indicate a likely response to hormonal therapy. Staining for the protein product of the oncogene *c-kit* in gastrointestinal stromal tumours and adenoid cystic carcinomas suggests a likely response with the targeted therapy inmatinib.

Immunohistochemistry can also be useful for the detection of various infectious agents, e.g. cytomegalovirus, herpes simplex virus, *Acanthamoeba*.

FLOW CYTOMETRY

Using this technique it is possible to identify, isolate and phenotype different cells within a mixed population. Cells in suspension are labelled with fluorescent markers, excited by a laser and counted electronically by passing them through a flow cytometer. This instrument determines the number of specified cells in a sample and the ratios between the different cell types. This is the technique employed for monitoring CD4+ counts in human immunodeficiency virus infection. It is also useful in the diagnosis of lymphomas and can be undertaken on vitreous fluid.

TUMOUR CYTOGENETICS

Chromosomal abnormalities are of fundamental importance in tumorigenesis. Karyotypic analysis of malignant tumours shows both numerical and structural chromosomal abnormalities when compared with normal cells. Translocations are important in haematopoietic malignances. In solid tumours amplifications and deletions of chromosomal regions are more common.

Chromosomal abnormalities within a tumour cell may fall into one of three categories:

- *Primary abnormality* – the aberration is thought to be essential to establish the tumorigenesis and tends to have strong correlation with tumour type, e.g. deletion of *Rb1* gene in retinoblastoma.
- *Secondary abnormalities* – these are a manifestation of tumour progression and clonal evolution and are not as tumour-specific as primary abnormalities, e.g. loss of *p53* and *DCC* in the progression of colonic adenoma to adenocarcinoma.
- *Cytogenetic noise* – this is a manifestation of the genetic instability of a tumour cell. These abnormalities are randomly distributed throughout the genome and are not tumour specific.

513

Cytogenetic abnormalities are also well recognized in tumours of the eye. Deletion of the *Rb1* tumour suppressor gene on chromosome 13q14 in retinoblastoma is one of the best known. Chromosomal abnormalities have also been extensively studied in uveal melanoma. In these tumours loss of an entire copy of chromosome 3 is associated with death from metastatic disease. Various aberrations, including numerical gains in chromosome 6p, are associated with a more favourable prognosis. There is loss of heterozygosity of the chromosomal regions containing the mismatch repair genes *hMSH2* and *hMLH1* in the sebaceous tumours associated with Muir–Torre syndrome.

These various chromosomal abnormalities may be detected using a variety of techniques including conventional cytogenetics, polymerase chain reaction techniques, fluorescence *in situ* hybridization and comparative genomic hybridization. Conventional cytogenetics has the disadvantage of requiring fresh tissue but allows examination of the entire chromosome compliment. In this technique disaggregated tumour cells are cultured and chromosomes are analysed in a metaphase spread.

POLYMERASE CHAIN REACTION

Polymerase chain reaction (PCR) involves the selective amplification of specific segments of DNA. The basic reaction involves repetitive cycles of DNA synthesis. Each cycle consists of three steps.

- *Denaturation* – the first step involves denaturation of the target nucleic acid, which renders it single stranded.
- *Annealing* – denaturation is followed by annealing of synthetic oligonucleotide primers specifically designed to hybridize to the target nucleic acid region.
- *Extension* – the third step involves extension from the annealed primer catalysed by a DNA polymerase enzyme. In a typical PCR analysis 20–40 cycles are carried out with successive products becoming templates for subsequent cycles such that there is exponential amplification of the target region.

The basic technique may be adapted for various applications.

Detection of genetic mutations and deletions
Following the amplification of various regions, mutations or deletions can be detected in various ways including:

- Direct sequencing of the PCR product
- Detection of single-strand conformation polymorphisms (SSCP) – the resulting PCR product is denatured and subjected to gel electrophoresis. Mutations or deletions can result in alterations in the folding pattern of the single-stranded DNA and thus in their electrophoretic mobility when compared with wild-type sequences.
- Detection of restriction fragment length polymorphisms (RFLP) – the resulting PCR product is subjected to digestion with various restriction enzymes. Loss or gain of RFLP sites as the result of mutations or deletion will result in larger or smaller product size detected by gel-electrophoresis

Detection of pathogens
PCR is useful for detecting various pathogens, particularly viral pathogens. Primers are designed to amplify conserved regions of the infecting organisms. This technique is useful for detecting hepatitis B, cytomegalovirus, Epstein–Barr virus, herpes simplex virus and human papillomavirus. It has also been used to detect various mycobacteria.

Detection of changes in gene expression
Reverse transcription–PCR is based on the comparison of the amount of PCR product generated with the amount produced from a known concentration or copy number of control amplification targets in the same reaction. This technique can be useful for studying cellular events occurring in neoplasia.

IN SITU HYBRIDIZATION

In this technique single-stranded complementary nucleic acid sequences can join with specific DNA or RNA sequences in cells or tissues and these hybridization sites can be identified by the addition of a fluorescent *in situ* hybridization (FISH) or enzyme-labelled probe.

FISH is utilized to detect chromosomal gains, losses and translocations that are important in the diagnosis and prognosis of certain malignancies. It is important in the diagnosis of lymphomas, which often have relatively specific chromosomal translocations. For example, a translocation (11;18) is present in the majority of extranodal marginal zone lymphomas whereas a translocation (14;18) is present in the majority of follicular lymphomas.

In situ hybridization may be used for assessing clonality for κ or λ light chains in plasmacytic lesions. It is also useful for detecting virus nucleic

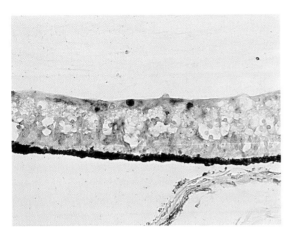

Fig. 9.41 *In situ* hybridization reveals cytomegalovirus in the large cells in the inner retina in a case of retinitis.

acids in infections with Epstein–Barr virus or cytomegalovirus (Fig. 9.41).

COMPARATIVE GENOMIC HYBRIDIZATION

In comparative genomic hybridization differentially labelled tumour and normal DNA samples are simultaneously hybridized to normal metaphase chromosomes. Regions of gains or losses within the tumour DNA can be identified by an increased or decreased colour ratio of the two fluorochromes used for the detection of hybridized DNA sequences along these reference chromosomes.

MICROSATELLITE ANALYSIS

Microsatellites are genetic polymorphisms that contain tandemly repeated sequences that are from one to four nucleotides in length. The number of times this sequence is repeated is highly variable and a characteristic that makes microsatellites a useful genetic marker. Since the majority of microsatellites occur in non-coding regions they generally do not cause disease but are used as a marker to identify a specific chromosome or locus and are a useful tool for chromosomal linkage and association studies.

MICROARRAYS

Microarrays are a powerful new technology for high throughput analysis of a large number of samples. Hundreds or thousands of samples (DNA, RNA, protein or tissue) are arranged on a single slide and then analysed by a single technique, e.g. Southern, Northern or Western blotting, immunohistochemistry or *in situ* hybridization.

FURTHER READING

Lee WR. Ophthalmic histopathology. London: Springer:2001.
Rao NA. Biopsy pathology of the eye and ocular adnexa. London: Chapman & Hall Medical:1997.
Reid R, Roberts F. Pathology illustrated. Edinburgh: Elsevier Churchill Livingstone:2005.
Sehu KW, Lee WR. Ophthalmic pathology: an illustrated guide for clinicians. Oxford: Blackwell Publishing:2005.
Shields JA, Shields CL. Atlas of intraocular tumors. Philadelphia: Lippincott, Williams & Wilkins:1999.
Shields JA, Shields CL. Atlas of eyelid and conjunctival tumors. Philadelphia: Lippincott, Williams & Wilkins:1999.
Shields JA, Shields CL. Atlas of orbital tumors. Philadelphia: Lippincott, Williams & Wilkins:1999.
Spencer WD, ed. Ophthalmic pathology, 4th edn. Philadelphia: WB Saunders:1998. (Available on CD-ROM.)
Yanoff M, Fine BS. Ocular pathology, 5th edn. London: Elsevier Mosby-Wolfe:2002. (Available on CD-ROM.)

INDEX

Note

Page numbers in *italics* refer to figures and tables.

517

523

529

533

photoreceptors (*cont'd*)
  renewal 241, 242, 247, 249, 254
    after dark adaptation 267–268
  responses with neural cells
    291–293
  resting potential 285
  retinal light stimulus detection 279
  synaptic events with inner nuclear
    layer cells 256–260
  turnover 242–243, 250–252
  visual stimuli 264
  see also dark adaptation; light
    adaptation
photosensitivity, retinal 268
photosensitization, systemic drug
  toxicity 350
phototransduction 252–253, 256, *257*
  cascade 256
  electrical response initiation
    277–278
  phosphoinositide metabolism
    253–254
phthisical eye 489
phthisis bulbi with ossification 475,
  489
pia mater *12*, 15–16
Pierre Robin syndrome 139
pigment epithelium-derived factor
  (PEDF) 248
pilocarpine 335, 336
  intraocular pressure control 341
pilomatrixoma 499
pineal tumour 505
pinguecula 489
pituitary fossa *9*, *10*
pituitary gland 8
  enlargement 73
  tumours *103*
pizotifen 345
place cells 295
plasma cells 354
  inflammatory reactions 471, 472,
    473
  monoclonal proliferation 490
  subretinal space leakage 475
plasma membrane 175, *176*
plasminogen activator inhibitor 1
  (PAI-1) 190
plasminogen activators 216
platelet-activating factor (PAF) 425
platelets 355
plectin 183
pleomorphic adenoma 510
plica semilunaris 90
Pneumocystis carinii choroidopathy 451
Pneumocystis carinii pneumonia (PCP)
  450
point mutations 149, 150
poly-A polymerase 146

polyarteritis nodosa 478, 479
polyclonal antibodies 375
polymerase chain reaction (PCR) 156,
  447, 501, *502*, 503, *504*
  fungal infections 454
polymixins 460
polymorphisms 153
  DNA 155–156
polymorphonuclear leucocytes (PMNs)
  429
polyols 236
polyploidy 148
pontine nucleus 82
positional changes 311, *312*
positron emission tomography (PET)
  304
posterior chamber *16*, 39
posterior pigment epithelium *31*, 32
posterior polymorphous dystrophy
  487, *488*
posterior uveitis
  Dalen–Fuchs nodule 392
  microgranulomas 390
pregnancy, rubella 448
premalignancy 496–497
prenatal diagnosis 159
preotic region 135
presbyopia 38
preservatives for drugs 334
prestriate cortex 264, 306
presumed ocular histoplasmosis
  syndrome 453, 493
pretectal nucleus 96
primitive streak 111
prochordal plate 135, *136*
profilin 182, *183*
promoters 146, *147*–148
Propionibacterium 442, 447
prostaglandin(s) 220–221, 343
  retinal blood flow 242
  trabecular meshwork synthesis 227
prostaglandin analogues 344
prostaglandin D_2 425
prostaglandin E_2 (PGE_2) 221
  retinal blood flow 242
prostaglandin $F_{2\alpha}$ 344
prostaglandin I_2 344
proteases 190
protein
  epitope mapping 413–414
  glycation 194–195, 196, *197*
  metabolism
    in lens 234–235
    in retina 240, 241
  synthesis 146–147, 148
    regulation 328
protein kinase C (PKC) 212, 213
protein synthesis inhibitors 460
proteinase inhibitors 452

proteoglycans 190–191, *192*
  scleral 217–218
proteomics 156, 157, 172–173
proteosomes 160
proton beam therapy 476
proto-oncogenes 497
protozoal infections 454–456
  inflammatory 470
pseudoepitheliomatous hyperplasia
  511
pseudoexfoliation syndrome 490
Pseudomonas 443
pterygium 489
pterygoid venous plexus 72
pterygopalatine ganglion *79*, 80, *91*
ptosis 87
  oculomotor nerve lesions 75
Pulfrich phenomenon 301, 302
pulley suspensions 65
pulvinar 314
pupil *16*, 27, 29, *30*
  functions 218–219
  light reflexes 276–277
  margin 29
    formation 120
  movements 32
  parasympathetic antagonists 337
  size 276–277
pupillary membrane 129
purine antagonists 346
Purkinje cells 315
Purkinje shift 288–289
pursuit 310
pyridoxamine *see* vitamin B6

quadrantanopia *104*

radiant energy damage 476
radiation vasculopathy 478
radiotherapy 476, 477
ranibizumab 347
RANK receptor 381
Ras activation 179
receptive fields 278, 280
RECK 359
recombinant DNA 155
recombinant DNA technology 155
  X-linked disorders 162
recombination rate 154
recoverin 253, *257*, *258*
red cells, inflammatory reaction 471
red–green differentiation 280, 283
reduction 195, *197*, 198
reflectance 303
Reis–Buckler dystrophy 485
release factor 147
repeat expansions 150
resin vascular casting 57, *58*
resolving power of eye 271, 275

535